Hyperbaric Facility Safety

A Practical Guide

– 2nd Edition –

Hyperbaric Facility Safety

A Practical Guide

– 2nd Edition –

Wilbur T. Workman

J. Steven Wood

Best Publishing Company

No responsibility is assumed by the publisher or editors for any injury and or damage to persons or property as a matter of product liability, negligence or otherwise, or from any use or operation of any methods, product, instructions, or ideas contained in the material herein. No suggested test or procedure should be carried out unless, in the reader's judgment, its risk is justified. Because of rapid advances in the medical sciences, we recommend that the independent verification of diagnoses and drug dosages be made.

All photos, images, and figures have been reproduced with permission. If not attribution is given, they have been provided by the chapter author(s).

Dedication photo courtesy of Joel Silverstein.

ISBN: 978-1-947239-21-0 (print)
ISBN: 978-1-947239-22-7 (ebook)

Library of Congress Catalog Number: 2020933985

Published by:
Best Publishing Company
631 U.S. Highway 1, Suite 307
North Palm Beach, Florida 33408

Printed and bound in the United States of America

Dedication

R. W. "Billy Bob" Hamilton, 1930-2011

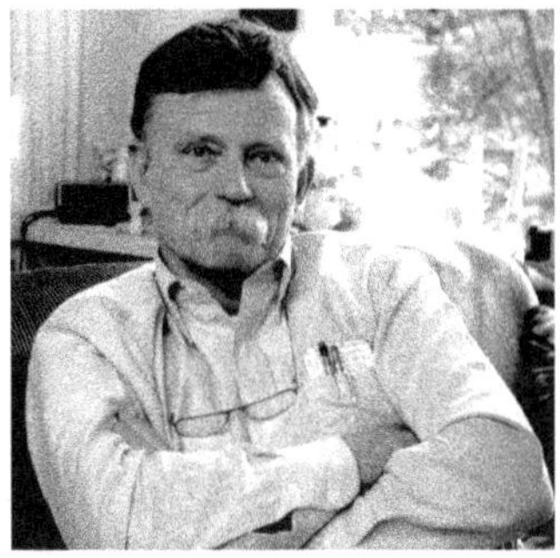

This second edition of *Hyperbaric Facility Safety: A Practical Guide* is dedicated to Dr. R.W. "Billy Bob" Hamilton. In the pantheon of hyperbaric luminaries, Dr. Hamilton's star is among the brightest. His contributions to the field covered the entire gamut of our field – his work with decompression tables (including developing algorithms that drive many dive computers), physiological effects of gases, and methods of managing exposure to oxygen were instrumental in the origination and development of the new field of "technical diving" as well as expanding the safety and efficacy of deep diving. Bill's work also translated directly to clinical hyperbaric medicine as well as space flight.

The hyperbaric community owes much to Dr. Hamilton's legacy, and he was an enthusiastic supporter of our profession. From serving as an officer of the Undersea and Hyperbaric Medical Society to educating much of the field, either directly, through his development of and participation in numerous workshops covering a broad range of topics, or to his consultations with government and civilian groups worldwide, Bill's influence continues to be felt. His contributions to the field have been recognized through awards from organizations representing the gamut of the diving and hyperbaric industry.

Bill was larger than life – fighter pilot, consummate professional, loving family man (particularly to his wife "Ruby Lips"), and a fine human being who encouraged everyone he met to be their best. The field has lost one of its rocks, but his legacy lives on. He will be missed.

Table of Contents

PART 2: A Practical Approach to Hyperbaric Safety

Preface

The fundamental premise of medicine embodied in the Hippocratic Oath, *Primum non nocere* ("First, to do no harm") is, at its core, an admonition to provide medical care that is safe.

The field of hyperbaric medicine has undergone a sea change since the publication of the first edition of this text. The number of facilities worldwide has increased substantially, yet the field faces monumental challenges. Economic pressures from health care funding agencies have placed a glaring spotlight on the accepted clinical conditions as the gimlet eye of evidence-based medicine has further challenged years of case experience that formed the foundation of the clinical condition lists. In the United States, the growth of wound treatment, using hyperbaric oxygen (HBO_2) as an adjunctive therapy, has further constricted the number of conditions treated, as most wound clinics are not structured to provide hyperbaric therapy for patients with serious or unstable conditions. But despite changes in the practice and application of hyperbaric oxygen therapy, the guiding tenant for providers of HBO_2 must be to deliver therapy safely.

There are two distinct aspects to the field of hyperbaric medicine that influence safety: technology (hardware) and the operators of that technology (software). HBO_2 is a technology-based therapy, supported by a long history of engineering and manufacturing refinement. The military and commercial diving roots of hyperbarics resulted in an initial pool of technologists who were trained to rigorous standards. Many of the pioneers in the field transitioned to the clinical and research sides of hyperbarics and brought a strong culture of operational safety.

Codes and standards related to the design, manufacturing, and installation of hyperbaric chambers are well-established and have broad distribution worldwide. Even in countries that don't have a mandatory regulatory scheme, end users can easily access and reference construction standards that will provide a chamber that is constructed in accordance with a proven safety record. One challenge posed by the existing standards is that due to the inherent inertia of the code/standard-writing process, the introduction of new materials and technologies often outstrips the code/standard process, resulting in the potential for stifling of innovation or the introduction of new technologies that might not be fully proven. Even in countries with a strong regulatory climate, it is not uncommon to see chamber designs that pose substantial risks due to their design or construction in widespread use. The bottom line is a chamber built, installed, operated, and maintained in accordance to accepted standards is rarely a factor in accidents.

Human factors—acts of omission or commission—play a role in the majority of hyperbaric safety-related incidents. The demographic change in the background of the people who operate chambers poses a great risk to the field. The growth of the field since the early 1990s resulted in a thinning of the experienced talent pool and the rise of a new generation of hyperbaric technologists. The risk- and cost-averse nature of modern health care has further restricted the use of HBO_2 predominately to medically-stable patients treated in an outpatient setting. The number of clinical facilities with the staff and equipment capability to manage seriously ill patients has dropped precipitously (at least in the United States), resulting in the need to transfer patients hundreds of miles to receive lifesaving treatment. Without a mandate to treat acute indications, facilities reduce technical staff, support equipment, and the specialized training necessary to provide high-level care is leading the hyperbaric field into a crisis of experience. The "old hands" (technologist and physician pioneers) in the field who set the bar for HBO_2 and were the fearless innovators who pushed the envelope of HBO_2 applications, are leaving the field due to retirement (or death). The challenge to the new generation of hyperbaric professionals is to preserve the institutional memory of the first generation and transmit it to the successors.

In developing the second edition of *Hyperbaric Facility Safety: A Practical Guide*, the editors have taken a more pragmatic approach to the organization of this edition, based on a conversation we had several years ago. We were discussing, with some vigor, an esoteric point within a subsection of NFPA code, when Tom commented on the small number of people in the industry who really cared about the minutia of regulatory code. That's the reality. Though chamber operators might find it useful to know the background of why they do what they do, they are more interested in how to do the job—the nuts and bolts of safety. With that concept in mind, this edition is divided into two major focus areas.

First, we look at the codes and standards that influence our field. Depending upon your location in the world, as many as 15 or more agencies' codes, standards, regulations, or laws may need to be conformed with in order for a facility to operate. Chapters cover the regulatory environment and take an in-depth look at the various systems that make up the modern hyperbaric chamber. We have also revamped information on the international aspects of the regulatory environment. Contributors from around the world completed a questionnaire that surveyed the practice of hyperbaric medicine in their respective countries. This data has been summarized in a table, with explanatory notes as required.

The second focus area takes a nuts-and-bolts approach to hyperbaric safety. Utilizing the expertise of key figures in the hyperbaric field, the reader will find a comprehensive compendium of resources that can be useful toward the development of a state-of-the-art hyperbaric safety program.

The editors express their sincere thanks to all of the contributors for their hard work and dedication to the production of this text. We hope that this edition will become a well-worn addition to your safety library.

Wilbur T. (Tom) Workman
J. Steven (Steve) Wood
Editors

Editors

Wilbur T. (Tom) Workman, BS, MS, CAsP, FAsMA, CHT-A, FUHM

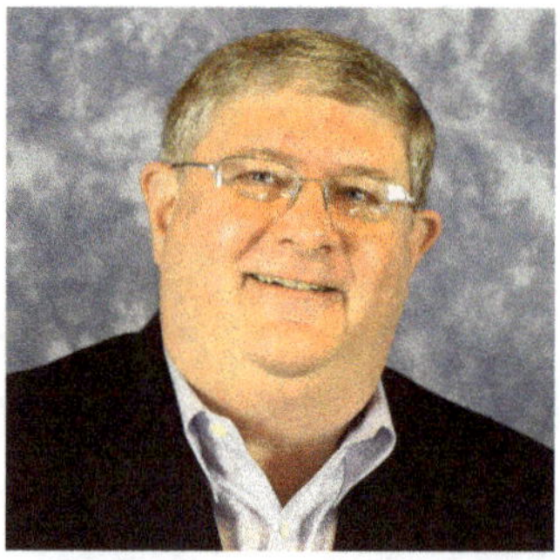

Tom Workman recently retired as the Director of Quality Assurance & Regulatory Affairs for the Undersea & Hyperbaric Medical Society. He was responsible for the development and management of the Society's Clinical Hyperbaric Facility Accreditation Program. He retired from the United States Air Force as a colonel after more than 23 years of service devoted to aerospace and hyperbaric physiology. From 1980 to 1992, Col. Workman was assigned to the USAF Hyperbaric Center, Brooks AFB, TX. During his last three years there, he was Chief of the USAF Hyperbaric Medicine Program. From 1992 until his retirement as Chief, Biomedical Scientist in 1995, he served as Commander, 9th Training Squadron, Beale AFB CA, where he was responsible for the worldwide physiological support for the only USAF-manned, high-altitude reconnaissance mission. In this capacity, he managed over 150 people and assets in excess of $47 million. He also served as Deputy Commander, 9th Medical Group, Beale AFB CA. Active in many professional organizations for over 45 years, Workman has served on the National Fire Protection Association's Technical Committee for Hyperbaric and Hypobaric Facilities since 1984 and the American Society of Mechanical Engineers Pressure Vessel for Human Occupancy Technical Committee for 30 years, among many other committee leadership positions.

Included in his many awards are the Undersea & Hyperbaric Medical Society's (UHMS) Craig Hoffman Memorial Award presented in 2001 for his contributions to diving safety and the first UHMS Gulf Coast Chapter Wilbur T. Workman Award named in his honor. He is also the recipient of the Aerospace Physiologist Society's Paul Bert Award for Physiological Research, the Wiley Post for Operational Physiology, and the Fred Hitchcock Award. Workman has more than 130 publications and presentations including editorship of *Hyperbaric Facility Safety: A Practical Guide* and the *UHMS Guidelines for Hyperbaric Facility Operations, 1st and 2nd Edition.* He is board-certified by the Aerospace Medical Association in Aerospace Physiology and by the National Board of Diving and Hyperbaric Medical Technology in Hyperbaric Technology and is a Fellow of the Aerospace Medical Association.

Editors

J. Steven "Steve" Wood

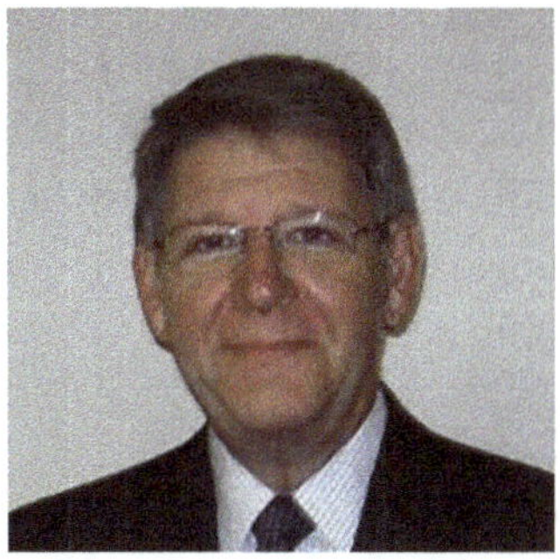

Steve Wood began his health care career at age 16, working in his hometown hospital as a respiratory therapy technician. At age 18, he successfully challenged the certified respiratory therapy tehnician (CRTT) examination and later completed the requirements to become a registered respiratory therapist (RRT). During his 13 years as a clinical respiratory therapist, Steve specialized in adult and neonatal critical care and also managed several hospital RT departments. He attained credentialing as an emergency medical technician (REMT) and was active as an instructor in various emergency medicine training programs ranging from EMT to advanced cardiac life support. Steve's hyperbaric career began in 1985 when he was introduced to hyperbaric medicine and was tasked with developing a hospital hyperbaric program. He was credentialed (with distinction) as a certified hyperbaric technologist (CHT) in 1993 and recertified in 2003 (also with distinction). Since that time, his career has taken him from a clinical caregiver role, to chamber manufacturing, consulting, and to cofounding one of the first hyperbaric contract providers. Steve has been a UHMS Associate member since 1986, Chair of the Associates, member of the Accreditation Council, and an accreditation surveyor since the program was introduced. In 2006, Steve received the Paul C. Baker Award, presented by the UHMS Associates for "outstanding contributions to the advancement of safety in hyperbarics worldwide." He has presented multiple papers on technical and safety aspects of hyperbaric therapy, served as an instructor in multiple introductory and specialty hyperbaric courses, and was recently granted a US patent for a hyperbaric safety device. Steve was a contributor to the first edition of this text.

Contributing Authors

A

Allen, Michael W.

B

Barry, Richard C., MS, STS, CHT-A
Beeson, Harold D., PhD
Bell, James, CHT, EMT, CFPS
Bird, Nicholas, MD, MMM, FAAFP, UHM/FUHM
Burman, Francois, BSc Engineering, MSc, IntPE
Butler, Glenn J.

C

Chiffoleau, Gwenael, PhD
Chipps, Mark
Cormier, Jolene, BSN, RN, CHT, CHRN
Corson, Kevan, CHT, CHWS, DMT-I

D

Davison, William J., CHT
Dixit, Ramesh K., PE

E

Evenson, Becky, RN, BSN, MBA, ACHRN, CWS

F

Fabus, Stephen, CHT Admin
Foreman, Christy, MBE

G

Garrett, Derall, CHT
Gearhart, William C., BS, CHT, EMT, CRT, RCP, CFPS, FI 1, FI 2
Geiser, Dennis, DVM, CHT-V
Godfrey, Greg, BS, MBA, RAC, CQE, CQA

Contributing Authors

H

Hamilton, R.W. "Bill", PhD (deceased)
Hardy, Sean, MD
Hoberg, Shelena, CHT, CHT-V
Hutson, Connie, RN, MS, ACHRN, CWCN, CHWS, STS

J

Jett, Noel A., DHA, MPH, CHT-A, CWS
Josefsen, Laura, RN, ACHRN

M

Mize, Jeff, RRT, CHT, CWCA

N

Newton, Barry E., PhD, PE

P

Peters, John, FACHE
Posey, John, CHT
Posey, Kevin I. "Kip", CHT

R

Raleigh, Greg, CHT,RCP
Reimers, Stephen D., PE
Richards, Guy, MA, CChem, FRSC
Robins, Marc, DO, MPH, FUHM, FAAFP

S

Sample, Richard (Dick), BSPH, RCP, RRT, CHT
Sheffield, Paul J., BS, MS, PhD, CAsP, CHT-A
Sheffield, Robert, BA, CHT
Sonnenrein, Regina
Subbotina, Nina, MD

Contributing Authors

T

Talati, Deepak, BSME, MSIE

Thurston, Sue, RN, Grad Cert (Acute Care), Grad Cert NS (Hyperbaric)

W

Weitershausen, Joanna, MSE

Wischhoefer, Larry L., PE (Ret.)

Wood, J. Steven

Workman, Wilbur T., BS, MS, CAsP, CHT-A, FAsMA, FUHM

Z

Ziemba-Diehl, Tina, RN, ACHRN, CHT

PART 1
Hyperbaric Chambers

CHAPTER 1
The History of Hyperbaric Chambers

Sue Thurston, RN, Grad Cert (Acute Care), Grad Cert NS (Hyperbaric)

There are many well-researched and documented histories of hyperbaric medicine.[1-7] However, as books, manuscripts, and articles are digitized and accessible via the internet, original references can more easily be reviewed and new information sourced in the early history of compressed air and hyperbaric oxygen therapy (HBOT).

From the 1600s, many have considered and explored using immersion in compressed air for various ailments and illnesses. Modern hyperbaric medicine began in the early 20th century with the introduction of breathing oxygen during hyperbaric exposures.

Hyperbaric Air

In his 1664 book *Aero-Chalinos, or, a Register for the Air in Five Chapters,*[8] Dr. Nathaniel Henshaw, an English physician practicing in Dublin, Ireland, suggested health is affected by the qualities and conditions of air. He proposed "a contrivance, by which any person may receive the benefit of a removal to another climate, at any season of the year, without removing from his own house or neglecting any employment." Henshaw describes how to construct a sealed brick room called a domicillium and use a bellow to increase inside pressures of air to "thrice" normal pressure and decrease the pressure by a "half." Pressure could be monitored using "a large weather glass or a tube of glass some forty inches long filled with quicksilver, after the torriecellian experiment." Treatment regime was to be two, three, or more hours "especially in the morning." For acute diseases, Henshaw suggested, "It should seem necessary that the patient continue in the said chamber during the whole course of the disease."

It is unknown if Henshaw's domicillium was ever built, but he did comment as follows: "There may, I doubt not, several other considerable conclusions be performed, by means of this contrivance. As also, that the thing itself is very capable of good improvement, as to the projection of it, far beyond that described by us. We leave for farther discovery, and confirmation, to practise and experience."

In 1820, Hamel, as well as Colladon, descended in a diving bell to a depth of 10 meters at Dublin Harbour, Ireland. They both proposed increased pressure inside a diving bell might be useful to treat deafness. Colladon also mentioned that one of the workmen "who had habitually breathed with great difficulty, was completely cured shortly after undertaking work in the bell."[9-10] In 1832, a pamphlet, "The Diving Bell as a Remedy for Certain Diseases," by Reverend Alden of New Hampshire, US, described the effect of increased pressure on the ears. He, too, suggested the use of a diving bell to treat deafness.[11]

Compressed Air Bath

Some conjecture remains about who was the first in France to use compressed air as a medical treatment. In 1834, Victor-Théodore Junod, a Parisienne physician, published the first report on the effects of breathing altered atmospheric air while inside a chamber (Figure 1). Emile Tabarie, a physician in Montpellier, southern France, published his findings six years later but stated he had commenced his research in 1832 [3,9] (Figure 2). Charles Pravaz in Lyon, France, soon followed in 1837 by publishing his results of using a *bain d'air comprimé* (compressed air bath).[1,13]

During the rest of the 19th century, many pneumatic centers using compressed air baths opened in Europe (Figures 3-4), Britain, and North America, with the majority in France and Germany. Many articles, pamphlets, and books were published extolling the benefits of using hyperbaric air. Most of these publications included case studies of

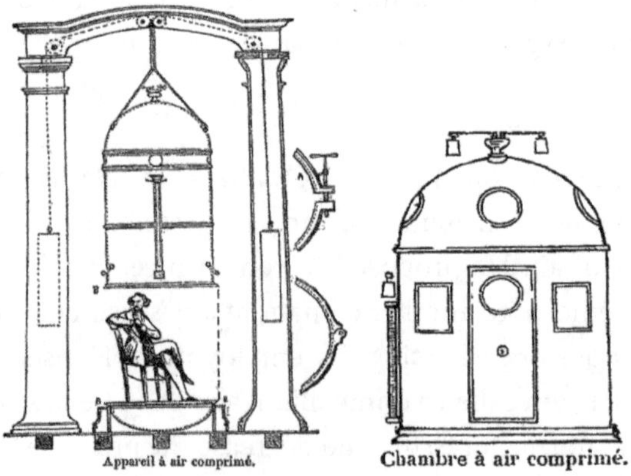

Figure 1. Junod; Paris, France.[12]

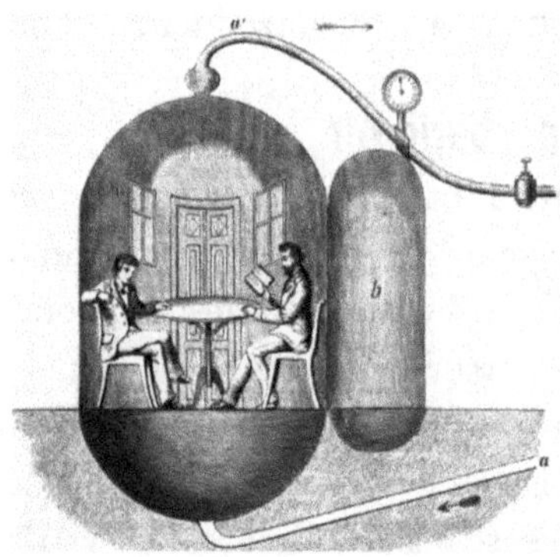

Figure 2. Tabarie; Montpellier, France.[13]

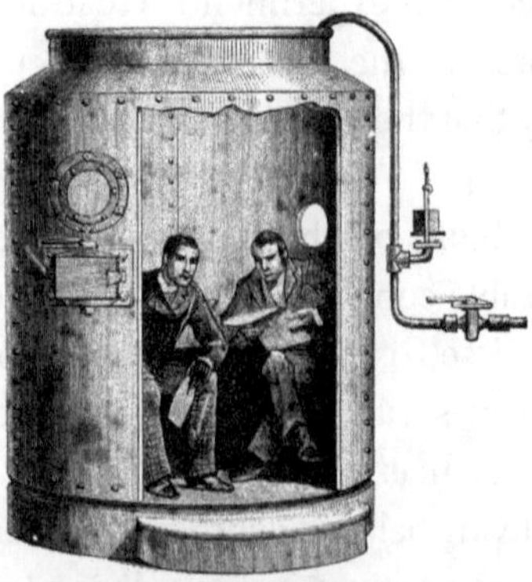

Figure 3. Arntzenius; Amsterdam, Netherlands.[13]

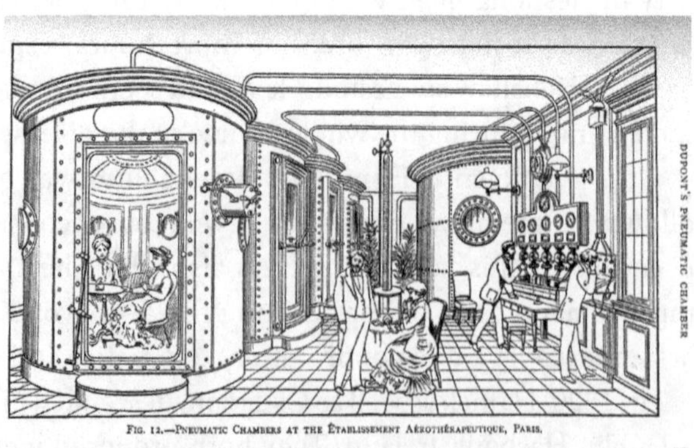

Figure 4. Dupont; Paris, France.[12]

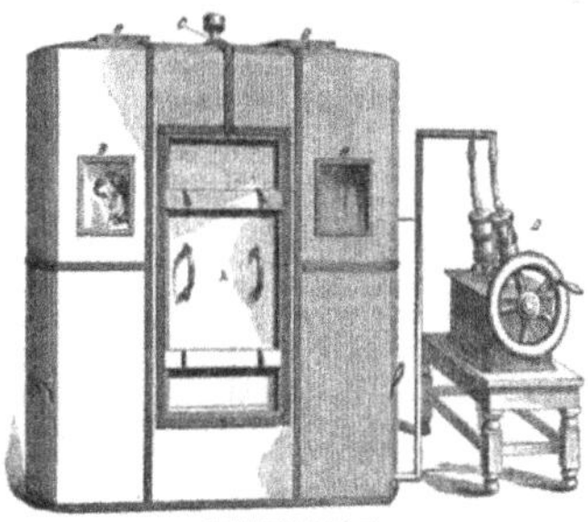

Figure 5.[18] Taylor; New York, NY.

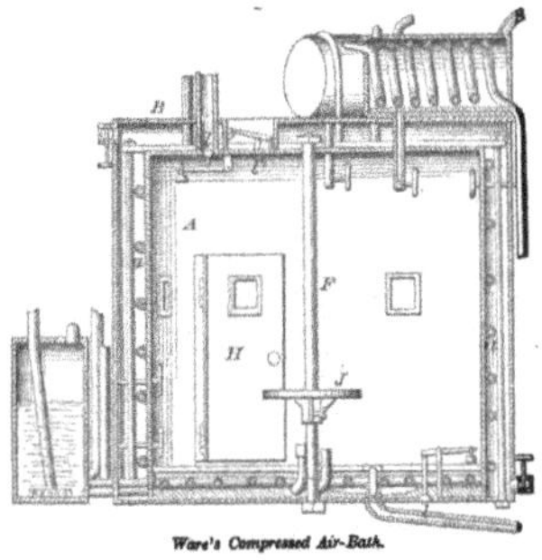

Figure 6.[17,20] P. T. Ware.

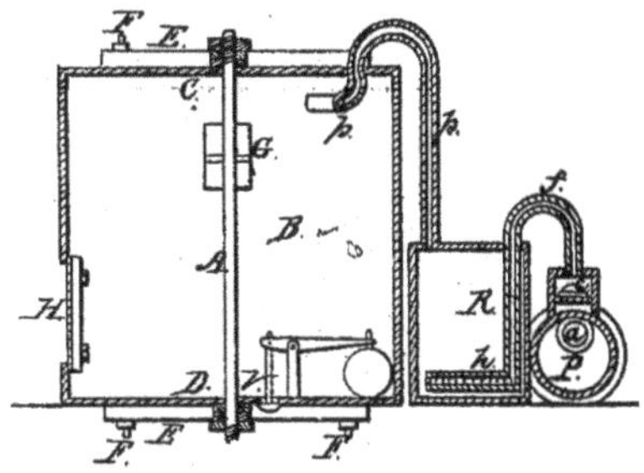

Figure 7. Othniel Stone.[21]

Figure 8. Bad Heustrich. Circa 1920. Courtesy of Staatskanzlei des Kantons Bern (State Archive of Bern) Switzerland, F1 Bad Heustrich 7/21.

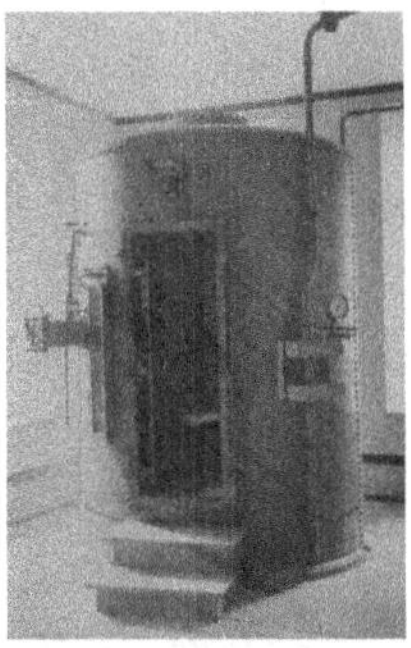

patients' successful outcomes. There is no evidence of application of a scientific approach other than the noting of changes in patients' respiratory and heart rates and symptom responses. A variety of conditions and diseases were treated, predominately respiratory, but also orthopedic, renal, various infective diseases, and nervous conditions. Not all at that time were convinced of the benefits of hyperbaric air treatments.[15]

In Canada, American-born Othniel Stone was granted a patent in 1857 for a "condensed atmospheric air bath with purifier and medicator to be called Stone's Atmospheric Air Bath."[16] Stone operated in Oshawa, Ontario, for approximately five years.[17] Also in 1857, Dr. George Taylor had a compressed air bath (Figure 5) in his rooms at 67 West 38th Street, New York.[18] He made the following declaration about his treatment in an April 1858 advertisement: ". . . the most successful treatment for Consumption, Dyspepsia, Constipation, Chronic Diarrhoea,[sic] General Weakness, especially with females and is particularly efficacious in spinal curvatures, paralysis and all those derangements in young people arising from neglect of physical education in boarding schools."[19]

Stone's compressed air bath was moved to Toronto, Canada, in 1862 where it was managed by Paul T. Ware[17,20] (Figure 6). In 1865, Othneil Stone patented his condensed atmospheric bath in the United States[21] (Figure 7) and operated it in Rochester, NY.[17] By 1867 others had opened in Buffalo, NY, and Clifton Springs, NY.[22]

The interest in compressed air baths waned toward the end of the 19th century. Some continued to be used until the 1920s, one in Switzerland (Figure 8), and several in spa towns in Germany and Austria (Figure 9).

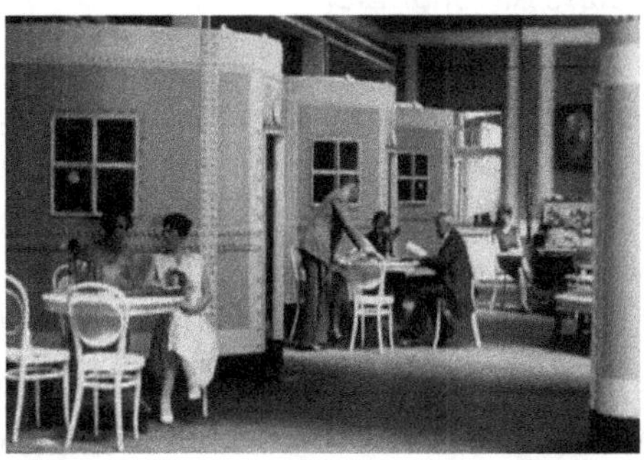

Figure 9. Dianabad Spa, Reichenhall, Germany. Postcard circa 1920.

Paul Bert

French physiologist Paul Bert researched respiratory physiology including hypoxia, barotraumas, air embolism, hyperoxia, and hypercapnia. He published numerous scientific papers, and in 1878 published a 1,178-page book titled *La Pression Barométrique: Recherches de Physiologie Expéerimentale* [*Barometric Pressure: Research in Experimental Physiology*]. As well as historical reviews, it contained detailed descriptions of hundreds of experiments, many conducted on himself in various pressure chambers in his laboratory at Sorbonne University, Paris, France[23] (Figure 10).

Through animal experiments, Bert discovered it was nitrogen bubbles that caused symptoms of what is now known as decompression illness (DCI). He noted that if decompression speed was slowed, less nitrogen would come out of solution and form bubbles. He suggested a decompression time of 10 minutes per atmosphere (14.7 pounds per square inch [PSI]).

Bert's work had some early critics[24] and was largely unknown except to a few scientists until 1943, when his work was translated into English. This was used to support altitude hypoxia research for Allied aircrew flying in unpressurized planes during World War II (WWII).

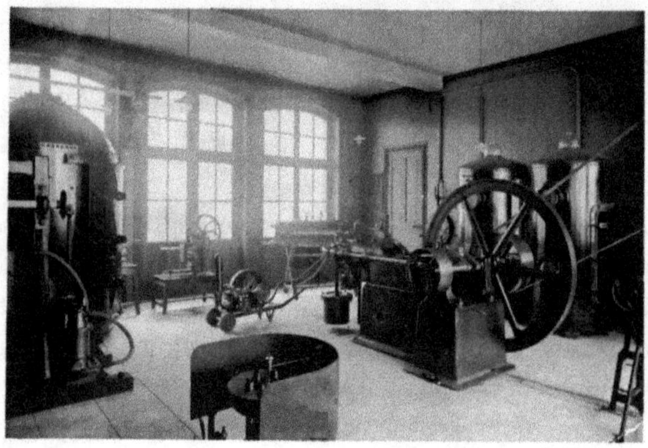

Figure 10.
Regnard, P., La Cure D'Altitude, Masson, Paris, 1897.

Mobile Hyperbaric Air Chamber

Paul Bert also researched the use of nitrous oxide as a safe anesthetic agent. The first human trial took place in February 1879 at Dr. Daupley's aerotherapeutic establishment in Paris, where Paul Bert, surgeon Leo Labbé, and others accompanied a patient inside a chamber to a pressure of 2.2 atmospheres absolute (ATA) (32.3 PSI). The patient received 85% nitrous oxide and 15% oxygen while having an ingrown toenail removed.[25-26] A month later, at the Pneumatic Institute of Dr. Joseph-Auguste Fontaine, Bert and five others accompanied a patient under pressure where a mastectomy was performed by surgeon Jules Pean. Again, recovery post-anesthesia was observed to be rapid and without signs of cyanosis or asphyxia. After these successes, Fontaine and

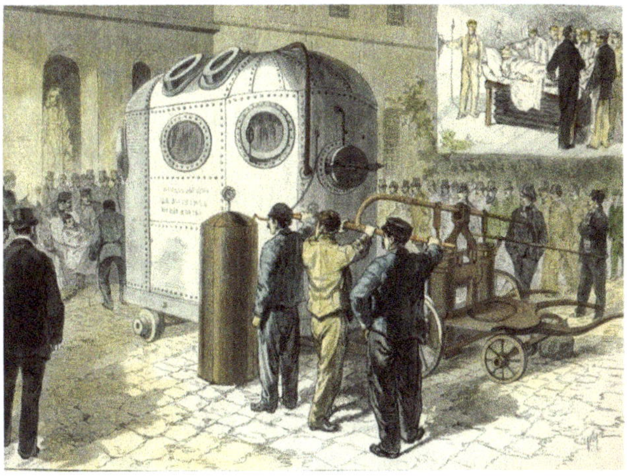

Figure 11.
Fontaine's Mobile Chamber. Drawing courtesy of Steve Goble.

Pean had constructed a mobile chamber which was pulled by a team of horses to various Paris hospitals for regular surgical lists[27] (Figure 11). The chamber was 2 meters wide by 3.5 meters long by 2.6 meters high and reportedly able to hold up to 12 people. It had what we now call a medical lock to allow articles to be passed inside or outside of the chamber without altering the inside pressure. Six men hand-pumped the pressure for the chamber using a mechanism similar to lever pumps employed to deliver compressed air for divers at that time.[4] According to Smith,[27] the mobile chamber continued to be used until 1913.

This method of applying nitrous oxide as an anesthetic was continued into the early 1900s by dentists in France, Switzerland, Belgium, Germany, and the United States.[7,27]

Caisson Disease

A caisson is a box-like structure commonly used in civil engineering projects where work is carried out in areas submerged in water. Pneumatic caissons are closed at the top but open at the bottom, with the water forced out by using compressed air, creating a working chamber, which is airtight in order for excavation to be carried out. These were often used in bridge pier construction. The deeper a project went, the higher the pressure of air was required to reduce water infiltration into the excavation site. Access to the increased air pressure area was via an airlock where pressure could be increased or decreased relative to the working pressure and to return to the surface pressure. The causes of arthralgia, paralysis, and sometimes death that workers experienced after returning to normal atmospheric pressure was unknown at the time. Later these symptoms were called caisson disease. Many authors have published detailed histories of compressed air work and its problems. [9-10, 28-31]

The first well-documented use of compressed air was by French Engineer Jacques Triger in a mine in 1839. Bert[9] describes how Triger noted the physiological effects in a caisson. Triger discussed the pain felt in ears during compression and change in tone of the voice. He commented on the difficulty experienced in attempting to whistle at pressure and remarked on the "fogging" and cooling of the air during a rapid decompression after a porthole rupture. Triger also noted the arthralgia some workers experienced after returning to surface pressure. It was not until 1854 that all the symptoms workers at a coal mine in Douchy, Northern France, were experiencing after exiting the caisson were monitored. French doctors Pol and Wattelle measured workers' respiratory and heart rate changes at increased pressure and listed workers' symptoms ranging from muscular and joint pains through to neurological changes, coma, and sometimes death. Further, Pol described "keen pains" he experienced after a visit to a caisson. They noted being under pressure was not dangerous in itself, but the return to normal pressure was, and that recompression relieved symptoms.[9] Pol quipped that "one only pays on leaving."[31]

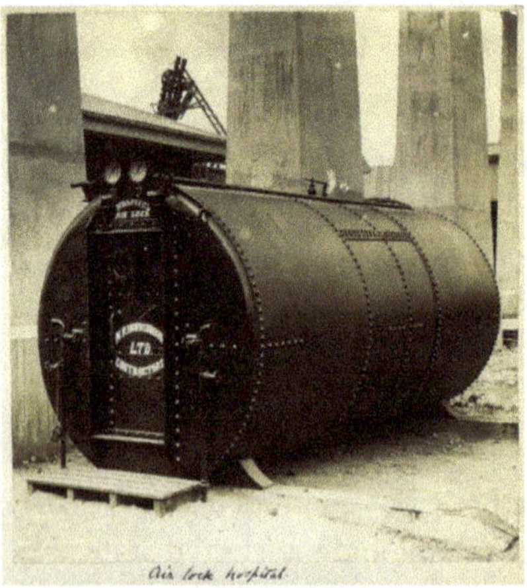

Figure 12. Hospital/medical lock used in the 1930s during the building of William Jolly Bridge, Brisbane, Australia. Photo courtesy of Dave King and the Hornibrook Family.

Many other compressed air projects took place all over the world, often referred to as the "Triger Method." Empirically, a slow return to normal pressure became the norm. Many projects employed doctors to monitor workers' health. Dr. Jaminet with the St. Louis Eads Bridge (1867-1874) and Dr. Andrew Smith with the Brooklyn Bridge construction (1869-1883) were just two to publish their findings. They could not agree on the causes of caisson illness, suggesting it was the increased humidity and/or carbon dioxide levels, but both stated that returning to pressure eased symptoms.[10, 28]

Sir Earnest William Moir, an English engineer with the Hudson Tunnel construction (1889-1908) linking Manhattan Island to New Jersey was the first to use a "medical lock," sometimes called a "hospital lock" (Figure 12). This was a boiler-like horizontal cylindrical chamber located near the entrance to the compressed air work. French Doctor Antoine Foley, in 1863, suggested using a separate air lock for symptom relief with recompression. Smith, at the Brooklyn Bridge construction, had one built but did not use it.[29, 31] At the Hudson Tunnel project, Moir had symptomatic workers return to a pressure of "half or two-thirds of that in which they had been working . . . the pressure was then lowered at the very slow rate of "one lb per minute or even less" (presuming this is one pound per square inch pressure, then this would be one PSI per minute). The mortality rate was reduced over the next 15 months from an appalling 25% down to 1.66%.[30]

Haldane

In the early 1900s, Scottish physiologist John Scott Haldane was asked by the British Admiralty to examine decompression procedures for Royal Navy divers. Haldane and Dr.

Arthur E. Boycott (senior researcher at Oxford University) and Lieutenant Guybon C. Damant, Royal Navy, first carried out this research using a recompression chamber located at the Lister Institute, London, England. Haldane had previously used a compressed air chamber at Brompton Hospital, London, while examining carbon dioxide and respiration in humans at increased and decreased air pressures.[32] The aim of the Royal Navy's decompression research was to explore safe decompression rates. Using both animal and human experiments, nitrogen uptake at various pressures, the rate of desaturation of nitrogen, and staging (holding at a certain pressures) to manage nitrogen offgassing were explored, based mainly on symptomatic effects. Carbon dioxide levels at different pressures were also measured. Boycott, Damant, and Haldane published their report in 1906.[33]

They tested their theories with in-water dives to many different depths at Loch Riddon in Western Scotland. This included two navy divers, Damant and Catto, diving to 35 fathoms (64 meters of seawater) with copper helmet diving apparatus and amazingly, hand-pumped compressed air. Six men were required for each air compressor pump with changeover relief required every five minutes.[33]

Worldwide navy divers, commercial divers, and caisson workers adopted the staged decompression dive tables published at the end of their paper.

Orval J. Cunningham

Anesthetist Cunningham commenced using compressed air in 1919 to treat large numbers of patients during the Spanish influenza pandemic.[34] Cunningham managed to borrow a hospital lock from a local bridge building contractor used with caisson work. The chamber, 2.1 meters wide and 6 meters long with two compartments, was installed at Bell Memorial Hospital, Kansas City, MO. Sellers[35] tells the sad story of a compressor failure causing an unknown number of patients to die after a rapid decompression with this chamber. Despite this, in 1920 Cunningham continued his pursuit and filed for a patent for "a certain new and useful improvement in therapeutic apparatus" which was granted in 1923.[36] He suggested having a trained nurse "familiar with the operation of the apparatus" to stay with patients in each compartment during treatment. The chamber would have showers and toilets as well as Pullman-type beds that could be raised when not in use. In 1920 he opened the Cunningham Sanatorium beside his house[35] (Figure 13), with a 30-meter-long chamber capable of treating up to 72 patients. It had two compartments divided by an

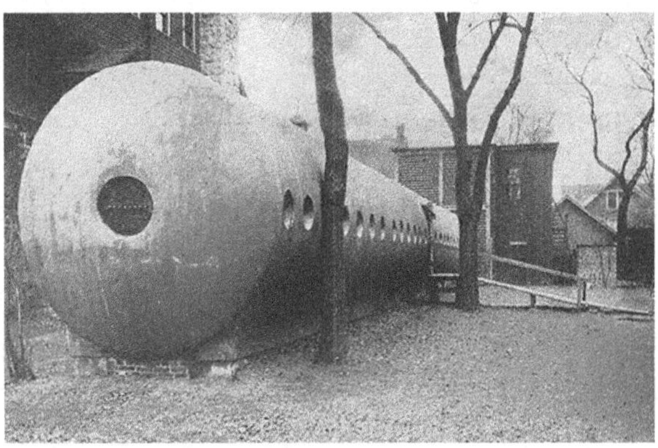

Figure 13. Cunningham's 2nd chamber, 1920. Kansas City, MO. Photo courtesy of Mary Jo Draper, Editor, *Midtown KC Post.*

airlock in the middle.[34, 37] Hyperbaric air pressures varied from 1.7 atmospheres absolute (ATA) (10 PSI) to 4.3 ATA (49.9 PSI) and lasted from 3 hours to 31 days. With the longer stays, decompression involved reducing the pressure by 49 PSI every 12 hours.[34] Smoke filled the chambers one night, when external heating caused inside furnishing to smolder; however, no one was hurt this time.[34]

Henry H. Timken, a grateful patient, apparently cured from uraemia, donated land and a million dollars to Cunningham to build a larger chamber in Cleveland, Ohio.[34,38] (Figure 14). Even before "Timken's Tank" was completed, questions were being asked about the science behind using compressed air as treatment for various medical conditions. Cunningham only published one paper on this subject in 1927.[39] In the *Journal of American Medical Association* (JAMA) 1928, Cunningham was criticized for lack of evidence of the science involved, along with queries regarding the financing of the treatment.[39]

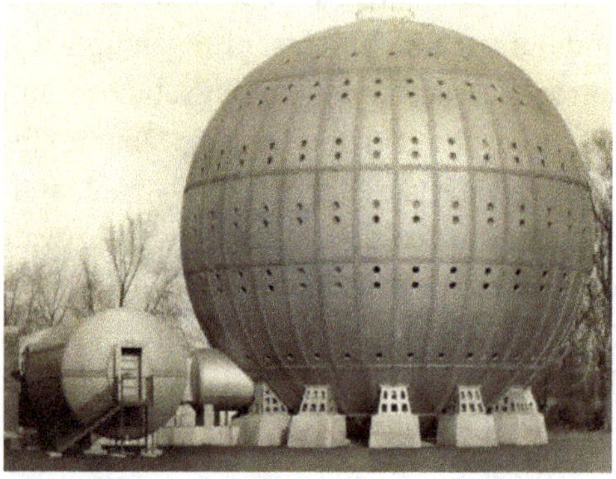

Figure 14. Cunningham's Sanitarium, Cleveland, OH. Photo courtesy of Best Publishing Company.

The compressed air chambers opened for business in December 1928. The ball chamber had 5 floors and 36 double bedrooms, each with private bathrooms, and an elevator in the center.[37] Working pressure was 2 ATA (29.4 PSI) and treatments were for seven days under pressure and seven days out, and then repeated. Two attached horizontal cylindrical chambers were used as airlocks and for decompression. According to Trimble,[34] it was not mounting medical criticism that caused Cunningham to eventually sell his interests in the steel ball chamber but the stock market crash of 1929 and the depression that followed. James Rand III took over running the chambers in 1934 but closed after only a year. Sadly, the chamber complex was sold for scrap metal and dismantled by 1942.[34-35]

Hyperbaric Oxygen (HBO_2)

Bert described the toxic effects of HBO_2 when he exposed animals to high pressures of oxygen in 1879.[9] In 1887, Dr. Francisco Venezuela in Madrid, Spain, treated several patients suffering from pneumonia with HBO_2 (unknown pressures) although he only reported on the antipyretic effects.[40] In 1889, Lorrain Smith re-explored Bert's animal experiments, looking more at lung changes while breathing at lower pressures of HBO_2.[41] Further research into oxygen at increased pressures was carried out by Hill and Macleod [42] and others.[43]

Bert advocated the administration of normobaric oxygen if minor symptoms of what we now call DCI appear, but if paralysis had occurred, to recompress with air immediately, then slowly decompress. In 1912, Hill suggested to treat caisson illness with normobaric oxygen for first aid, not during recompression.[10] According to Elliott,[44] Austrian physiologist von Schrötter also suggested the use of oxygen with DCI treatment.

In the 1930s, Brazilian doctor and scientist, Dr. Álvaro Osório de Almeida, published his research with hyperbaric oxygen, although apparently many of these works were animal experiments only. He reported on the toxic effect of HBO_2 and then the application of HBO_2 for the treatment of Hansen's disease (leprosy), gas gangrene, and combining HBO_2 with radiation for cancer treatments. As Clarke comments,[1] despite publishing in several languages, Osório de Almeida's work remains mostly unknown.

In the 1930s Albert Richard Behnke Jr., of the U.S. Navy, began his research into DCI. In 1937 he suggested HBO_2 during recompression for the treatment of DCI [45] and in 1939, with Yarbrough, published their research.[45] Despite the reduction in treatment time and improved outcomes, oxygen usage combined with hyperbaric pressure was not common practice until the 1960s.[44]

During WWII, Dr. Kenneth Donald, medical officer in the Royal Navy, looked into the use of closed circuit oxygen rebreathers for Royal Navy divers. Although Haldane and Hill had earlier researched divers breathing oxygen via a self-contained unit,[10] Donald investigated oxygen toxicity using Royal Navy divers at increased pressure both in water and in recompression chambers.[46-47]

Churchill Davidson et al. published a paper in 1955, "High Pressure Oxygen and Radiotherapy,"[48] which reported the results of eight patients with carcinomas receiving radiation treatment while breathing oxygen at 3 ATA (44.1 PSIA) in a chamber which was a modified naval diving recompression chamber. The chamber was 2.8 meters long and 0.76 meters wide, with one 25 centimeter (cm) diameter Perspex porthole on the top and 2 more on the door.[49] This method of treatment came to be used worldwide, although by the mid-1970s interest declined due to mixed patient outcomes and new directional radiation equipment.[1-2] One legacy of this period was the introduction of the cylindrical acrylic tube monoplace chambers which were designed to have better access for patient irradiation (Figure 15). The first acrylic shell monoplace chamber was manufactured by the British company Vickers in 1960.[50] Today manufacturers from various countries make monoplace chambers in a range of shapes and designs.

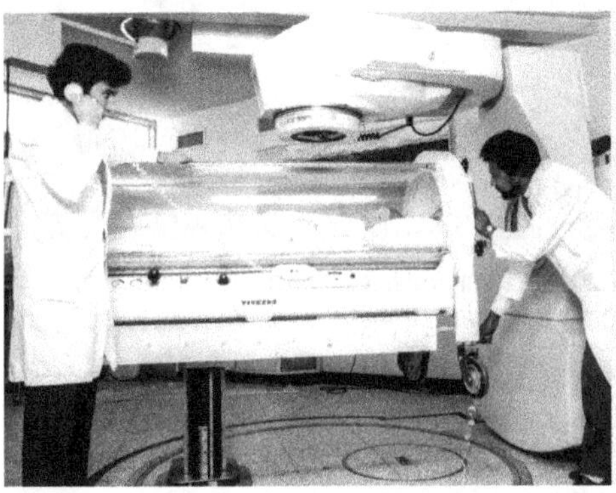

Figure 15. Delivering radiation to a patient in a Vickers monoplace chamber. Royal Perth Hospital, Australia, circa 1971. Photo courtesy of Royal Perth Hospital Museum.

Ite Boerema

In the mid-1950s, Dutch surgeon Ite Boerema investigated ways to increase operation time during cardiac surgery. He looked first at patient hypothermia and then operating while in a hyperbaric chamber delivering HBO_2 at 3 ATA (44.1 PSIA) to the patient. After encouraging trials with a Royal Dutch Navy chamber, Boerema had a large chamber built big enough to hold a full operating team inside[1-3] (Figure 16). A colleague of Boerema's, W. H. Brummelkamp, published in 1961 that anerobic infections could be inhibited with HBO_2.[1-3] Shortly after, a large chamber was installed at the Glasgow Infirmary, Scotland. In 1961 at Glasgow, Smith and Sharp reported the benefits of HBO_2 in carbon monoxide poisoning (COP).[1]

From the late 1950s, large chambers (of all shapes and sizes) for cardiac surgery were installed internationally, including Austria, Australia, USSR, Japan, and more than five in the United States[3] (Figure 17). In 1963, Boerema and his colleagues at Amsterdam, Netherlands, hosted the first International Congress on Clinical Application of Hyperbaric Oxygen.[51] Delegates came from many countries including the Netherlands, Scotland, England, United States, Canada, Australia, Sweden, South Africa, Antilles, Italy, and France.

Staffing for these first chambers mainly came from the operating room area but soon expanded to include interested staff from all fields of medicine and nursing along with military personnel, as HBO_2 extended its scope.[5]

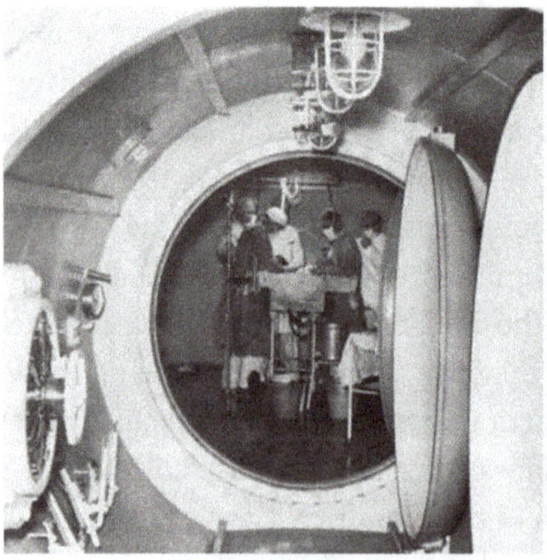

Figure 16. Professor Boerema's Chamber. Amsterdam, Netherlands. Circa 1955. Photo courtesy of Best Publishing Company.

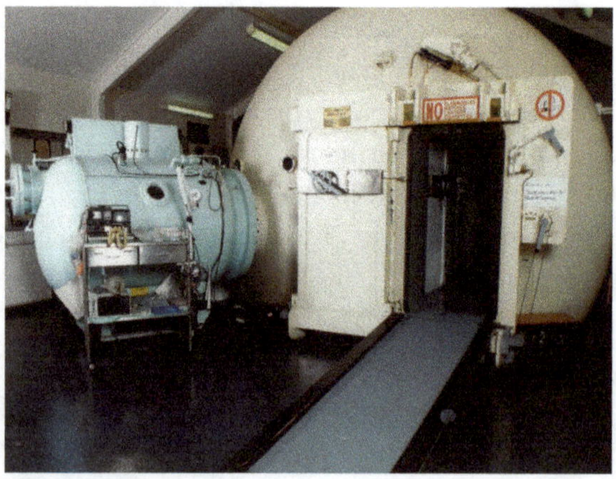

Figure 17. Prince Henry Hospital, Sydney, Australia. Circa 1985. Photo courtesy of Dr. Harry Oxer.

Cardiac surgery under hyperbaric conditions declined after cardiopulmonary bypass pumps became more available. For the next 30 years, numerous papers were published suggesting a wide variety of various patient conditions and diseases that might benefit from HBO_2. Boerema, in 1964, urged that future research for patients to receive HBO_2 there should be a rational medical indication for treatment.[51]

Meanwhile in the 1960s, the field of commercial diving grew with increasing subsea oil and gas exploration and production worldwide.[44] A number of clinical hyperbaric centers started with ex-commercial diving recompression chambers available in abundance. Many hyperbaric technicians and medics came from the oil and gas exploration field. A common commercial diving chamber, known as a "deck chamber," was often used in clinical HBO_2. These twin lock chambers were not designed for clinical and critical care patients, having small floor space and round door entrances. The need for purpose-built chambers was soon taken up by chamber designers, many from the oil and gas exploration industry. Changes implemented for purpose-built chambers included rectangular doors, larger floor space, and the development of upright cylindrical chambers.[4]

Several manufacturers now supply rectangular chambers. These hyperbaric rooms are large rectangular chambers (Figure 18). Despite the improvements in multiplace chambers, due to their high cost, complexity of operation, and increased staffing requirements, many clinical hyperbaric centers, particularly in the United States and Japan, only have monoplace chambers (Figure 19).

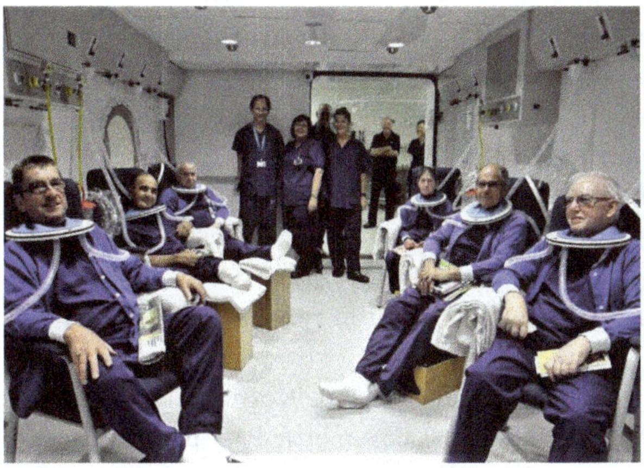

Figure 18. Fink Engineering triple lock chamber at Fiona Stanley Hospital, Perth, Australia, 2014. Photo courtesy of Fiona Stanley Hospital.

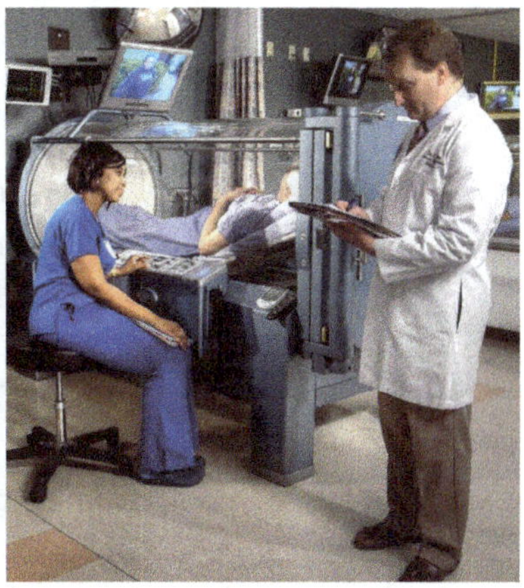

Figure 19. Monoplace hyperbaric unit. Photo courtesy of Prisma Health Richland Hospital, Columbia, SC.

The over 350-year journey of the use of increased pressure to treat medical conditions has had many pioneers and false starts. There are many HBO_2 centers in many countries around the world. The majority of patients receiving HBO_2 nowadays is based on an international evidence-based approach for conditions that are known to benefit from HBO_2.[52] Despite this, HBO_2 is still being used for patient conditions with limited research and anecdotal symptom response.

References

1. Clarke D. History of Hyperbaric Therapy. In: Neuman TS, Thom, SR, editors. Physiology and medicine of hyperbaric oxygen therapy. New York, NY: Elsevier Health Sciences; 2008:3-23.
2. Bakker DJ. History of Hyperbaric Medicine and Surgery. In: Bakker DJ, Cramer FS, editors. Hyperbaric surgery. Flagstone, AZ: Best Publishing Co.; 2002.
3. Kindwall EP. A History of Hyperbaric Medicine. In: Kindwall EP, Whelan, HT, editors. Hyperbaric Medicine Practice 3rd edition. Flagstaff, AZ: Best Publishing Co.; 2008.
4. Haux GF. History of Hyperbaric Chambers. Flagstaff, AZ: Best Publishing Co.; 2000.
5. Handley S, Clarke D. Hyperbaric History and the Nursing Evolution. In: Valerie Larson Lohr, Helen Norvell LJ, Jim Wilcox, editors. Hyperbaric Nursing and Wound Care. Palm Beach Gardens, FL: Best Publishing Co.; 2011:1-11.
6. Colin J. PAUL BERT -Translation of "Paul Bert", Science (French Edition of Scientific American), No. 12, Oct. 1978): NASA TM - 75599; 1978. [Available from: http://ntrs.nasa.gov/archive/nasa/casi.ntrs.nasa.gov/19790005516_1979005516.pdf.
7. Jacobson JH, Morsch JHC, Rendell-Baker L. The Historical Perspective of Hyperbaric Therapy. Annals of the New York Academy of Sciences. 1965;117(2):651-70.
8. Henshaw N. Aero-Chalinos, Or, a Register for the Air in Five Chapters. 1st ed. Dublin: Samuel Dancer; 1664.
9. Bert P. La Pression Barométrique: recherches de physiologie expérimentale 1879. In: Hitchcock MA, Hitchcock FA, editors. Bert P, Barometric Pressure: researches in experimental physiology. Columbus OH: College Book Company; 1943.
10. Hill L. Caisson sickness and the physiology of work in compressed air. London: Arnold; 1912.
11. Reverend TA. An account of several descents in a diving bell at Portsmouth NH. American Journal of Science. 1835;XXII(2):325-6.
12. Junod V-T. Considérations sur un nouveau et puissant moyen curatif- Méthode hémospasique, appareils du Dr. Junod 1841.
13. Tissier PL. Pneumotherapy including aërotherpy and inhalation methods and therapy. Cohen SS, editor. Philadelphia PA: Blakiston's Son & Co; 1903.
14. Arntzenius AKW. De geneeskundige pneumatische inrichting te Amsterdam: ervaringen op het gebied der pneumatische therapie. Amsterdam: Scheltema & Holkema's Boekhandel; 1889.
15. Chirurgus. The compressed air-bath into corresponents. Medical Times and Gazette. 1860.
16. Canadian Patents. Ottawa, Canada: Library and Archives Canada. 1857.

17. Lee C. Extract from a lecture on the physiological and remedial effects of increased pressure of the atmosphere: Joseph Warren & Co., Printers; 1867:6(199-211). Available from: http://books.google.com.au/books?id=lVUBAAAAYAAJ.
18. Taylor GH. Medical Hygiene in Pulmonary Disease, The Compressed Air Bath. Boston Mass. 1857:2(262-265). Available from: http://hdl.handle.net/2027/mdp.39015070245025. 1856-57:Vol 1-2.
19. Taylor GH, Taylor, CF. The Movement Cure on Swedish Method of Curing Disease (Advertisement). New York: Theodore Foster; 1857-58;47-49:317. Available from: http://books.google.com.au/books?id=hrgrAAAAYAAJ.
20. Knight EH. Knight's new mechanical dictionary. Boston MA: Houghton, Mifflin and Company; 1884. Available from: http://www.archive.org/details/knightsnewmechan00knigrich.
21. Stone O. Improvement in treating diseases by condensed air 1865. Available from: www.google.es/patents/US50641.
22. Baldwin DA. Compressed Air as a Therapeutic Agent. Moffat JL, Wilcox DWG, Paige HW, editors; 1867.
23. Regnard P, Dr. La cure d'altitude. Cie Me, editor. Paris;1897.
24. Kellogg RH. La pression barométrique: Paul Bert's hypoxia theory and its critics. Respiration Physiology. 1978;34(1):1-28.
25. Rottenstein JB. Traité d'anesthésie chirurgicale: contenant la description et les applications de la méthode anesthésique de M. Paul Bert: G. Bailliére; 1880.
26. Brown WE, Lucas GHW, Henderson VE. The anesthetic value of nitrous oxide under pressure. *Journal of Pharmacology and Experimental Therapeutics.* 1927;31(4):269-89.
27. Smith W. D. A history of nitrous oxide and oxygen *anaesthesia. IX. The introduction of nitrous oxide and oxygen anaesthesia.* Br J Anaesth. 1966;38(12):950-63.
28. Snell H. Compressed Air Illness or So-called Caisson Disease; 1896.
29. Elliott DH. Early decompression experience: compressed air work. *SPUMS Journal.* 1999;29(1):28-34.
30. Copperthwaite WC. Tunnel shields and the use of compressed air in subaqueous works. London: Archibald Constable &Co Ltd; 1906.
31. Phillips JL. The bends: compressed air in the history of science, diving, and engineering. New Haven CT: Yale University Press; 1998.
32. Haldane JS, Priestley, JG . The regulation of the lung ventilation. *J Physiol.* 1905;32(3-4):225-66.
33. Boycott A, Damant, GCC, Haldane, JS. The prevention of compressed air illness. 1908; 8:342-443. Available from: http://archive.rubicon-foundation.org/7489.
34. Trimble VH. The Uncertain Miracle. New York: Doubleday; 1974.

35. Sellers LM. The fallibility of the forrestian principle: "semper primus pervenio maxima cum VI." *The Laryngoscope.* 1964;74(5):613-33.
36. Cunningham OJ. Therapeutic Apparatus 16 Oct 1923. Available from: www.google.com/patents/US1471144.
37. Sick people cured by compressed air New York, NY: Modern Publishing Company. 1920:97(2);54. Available from: http://books.google.com.au/books?id=7CkDAAAAMBAJ&source=gbs_all_issues_r&cad=1.
38. Bureau of Investigation. The Cunningham "Tank Treatment." 1928;90:1494-98.
39. Cunningham OJ. Oxygen therapy by means of compressed air. *Anesth Analg.* 1927;6:64-6.
40. Anon. Oxygen as an Antipyretic. The Lancet. 1887;129(3327):1144-5.
41. Lorrain Smith J. The pathological effects due to increase of oxygen tension in the air breathed. *J Physiol.* 1899;24(1):19-35.
42. Hill L, Macleod, JJ. The influence of compressed air on the repiratory exchange. *J Physiol.* 1903;29(6):492-510.
43. Binder CA, Faulknenr, JM, Moore, RL,. Oxygen poisoning in mammals. *J Exp Med. 1927*;45(5):849-64.
44. Elliott DH, Vorosmarti, J. An outline History of Diving Physiology and Medicine. In: Brubakk A, Neuman, TS., Bennett, P B., Elliott, DH., editor. Bennett and Elliott's physiology and medicine of diving. Philadelphia PA: Saunders; 2003:4-16.
45. Yarbrough OD, Behnke, AR. The treatment of compressed air illness using oxygen. *Journal of Industrial Hygiene and Toxicology.* 1939;21:213-8.
46. Donald K. Oxygen poisoning in man part 1. *BR MED J.* 1947;1(4506):667-72.
47. Donald KW. Oxygen poisoning in man part 2. *BR MED J.* 1947;1(4507):712-7.
48. Churchill-Davidson J, Sanger, C, Thomlinson, RH. High pressure oxygen and radiotherapy. *Lancet.* 1955;1:1091-5.
49. Sanger C, Churchill-Davidson I, Thomlinson RH. Anaesthesia for radiotherapy under high-pressure oxygen. *Br J Anaesth.* 1955;27(9):436-46.
50. Williams K, Hopkinson, WI,. Small Chamber Techniques in Hyperbaric Oxygen Therapy. In: Ledingham IM, editor. Hyperbaric Oxygenation - Proceedings of the Second International Congress. Glascow Scotland: E & S Livingstone Ltd; 1964.
51. Clinical application of hyperbaric oxygen: Proceedings of First International Congress Amsterdam, 1963. Flagstaff, AZ: Best Publishing Co.; 1964.
52. UHMS Hyperbaric Oxygen Therapy Indications. Weaver LK, editor. North Palm Beach, Florida: Best Publishing Co.; 2014.

CHAPTER 2
Hyperbaric Chambers: Definition, Types, Future Directions

J. Steven Wood

In this chapter, we will review the classes of hyperbaric chambers, discuss typical design components, and consider what the future may hold for human (and animal) pressure vessels.

In many respects, today's hyperbaric chambers are identical to systems that were deployed 50 or 100 years ago. It is not uncommon to encounter chambers in use that, due to careful design and diligent maintenance, have provided yeoman's service for decades.

A hyperbaric chamber is a device which is pressurized to some pressure above the local ambient pressure. A chamber may accommodate single or multiple occupants, dependent upon design. Chambers may be pressurized by a variety of gases, with air and 100% oxygen being the most common for clinical use. Specialty gas mixes may be utilized in certain applications, such as the prevention or treatment of decompression illness.

Hyperbaric chambers are classified by their occupancy, utilizing the categories established by the U.S. National Fire Protection Association. There are three classes: Class A (multiplace), Class B (monoplace), and Class C (animal).[1] Chambers are typically constructed in accordance with standard engineering codes (discussed later in this text), and as a result, there is little variation in the design of the pressure vessel itself. Control systems, viewports, and interior/exterior finishes are the primary differentiating factors between chambers.

Components

A hyperbaric chamber system consists of the following multiple components: the pressure vessel, with its attendant doors, viewports, and hull penetrations; gas supplies and attendant piping; control and life support systems; and internal fixtures for occupant comfort and care.

The Pressure Vessel

Modern hyperbaric chambers have direct engineering roots to boilers and pressure vessels that powered the Age of Steam. Hard lessons, written in the blood of victims of boiler explosions and other mishaps, led to the development of strict design rules designed to protect the lives of those who worked with and lived around these devices. By the early 20th century, safe designs had been promulgated. As a result, pressure vessel designs today, though refined somewhat in design and materials, bear striking similarities to vessels of our grandparents' days. The "if it works, don't mess with it" school is the mantra of the mass-market pressure vessel manufacturer, whose designs strictly follow accepted engineering codes. Deviation from codes can result in substantial investments in time and money to convince regulatory authorities that a new design or material can provide a comparable level of safety to existing approved design standards.

Though there have been some innovations in materials, most chambers are manufactured from steel or aluminum. Advances in design and analysis tools (computer-aided design, finite element analysis, nondestructive testing, and failure analytics) have allowed designers to produce extremely strong vessels made of unusual materials. Chambers have been constructed of titanium, concrete, Kevlar, and carbon composites; however, attaining approval of these innovative materials by regulatory authorities can require extensive testing and documentation. The time and cost burden imposed on manufacturers who wish to introduce new designs or materials to pressure vessel construction that are compliant to accepted engineering code is often so high that an economic case cannot be made to innovate.

Human-occupied pressure vessels that do not conform to accepted standards, such as the *American Society of Mechanical Engineers (ASME) Pressure Vessels for Human Occupancy (PVHO)*, are built and sold. Some nonconforming chamber designs have received approval for sale as medical devices by the U.S. Food and Drug Administration. In locales that have adopted ASME standards as part of their building codes, the operation of a noncode pressure vessel may be illegal, and the operator subject to civil penalties or even criminal charges in the event of an accident that results in injury.

Hull shapes are commonly horizontal or vertical cylinders, hearkening back to traditional boiler designs. Rectangular shapes are becoming more common in multiplace clinical chambers as these designs provide a more "room-like" environment for patients. Multiplace chambers usually are designed with two or three internal compartments that can be independently pressurized and depressurized, allowing occupants and workers to enter and leave the chamber as necessary. Monoplace and animal chambers are typically single compartment designs.

Access to the chamber may be accomplished via doors or hatchways. Due to the high-imposed stresses and need to provide a gas-tight seal, door/hatch design is vital for safety. In a large Class A chamber, the door alone may weigh in excess of 500 kg (1,100 lbs). The closure mechanism must be robust enough to tolerate the high loads from chamber pressurization, yet balanced appropriately to allow easy opening and closing. A multiple-compartment vessel may be equipped with a variety of door designs, from large rectangular doorways that allow gurney-bound patients to be rolled into the chamber to circular hatchways between the compartments.

Gas Supplies/Piping

All chambers will require gas supplies for chamber pressurization and patient breathing. Gases will be piped to and from the chamber via piping systems. Depending upon chamber design, the gas supply required may be a single gas, utilized for both chamber compression and patient breathing, as in a Class B chamber utilizing 100% oxygen. Class A chambers are typically supplied with multiple gas systems: air for compression, oxygen for treatment, and air for breathing. Class A chambers utilized for treatment of decompression illness may be equipped with mixed-gas compression and breathing systems utilizing specialized mixes of oxygen, nitrogen, helium, and other gases.

Oxygen is usually supplied from liquid oxygen (LOX) systems, backed up with high-pressure cylinders. LOX may be stored in fixed tanks of 1,000-100,000 liter capacity, which are filled from tanker trucks. For remote locations, or systems with more modest oxygen demands, smaller portable LOX tanks (80-200 liter) or high-pressure cylinders may be utilized. Though not yet approved for health care use in the United States, there is growing use of molecular sieve technology which can provide a continuous oxygen supply by separating oxygen from air.

Air utilized for chamber compression and breathing is usually supplied by dedicated compressor systems with backup by high-pressure cylinders. Compressed air must meet stringent standards for cleanliness and purity, with attendant filters, dryers, and monitoring equipment. Some Class B facilities may utilize small quantities of compressed air for air break breathing, supplied by high-pressure cylinders.

In hyperbaric facilities that treat complicated decompression illness or conduct research, other gases, such as helium, nitrogen, or argon may be utilized. Specialty gases are typically stored in banks of high-pressure cylinders controlled by automated switching systems.

Piping systems conduct gases to the chamber(s) for pressurization and patient breathing and may also provide water for fire protection, environmental control, and sanitary services. During ventilation and decompression, gases must be conducted from the chamber to the outside of the hyperbaric facility. The piping system must be designed to conform to standards for materials and fabrication to assure that the system provides passages for gases and fluids that are secure and safe. Supply piping is typically fabricated from specially cleaned copper, assembled by pipe fitters who have been trained in gas system construction, then tested to assure pressure integrity, cleanliness, and that the installed lines deliver the gases that they are supposed to deliver. Exhaust lines must be designed to accommodate high flows encountered during emergency decompression as well as standard ventilation flow. Codes require that exhaust lines be protected from intrusion from insects, debris, water, and located to ensure that gases cannot re-enter the hyperbaric facility.

Control Systems

In early chambers, control systems were rudimentary: a valve to control the flow of gas into the chamber; a valve to control the flow of gas out of the chamber; and a pressure gauge indicating pressure within the chamber. By adjusting in- and outflow, the chamber operator could pressurize, maintain, or depressurize the chamber. Though control systems have evolved over the years, in reality, the role of a modern control system is to do those three functions, while reducing operator workload.

By the mid-20th century, control systems utilized pneumatically powered regulator and valve sets to pressurize and depressurize the chamber at prescribed rates and maintain the chamber at a determined pressure. The majority of monoplace chambers in use worldwide utilize these simple control systems. The growing complexity of multiplace chambers led to the development of analog electronic control systems that integrated pressure and flow sensors to allow automation of pressurization/depressurization operations. However, due to cost and the custom nature of these systems, few were deployed.

Microprocessor-based control systems were first introduced for monoplace chambers in the mid-1980s by Environmental Tectonics Corporation, utilizing control architecture developed for steam autoclaves. Multiplace chamber manufacturers soon followed suit, and today, most clinical multiplace chambers utilize digital control systems. With microprocessor-based control systems, operators can program the entire treatment profile into the master computer, which utilizes a series of pressure and flow sensors coupled with digitally-controlled valves to automate the treatment pressurization/hold/decompression profile. Digital control systems often also include data logging and patient record-keeping functions, which streamline documentation.

With an increase in control system complexity comes a potential for failure within the system, so backup manual systems are still integrated into modern chambers. It is vital that the chamber operators have a thorough understanding of the control architecture and extensive training in the use of manual backup systems, in order to promptly respond to emergencies arising from a failure of the automated control system.

Safety Systems

Safety in a hyperbaric chamber begins with design and specifications that are incorporated in construction codes such as the *ASME Boiler and Pressure Vessel Code*. *ASME* and related codes establish minimum standards for materials utilized in the construction of a chamber and how those materials are fabricated.[2] Subcodes address specific requirements for pressure vessels intended for human occupancy and the viewports utilized in the chamber.[3] ASME codes focus on maintenance of the structural integrity of the chamber during routine operations as well as providing safety components such as pressure relief valves to reduce the potential for catastrophic failure of the chamber in the event of overpressure resulting from fire or other mishap. A chamber will undergo inspection, testing, and be stamped to indicate that it has been manufactured in compliance with the applicable pressure vessel code. In many locales, only stamped pressure vessels are allowed to be utilized.

Chamber construction codes focus on structural integrity of the pressure vessel, but that is not the limit with respect to chamber safety. Other codes (*National Fire Protection Association [NFPA] 99* and related) impose additional requirements for protection of the facility that houses the chamber, safe operation of the chamber, and protection of occupants. More detailed discussions of these code requirements will follow in this text.

Environmental and Life Support Control Systems

In operation, the characteristics of the chamber environment can vary dramatically. Temperatures rise and fall with pressurization and depressurization. Chamber occupants emit heat, water, carbon dioxide (CO_2), and waste products into the chamber environment that must be managed to provide a safe and comfortable space for the occupants. Chamber type and treatment/mission requirements will influence the complexity of the environmental control system. Internal environmental monitoring may range from nothing more than a pressure gauge, to asking the occupant how they feel, to a complete suite of sensors that display pressure, temperature, humidity, oxygen, and other gas percentages, volatile agent sensors, and smoke detectors. Simple chambers may only require ventilation adjustment to maintain a safe, comfortable environment, while complex, pressurized habitats will be equipped with multiple gas mixes, heat exchangers, sanitary facilities, and other systems.

Monoplace chambers are typically pressurized with oxygen, and the occupant simply breathes the pressurization gas. In a monogas system, carbon dioxide levels, temperature, and humidity are managed by adjusting gas flow through the chamber. *ASME PVHO* requires a minimum ventilation flow of one cubic foot per minute per occupant of the chamber for CO_2 removal.[3] Additional ventilation flow may be required for occupant comfort. Some monoplace chambers are designed to be pressurized with air, with oxygen delivered through a mask or hood system. Air-pressurized monoplace chambers may be subject to similar monitoring requirements of multiplace chambers.

Multiplace chambers are typically pressurized with air, with occupants breathing oxygen or gas mixes through mask or hood systems. Some chambers used for the treatment or prevention of decompression illness may be pressurized with other inert gas mixes such as helium/oxygen or helium/nitrogen/oxygen. Monitoring and maintenance of oxygen levels within the chamber is necessary to reduce fire hazards, with a typical maximum allowed oxygen concentration of 25% in the chamber pressurization gas. Chambers utilized in deep saturation diving may operate with very low oxygen percentages (5% or less) in order to reduce oxygen partial pressures enough to reduce the risk of oxygen toxicity in these extreme environments. Though there are some systems that automatically maintain chamber atmospheres via closed-loop control systems, the more common practice is to have a highly trained operator monitor the sensor systems and manually adjust gas flows to maintain the proper atmospheric gas mix.

Ventilation flow alone may not be enough to provide efficient management of temperature and humidity in larger chambers. Though fans may be utilized to provide cooling in some chambers, they may be coupled with heat exchangers supplied with conditioned water pumped from outside the chamber.

Communications, Physiologic Monitoring, and Support

Communications between the chamber occupants and outside operators is typically provided by an intercom system. Most communications systems include provisions for providing audio feeds for occupant entertainment. Entertainment video displays may be mounted outside a chamber viewport (particularly in monoplace chambers). Other options for providing entertainment video include projecting images through a viewport or installing individual video displays that have been modified with inert gas purging or other features to enhance safety.

Redundant audio communications are typical in multiplace chambers, with speakers and microphones in each compartment. Typical backup communications include the use of sound-powered phones which do not require external power. Monoplace chambers typically have a single communications system installed, so alternate communications provisions should be implemented and ready in the event of failure of the primary communications system. Backup communications can range from having a pad of paper or erasable marker board to a set of pre-printed cards that can be held up to a viewport.

Visual contact with chamber occupants is important for safety. The large cylindrical viewport of monoplace chambers provides unobstructed visibility of the patient. Video monitoring is common in multiplace chambers, as visibility of the chamber interior may be impeded by smaller viewports and multiple compartments. Monoplace facilities that operate multiple chambers may benefit from closed circuit video, particularly if the facility is designed with a central work station rather than chamber-side work stations for staff.

The current trend toward outpatient hyperbaric facilities that focus on the treatment of nonhealing wounds has resulted in a proliferation of facilities that limit their patient acceptance to low-acuity, physiologically-stable patients. The downward spiral in numbers of facilities with the capability to provide high-acuity patient treatment is further exacerbated by the outpatient-focused facilities that have little or no equipment, staff, or desire to treat the full gamut of disorders that are amenable to adjunctive HBO_2. In some areas of the United States, a critical patient with acute decompression illness, carbon monoxide poisoning, or a necrotizing soft tissue infection may require transport to a facility hundreds of miles away to a facility that is staffed and equipped to treat such cases, despite the referring facility having hyperbaric capability. Without a fundamental change in philosophy, in many parts of the world, hundreds of patients face suffering, disability, or death due to lack of access to a proven therapy.

Though there has been a steady decrease in the number of hyperbaric facilities that treat high-acuity patients, some level of physiologic monitoring or assessment is conducted in most hyperbaric facilities. Electrocardiograms, indirect tissue oxygen assessments (tcpO2), and arterial/venous blood pressures (invasive and noninvasive), are among the most common monitored variables. As few monitoring systems are designed for the hyperbaric environment, common practice is to provide specialized hull penetrations that allow placement of a wired sensor inside the chamber, with processing and display of the data done outside the chamber.

Support for the high-acuity patient is even more problematic. With fewer facilities treating such patients, there is less demand for support equipment that is designed for use in or with the hyperbaric environment, which disincentives manufacturers from developing this equipment. Many hyperbaric programs have been forced to modify devices on their own, which raises medico-legal issues, particularly if a patient or staff injury arises subsequent to such a modification.

Chamber design introduces a compounding factor in supporting the acutely-ill patient. Monoplace chamber's confined space, lack of hands-on access, and 100% oxygen environment imposes substantial restrictions of support devices. The compressed air environment of the multiplace chamber does allow the use of standard infusion pumps and ventilators. However, there should be rigorous, documented evaluation of any device under operational hyperbaric conditions before utilizing the device for patient care.

Intravenous fluid administration may be provided with the pump situated outside the chamber, if the pump is capable of overcoming the pressure differential, though few, if any, pumps have the pressure capability to be utilized outside the chamber. Accuracy of volume administration should be assessed to ensure that the pump can provide the fluid volumes desired at pressure. Fluids may also be administered as a bolus or small volume dose from outside the chamber through a stopcock system. If a small volume of drug is administered, it should be flushed to prompt administration of the drug. Pumps taken inside the multiplace chamber should be evaluated prior to use to ensure proper and accurate function under pressure.

Mechanical ventilators purpose-designed for hyperbaric use are, for the most part, frozen at a design phase approximately 50 years old. These ventilators have limited flexibility and may be incapable of supporting a patient with substantial pulmonary dysfunction. Most hyperbaric ventilators are time-cycled, pressure-limited units that cannot even provide patient-triggered ventilation. For patients with severe pulmonary issues, it may be necessary to utilize paralytic agents in order to maintain adequate ventilator support.

In the multiplace environment, the options for mechanical ventilation are more flexible, as there are several more modern ventilators that can be utilized inside the chamber. Advanced pneumatic/fluidic ventilators are desirable for their lack of dependence on electrical supply, but, as noted, extensive performance testing should be conducted prior to use of any device.

Access and Internal Fixtures

In the early days of hyperbarics, when the primary occupants of the chamber were young, fit divers, little consideration was given to chamber ingress and egress and occupant comfort. Small circular hatchways would force the divers to crawl through the hatch, and if an injured diver was being treated, movement was difficult. Occupants sat on the floor of the chamber, with, at best, a thin pad separating the person from the chamber hull.

Over the years, with the growth of medical hyperbarics, patient handling and occupant comfort considerations have led to the installation of larger hatchways and, in multiplace chambers, rectangular doors wide enough to allow passage of gurneys. Monoplace chambers are typically equipped with gurney/stretcher systems that allow easy transfer of the patient in and out of the chamber. Modern multiplace chambers are equipped with removable seating systems that allow reconfiguration of the interior to accommodate varying patient loads and acuity.

As noted earlier, environmental control is becoming a desirable feature in chamber designs. Providing the patient with a comfortable environment is conducive to patient treatment compliance. Entertainment systems are pretty standard across the board. Video and music can be provided. In some multiplace designs, each patient station is equipped with a multichannel entertainment device, similar to airliner inflight systems.

The Hyperbaric Facility

With the exception of chambers utilized for the treatment of decompression sickness in remote areas, shipboard chambers, or mobile/trailer mounted units, most hyperbaric facilities are fixed installations that are located in buildings that have been constructed or modified to house the chamber. The facility design and construction may be influenced by local conditions and codes enforced by the local authority having jurisdiction (AHJ). The facility design must provide for safe and rapid evacuation of the staff and patients in the event of an emergency. The facility must provide protection for the hyperbaric facility from outside threats and be designed to protect the surrounding facility from mishaps that could occur within the hyperbaric unit.

Specific housing rules may vary with locale and chamber type, but in general, the room housing the hyperbaric chamber should be constructed of materials that will protect the room and chamber occupants from external fire, smoke, and other combustion products for a time interval that is adequate to allow safe decompression of the chamber and egress from the area. Area-specific rules may mandate additional precautions. In areas with a history of seismic events, AHJs may require additional reinforcement as well as the addition of restraint systems to securely anchor the chamber.

Walls and doors must be constructed to specific fire ratings (typically up to 1½ hours) and heating, ventilation, and air conditioning (HVAC) systems designed to protect the room from smoke/fume infiltration. Chamber operators must be protected from smoke/fume infiltration so they can continue to operate the chamber in the event of a fire in the facility. Most facilities are equipped with self-contained breathing apparatus or smoke hoods for staff respiratory protection.

The facility that houses the hyperbaric chamber must also be protected from fires that might occur in the chamber or the housing room. Chamber exhaust must be vented outside of the building to prevent the buildup of excessive oxygen levels within the chamber room. The chamber exhaust line must also be sized to allow rapid decompression of the chamber from working pressure (typically two to six minutes, depending upon chamber class). In some locales, additional exhaust lines may be required to exhaust gases from overpressure relief valves, reducing the potential for release of smoke or gases into the chamber room. Exhaust lines should be fabricated from heat-resistant materials, as hot exhaust gases resulting from a chamber fire could broach the exhaust line and contaminate the atmosphere of the chamber housing room.

Following best practices as well as design and construction guidelines can help protect the facility from external fires, but in the event of a fire within the hyperbaric chamber or the chamber housing room, active suppression measures are prudent, and may be required by the AHJ. Water-deluge and hand hoses are required under code for fire suppression in multiplace chambers but are not currently mandated in oxygen-pressurized monoplace chambers. Effective fire suppression systems that generate a high-density water fog have been designed and prototyped for monoplace chambers, but to date, have not been introduced into the market.

A layered approach to fire protection is common in the chamber housing room. A means of generating a fire alarm and receiving fire alerts should be installed. Multipurpose hand-held fire extinguishers should be located within the chamber room. In some locales, automatic sprinkler systems may be required to further protect the facility.

A well-built chamber in a well-built room goes a long way toward safety, but the most important component of a safe chamber is the staff that operates the facility. A staff composed of well-trained professionals who undergo a regular program of emergency drill practice and continuing education can make the difference between a safe program and disaster.

The Future

Hyperbaric oxygen therapy is at a crossroads. Since the early 1990s, the number of hyperbaric chambers in use worldwide has grown exponentially. The field has shifted from a few, highly complex multiplace chamber programs based in research institutions, to small treatment facilities in shopping centers where hyperbaric therapy (HBOT) is simply another option on a menu. Formerly accepted indications for the use of HBO_2 face increasing scrutiny from the medical community, while other indications are touted with little strong evidence of efficacy. The technology of HBOT has a stable engineering and regulatory base, but the inherent inertia within the regulatory environment, coupled with the huge costs associated with obtaining regulatory approval for innovative approaches to design and materials, has slowed the pace of innovation in the hyperbaric industry. Considerations for the future include accepted indications for HBO_2, medical oversight, technologic innovation, training, professional organization, and staffing.

The challenge facing all hyperbaric professionals is to provide the necessary leadership to help those new operators provide therapy in chambers that are manufactured to accepted standards and operated in a safe fashion. There are great opportunities for growth in the field of HBOT but many challenges. A few of the major challenges for the future are discussed below.

Accepted Indications

Despite its ubiquity in nature and use in many industrial processes, when used in medical settings, oxygen is classified as a drug and must be prescribed by an appropriately licensed provider. In the United States, oxygen for medical use is subject to regulation by the Food and Drug Administration (FDA). Though the primary regulatory focus of the FDA is on the assurance that medical oxygen is produced to specific purity standards, oxygen is also listed as a drug, with an indication of treatment of hypoxia. In many respects, HBO_2 is simply high-dose oxygen therapy, and one can make a case that at their root, many, if not all of the uses of HBO_2 are to correct hypoxia and utilize the additional delivered oxygen to stimulate various biologic processes.

One of the first attempts to define appropriate use of HBO_2 was the *UHMS Hyperbaric Oxygen Therapy Committee Report.*[4] Since its introduction over 30 years ago, the number of listed indications has stayed relatively stable, though the list has been subject to criticism as many of the indications have not been subjected to the same level of scrutiny (double-blind, placebo-controlled studies) as modern drugs. Some critics of HBO_2 believe that the lack of modern proof means that HBO_2 is a scam perpetrated on a gullible public, despite strong clinical evidence of efficacy. Given that oxygen is cheap and not patentable, there is little incentive for drug companies to fund studies to support research into new indications, so research is limited to some government and private funding into clinical applications.

Despite the challenges to accepted indications, much of the growth of HBO_2 has been as an adjunctive therapy in the treatment of problem wounds typically associated with diabetes. Since most wound treatment is provided in outpatient clinic settings, HBO_2 has become a treatment of low-acuity patients. The number of clinical hyperbaric facilities that provide treatment coverage 24/7 continues to drop; as a result, acutely ill patients with disorders shown to be responsive to HBO_2 often face long transports or no treatment at all. The reliance of the HBO_2 industry on a limited set of disorders puts the field at risk of collapse if a cheaper or more effective treatment were to be developed.

Economics plays a role in this contraction of the field. Since most health care is paid for by the government or insurance companies, the organizations that pay the bills want to know that their money is spent on an effective therapy. Cost controls by the bill paying groups have forced hyperbaric program operators to provide extensive documentation prior to initiation of treatment, and extensive audits are conducted by many payors.

Some HBO_2 providers have been subject to criminal charges resulting from fraudulent billing practices, and one can expect to see higher levels of scrutiny in the future.

Concurrent with the narrowing of accepted conditions, there has been a growth in the off-label use of HBO_2. Entrepreneurs, driven in many cases by financial motives, tout the use of HBO_2 for a range of disorders, with minimal or no scientific evidence to support the use. In addition to traditional HBO_2, most of the growth in the alternative arena has been the proliferation of mild hyperbarics, which is low-pressure treatment (typically limited to 1.4 atmospheres absolute pressure [ATA]) with compressed air (sometimes with supplemental oxygen, prohibited by the FDA), using chambers that do not conform to accepted industry construction standards. See Technological Innovations section. Mild chambers are popping up in the offices of alternative health practitioners (chiropractors, naturopaths, etc.), in freestanding cash-pay clinics and in the home. To date, there has been little regulatory interest in the alternative side of the hyperbaric industry, and many industry insiders feel that none will be forthcoming unless a major accident occurs that results in multiple deaths or injuries.

Medical Oversight

HBO_2 requires a prescription and medical oversight. Few physicians receive exposure to HBO_2 during their primary training and there are only a few civilian medical residency programs in hyperbaric medicine. Physicians interested in HBO_2 must take short courses of various types, but there are no mandated training qualifications or oversight standards for HBO_2. The UHMS Facility Accreditation Program standards do call out for a minimum of physician training, case review, and continuing education, but since the program is not mandated, less than 25% of the hyperbaric facilities in the United States are currently accredited. Unless a facility chooses to establish an educational minimum for physicians, it is possible for a physician to begin practicing hyperbaric medicine without any formal training. Such a situation is rare, as few facilities would take the medico-legal risk associated with the practice of an untrained provider.

Hyperbaric medicine has increasingly become a field for physicians who are transitioning toward retirement, looking for a job that has stable patients, no emergency call, and a reasonable income. As professional reimbursement for supervision of HBO_2 is not stratified by patient acuity, there is little financial incentive for physicians to consider treating critically ill patients in the middle of the night.

In recent years there has been a substantial increase in the use of physician extenders, physicians' assistants (PA), and nurse practitioners (NP), particularly within the wound care/hyperbaric segment of the industry. Though these paraprofessionals can provide extension of physician services, they cannot independently provide oversight of hyperbaric treatment. It is likely that there will be cost control pressures from reimbursement agencies that will result in more widespread use of physician extenders.

Technologic Innovation

As discussed earlier in this chapter, the inertia of change within chamber design codes, coupled with the adoption of those codes into law, has essentially frozen chamber design. Innovations in chamber design and materials are unlikely to be seen within the code compliant, i.e. the accepted indications component of the hyperbaric industry, which typically requires chambers designed to operate at pressures greater than 1.4 ATA. Growth of the mild hyperbaric/off-label market segment has resulted in a growing pool of chambers constructed of materials that have not undergone the rigorous level of evaluation that traditional chambers have been subject to.

Absent an expansion in the number of accepted indications for HBO_2, it is unlikely that there will be a substantive change in the design or materials of traditional monoplace or multiplace chambers. The most likely scenario will result in incremental refinements in control systems, with an increase in digital control systems that include interconnections to electronic medical records systems, allowing chamber operational data to directly entered into the patient record.

With fewer high-acuity patients undergoing HBO_2, there is less demand for ancillary support devices such as ventilators, intravenous fluid pumps, and physiologic monitors that are designed for use with or in the hyperbaric chamber. As demand drops, fewer manufacturers will be willing to invest in the research and development necessary to bring these devices to market. It is conceivable that sometime in the near future, it may be nearly impossible to provide treatment for acutely-ill patients due to a lack of this necessary equipment.

In summary, the hyperbaric chamber of the future will likely look much like the chamber of today but may only be used to treat only a fraction of the disorders that have been treated to date.

Safety

As stated in Chapter 5.1: Hyperbaric Fires: What is the Extent of the Problem?, Paul Sheffield documents that compared to other medical specialties, the incidence of fire is relatively low. However, Sheffield's 50 years of data offers a stark truth. In the latter 25-year period (1992-2016) analyzed, the number of reported fires and fatalities rose 75% and 264% respectively. This time period also correlates to the period of great expansion in the number of clinical hyperbaric facilities worldwide. This growth poses many challenges for the field of hyperbaric medicine.

In pure economic terms, the development of the oxygen pressurized monoplace chamber drove the growth of the field. A monoplace-based hyperbaric facility could be established at the fraction of the cost of a multiplace chamber facility. The lower economic bar to entry, coupled with (at least in the period from the late 1980s through the early 2000s) stable reimbursement, fed the increase in the number of clinical facilities, particularly in the United States. This rapid growth had an impact on personnel, training, and safety.

In the early days of hyperbarics, the pool of experienced technical personnel was very small. Most of the acknowledged experts came from what were not considered to be clinical backgrounds, i.e. diving and aerospace, which were somewhat narrowly focused to the unique aspects of those areas. The predominance of multiplace chamber systems, with their complex systems, required personnel to have strong technical backgrounds and the ability to do much of their own repair and maintenance (wrench skills). The introduction of monoplace chambers, with their relatively simple pneumatic control systems, resulted in an influx of chamber operators with a strong clinical background but with less of a technical focus. Passing on the knowledge of the pioneers of the field is critical to having a safe field.

Training is the foundation of safety. When the author began his hyperbaric career in 1985, there were few basic training courses offered. Today, there is a robust training community that offers introductory 40-hour training programs and advanced training in hyperbaric safety. The UHMS Hyperbaric Facility Accreditation program's requirements of training and ongoing education of technical staff have helped facility operators to strengthen staff education and competency testing.

Despite the growth in training and related educational resources (including this text), we still face the fact of increasing accidents. Though equipment malfunctions do occur, human factors are still the big killer in the field. Some may say that the operational simplicity of modern monoplace chambers has resulted in a dumbing down of the technical side of the field. Rather than having a dedicated technical staff to maintain and operate a large multiplace chamber, some facility operators consider chamber technologists as an afterthought, particularly in those facilities that utilize monoplace chambers and hyperbaric therapy as an adjunct to treatment of problem wounds.

Compounding the future safety picture is the increasing growth of the so-called mild hyperbaric chamber. Constructed of flexible material with zippered closures, and typically limited to 1.4 ATA, these devices are based on a design of a similar chamber that was originally approved by the FDA for use in the treatment of altitude decompression sickness. Health benefits claimed for mild hyperbaric treatments by alternative health care practitioners (chiropractors and naturopaths), athletes, and celebrities have resulted in a proliferation of these devices that are sold for use in clinics and the home. Despite not having FDA approval for use with oxygen, flexible chambers are regularly sold with oxygen concentrators. It is not uncommon to see social media posts by individuals undergoing treatment in "mild" chambers with supplemental oxygen while using electronic devices that could serve as ignition sources (cell phones, personal entertainment consoles, etc.). Though there is no comprehensive database of accidents associated with these devices, deaths associated with improper use of these chambers have been reported in the United States and Canada.

Gazing into the crystal ball, the future for hyperbaric safety is cloudy. Economic pressures within the traditional hospital-based hyperbaric facilities may result in closure of some facilities and downsizing of others. It is vital that hyperbaric professionals continue to advocate for implementation of the safety procedures delineated in this text, and to encourage the adoption of comprehensive safety programs in any setting in which HBOT is provided. The only way that the upward spike in accidents can be stopped is to work for a world in which HBOT is administered in chambers that are constructed and maintained in accordance with proper engineering and manufacturing standards, operated by personnel who are properly trained to practice safe operations of their facilities, and supported by management that places a premium on the provision of a safe environment for patients and staff. The challenge to all of us in the industry is there. We must accept it and do all we can to protect our patients.

References

1. National Fire Protection Association. NFPA 99: Health care facilities code. Quincy, MA: NFPA. 2018.
2. American Society of Mechanical Engineers. ASME Boiler and Pressure Vessel Code (BPVC), Section VIII: Rules for Construction of Pressure Vessels, Division 1. ASME Standard: BPVC-VIII-1. 2017.
3. American Society of Mechanical Engineers. Safety standard for pressure vessels for human occupancy (ASME-PVHO-1). ASME Standard: PVHO-1. 2016.
4. Weaver, LK ed. Hyperbaric Oxygen Therapy Indications 13th Edition. Undersea and Hyperbaric Medical Society. North Palm Beach, FL: Best Publishing Company; 2013.

CHAPTER 3
Codes, Standards, and Regulatory Compliance

CHAPTER 3.1
Things You Should Know about *NFPA 99* Health Care Facilities Code

Robert Sheffield, BA, CHT

Since 1968, the National Fire Protection Association (NFPA) has published a standard for hyperbaric facilities. This guidance currently exists as a chapter in *NFPA 99: Health Care Facilities Code.* There are other fire codes and building codes in the United States, but *NFPA 99* is the only code to specifically address hyperbaric facilities. Documents that do not apply in a regulatory context can still be very useful as sources of information. This is certainly the case with the hyperbaric facilities chapter of *NFPA 99.* This chapter contains guidance on design of hyperbaric chambers, design of hyperbaric facilities, and hyperbaric facility operations.

Although NFPA is a United States organization, *NFPA 99* has been referenced in the standards of other countries. Each country has its own regulatory system in place and how these different systems operate varies. Discussion of code adoption, compliance, and authorities having jurisdiction (AHJ) in this chapter are based on the U.S. regulatory system.

Must I comply with the *NFPA 99* code?

Maybe. If your hyperbaric facility is in a hospital, clinic, doctor's office, or any other business occupancy in the United States, then the answer is probably. The answer is not necessarily "yes" because fire codes are not federally mandated. They are chosen by individual states, counties, or municipalities (for the purpose of this discussion the generic term "jurisdiction" is used), and *NFPA* is not the only fire code to choose from. There are different fire codes in force in different jurisdictions across the United States. *NFPA 99* is the most widely used fire code for health care facilities in the United States. It probably applies to you. Even if compliance with *NFPA 99* is not mandatory in your jurisdiction, the Hyperbaric Facilities Chapter is an excellent source of information on hyperbaric safety.

Am I meant to follow the most recent edition?

This will vary by jurisdiction. Each jurisdiction will periodically re-address their choice of fire codes and potentially update the edition they choose to enforce. This decision process does not operate on the same timeline as the revision cycle for *NFPA 99*. Therefore, a particular jurisdiction may be enforcing the most recent edition, or it may be enforcing one of several older editions. Different jurisdictions do not necessarily coordinate with one another. Various editions of the code are in force across the United States. Even though you might be legally required to comply with a certain edition of *NFPA 99*, you should look at the newest edition as a source of information. It has incorporated more experience and contains the most current thinking.

Who enforces *NFPA 99*?

The policing authority for the fire code is called the Authority Having Jurisdiction (AHJ). This is usually the local or state fire marshal. This individual is mandated by his or her jurisdiction to enforce whichever edition of whichever fire code has been adopted by that jurisdiction. Fire marshals interpret *NFPA 99* (or whichever fire code has been adopted) as they believe applies to you. Fire marshals have the authority to mandate changes or close a facility if they deem something to be a hazard to life.

If you ever meet your AHJ, it is a good idea to be aware of the regulations he or she is trying to enforce upon you. If compliance with *NFPA 99* is mandatory in your jurisdiction, you should know what is required and be able to demonstrate how you are in compliance.

How are NFPA standards generated?

NFPA is a standard-making organization governed by the American National Standards Institute (ANSI) process. One of the governing principles of NFPA is openness. Any action taken by NFPA or one of its committees is public information.

For each NFPA document, there is a technical committee (TC) responsible for the content of the document. Another governing principle of NFPA is balance. The composition of NFPA committees is regulated to ensure no one company or group of interested parties has undue influence on the content of the document. Applications for TC membership are scrutinized by the NFPA standards council. In the case of *NFPA 99*, there are several TCs, each responsible for a particular chapter and a technical correlating committee (TCC) responsible for issues of coordination among chapters. The TC responsible for the Hyperbaric Facilities Chapter is the Healthcare – Hyperbaric TC (HEA-HYP).

Is the Hyperbaric Facilities Chapter the only part of *NFPA 99* relevant to me?

No. For the purpose of this discussion, the chapter numbers in the 2018 edition of *NFPA 99* are used. Chapter numbers may change among different editions of *NFPA 99*. You will find useful information in the following chapters of *NFPA 99*:

- Definitions (Chapter 3)

- Gas and Vacuum Systems (Chapter 5)
- Gas Equipment (Chapter 11)
- Hyperbaric Facilities (Chapter 14)
- Annex A
- Annex B

Annex A contains additional guidance and explanatory information. Each note in Annex A refers back to a specific requirement in the body of the code. There are many notes in Annex A related to the Hyperbaric Facilities Chapter. Annex B contains general safety information (not related to a specific requirement). There are several notes in Annex B relevant to hyperbaric facilities.

Although not part of *NFPA 99*, guidance on the liquid oxygen supply systems utilized by most hyperbaric facilities can be found in *NFPA 55: Compressed Gases and Cryogenic Fluids Code.*

Can I request a change to *NFPA 99*?

Yes. Changes to NFPA documents are driven by input from the public. You do not need to be a member of NFPA or a member of a TC in order to participate. The revision cycle of a NFPA document has three stages: input stage, comment stage, and NFPA technical meeting. You have an opportunity to make your voice heard by NFPA in each of these stages. Information about submitting input to NFPA can be found in the back of the *NFPA 99* code book and on the NFPA website: www.nfpa.org. The following is a description of the revision cycle for *NFPA 99* (Figure 1).

Figure 1. The revision cycle for *NFPA 99.*

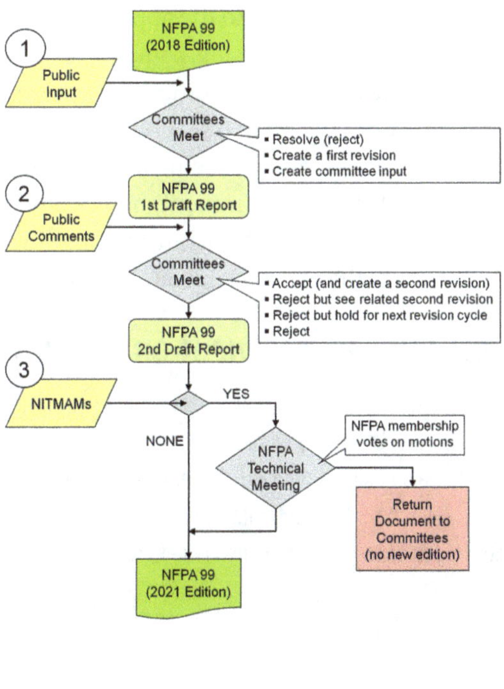

The First Draft

Shortly after a new edition of *NFPA 99* is released, work begins on the next edition by opening a public input period of approximately six months. Anyone can submit public input within the prescribed period. These suggested changes will help create the first draft of the next *NFPA 99*. At the end of the public input period, the suggested changes are distributed to the appropriate TC, who must meet and address all the suggested changes. Any input for the Hyperbaric Facilities Chapter is directed to the HEA-HYP committee. When addressing public input, the TC has three possible actions: resolve the public input (i.e. choose not to use the input in the first draft), create a first revision, or create a committee input with the intent of collecting public comments. With any of these actions, the TC must generate a statement explaining the TC action. Before the first draft is finalized, there is a ballot of TC members to vote and comment on each of the TC actions. At the end of this input stage, NFPA publishes a first draft report which contains all pertinent information about this stage of the revision cycle, including first draft, public input, committee input, TC and TCC statements, and ballot statements. The first draft report is available to the public so you can see what was proposed, what the TC did with it, and why.

The Second Draft

When the first draft report is published, this opens a comment period of approximately two months. The comment period is an opportunity for the public to suggest changes to the first draft. You can only submit comments related to TC actions in the first draft (i.e. first revisions, committee input, or public input that was resolved by the TC). This is your chance to "straighten out" the TC if you feel something in the first draft is not appropriate, but you may not introduce new input at this stage. At the end of the comment period, comments are distributed to the appropriate TC, who must meet and address all public comments. When addressing comments, the TC has four possible actions: accept the comment (the comment becomes a second revision exactly as it was submitted); reject the comment but see related second revision (the TC agrees with the comment in principle but has already made one or more second revisions addressing the issue with language different than the comment); reject but hold the comment (the comment will not be used in the second draft but will automatically become public input in the next revision cycle of the code); or reject. With any of these actions, the TC

TIPS FOR SUBMITTING PUBLIC INPUT OR COMMENTS TO NFPA

Public input and comments are meant to be the exact text in the exact place you want it to appear in the next edition of ***NFPA 99***. Be precise in the language you choose. Vague language might be misinterpreted by the TC. You should also include detailed rationale and technical substantiation (e.g., data, references) for your proposal. Give the TC enough information to understand your intent and appreciate the value of your suggestion. If you have more than one issue to address, submit each one as a separate input/comment.

must generate a statement explaining the TC action. Before the second draft is finalized, there is a ballot of TC members to vote and comment on each of the TC actions. At the end of this comment stage, NFPA publishes a second draft report which contains all pertinent information about this stage of the revision cycle, including second draft, public comments, TC and TCC statements, and ballot statements. The second draft report is available to the public so you can see what was proposed, what the TC did with it, and why.

If a member of the public is not satisfied with a TC action in the second draft, he or she can submit a comment on the second draft, but at this stage in the process it is called a notice of intent to make a motion (NITMAM). The window of opportunity to submit a NITMAM is approximately one month from the release of the second draft report. New input cannot be introduced at this stage, so NITMAMs must be related to issues from the second draft. If the NITMAM is certified as appropriate by NFPA, it becomes a certified amending motion. The motion would occur on the floor of the main NFPA technical meeting prior to the vote on adoption of the second draft as the new edition of *NFPA 99*. The individual making the motion must appear at the main meeting and state his case to NFPA membership. The NFPA membership will then take a vote to determine if the motion carries or not. If the motion carries, the second draft is amended to include the content specified in the NITMAM. It is possible to have a certified NITMAM proposing rejection of the entire second draft of *NFPA 99*. If this motion carries at the main NFPA technical meeting, *NFPA 99* is returned to committee for another revision cycle and a new edition is not released. If there are no certified NITMAMs to modify or reject the document (or these motions fail by vote of NFPA membership), the second draft of *NFPA 99* becomes the new edition of *NFPA 99*.

Note: The author has been a long-standing member of the NFPA HEA-HYP for more than 20 years, is past-chairman of the committee, and has a strong command of the contents of the code on hyperbaric facilities. As a result of his content knowledge, he provided the reader with a bibliography in lieu of a formal reference list.

Bibliography

1. Workman, WT. Understanding the Regulatory Environment Lecture. In: Hyperbaric Safety Director Course. San Antonio, TX: International ATMO; 2018.
2. NFPA 55: Compressed Gases and Cryogenic Fluids Code. Quincy, MA: National Fire Protection Association; 2016.
3. NFPA Standards Directory. Quincy, MA: National Fire Protection Association; 2018.

CHAPTER 3.2
The Regulatory Landscape in the United States (Who Is the Authority Having Jurisdiction?)

Wilbur T. Workman, BS, MS, CAsP, CHT-A, FAsMA, FUHM

Introduction

In my opinion, the regulatory environment with regard to oversight over the field of hyperbaric medicine in the United States can best be described as a quagmire. Based on my personal assessment, there are at least 18 agencies and organizations that have some sort of relationship with the hyperbaric medicine community. This creates a problem in that most of them do not fully understand the role they play nor do they communicate among themselves.

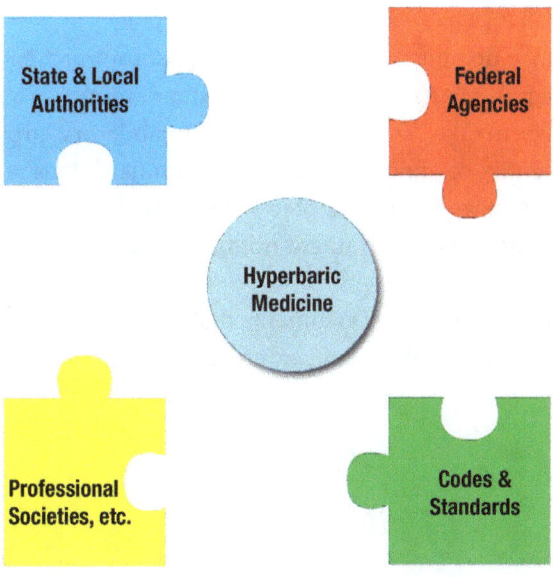

As I travel around the country, I am constantly amazed at the low level of knowledge of just who has oversight over hyperbaric medicine and who does not. This knowledge deficit is not just limited to hyperbaric practitioners but within the agencies themselves who are responsible for regulation. In this chapter I will attempt to identify these agencies and organizations, define where they fit into the jurisdictional hierarchy, and suggest how you can help eliminate some of the educational gaps related to these deficits.

Definitions

To help set the foundation for many of the concepts that will be addressed, I believe defining some terms will be helpful. Having been affiliated for over 45 years with most of the organizations that will be addressed in this chapter, I have developed my own definitions of key terms and concepts, namely, laws, code, standards, guidelines, and recommended practices.

Authority having jurisdiction (AHJ): A government agency (local, state, or federal) that has the authority to enforce laws, codes and standards.

Law: A rule that must be obeyed or some form of punishment will follow (if caught!). Enforcement of a law is by a governmental agency (local, state, or federal).

Code: A compliance document that contains only mandatory provisions using the word “shall” to indicate requirements. Codes are generally written in a manner that they can be adopted into law by a governmental agency (local, state or federal). In the absence of a government agency adopting a code into law, they are nothing more than a “best practice” document and might not be enforceable.

Standard: A compliance document that contains mandatory provisions using the word “shall” to indicate requirements. Unlike a code, a standard may also contain additional provisions using a term like “should.” These nonmandatory provisions are usually contained in an appendix or annex. Like a code, a standard does not have the force of law unless a government agency has adopted the standard into law and is nothing more than a “best practice” document and might not be enforceable.

Guidelines and recommended practices: Documents that contain information that is advisory or informative in nature and contains only nonmandatory provisions.

The Hierarchy of Jurisdiction

Primary Regulatory Agencies

There are three categories of agencies that have the highest degree of oversight of the hyperbaric medicine community: federal, state, and local AHJs.

At the federal level there are the Centers for Medicare & Medicaid Services (CMS) and the Food and Drug Administration (FDA). At the state and local levels there are state departments of health, state medical boards, state pressure vessel inspectors, fire marshals, and building code inspectors. Each of these organizations has a different focus and is one of the components that contribute to the quagmire.

The Centers for Medicare & Medicaid Services

CMS establishes a National Coverage Determination (NCD) policy regarding the reimbursement policy for hyperbaric oxygen therapy (HBOT). This federal policy (you can read that as law) is implemented by a network of seven medicare administrative contractors (MACs). Each of the MACs has the option of developing its own local coverage determination (LCD) regarding how it intends to implement CMS guidance. Not every MAC has an active LCD for HBOT. In such cases, the NCD takes precedent.

It is important to know that CMS uses the Undersea & Hyperbaric Medical Society's (UHMS) recognized indications of use as a guide to establish its reimbursement policy. However, it does not accept all of the indications as listed by the UHMS.

If you do not know how your MAC intends to implement CMS reimbursement policy, you should research their position, since as LCDs are updated, the requirements that must be met for training, documentation, etc., are becoming increasingly stringent.

One of the requirements for a health care facility to receive Medicare reimbursement for services is to comply with the 2012 edition of the *NFPA 101, Life Safety Code.*[1] It should be noted that this declaration also included specific language regarding the requirement for health care facilities that provide HBOT services to comply with the hyperbaric facility requirements cited in *NFPA 99.* The question that immediately comes to mind is, "Who is going to enforce this targeted requirement?"

The Food and Drug Administration

It is important to remember that the FDA does not regulate the practice of medicine. However, the FDA does regulate the manufacture and marketing of hyperbaric chambers. In 1976 they defined a hyperbaric chamber as a Class II medical device in the Safe Medical Device Act of 1976 (21 CFR Part 868, Section 868.5470 Hyperbaric Chamber).[2]

In addition to establishing the requirement for a manufacturer of a hyperbaric chamber to seek approval via the FDA's PreMarket Notification (510k) process before they legally place their chamber system into commercial distribution in the United States, the FDA has classified a clinical hyperbaric chamber as a prescriptive device. This means that its use must be based upon the issuance of a prescription from a licensed practitioner such as MD or DO. Based upon my personal experience, this federal mandate is being ignored daily all over this country with the appearance of hyperbaric chambers in settings like health spas, etc.

Like CMS, the FDA has adopted the UHMS recognized indications to establish their listed indications of use. That said, when the FDA set the list, they used the UHMS recommendations that were in place in 1978 and has not been updated since.

In an effort to close the communication gap among the various organizations with some degree of oversight over the practice of hyperbaric medicine, the FDA and the UHMS jointly sponsored a one-day conference in April 2000 to discuss areas of responsibility. Thirteen different groups were represented, including CMS (Life Safety), FDA, UHMS, National Fire Protection Association (NFPA), American Society of Mechanical Engineers (ASME), The Joint Commission (TJC), the National Board of Diving & Hyperbaric Medical Technology (NBDHMT), the Baromedical Nurses Association (BNA) and others. In spite of unanimous agreement among all attendees that the conference was a success and should be held on some recurring basis, unfortunately there has been virtually no follow-through since.

The most obvious method of FDA oversight is through the issuance of warning letters to hyperbaric chamber manufacturers and in rare instances, users of hyperbaric chambers. According to my personal records, 14 warning letters have been issued since 2000 to 10 different companies and treatment facilities. These warnings were based on a variety of issues including premarket notification violations, off-label use, quality systems violations, lack of medical device reporting systems, and misbranding. The FDA even issued a formal consumer notice in August 2013 warning consumers not to be misled by claims of the efficacy of HBOT for a growing list of off-label indications.[3]

Authorities Having Jurisdiction (AHJ)

In addition to CMS and the FDA, there are other AHJs that have direct oversight of various aspects of hyperbaric medicine. As noted above, there are state departments of health, state medical boards, state pressure vessel inspectors, fire marshals, and building code inspectors, etc. Even though state departments of health and their respective medical boards do have oversight on primarily medical and quality of care issues, their level of activity is generally low. For that reason, I will focus on the state pressure vessel inspector and the local fire marshal.

In the United States, each state has an office responsible for oversight of boilers and pressure vessels. This office is typically organized under the state's Department of Labor. A primary responsibility of this office is to periodically inspect boilers and other pressure vessels for certification and continued safe use. Hyperbaric chambers are pressure vessels designed specifically for human occupancy and may fall under the jurisdiction of this office. I say "may" since compliance to the engineering codes for pressure vessels for human occupancy is not separately mandated in all 50 states. At the time of this writing, compliance to *ASME Boiler and Pressure Vessel Code*, Section VIII and

ASME PVHO-1 is only mandated by 11 states and 3 cities.[4] They are:

- Arkansas
- California
- Delaware
- Georgia
- Hawaii
- Minnesota
- North Carolina
- Oregon
- Tennessee
- Washington
- Wisconsin
- City of Denver
- City of Seattle
- District of Columbia

Until recently, pressure vessel inspectors in the above states had not focused resources on the routine inspection of clinical hyperbaric chambers. This is slowly changing. More specifically, pressure vessel inspectors in Delaware, Georgia, and North Carolina are becoming more engaged with oversight of clinical hyperbaric chambers.

One of the most direct lines of oversight of the field of hyperbaric medicine falls under the jurisdiction of the state and local fire marshal and to a lesser degree that of the local building code inspector. Since the state fire marshal does not routinely get directly involved in local matters, I will limit this discussion to the responsibilities of the local fire marshal.

There are two primary codes that fall under the purview of the fire marshal's office (frequently referred to as the Office of Fire Prevention). The most directly applicable is *NFPA 99, Health Care Facilities Code* of which the 2018 edition is the most current at the time of this writing. The second is *NFPA 101, Life Safety Code* of which the 2018 edition is also the most current at the time of this writing. A more in-depth discussion of these two codes follows below.

Codes and Standards

It is important to know that codes and standards are not haphazardly developed. For the most part, they are developed as a result of some sort of catastrophic event such as loss of life, property, or both. Just under 10,000 such documents have been developed under the American National Standards Institute's (ANSI) standardization and conformity procedures known as essential requirements.[5]

ANSI is a private, nonprofit (501(c)3) that administers and coordinates voluntary standardization and conformity assessment systems. It was established in 1918 by engineering societies and government agencies. Over 200 organizations that develop codes and standards are accredited by ANSI. These include ASME and the NFPA.

ANSI's essential requirements consist of four key elements:

- Openness
  - Allows for public review and comment

- Balance
  - No one industry segment can dominate the process
- Consensus
- Due process
  - Allows for differing opinions to be expressed
  - Provides a process for appeal

American Society of Mechanical Engineers

One of the basic building blocks for hyperbaric chamber safety is the appropriate design, fabrication and testing of these devices. As mentioned above, the majority of codes and standards are developed as the result of some sort of catastrophic event. Such was the case when the American Society of Mechanical Engineers established the Boiler Code Committee in 1911. The committee was formed in response to a series of boiler and pressure vessel accidents, one of which was the tragic failure of a boiler at a shoe factory in Brockton, MA, in 1905 which killed over 50 workers and injured approximately 150. The committee completed their work to develop standards related to the construction and care of boilers and pressure vessels and approved the Boiler Construction Code in 1915. The code is now known as the *Boiler and Pressure Vessel Code (BPVC)*. In the United States, most hyperbaric chambers are designed, fabricated, and tested in accordance with Section VIII, Division 1 or Division 2. To simplify matters, Section VIII deals primarily with the metallic portions of a hyperbaric chamber. For a multiplace chamber, this means the actual pressure vessel and associated piping. For a traditional monoplace chamber, this means the metallic portions of the pressure boundary such as the metal end plates and tie rods. Once a hyperbaric chamber is fabricated, tested and inspected by a third-party inspector, a "U" stamp is affixed to the vessel to certify compliance to the code.

For nearly 45 years, hyperbaric chambers were compliant to the above code. However, in the late 1950s and early 1960s hyperbaric chamber systems used to support the commercial diving industry's involvement in offshore oil exploration demonstrated that reliance solely on the *BPVC* was insufficient. When the contents of a pressure vessel are humans instead of water or other liquid or gas, the stakes are higher. There were several areas where stricter standards were needed: quick opening hatches, lighter metals, lower allowable temperatures for metal selection, and the use of acrylic viewports instead of tempered glass.

In response to this industry need, the ASME established the Technical Committee on Pressure Vessels for Human Occupancy (ASME PVHO) in 1971. The committee published its first consensus standard under ANSI requirements in 1977 known as *ASME PVHO-1*. It was not until the 2007 edition of the code that the committee included rules specifically for hyperbaric chamber intended for medical treatment.

The scope of *PVHO-1* relates to new construction, design (for any pressure vessel that is designed for a pressure differential across the pressure boundary ≥ 2 pounds per square inch [PSI]), fabrication, inspection, testing, and stamping in addition to criteria for welding, piping, and acrylic viewports/tubes. It is applied to both to hypobaric (external pressure) and hyperbaric chambers (internal pressure).

Unlike the *BPVC*, compliance to *ASME PVHO-1* is not verified by third-party inspection. Instead, it is a self-certification that is claimed by the manufacturer of the chamber. Also, I describe it as a layered code. A chamber manufacturer can have a "U" stamp issued for a chamber without also being self-certified as compliant to *ASME PVHO-1*. The reverse is not true. A hyperbaric chamber cannot be self-certified as compliant to *ASME PVHO-1* UNLESS it possesses a valid "U" stamp certifying compliance to the *BPVC*.

Beginning in 1998, the *ASME PVHO* Technical Committee created a task group to begin work on a new code that is probably the most significant and financially beneficial to the end user: *ASME PVHO-2, Safety Standard for Pressure Vessels for Human Occupancy: In-Service Guidelines*. While *ASME PVHO-1* is a new construction code, *PVHO-2* is a post-construction code that provides guidance for the operation and maintenance of hyperbaric chambers designed and manufactured in accordance to the ASME codes referenced above. The benefit to the user is that the service life of acrylic viewports and monoplace chamber tubes can be doubled if the daily inspection and documentation requirements are being met by the end user. This translates directly to a significant reduction in long-term maintenance costs.

As noted above, the ASME per se has no authority. The codes and standards developed by them only have the force of law in those jurisdictions that have formally adopted them into law.

National Fire Protection Association

Like ASME, the NFPA has no authority. The codes and standards developed by them only have the force of law in those jurisdictions that have formally adopted them into law except as described below.

The NFPA has long been a prominent force in the hyperbaric medicine community. The first hyperbaric facility safety standard was published in 1968 as a tentative standard (*NFPA 56D-T*). It became a full standard in 1970 and was integrated into *NFPA 99, Safety Standard for Health Care Facilities* in 1984. Beginning with the 2012 edition, *NFPA 99* was elevated from a standard to a code.

As is usually the case with the creation of codes and standards, the first hyperbaric safety standard came about as a result of two catastrophic events. The first accident is common knowledge to many—the *Apollo 1* Command Module fire on January 27, 1967, that was fatal to three astronauts: Lt. Col. Virgil (Gus) Grissom, Lt. Col. Edward White, and Roger Chaffee. The second accident which occurred four days after the *Apollo 1* fire is much less known. On January 31, 1967, two USAF airmen Richard Harmon and William Bartley Jr. were killed at Brooks AFB, San Antonio, Texas, while tending research animals in an oxygen-filled research chamber fire. As a result of these two tragic events both occurring in an oxygen-enriched environment, the NFPA began to develop what has become the de facto international fire safety code for the hyperbaric medicine community.

The scope of the hyperbaric chapter of *NFPA 99* applies both to the construction of new hyperbaric facilities and the day-to-day operation of new and existing hyperbaric facilities. Historically, the *NFPA 99* has been applied to health care occupancies (hospitals, clinics, outpatient locations, doctor's offices, etc.). One of the most dramatic changes to the code in decades is that beginning with the 2018 edition, the hyperbaric code is now applicable to residential occupancies (*NFPA 99*, 14.1.4).[6] However, with this change comes the challenge of enforcement. It will be difficult for AHJs to enforce this new requirement on home-based hyperbaric chambers even though the risks association with the operation of home-based chambers are greater than in established health care facilities.

I believe that the authors of the 1968 standard were visionary in that they recognized from day one the importance of code compliance and operational responsibility. With creation of *NFPA 56D-T*, they identified the requirement to comply with ASME codes for hyperbaric chamber design and fabrication and established the need for a unit-specific safety director.

The NFPA is also responsible for the publication of another code that has been adopted into law in all 50 U.S. states: *NFPA 101, Life Safety Code*. The scope of *NFPA 101* is to classify structures according to general purpose (such as business occupancies, etc.) and to establish requirements to facilitate prompt egress should there be a fire in said occupancy.

Many do not realize that there is a direct link in the *Life Safety Code* to hyperbaric facilities. Beginning with the 2000 edition of the code, compliance to the requirements found in the hyperbaric facilities chapter of *NFPA 99* was mandated.[7] Even though *NFPA 99* is not invoked in all 50 U.S. states, it becomes a national requirement by virtue of the link in *NFPA 101*.

The importance of CMS as an AHJ is described above. As it relates to hyperbaric facilities seeking reimbursement from CMS for hyperbaric treatment services, CMS requires the treatment facility to comply with the *Life Safety Code*. (At the time of this writing it was the 2012 edition.) *The Life Safety Code* requires compliance to the hyperbaric requirements of *NFPA 99*, thus establishing the hyperbaric requirements as found in *NFPA 99* as a national mandate in the United States.

Guidelines

Similar to organizations and agencies that produce codes and standards, those who produce industry-specific guidelines generally have no authority. There are two organizations that are perhaps the most relevant to the hyperbaric community: the American Society of Testing and Materials (ASTM) and the Compressed Gas Association (CGA).

The ASTM, founded in 1898, is one of the world's largest organizations devoted to the development of voluntary technical standards and guidelines for materials, products, systems, and services. The most relevant to the hyperbaric community is the scope of what is known as the G-04 Committee. This group of industry experts is responsible for developing technical guidance on the compatibility and sensitivity of materials in an oxygen-enriched environment. Their publication of the *Safe Use of Oxygen and Oxygen Systems* should be part of the reference library at every hyperbaric treatment facility.

Similar to the ASTM, the CGA was formed in 1913 and focuses their technical expertise on the safe use of gases. CGA guidelines important to the hyperbaric community deal with oxygen, oxygen-enriched environments, cleaning equipment used for oxygen service, use of medical gases, the safe handling of gases, etc. Publications of the CGA should also be a frequently consulted part of a hyperbaric facility's reference library.

Neither the ASTM nor the CGA have any regulatory oversight.

Professional Societies and Organizations

In the United States there are several formal medical societies and organizations that help establish "best practice" standards and guidelines for the field of hyperbaric medicine.

Regulatory Weaknesses

The fact that there are multiple agencies and organizations that have some relationship to the practice of hyperbaric medicine and for which there is little coordination or communication among them should come as no surprise to anyone. The following are just a few examples of weaknesses that are a result of this quagmire:

- Compared to other medical specialties, the hyperbaric medicine community is small.
    - AHJs such as CMS and the FDA have higher priorities for resource allocation.
- There are no mandatory minimum staffing or training criteria.
    - The exception is when hospitals apply minimum training and other credentialing requirements for the medical staff.
- There is no requirement that hyperbaric facilities be licensed.
    - This is especially true for nonhospital-based, freestanding hyperbaric facilities.
- A mechanism for mandatory notification to the AHJ of questionable hyperbaric facility operations does not exist.
- Oversight of gas vendors who supply oxygen to users of nonhospital-based, freestanding hyperbaric facilities do not exist.
- Resources to educate the greater regulatory community are extremely limited.

Conclusion

The defined AHJs discussed above do not have a fundamental working knowledge of hyperbaric medicine or the requirements to operate a hyperbaric facility safely. As a result, maintaining a high level of quality of care and operational safety is left up to you! I am a strong believer in a person controlling what they can control because there are so many things that a person cannot control. So, what can the hyperbaric physician, nurse, technician, etc., do to help close the gap?

Well, for starters, get to know your community. Establish a working relationship with other hyperbaric facilities in your geographical area whether they are your competitor or not. Local networking is a good thing. Also, identify those facilities in your area that might not be operating according to "best practice" and try to help them raise their bar for quality and safety.

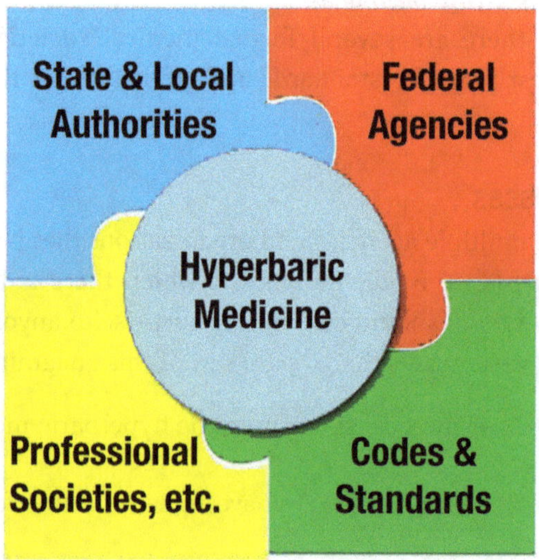

Next, educate when you can. Get to know your local AHJ (fire marshal) and the fire department that will respond to your facility should there be an accident. Bring them into your center and conduct joint drills with them to help them better understand the unique environment that you are part of every single day. These people are just as professional as you are and should be given the opportunity to improve their game.

You should also look for ways to differentiate your program from those in your area that might be up to standards. One way to do this is to seek hyperbaric facility accreditation by the UHMS. See Chapter 10: Hyperbaric Facility Accreditation for more information on accreditation for more information.

An equally important element in helping close this gap is to consider what you do as a profession instead of a job. If you think of your position as just a job, you approach your tasks in a very different manner; you punch the clock in the morning and again in the afternoon. And, for the most part, you check your hyperbaric life at the door. If you perceive your involvement in hyperbaric medicine as a profession, you treat your involvement in a very different way – you do not check your hyperbaric life at the door. Instead, you are constantly striving to be a better member of your hyperbaric team.

So, in the absence of meaningful oversight, establishing and maintaining high quality of care in the safest manner possible is up to you. At the end of the day, the objective is to bring the pieces of the puzzle together for a better hyperbaric medicine community. If we can achieve that, we all win, especially the patient!

References

1. https://www.cms.gov/Medicare/Provider-Enrollment-and-Certification/CertificationandComplianc/LSC.html (sourced Dec 3, 2018).
2. Foreman, C, Weitershausen, J. Regulation of Hyperbaric Chambers as Medical Devices, Hyperbaric Facility Safety: A Practical Guide, W.T. Workman (editor). Flagstaff, AZ:Best Publishing Company; 1999;135-147.
3. https://www.fda.gov/forconsumers/consumerupdates/ucm364687.htm (sourced Dec 3, 2018).
4. Swanson, RP. Governing Directives, Hyperbaric Facility Safety: A Practical Guide, W.T. Workman (editor). Flagstaff, AZ: Best Publishing Company; 1999;25-37.
5. https://share.ansi.org/shared%20documents/Standards%20Activities/American%20National%20Standards/Procedures,%20Guides,%20and%20Forms/2015_ANSI_Essential_Requirements.pdf (sourced Dec 3, 2018).
6. NFPA 99, 14.1.4, Health Care Facilities Code, 2018 Edition. Quincy, Mass: National Fire Protection Association; 2018.
7. NFPA 101, 8.4.5, Life Safety Code, 2000 Edition. Quincy, Mass: National Fire Protection Association; 2000.

CHAPTER 3.3
Pressure Vessels: An International View

The Challenge of Selecting from the Multiple Codes and Standards Available for Designing and Fabricating Pressure Vessels for Hyperbaric Systems Intended for International Sale

Francois Burman, BSc Engineering, MSc, IntPE

Reader Notes

This section is a perspective based on the author's practical experiences and on the views expressed by other international manufacturers, service and sales agents, designers, and regulatory authorities, with whom the author has had regular contact.

Of specific note is that South Africa is an example of a country where the regulatory authority has elected to invoke several international codes and standards that cover the design and construction of pressure vessels. Here, the user is granted the freedom to select an applicable code or standard from an approved, comprehensive list rather than being instructed to use a local standard or to select one only from a restricted list.

The term "codes and standards" used throughout this section follows the generally-accepted concepts of codes of construction and safety standards. It applies specifically to the category of codes and standards that has been compiled and introduced for the design, construction, testing, certification, and maintenance of pressure vessels, including hyperbaric chambers.

Introduction

The dilemma facing most design and manufacturing companies preparing to target the export market is how to address the issue of compliance with the various codes and standards applicable to design and construction within the destined country or state.

As yet, no truly international hyperbaric safety standard has been published that would allow a prospective purchaser, designer, manufacturer, or service supplier to either invoke the standard or refer to it.

Each country and, in some instances, each state within a country has its own specific requirements. These might incorporate the local statutes, bylaws, and other regulations together with either one, or as in some cases, several, internationally acknowledged codes of construction.

Intertwined with this often-intricate set of controlling instruments is an overall commitment to the process of rendering the industry safe. This process may therefore incorporate several additional parameters, such as:

1. The level of skills and competence in a country's manufacturing industry extending to the following:
   - available fabrication methods
   - confidence in build-quality
   - ability to work within a defined quality regimen
   - status of nondestructive testing (NDT)
   - availability of qualified design personnel
   - available inspection agencies
   - local regulating bodies, etc.
2. The attitude toward greater or lesser degrees of self-regulation
3. The propensity toward civil litigation as an effective control measure within the country
4. The overall attitude toward training and continuing education
5. The general level of skills of operators of regulated equipment
6. The attitudes toward post-construction, maintenance, and regular testing

These elements are among the issues that a regulating authority would consider when assessing the level of control necessary to ensure operational and occupational health and safety within the country.

Obviously, a designer and/or manufacturer cannot be expected to be aware of all these considerations or to embody them all within the design, build-quality, and final product. However, what is imperative is that this manufacturer imparts a message of confidence to the importer that the system will comply with both the printed and the implied control regulations.

The following sections are intended to give the reader an insight into the process of providing equipment that complies with foreign regulations, while acknowledging the problems and dangers associated with a patchwork approach.

The Immediate Challenge

The immediate challenge is to produce a hyperbaric chamber system meeting the client's existing or intended operational, contractual, and statutory requirements, within the initial region or country of installation.

Typically, a manufacturer would need to consider the following aspects:

- the *minimum disruption* to the existing quality management systems
- the *minimum cost impact* to effect code or standard changes (including any re-qualification of welding and NDT procedures, additional design reviews and resulting design and drawing changes, appointment of a different or additional inspection authority, accreditation or local design registration fees, etc.)
- the *minimum delay*, etc.

Due cognizance of possible legislative changes within the client's area of operation should also be taken (e.g., requirements for CE Marking, US Food and Drug Administration (FDA) 510K Clearance, Canadian Therapeutic Products Directorate, Australian Therapeutic Goods Administration, registration of plant, compulsory industry accreditation schemes, etc.).

The Longer-Term Challenges

There are essentially three additional challenges that should be considered within the manufacturer's sales strategy or the prospective buyer's decision to purchase:

1. **Value:** The *international resale value* of the hyperbaric chamber or complete facility. This, while not always an immediate consideration, may affect a client's ability to finance the acquisition of such equipment, especially where the asset base-value is increased if the system can possibly be sold within a much wider market.
2. **Consent:** *Acceptance* within the medical industry. The chamber must meet the minimum requirements for registration as a medical device, thus ensuring that the facility is able to operate as a reimbursable medical service.
3. **Credibility:** The credibility of scientific research emanating from a clinical facility (in the materials and methods) is related to the sophistication and reputation of the treating facility. As such, the perceived quality of any research work submitted is enhanced by accreditation within programs, such as those offered by the classification societies, insurance companies and certification authorities, and other more holistic schemes available.

In the United States, for example, the combined guidance offered by the National Fire Protection Agency (NFPA), the FDA, the American Society of Mechanical Engineers (ASME) Committee for Pressure Vessels for Human Occupancy (PVHO), and the Undersea and Hyperbaric Medical Society (UHMS) all confer additional credibility.

Similarly, in Europe the following of the Directives for Medical Devices (MDD) and Pressure Equipment (PED), as well as the European Standards organization (EN) hyperbaric medicine specific standards provide the equivalent level of credibility.

In general, though, the medical fraternity recognizes a minimum level of fit-out and safety, as well as conformance to a more generally used (or in most cases, local) code and/or standard.

All of these challenges imply that the consideration of the codes and standards needs to be taken a step further, especially where a country of destination allows a choice.

The Hazards of Cut-and-Paste: A General Exposè

Codes and standards of construction are generally designed to be *self-sufficient* within the defined scope of application. In other words, the philosophy of safety and the acknowledgment of risks are consistently addressed throughout. This applies to both the factors of safety provided or allowed for, as well as the degree of assurance required through NDT (e.g., acceptance criteria, degree of testing required, testing methods to be applied, and training of operators and interpreters), material certification requirements, training, quality control requirements, and design calculations.

Furthermore, codes and standards are developed over many years, consistently validated, reviewed, and revised through industry feedback, specialist evaluation, and focused research programs. The outstanding safety records achieved over the years, where specific codes and standards have been applied consistently, bear testament to the fact that they can stand on their own.

Therefore, it is never advisable for anyone, without specialist in-depth knowledge, to decide for themselves which subset or part of the code or standard they would like to apply to a given aspect of a pressure vessel under design or manufacture. It is too tempting to select the least stringent control measures from each of a list the codes and standards considered, thereby negating the overall safety-philosophy incorporated and thus compromising the safety of the critical design elements.

Generally, codes or standards offer a balance in terms of the degree of design analysis, the amount of manufacturing quality control, the requirement for certification of materials, the amount of NDT utilized, etc. If any one aspect is decreased in terms of either control or measurable results, then another must be increased accordingly to compensate.

To illustrate this, a good example of this teeter-totter effect within a specific code or standard is the aspect of full (or 100%) radiographic testing of all butt weld seams. The amount of examination can be reduced to spot (or 10%) radiography if the joint efficiency factor used is decreased, thereby allowing a slightly heavier plate section to be considered to compensate for the assumed lower strength of the welded joint. (Note: This example does not apply to a PVHO where 100% testing is a mandatory requirement.)

An example of using more than one code and/or standard would be the optimizing of the required thickness of a dished end using British Standard (BS) Published Document (PD) 5500, followed by the selection of the *ASME: Boiler & Pressure Vessel Code* Section VIII. *ASME* VIII allows for a manway to be placed within the knuckle. This application of two codes within a single construction compromises the vessel under both codes. The *ASME* code compensates for the reduction in the strength of the end where the manway material is removed, so the dished head needs to be thicker. The BS PD standard allows a thinner dished head, as it assumes all the material will be present to support the intended pressure. You cannot simply draw the benefits of both without accepting that there is sound reasoning behind the decision to allow less material to be used.

The principle to consider is *balance.* Few manufacturers would have access to the expertise required to achieve this when multiple codes and standards are being used. On the other hand, the future user may be oblivious to the code implications of his or her requests for a more functional design, producing inevitable tension between code compliance and design for the manufacturer.

The Historical Approach: Diving Industry Rules

Pressure vessels and habitat systems designed for human occupancy have been produced for the diving industry over many decades. The classification societies have developed their series of rules that govern such systems in order to do the following: provide a holistic and sound approach; provide owners with the assurance of safety; limit liability; quantify insurable risks; and include the post-construction aspects of ongoing inspections and maintenance. A list of classification society rules is provided in the next section.

A pressure vessel intended for human occupancy is considered to be a subsection of a complete diving or submersible system. As a subsection, more than one internationally acknowledged code or standard may be considered for the design of such a pressure vessel. In other cases, only the code or standard incorporated by the specific country in which the system is to be operated needs be considered.

However, the advantage offered by these classification society rules is that guidance and regulations on all the appurtenances, viewports (transparent pressure boundaries), life-support systems, gas supply systems, power interfaces, ongoing maintenance, and inspection is provided in one compendium.

Diving contractors often contract to work in the waters of other sovereign countries and states. This has led to the situation where the classification society rules have been adopted by many of these contractors, specifically where the regulatory authorities in the countries involved (the Port States) have been prepared to accept systems complying with the rules of class of shipping. This approach is very practical when considering that such diving systems are generally installed on vessels, that vessels usually have to be maintained in class for insurance purposes, and that vessels are generally accepted into most territorial waters.

However, not all diving systems are installed on such vessels and the classification society option is not the only route available. In terms of internationally recognized guidance schemes, the International Maritime Contractors' Association (IMCA), an industry association, offers guidance in the form of a similar holistic program. The approach offered is more self-regulatory where specific design and construction requirements are concerned and focuses on working within a specific country's regulations while only mandating a few relevant and safety-proven considerations.

Where does this leave the prospective designer and/or manufacturer in the quest for guidance in the selection of a suitable set of codes and standards in order to render a hyperbaric facility compliant with a host of requirements? History provides us with the inevitable and invaluable lessons with which we can predict (albeit to some limited extent) the safety outcome of new trends and developments. In essence, we strive for a path that will maintain the advantages of international acceptability and credibility, while at the same time, offering a solution that is cost effective so as to remain financially viable.

Available and Complimentary Design and Safety Publications

The following list of codes, standards, and publications is not exhaustive. It also includes many publications originally intended for application to diving systems but have eventually applied, to a greater or lesser extent, to the design and construction of hyperbaric chamber facilities. In general, however, the list should provide the reader with an idea of the range of *instruments* historically available to the hyperbaric system designer and manufacturer.

Pressure Vessel Codes and Standards

Australia: AS/NZS 1200: Pressure Equipment. Standards Association of Australia.

Canada: CSA B51: Boiler, Pressure Vessel & Pressure Piping Code. Canadian Standards Authority.

China: GB 150: Steel Pressure Vessels. National Standard of the People's Republic of China.

European Union: EN 13445: Unfired Pressure Vessels. Specifically, parts 1-5 and 8.

France†: CODAP: Code for the Construction of Unfired Pressure Vessels. National Union of Boilers, Piping & Maintenance (SNCT).

Germany†: DIN 13256 Part 2: Pressure Vessels for Human Occupancy; Accessible Pressure Vessels for Hyperbaric Therapy; Safety Requirements and Testing. German Institute of Standards.

AD2000-Merblatt: Technical Rules for Pressure Vessels (TRB). German Institute of Standards.

India: IS 2825: Code for Unfired Pressure Vessels. Bureau of Indian Standards.

Italy†: VSR Rules: Concerning Design Rules for Pressure Vessels. Higher Institute for Accident Prevention and Safety at Work (ISPESL).

Japan: JIS B8243: Construction of Pressure Vessels. Japanese Industrial Standards.

Russia: GOST-R: Russian Code for Pressure Equipment. Euro-Asian Council for Standardization.

Sweden†: Swedish Pressure Vessel Code (Calculation of the Strength of Pressure Vessels). The Swedish Pressure Vessel Commission.

UK[†]: (BS) PD 5500: Specification for Unfired Fusion Welded Pressure Vessels. British Standards Institute.

USA: *ASME* VIII: Rules for Construction of Pressure Vessels. American Society for Mechanical Engineers.

[†]Initially the European Community enforced harmonization of all country-specific codes and standards with the Pressure Equipment Directive (PED) 97/23/EC by 2002. More recently, it has phased out individual country codes and standards for pressure vessels, to be replaced with the EN 13445, Unfired Pressure Vessels. However, as pressure vessels are often reused, the older, country-specific codes are still maintained and found to be used in practice.

System Standards

ASME PVHO-1 *Pressure Vessels for Human Occupancy, Safety Standard.* This standard only recognizes the *ASME* VIII Code.[1]

CSA Z275.1 Hyperbaric Facilities, Canadian Standards Association. This standard recognizes the *CSA B51 Pressure Vessel Code.*[2]

EN 14931 *Pressure Vessels for Human Occupancy, European Standard.* This standard requires registration and conformity assessment with the Medical Device Directive (93/42/EC) and PED (97/23/EC).[3]

Classification Society Rules

ABS American Bureau of Shipping: Rules for Building & Classing Underwater Systems & Vehicles. These rules provide design guidelines and specifically recognize the *ASME* Code, viz. Section VIII, and the *PVHO-1* Standard.[4]

BV Bureau Veritas: Rules and Regulations for the Classification of Submersibles.

CCS China Certification Society: Rules for Offshore Engineering. Rules for the Construction and Classification of Diving Systems and Submersibles.

DNV Det Norske Veritas: Offshore Standard for Diving Systems. [†]These rules allow any international code or standard of construction, accepted within a specific country's applicable regulations, to be used.[5]

GL Germanischer Lloyd: Rules for Classification & Construction, Offshore Technology. [†]These rules provide guidelines to be used in conjunction with the German Standard: DIN 13256 Part 2.[6]

LR Lloyd's Register of Shipping: Rules & Regulations for the Construction & Classification of Submersibles & Diving Systems. These rules provide design guidelines and allow any international code or standard of construction, accepted within a specific country's applicable regulations, to be used.[7]

NK Nippon Kaiji Yokai: Rules for Installation of Ships. Rules & Guidance for Diving Systems.

RINA Registro Italiano Navale: Rules for the Construction & Classification of Underwater Vehicles & Diving Systems.

RM Russian Maritime Register of Shipping: Rules for the Classification & Construction of Manned Submersibles, Ship's Diving Systems & Passenger Submersibles.

Note: The above classification society rules are listed alphabetically; however only ABS, DNV, GL, and LR are generally referred to in the design of hyperbaric treatment chambers.

†The merger of DNV and GL, now known as DNV GL, has had an impact on their rules for manned pressure vessel design. However, while not always subject to regulation or enforcement, applicable editions of both rules provide applicable requirements that are not necessarily replicated and serve to provide details on specific aspects of design and construction.

Additional System Guidance Documents

AS 2299 *Occupational Diving, Australian Standard. AS 2299* recognizes the AS 1210 and *ASME* VIII Codes.[8]

NFPA 99 Health Care Facilities, American National Standard. *NFPA 99* only recognizes the *ASME* and *PVHO* Codes of Construction.[9]

SANS 10377-1 *Pressure Vessels for Human Occupancy, Part 1, Hyperbaric Chambers (Therapeutic), South African National Standard Code of Practice. SANS* 10377-1 recognizes any nationally approved pressure vessel design and construction code.[10]

UHMS *Guidelines for Clinical Monoplace & Multiplace Hyperbaric Facilities,* Undersea & Hyperbaric Medical Society. *The UHMS Guidelines* only refers to the *ASME* VIII Code of Construction and the BS (PD) 5500 Safety Standard.[11]

Regulatory Instruments

Countries tend to regulate the operation of hyperbaric equipment through their respective departments, ministries, or directorates of labor, health, or occupational health and safety.

The applicable publications therefore tend to originate from a country's governmental regulations with further control measures expressed in the appropriate regulations and are finally published as guidance documents, codes of practice, safety standards, and requirements for registration.

The name, nature, and extent of such publications are unique in each country, and any attempt to list these is not considered practical within the scope of this section.

The Multifaceted Role of the Inspection Authority

The majority of codes and standards require that safety or quality critical inspections be performed, or at the very least be witnessed, by a party who is able to remain relatively impartial to the performance of the contract. This party is known as the authorized or approved inspection authority or agency (the AIA), or in European terms, the notified body.

In many countries, the AIA also performs the necessary regulatory functions due to the body's implied access and presence during initial design, construction, testing, installation, commissioning and in-service inspections and tests.

Codes and standards place the full responsibility for design and build-quality with the manufacturer. Statutory regulations make the user and/or owner responsible for acquisition, installation, operation, maintenance, and post-construction inspections. However, in many cases, the AIA is expected to fulfill both these roles. It is common to hear a client, manufacturer, or even a regulator refer all matters to the AIA, including selection of a suitable code or standard.

Instead of thus being capable of remaining impartial, serving both the client and the regulatory authority, the AIA is expected to lead all parties toward a state of compliance. This was not the original intent. However, it is a valid presumption for the foreign manufacturer that the AIA is an invaluable source of knowledge regarding accepted codes and standards, systems standards, marking, certification, and accreditation requirements, design registration, and the registration of the plant and equipment for each specific country.

Aspects that Affect Economy of Construction, Simplicity, and Post-Construction

1. There are several considerations in the selection of a code or standard that affect the economy of construction (i.e. the price) and simplicity of the system. The more simple and foolproof the design process, the less expensive the NDT and welding qualifications, the lesser the degree of testing and product qualification, the easier the material certification and testing requirements, and the thicker the plate size needs to be. A balance is once again achieved.

   However, where price is a lesser consideration, and where weight or material selection are more important determining factors, it is often more prudent to make the selection based on the design allowances within the code or standard that would provide the designer with the necessary flexibility and fine-tuning benefits.

   Once again, a knowledgeable and experienced AIA will be in a position to offer an opinion as to a suitable and applicable code or standard, where such additional considerations are called for.

2. Post-construction is where we find the biggest void in most of the current codes and standards available to the designer, manufacturer, or the system purchaser. Few, if any, offer any real guidance on post-construction inspection, maintenance, or testing, as the emphasis is generally placed on a new-build only.

A manufacturer should consider the client's capabilities, and especially where such work is generally contracted out, what codes and standards the manufacturing industry is generally competent to comply with. It is not sensible to offer a code or standard for which there is little known expertise or capability within that region. The cost of additional qualification (welding, NDT, manufacturing, and design) could be prohibitive.

How To Select?

The selection process is essentially an exercise in technical and marketing decision making.

The responsible marketer, designer, or manufacturer must list the applicable criteria covered above. These specifically include regulations and import considerations, unique requirements of the country of final destination, available inspection authorities, applicable or accepted codes, standards, classification society rules and general system standards, regulatory clearance requirements, contractual requirements, and the target price. Finally, the decision makers must match these to their own abilities, competencies, and knowledge of the selected codes and standards.

Finally, information and any guidance relating to the country of final destination, including the level of awareness, competence, and service industry skills will ensure a choice that offers both the seller and the buyer the best technical and economical compromises within an acceptable safety envelope.

Concluding Remarks

Upon review, there are a great many publications available to both manufacturers and users of hyperbaric chambers. As wide and diverse as the variety is, there are equally as many considerations that need to be addressed prior to selecting a final publication or set thereof.

It is indeed too simplistic to expect the international hyperbaric community to agree to any one course of action and unrealistic to interfere with the sovereignty of a country's regulatory authority. Perhaps this edition can serve as a definitive publication containing the crucial elements required to make the final choice less daunting and more informed.

References

1. ANSI/ASME PVHO-1-2016. Safety Standard for Pressure Vessels for Human Occupancy. New York: American Society of Mechanical Engineers. 2016. (www.asme.org).
2. Z275.1-16, Hyperbaric Facilities. Ontario, Canada: Canadian Standards Association. 2016. (www.csa.ca).
3. EN 14931: 2006. Pressure Vessels for Human Occupancy (PVHO); Multiplace Pressure Chamber Systems for Hyperbaric Therapy, Performance, Safety Requirements, and Testing. Brussels, Belgium: European Committee for Standardisation. 2006. (www.cen.eu).
4. ABS. Rules for Building and Classing Underwater Vehicles, Systems, and Hyperbaric Facilities. New York: American Bureau of Shipping. 2018. (www.eagle.org).
5. DNV-OS-E402. Offshore standard for diving systems. Hovik, Norway: Det Norske Veritas; 2010. (www.dnv.com).
6. DNV GL-2015, Part 5 Chapter 1 Section 1: Manned Hyperbaric Systems. Electronic version: http://www.dnvgl.com.
7. LR, Rules and Regulations for the Construction and Classification of Submersibles and Diving Systems. London, UK: Lloyd's Register Group. 2016. (www.lr.org).
8. AS/NZS 2299.1: 2015. Occupational Diving Operations. Sydney, Australia: Standards Australia. 2015. (www.standards.com.au).
9. NFPA 99, Health Care Facilities Code, Chapter 14. Hyperbaric Facilities. Boston, Mass: National Fire Protection Association. 2018. (www.nfpa.org).
10. SANS 10377-1, Pressure Vessels for Human Occupancy: Part 1: Hyperbaric Chambers (Therapeutic). Pretoria, South Africa: South African Bureau of Standards. 2002. (www.sabs.co.za).
11. UHMS. Guidelines for Clinical Multiplace Hyperbaric Facilities. Report of the Hyperbaric Chamber Safety Committee of the Undersea and Hyperbaric Medical Society. Kensington, Maryland: Undersea and Hyperbaric Medical Society, Inc.; 1994. (www.uhms.org).

Bibliography

1. AD 2000 Merkblatter. Technical Rules for Pressure Vessels. Berlin, Germany: German Institute for Norms (DIN). 2002 (www.din.de/en).
2. ASME Boiler & Pressure Vessel Code Section VIII. Rules for Construction of Pressure Vessels. New York: ASME. 2015. (www.asme.org).
3. CODAP 2005, Div. 1 & 2. Code for Construction of Unfired Pressure Vessels. Courbevoie, France: SNCT. 2015. (www.snct.org).
4. DIN 13256 Parts 2 (multiplace pressure chambers: 2002 – withdrawn) and 4 (monoplace pressure chambers: 2002). Pressure Vessels for Human Occupancy. Berlin, Germany: German Institute for Norms. 2002. (www.din.de/en).

5. IMCA Diving Division. Codes of Practice and Guidance Notes for the Offshore Diving Industry. London, UK. (www.imca-int.com).
6. Nuckols ML, Sarich AJ, Marr WJ, Robillard DJ. Life Support Systems Design, Diving, and Hyperbaric Applications, 2nd Edition. Annapolis, Maryland: Ace Sarich Publishing. 2015.
7. Naval Sea Systems Command. U.S. Navy Diving Manual, Revision 7, 2017. Washington, DC: US Navy. 2008.
8. PED. Pressure Equipment Directive 97/23 / EEC, Directive 97/23 / EC of the European Parliament and of the Council. 29 May 1997.
9. SANS 347, Categorization and Conformity Assessment Criteria for All Pressure Equipment. Pretoria, South Africa: South African Bureau of Standards; Edition 2. 2012. (www.sabs.co.za).

CHAPTER 3.4
Summary of International Regulatory Landscape

J. Steven Wood and Wilbur T. Workman, BS, MS, CAsP, CHT-A, FAsMA, FUHM

Hyperbaric chambers are manufactured and utilized around the world. Compared to other medical specialties, hyperbaric medicine is relatively small, but there is a vibrant international community that contributes to an ongoing exchange of research and clinical experience. Each country establishes a regulatory framework for their health care system that is unique, yet there are common denominators that arise, particularly with respect to regulation of chambers as pressure vessels and medical devices. The actual practice of hyperbaric medicine in each country may be informed by international "best practices" that are routinely shared, but the way in which the therapy is delivered will be influenced by the structure of the country's health care delivery system.

Regulation within the hyperbaric industry follows a similar pattern not uncommon to other industries worldwide. First, consider the safety of the device/therapy, then establish oversight or controls on its use. Levels of proactivity vary by country, ranging from those who take a comprehensive approach to the regulatory scheme to those with little or no interest in what is done in the field. It is often the countries with nascent hyperbaric communities that have attempted to set standards approaching international best practices. These new hyperbaric medicine centers often utilize outside consultants to advise them and their government on which standards and guidelines to implement, which provides a strong framework for additional hyperbaric medicine programs to be established within the health care network. Yet, even in those countries with a robust hyperbaric community, they often have little to no regulatory oversight of the field.

Given the inherent hazards associated with the use of pressure vessels, it is not unexpected that industrialized countries would establish design and manufacturing guidelines to enhance public safety and even adopt those standards into law. Though pressure vessel technology is still innovating (albeit slowly), the safety, design, and manufacturing basis is now well into its second century of evolution. With few exceptions, regulatory and statutory controls over various types of pressure vessels are common worldwide, and it is not uncommon for countries with strong export manufacturing infrastructure to produce pressure vessels compliant with both internal standards as well devices constructed to compliance with market standards.

With their unique straddling of the industrial and medical spaces, hyperbaric chambers are also subject to regulation as medical devices, in addition to the basic pressure vessel regulation. Medical device regulation ranges from strict to nonexistent, and, again, many countries have policies that allow the use of almost any type of medical device as long as it conforms to the standards of some (typically US/EU).

Though some of our American colleagues may disagree, it is the actual practice of hyperbaric medicine that has the least regulatory oversight. Despite the exponential growth in the use of hyperbaric medicine worldwide, health care providers have little restrictions on their practice (beyond limits on payment for treatment services). There are few specific rules governing the use of hyperbaric oxygen therapy (HBOT) or establishing legal standards of training and operational oversight for hyperbaric programs. As human factors play a major role in accidents, the development and implementation of operational, training, and maintenance standards is vital for the growth of a safe industry.

In producing this section, the editors developed a 15 question survey that explored the regulatory environment governing the practice of hyperbaric medicine. Questions covered the gamut of the field, from design/construction standards for chambers and the facilities that house them, through the degree of official oversight of the practice of hyperbaric medicine, the economics of providing therapy, and the degree of professional organization in each country. Utilizing personal and professional contacts, the editors attempted to identify international leaders in each country who could provide a comprehensive picture of the practice profile. Though we were not successful in obtaining reports from each country polled, we believe that this chapter is the most complete compilation of its type. Survey questions and our general comments on the responses are listed below.

INTERNATIONAL CONTRIBUTORS STANDARDIZED QUESTIONS

1. Are pressure vessels for human occupancy (hyperbaric chambers) designed, fabricated, and tested in accordance to a national mandatory pressure vessel code? If so, please identify the code they must comply with.

   Some form of pressure vessel code is utilized in most countries, though a number of countries do not have specific statutory codes regulating human-occupied pressure vessels. In countries that do not have code coverage of human-occupied chambers, end-users commonly specify compliance with some established codes, typically ASME or EU codes.

2. Are pressure vessels for human occupancy (hyperbaric chambers) used for medical treatment considered as a regulated medical device in your country? If so, please describe the government regulatory requirements that they must meet before they are marketed for sale.

Medical device regulation varies widely across the globe. Regulation of chambers as medical devices is spotty, and some countries that have agencies that regulate medical devices do not have the expertise to fully evaluate hyperbaric chambers.

3. Do medical hyperbaric facilities in your country have to comply with mandatory fire safety regulations? If so, please describe the safety codes they must comply with.

   Few countries have established hyperbaric-specific fire codes. Statutory regulation is typically limited to general fire codes for health care facilities. Voluntary compliance with accepted international standards such as NFPA is common.

4. Are there mandatory hyperbaric medicine training standards in your country for the staff that conduct hyperbaric medicine treatments? If so, please describe.

   Few countries require mandatory training for staff.

5. Are there mandatory hyperbaric medicine staffing standards in your country for the staff that conducts hyperbaric medicine treatments? If so, please describe.

   Few countries have established staffing standards.

6. What medical indications are treated with HBOT in your country?

   UHMS and EUBS indication lists are common worldwide as the core of treated indications, but there is a wide range of disorders reported. In general, reimbursement for treatment under national health care plans and private insurers tends to track with the "accepted" indications lists, but in the private pay arena, therapy may be provided for literally hundreds of disorders.

7. Describe the payment system for HBOT in your country.

   Reimbursement for treatment falls into three categories: national health care plans, private insurance, and self-pay, though in reality there is a mix of all three. National plans and private insurance typically are more restrictive in the conditions that are covered (in those countries that have such plans).

8. Who has regulatory oversight over the safe operation of medical hyperbaric facilities in your country? If there is an organization with such oversight authority, please describe their authority.

   Few countries have established specific oversight criteria for hyperbaric facilities and providers. If there is oversight, it is typically related to general provider licensure.

9. Approximately, how many medical hyperbaric treatment centers are there in your country?

   Facility counts range from as few as one, to over 5,000 centers. It appears that there is a higher level of regulation at both ends of the spectrum.

10. Is there a professional hyperbaric medical society in your country? If so, please describe their scope, goals, and objectives.

    Most countries have some professional hyperbaric society, but there is a strong international community, and it is not uncommon for members of local societies to hold membership in broader-based groups as well.

11. If your country has a profession hyperbaric medical society, does it conduct periodic medical/scientific conferences?

    If a country reports having a professional society, they report having regular conferences, and many publish newsletters and journals.

12. Is there a requirement for continuing education in hyperbaric medicine in your country? If so, please describe.

    Few countries require mandatory continuing education.

13. Please describe the typical staff makeup (physician, nurse, technician, etc.) in a clinical hyperbaric facility in your country.

    Staff composition is one of the few areas of commonality worldwide. Programs operate under medical direction, with nursing participation as required for care (in some locales, nurses also act as chamber operators), and technicians serving as chamber operators, particularly in multiplace facilities.

14. Is there a clinical hyperbaric facility accreditation program in place in your country? If so, please describe.

    Few countries have mandatory accreditation programs, though there is a growth in voluntary accreditation, based on the UHMS model.

15. Are inspections or permits by national, regional, or local authorities having jurisdiction required prior to the initiation of operations or periodically following initiation of operations of the hyperbaric facility? If so, please describe the scope of the inspections or permits, including the agencies responsible for such inspections or permits.

    Most countries have established general inspection requirements for health care facilities, though there are few that have hyperbaric-specific inspections. Some countries require inspection prior to facility opening but have no ongoing inspection requirements.

Results of the survey are presented in the table below, followed by country-specific explanatory sections. Though there is much commonality between the standards utilized in many countries (typically, standards developed in "early adopter" countries often spread across a continent), there may be specific local variances that must be considered. One commonality across the world is staffing. All countries report medical direction by a physician, chamber operators with varying degrees of training, and involvement of nurses or allied health professionals such as dive medics. As a result, responses to question #13 were omitted from the table. Each country-specific section will address unique aspects of hyperbaric medicine, following a standard format.

	Argentina	Australia/ New Zealand	Bahrain	Brazil	Canada	People's Republic of China
Mandatory Nat'l Pressure Vessel Code?	No	*ASME PVHO*, Australian Stds	No	National Stds	*ASME PVHO*	National Stds
Regulated Medical Device?	Yes	Class IIb	Yes	Yes	Yes	Yes
Mandatory Facility Fire Safety Regs?	No	References to NFPA	Yes	Yes	NFPA, Provincial Regs	Yes
Mandatory Training Stds?	No	National Std	No	No	No	Yes
Mandatory Staffing Stds?	No	National Std	No	No	No	Yes
Indications Treated?	UHMS	ANZCA Sig./ ANZHMG	UHMS, OL	UHMS Plus Others	UHMS	62 Listed
Payment System?	Govt/Private Insurance	Gov/Pvt Insurance	Gov/Pvt	Gov/Pvt	N/A	National Insurance
Regulatory Oversight?	No	No	No	Limited	Health Canada	National Standards
Number of Facilities?	23	17	1	150	Unknown	Approx 5000
Professional HBO_2 Society?	Yes	HTNA/SPUMS	UHMS/ SAUHMA	Yes	Yes	Yes
Prof Society Conferences?	Yes	Yes	No	Yes	Yes	Yes
CE Required?	No	No	Yes	No	NA	Yes
Accreditation Program?	No	No	Yes, SAUHMA	No	NA	Yes
Inspecton Required?	No	Yes	Yes	Limited	No	Yes

	Egypt	France	Greece	Hong Kong	India	Italy
Mandatory Nat'l Pressure Vessel Code?	Not for Human Occupancy	Yes	National Stds	EU Stds	No	Yes
Regulated Medical Device?	No	Yes	Yes	No	No	Yes
Mandatory Facility Fire Safety Regs?	Not HBO_2 Specific	Yes	Yes	Not HBO_2 Specific	No	Yes
Mandatory Training Stds?	No	Yes	Yes	No	No	Yes
Mandatory Staffing Stds?	No	Yes	Yes	No	No	Yes
Indications Treated?	Mix	EUBS/ECHM	UHMS/ECHM	ECHM+	No Limits	ECHM
Payment System?	Varies by Program	National Insurance	Various	National Insurance	Cash	National Insurance
Regulatory Oversight?	No	National/ Regional	Yes	No	No	Yes
Number of Facilities?	12+	20	9	1	Unkown	50
Professional HBO_2 Society?	No	Yes	Under Development	No	Yes, 2	Yes
Prof Society Conferences?	No	Yes	By Navy	CE By Facility Only	Yes	Yes
CE Required?	No	Limited	No	No	No	Yes
Accreditation Program?	No	Limited	No	No	No	Yes
Inspecton Required?	Limited, Not Specific To HBO_2	Yes	No	Yes	Limited, By Region	Yes

	Israel	Japan	Korea	Mexico	Phillipines	Russia
Mandatory Nat'l Pressure Vessel Code?	Yes, similar to EU	Yes	No	No	No	Yes
Regulated Medical Device?	Yes	Yes	Yes	Yes, Partial	No	Yes
Mandatory Facility Fire Safety Regs?	Yes	Yes	Chamber Only	No	No	Yes
Mandatory Training Stds?	Yes	No	No	No	No	Yes
Mandatory Staffing Stds?	Yes	No	No	No	No	Yes
Indications Treated?	UHMS + Additional	UHMS + Additional	Limited	No Limits	UHMS + Off-Label	Wide Range of Conditions
Payment System?	National Insurance, Pvt Insurance, Self-Pay	Natiional Insurance	National	Cash	Cash	National Insurance, Cash
Regulatory Oversight?	Yes	Yes	No	No	No	Yes
Number of Facilities?	3	443	24	5-10 Hospital, Approx 750 Freestanding	Unkown	900
Professional HBO_2 Society?	Yes	Yes	Yes	Yes	No	Yes
Prof Society Conferences?	Yes	Yes	Yes	Yes	No	Yes
CE Required?	Yes	No	No	No	No	Yes
Accreditation Program?	Yes	Yes	No	No	No	Under Development
Inspecton Required?	No	No	No	Limited, Not HBO_2 Specific	No	Yes

	Saudi Arabia	Singapore	South Africa	Spain	Taiwan	Thailand
Mandatory Nat'l Pressure Vessel Code?	No	Multiple International Stds	Yes	Limited to Multiplace	Yes	Yes, *ASME PVHO*
Regulated Medical Device?	No	Yes	No	Limited	Yes	Yes
Mandatory Facility Fire Safety Regs?	No	Yes	Not HBO_2 Specific	Limited	Yes	Yes
Mandatory Training Stds?	No	Yes	Under Development	No	Yes	No
Mandatory Staffing Stds?	No	No	Commercial Diving Only	No	Yes	No
Indications Treated?	UHMS	UHMS	UHMS/ECHM	ECHM + Additional	UHMS + Additional	UHMS
Payment System?	Government, Self-Pay	Private Pay	Multiple	National System, Private Insurance, Out of Pocket	National Health Insurance Covers Some Indications	Range From National Insurance to Private Pay
Regulatory Oversight?	No	Yes	Under Development	No	Limited	No
Number of Facilities?	10 - 15	3	10 Accredited, Multiple Diving-Focused	10+	Approx 50	25
Professional HBO_2 Society?	Under Development	No	Yes	Yes	Yes	Yes
Prof Society Conferences?	No	No	Yes	Yes	Yes	Yes
CE Required?	No	Yes	Yes	No	Yes	No
Accreditation Program?	No	Through UHMS	Yes	Yes	Yes, Limited	No
Inspecton Required?	No	Yes	Yes	Yes	Yes, Limited	Initial

	Turkey	United Kingdom	Vietnam
Mandatory Nat'l Pressure Vessel Code?	No	Yes	Yes
Regulated Medical Device?	Yes. CE	Yes	Yes
Mandatory Facility Fire Safety Regs?	Limited	Yes	Yes
Mandatory Training Stds?	Limited to Physicians	No	Yes
Mandatory Staffing Stds?	No	No	Yes
Indications Treated?	Ministry of Health, Similar to UHMS	Limited by National Health Service	48 Approved by Ministry of Health
Payment System?	Social Security System to Private Pay	National Health Service, Some Self-Pay	Covered by State Insurance
Regulatory Oversight?	Ministry of Health	Yes, National Health Service	Yes
Number of Facilities?	60	14-15 Regulated by NHS, Unknown # of Unregulated	30
Professional HBO_2 Society?	Yes	Yes	Yes
Prof Society Conferences?	Yes	Yes	Yes
CE Required?	No	Yes	Yes
Accreditation Program?	No	Yes	Yes
Inspecton Required?	Yes	Yes	Yes

Argentina

Number of facilities reported: 23

Respondent: Nina Subbotina, MD, PhD

There are no national standards for human-occupied chambers, though ASME code is used unofficially. La Administracion National de Medicamentos, Alimentos y Technologia Medica (ANMAT) regulates medical devices, including chambers. There are no hyperbaric-specific fire regulations under law, but *NFPA 99* is commonly followed. There are no mandatory requirements for staffing or training. The UHMS accepted indication list is followed. Reimbursement for treatment is through the government health system and private medical insurance. There is no official governmental oversight of hyperbaric facilities. The Argentinean Society for Hyperbaric and Diving Medicine—Sociedad Argentina de Medicina Hiperbárica y Actividades Subacuáticas, Asociación Civil (SAMHAS) was established in 1986 and conducts regular conferences on diving and hyperbaric medicine. Though there is no national requirement for inspections, SAMHAS provides inspections that focus on *ASME PVHO-2* requirements.

Australia/New Zealand

Number of facilities reported: 17

Respondent: Steve Gobel

Chamber construction is regulated by Standards Australia which requires adherence to *ASME PVHO*. Chambers are considered medical devices and are regulated under the Australian Register of Therapeutic Goods. Facilities that house hyperbaric facilities must comply with *NFPA 53* and *NFPA 99*. Inspections of the facility and chamber are conducted prior to the start of operations and annual inspections of chambers by state pressure vessel inspectors are required. There is no hyperbaric-specific accreditation program in place, but hospitals may be accredited by the Australian Council on Healthcare Standards.

AS4774.2 describes all staffing standards and minimum staffing requirements. Staffing patterns are influenced by patient acuity, numbers of patients, and chamber type. The standard delineates job responsibilities for the various positions that might be filled in a given facility. There are no specific initial or continuing education requirements mandated by law and no specific regulatory oversight of the practice of hyperbaric facilities.

A list of accepted indications has been produced by a joint Australia/New Zealand hyperbaric group. This list is similar to the UHMS and EUBS indications lists. Hyperbaric treatments are covered by the Australian Medicare system and private insurers, but not all of the indications on the published list are covered for reimbursement.

Two professional organizations operate in the region: Hyperbaric Technicians and Nurses Association (HTNA) and South Pacific Underwater Medicine Society (SPUMS). HTNA focuses primarily on technical and nursing issues specific to hyperbaric therapy while SPUMS is geared toward physicians. Both organizations conduct annual meetings.

Bahrain

Number of facilities reported: 1

Respondent: Chaitanya Kodange, MD

With only a single hyperbaric facility, Bahrain is virtually unregulated. The National Health Regulatory Authority (NHRA) exercises little oversight over chambers or facilities, though there is acceptance of various international standards (typically US/EU). The NHRA has established limited standards for health care facilities and has established general CME requirements for renewal of medical, nursing, and paramedical licenses. Initial and ongoing training as well as accreditation follows South African guidelines. UHMS treatment guidelines are generally followed, and payment is covered by the government for Bahraini nationals. Non-Bahrainis and those treated for off-label disorders are considered "private" patients and must pay out of pocket unless they have private insurance that will provide reimbursement for a particular indication. Facility inspections are conducted by NHRA and the military (as the chamber is used as a backup for management of diving disorders and for training) and supplemented by manufacturer-supplied preventive maintenance.

Brazil

Number of facilities reported: 150

Respondent: Roberto Bammann, MD

Chambers must be constructed in conformance with Associação Brasileira de Normas Técnicas/Brazilian National Standards Organization (ABNT) NBR 15949, which also establishes fire safety regulations for facilities. Chambers are regulated as medical devices under the RDC 59-2000 (Good Practices for Manufacturing of Medical Devices) and must be registered and cleared for sale. There are no statutory requirements for training (though completion of an introductory course is required for membership in the Brazilian Hyperbaric Medicine Society) or staffing beyond the requirement to have a medical director and registered nurse. Indications treated include the UHMS list along with some off-label uses, with limited reimbursement provided by some governmental programs, though not through the national health system. Inspections of facilities are not specific to hyperbaric units but more generally focused on fire safety and sanitation. There is no local accreditation program; however one facility has been accredited by the UHMS. The Brazilian Society of Hyperbaric Medicine supports hyperbaric practice through regular educational programs and conferences.

Canada

Number of facilities reported: Unknown

Respondents: Ron Linden, MD and Andrew Hawel, BSc

Sale of chambers requires Canadian Medical Device license through Health Canada's Medical Device Bureau. Requirements for review include a valid QMS Certification and providing safety and effectiveness information, which includes device description, design philosophy, indications/contraindications, marketing history, labeling/IFU, standards, pre-clinical bench testing, biocompatibility testing, clinical studies, software verification, and validation studies. Health Canada provides regulatory oversight related to chamber use (adverse events, complaints, incidents, recalls, etc.) and recognizes the UHMS indication list as part of device licensure. Physician specialty credentialing (includes required continuing medical education) in hyperbaric medicine is available through the Royal College of Physicians & Surgeons of Canada. Facility standards are set by Health Canada and some provinces have established additional requirements for facilities as well. The Canadian Undersea and Hyperbaric Medical Association (CUHMA) sponsors an annual professional conference and a facility accreditation program similar to the UHMS program.

People's Republic of China

Number of facilities reported: 5,000

Respondent: Lu Shi, PhD

National standards have been established for both air and oxygen pressurized chambers, with design standards approved by the Boiler and Pressure Vessel Safety Supervision Bureau of the State Bureau of Quality and Technical Supervision. The Bureau issues licenses for companies that manufacture or repair chambers. Medical facilities that wish to add hyperbaric therapy must obtain permission from the local and provincial health administrations. Mandatory fire safety regulations are established for facilities. Inspections to assure conformance to various national standards are required before a facility begins operation. Prior to starting clinical operations, physicians, nurses, engineers, and technicians must obtain the Qualification of Medical Oxygen Compartment Training (Employment) Certificate and Special Equipment Operator Certificate accreditation. Training standards are enforceable for the relevant staff who conduct hyperbaric medicine treatments. The safety management of hyperbaric oxygen chamber and employee trainings are organized and implemented by the medical administrative departments of the provincial health administrative departments. We mainly follow the "Safety Management and Application of Medical Hyperbaric Oxygen Chamber" (the latest version is 2015), which was promulgated and implemented by the professional hyperbaric society in China, Hyperbaric Oxygen Medicine Branch of the Chinese Medical Association. Staffing is also mandated according to this. Over 60 indications for treatment are recognized, with reimbursement covered by the national basic medical insurance system.

The aim of the Hyperbaric Oxygen Medicine Branch of Chinese Medical Association is to provide a platform for academic exchanges in clinical and basic research, experience summary, nursing experience, literature review, equipment maintenance and renovation, safety management, and discipline construction of hyperbaric oxygen medicine. An annual conference is held which draws more than 300 participants.

The clinical hyperbaric facility accreditation program in China is described by the national special equipment specification document, "Supervision Regulation on Safety Technology for Hyperbaric Oxygen Chambers" (TSG 24-2015), which is issued by the General Administration of Quality Supervision, Inspection and Quarantine of the People's Republic of China. (NOTE: Te Zhong She Bei Gui Fan (TSG) means special equipment specification.)

Egypt

Number of facilities reported: 12+

Respondent: Adel Taher, MD

There is no regulation of chambers or facilities in Egypt beyond basic standards for nonhuman occupied pressure vessels and general fire safety standards for health care facilities. A wide range of disorders are treated, but there is no standardized system of reimbursement. The practice of hyperbaric medicine is not regulated nor are there any minimum training standards for providers. Most providers receive initial training in Europe or the United States. There is no local professional society.

France

Number of facilities reported: 20

Respondent: Daniel Matthieu, MD

As a member of the EU, France follows EU standards for construction of chambers, medical device regulation, and fire safety standards as part of EN 14941. EN 16081 focuses on fire safety/extinguishing standards for multiplace chambers. The Ministry of Labor in France has established training requirements for physicians and chamber operators who oversee chambers that have attendants working under pressure in a chamber. Reimbursement for treatment under the Securité Sociale System requires the supervising physician to hold a specific diploma in diving and hyperbaric medicine. Both the Ministry of Labor and Securité Sociale System have established staffing requirements for hyperbaric facilities. Disorders treated follow ECHM-accepted indications, with additional disorders treated under research protocols or compassionate use. Reimbursement under the national health care system is limited to disorders on the ECHM list. There is no hyperbaric-specific oversight beyond general oversight provided at the local and regional level. The Societe Française de Physiologie et de Medecine Subaquatiques et Hyperbares conducts two annual meetings and ongoing medical education, in addition to liaison with the EUBS. There are no hyperbaric-specific continuing education requirements, but physicians have to meet national standards for recertification. There is no hyperbaric-specific accreditation program, but facilities are inspected under the general hospital accreditation program. Facility inspections are conducted prior to opening, at five-year intervals, and at other times as desired by the national and regional health authorities.

Greece

Number of facilities reported: 9

Respondent: Vasileios Kalentzos, MD, MPH

As there are no local chamber manufacturers in Greece, chambers must comply with European standards for construction and medical devices. Fire safety standards are established by a ministerial act adopted in 2005. This act also sets initial training requirements for physicians and nurses. There is a list of indications set by the Ministry of Health in 2010. These indications are partially included in the UHMS and the ECHM list of indications. All indications included in these three lists (ministerial act, ECHM, and UHMS) are accepted and treated in that order of acceptance. Reimbursement is tiered according to location of treatment. Public sector hospital treatment is covered by the public insurance fund. Private hospital and stand-alone units are paid out of pocket or by private insurance. Oversight of civilian facilities is provided by the Ministry of Health. Military facilities are regulated by the Hellenic Navy, which operates two of the four hospital-based facilities in the country. A professional organization is under development, and there is an ongoing annual seminar on diving and hyperbaric medicine organized by the Athens Naval Hospital Department of Hyperbaric and Diving Medicine. An accreditation program is under development.

Hong Kong

Number of facilities reported: 1

Respondent: Jeffrey Chau, MD

There are no mandatory pressure vessel codes in Hong Kong for designing and fabricating hyperbaric chambers. However, we have complied with the same installations in European countries with the respective requirements laid down by the European Union. In particular for PVHO, our chamber system must conform to "Medical Device Directive 93/42/EEC" and "Pressure Equipment Directive 2014/68/EU." The relevant standards for chamber system would be EN 14931 (performance and safety for PVHO) and EN 16081 (performance and testing requirement for fire-fighting system of PVHO).

Although PVHO intended for medical treatment is regarded as a medical device in Hong Kong and other parts of the world, currently there is no regulation nor applicable law requirement on medical devices in Hong Kong. There is no requirement on marketing/sale activities on equipment intended for medical treatment. However, there are some indirect requirements on the pressure vessels which are overseen by pressure vessels division of the Labour Department of HK Gov. Any pressure vessels/receivers involved in the chamber system shall comply with these basic requirements, although they are not specific to PVHO. Also, any pressure vessel must be inspected by recognized inspectors in Hong Kong and registered in the Labour Department. There are no specific standards for facility housing, training, nor staffing, though UHMS and Australian standards are followed. Disorders treated follows the UHMS-accepted list and reimbursement is covered for Hong Kong citizens as part of the public hospital program. Though there is no professional organization in the country, the sole hyperbaric program conducts a regular symposium bi-annually. Annual inspections are conducted by the fire service and the pressure vessel branch of the Labour Department (with a focus on compressed air tanks).

India

Number of facilities reported: Unknown

Respondent: Ravi Patel, MD

There is essentially no regulation of chambers or practice in the country. Some facilities are operated by US-based management companies that typically follow NFPA and UHMS accreditation guidelines. With the exception of US-managed programs and some major hospital systems, which typically follow UHMS, CMS, EUBS, Russian, Chinese, and other published indication lists, there is no limitation on the use of HBO_2. Off-label use is rampant. Reimbursement is cash, with no coverage by insurers. There are two professional organizations: Wound and Hyperbaric Medicine Society of India and Hyperbaric Society of India, which conduct periodic meetings.

Italy

Number of facilities reported: 50

Respondents: Pasquale Longabardi, MD, Marco Bellomo, and Jurg Wendling, MD

Chambers are regulated under European standards for construction and as medical devices. Facility housing is also regulated under EU standards. Chamber fire safety is regulated under both EU and Italian statutes. The national health system via local authorities provide regulatory oversight, including establishing specific continuing medical education requirements for physicians and nurses, facility accreditation, and regular inspections. The professional hyperbaric medical society, Societa Italiana Medicina Subacquea e Iperbarica (SIMSI), has established a list of medical indications that is similar to the ECHM indications list. Reimbursement for treatment is provided by the national health system, but there are variations in reimbursement across regions. SIMSI conducts regular training programs across the country.

Israel

Number of facilities reported: 3

Respondent: Shai Efrati, MD

Israel has established construction codes for chambers which are similar to CE code. Chambers are regulated as medical devices by the Minister of Health, which also provides oversight of facilities. Training and staffing standards are established by code. Conditions treated generally follow the UHMS indications list, with some additional disorders added, based on current research. Reimbursement for most conditions is covered by national insurance, with additional disorders covered by private insurance or self-pay. The Israeli Society for Hyperbaric and Diving Medicine (ISHDM) offers ongoing educational opportunities, though there are no mandated continuing education requirements.

Japan

Number of facilities reported: 443

Respondent: Mahito Kawashima, MD

Chamber construction rules are incorporated into Japanese Industrial Standards, which address the pressure vessel as well as associated control and communication devices. Chambers are regulated as medical devices by the Pharmaceuticals and Medical Devices Agency and the Ministry of Health, Labor and Welfare. General fire safety regulations are incorporated into law, which are referenced by the Japanese Society of Hyperbaric and Medical Society (JSHUM). There are no mandatory staffing or training standards. Indications treated include most of those listed by the UHMS with additional disorders included. Reimbursement for treatment is provided by national public medical insurance, with copays influenced by patient age and income. Oversight of hyperbaric facilities is by the Ministry of Health, Labor and Welfare. The JSHUM and its subsidiaries serves the profession and conducts annual conferences and workshops and publishes journals and books. JSHUM also offers certification for physicians and technicians as well as a voluntary facility accreditation program. There are no legally mandated inspections.

Korea

Number of facilities reported: 24

Respondent: Yong Sung Cha, MD

There are no national codes governing chamber construction, but *ASME PVHO* is generally followed. Chambers are regulated as medical devices by the Korea Food and Drug Administration (KFDA). KFDA has specific requirements for chamber windows to be compliant with PVHO and for chambers to be equipped with a fire safety system. There are no specific rules for chamber housing. Though there are no mandatory requirements for staffing and training, the Korean Academy of Undersea and Hyperbaric Medicine (KAUHM) conducts annual training for physicians and non-MDs. Disorders treated are similar to those on the UHMS indications list.

Mexico

Number of facilities reported: 5-10 hospital-based, approx. 750 freestanding

Respondent: Cuauhtemoc Sanchez, MD

Beyond requiring approval by COFEPRIS (Mexican FDA) for chambers used in hospitals, there are no mandatory requirements for chamber construction, housing, training, or staffing of hyperbaric units. Conditions treated generally follow the UHMS-accepted indications list, with extensions. Reimbursement is out of pocket, with limited private insurance coverage. A professional society was re-formed in 2017, and meetings are held at least once per year.

Philippines

Number of facilities reported: Unknown

Respondent: Jeffrey Ramos, MD

No mandatory regulation with respect to chambers, housing, staffing, training, practice oversight, or uses of HBO_2. There is no professional organization.

Russia

Number of facilities reported: 900

Respondent: Larisa Polyakova, MD

Chamber construction is regulated under various orders and rules issued by the Federal Service for Environmental, Technological and Nuclear Supervision. In addition to general requirements for medical hyperbaric chambers, there are specific rules for both monoplace and multiplace systems as well as diving chambers. As medical devices, chambers are also regulated by the Federal Service for Supervision of Healthcare, which approves chambers for use within the Russian Federation. Facilities are subject to inspection prior to beginning operations, and regular inspections are also required that cover the operation and the physical plant. A separate accreditation program is under development. Physicians, nurses, and engineers who wish to work in hyperbaric medicine undergo special training of 288 hours and pass an exam before beginning practice. After five years of work, an additional 144-hour training course is required for continued employment. The All-Russian Association of Specialists in Hyperbaric Medicine and Technique was formed in 1998. The Association has more than 70 regional branches and sponsors conferences, symposiums, and seminars throughout the Federation. There is no definite list of indications for HBO_2. Each region of the country has developed approved standards for the use of HBO_2. Conditions on the approved list are covered by insurance; unlisted uses must be paid for by the patient.

Saudi Arabia

Number of facilities reported: 10-15

Respondent: Sultan Alturkistani

There is little regulation of hyperbarics in the Kingdom. There are no codes specific to chambers, and chambers are not regulated as medical devices. Imported chambers typically are constructed in conformance to rules of the country of origin. There are no standards for facility housing, training, or staffing, though voluntary conformance to UHMS and NFPA standards is common. The UHMS-accepted indications are typically followed, with reimbursement via government programs or self-pay. A professional organization is under development.

Singapore

Number of facilities reported: 3

Respondents: Edwin Low, MD and Elton Goh, RN, ME4

Singapore requires that chamber construction conform to one of five code standards *(ASME/BE EN/JIS/DIN/AD2000)*. Inspections by independent-approved inspection agencies are required for all chambers. Fire safety regulations for facilities are in place and are based on *NFPA 99* standards. Inspections of facilities are carried out by the Ministry of Manpower (civilian chambers) and the military (for military chambers). Some practice standards are in place but are focused more toward compressed air work (tunneling, diving) rather than clinical hyperbaric medicine. Physicians are required to have specialist qualifications, i.e. occupational health, anesthesia, surgery, and emergency medicine. There are no mandated staffing standards. Indications treated follow UHMS guidelines. Reimbursement for treatment is by cash or the national medical savings scheme (Medisave). There is no professional hyperbaric medicine society, but one facility in the country has undergone UHMS facility accreditation.

South Africa

Number of facilities reported: 10+

Respondents: Francois Burman, BSc Engineering, PE, MSc and Jack Meintjis, MD

South Africa has promulgated standards for the construction of pressure vessels that incorporate various national and international standards, including various ASME standards. Chambers are not regulated as medical devices, but the standards governing pressure vessels are applied, and these standards also regulate marketing and importation. Facilities are subject to general health care facility standards. There are no hyperbaric facility-specific standards. The South African Undersea and Hyperbaric Medical Association (SAUHMA) has actively developed various standards for training, staffing, and facility accreditation. The accreditation program developed by SAUHMA is referenced in national regulations and thus is a requirement. SAUHMA has adopted UHMS and ECHM lists of indications, though other indications are considered under a peer review/hospital ethics process. There are various mechanisms for funding treatment, ranging from private insurance to compensation for occupational injury (e.g., decompression illness) through cash payment. SAUHMA conducts a biennial conference and multiple short courses focusing on updates or specific needs (precordial Doppler, transcutaneous oximetry, etc.).

Spain

Number of facilities reported: 10+

Respondent: Jordi Desolo, MD, PhD

Spain follows EU guidelines for multiplace chamber construction and regulation as medical devices, but there is little specific regulation for monoplace chambers. As a result, there are approximately 10 multiplace hospital-based facilities (Centers of

Hyperbaric Medicine) that voluntarily base their practice on EUBS standards and guidelines, but there is much variability in practice within the monoplace chamber community. The multiplace facilities are subject to substantial inspections prior to beginning operations and at regular intervals thereafter. Given that there are no statutory standards for training, staffing, or practice, adherence to accepted standards is up to the facility. Centers for Hyperbaric Medicine typically operate in a structured fashion, following EUBS standards and treatment indications. Reimbursement for treatments conducted in a Center for Hyperbaric Medicine is provided under either the national Social Security System, some private insurers, and rarely out of pocket. Treatments provided by monoplace chamber facilities are predominately reimbursed by patients out of pocket. The Comite Coordinador de Centros de Medicina Hiperbárica (CCCMH) is the principal professional organization for hyperbaric medicine in Spain (there are other organizations supported by chamber manufacturers) and regular conferences are conducted.

Taiwan

Number of facilities reported: Approx. 50

Respondents: Ben Tsai, BS, RPh and Rick Shu, PE

Construction standards for pressure vessels are mandated by law. Chambers rated for 1.4+ atmospheres absolute (ATA) and 100% oxygen administration are classed as medical devices and regulated by the Taiwan Food and Drug Administration. There are no hyperbaric-specific facility fire safety standards, but facilities are rated as Class A locations under the "Standard for Installation of Fire Safety Equipment Based on Use and Occupancy." Staff qualification and chamber safety are mandatory and regulated by law. Training is conducted by the Association of Hyperbaric and Undersea Medicine (AHUM). The training program includes a 40-hour basic course in HBOT and three months of clinical practice in an AHUM-designated hospital. The 18 indications treated generally follow the UHMS indication list. Reimbursement is through the Bureau of National Health for nine of the AHUM-listed indications. AHUM is the professional hyperbaric organization for Taiwan. The organization publishes a magazine, conducts training classes, acts as an advisor to local AHJs, and conducts regular academic lectures and seminars. Accreditation is limited to AHUM-designated HBO_2 course-training hospitals. Inspections are required prior to facility operation, but subsequent inspections are limited to the initiation of a new device into service.

Thailand

Number of facilities reported: 25

Respondent: Prawin Yanapirak, MD

The Thai Navy has been the leader in establishing hyperbaric medicine in the country, consequently, much of the regulation in place is based on naval requirements. The navy specifies chambers to be compliant with *ASME PVHO-1* and *DIN 13256*. Though chambers are considered medical devices, no specific standards have been established by the Thai Food and Drug Administration. Fire safety standards for facilities are based on NFPA guidelines. Other than a requirement to have permission from the Ministry of Public Heath before beginning operations, there are no legal standards governing staffing, training, or facilities. UHMS guidelines for treatment are followed. Reimbursement for treatment may be covered by various government programs, personal insurance, or cash. The Thai Underwater Medical Society (TUMS) conducts an annual conference. There is no local accreditation program, but the Naval Medical Department has completed UHMS accreditation and is planning to set up a national standard for hyperbaric unit accreditation for other facilities in the country.

Turkey

Number of facilities reported: 60

Respondent: Dreylem Koca, MD

Turkey follows EU standards for chamber construction and regulation as medical devices (EN14931). A company that claims to sell hyperbaric chambers as medical devices is required to employ a product manager and a sales director who have passed a certain exam about medical devices. There are limited chamber-specific fire regulations, focusing mainly on the use of nonflammable or fire-retardant materials and a requirement for fire extinguishing systems. Hyperbaric-specific training is required for physicians and chamber operators but not for nurses. Physician training is under the regulation of the Ministry of Health. Nonphysician training is partially standardized by the university and Council of Higher Education and chamber operators must hold a chamber operator certificate approved by the appropriate government authorities. The Ministry of Health has a defined list of indications that are similar to UHMS/EUBS. The Social Security System provides reimbursement for the accepted indications; however, some private HBO_2 centers impose additional charges that are paid out of pocket. Inspections of facilities that put an emphasis on safety are conducted prior to facility opening by the Ministry of Health and every six months, but since there are not detailed specifications and most inspectors have limited knowledge about hyperbarics, inspections are not sharply focused. A professional organization is in place that advocates for hyperbaric medicine and conducts an annual conference.

United Kingdom

Number of facilities reported: 14-15 regulated by NHS, unknown # unregulated

Respondents: Martin Sayer, PhD; Lee Griffiths, MSc, CMIOSH; Roly Gough-Allen, CHT, ECHCO, ECHSM; Peter Atkey, CMIOSH, MInstNFT; and Jurg Wendling, MD

Editor's note: This response was received prior to the Brexit vote, and the impact of that action is unknown at this time. The UK follows EU standards for chamber construction and medical device regulation, though British Standards Institution BS coding is used to fit current UK legislation nomenclature. Facilities must conform to fire safety standards based on EN 16081:2011+A1:2013: "Hyperbaric Chambers. Specific Requirements for Fire Extinguishing Systems. Performance, Installation, and Testing." The National Health Service (NHS) has oversight of the operation of all the hyperbaric facilities that are members of the British Hyperbaric Association (BHA). Accepted indications are determined by the NHS, which also provides reimbursement for much of the clinical therapy provided, and funding may be available for indications that fall outside the NHS list. Private payment may be done for treatments not funded by the NHS and/or those currently considered as off-label, such as multiple sclerosis. The BHA serves as the primary advocate for hyperbaric therapy in the UK and provides a forum for the dissemination of information. An annual scientific meeting is conducted. Every second year, the BHA meeting is held jointly with the UK Diving Medical Committee. Though there are no general continuing medical education requirements, some oversight agencies may have specific requirements mandated by reimbursement agencies. The BHA operates two accreditation programs: one for Scotland (three-year cycle) and the other for non-Scottish chambers (five-year cycle). Accreditation is required for full BHA membership and reimbursement by the NHS. Beyond the basic inspections required for any business, the number and level of hyperbaric-specific inspections and permits depends very much on whether the facility will be treating NHS patients and obtaining NHS funding.

Vietnam

Number of facilities reported: 30

Respondent: Nguyen Truong Son, MD, PhD

Chambers must be built and housed in conformance with either Chinese or Australian standards and are considered medical devices. Training is mandated for physicians and nurses (basic classroom training + field experience). A certificate of training is required to work in the field. The Ministry of Health recognizes 48 indications for hyperbaric treatment, which are reimbursed by the state insurance program. Facilities are inspected annually by the Department of Measurement and Quality Management. In 2017, the Association of Medical Underwater and Hyperbaric Oxygen Therapy was founded. The Association advocates for the field, produces a journal, and conducts ongoing conferences.

Chile

CHAPTER 3.5
The Regulation of Hyperbaric Chambers as Medical Devices

Christy Foreman, MBE and Joanna Weitershausen, MSE

The Food and Drug Administration (FDA) regulates medical devices. The congressional mandate is to promote and protect the public health by ensuring their safety and effectiveness when used as indicated. Since 1976, the FDA has regulated hyperbaric chambers as medical devices. In that time, the agency has cleared 66 chambers or chamber accessories, such as hood drivers or ventilators, for marketing. Most of those clearances have occurred in recent years, illustrating the growth in the hyperbaric industry. To view a list of chambers that have been cleared for commercial distribution by the agency, the releasable 510(k) database may be searched at the website, https://www.accessdata.fda.gov/scripts/cdrh/cfdocs/cfPMN/pmn.cfm. Searching under the product code CBF will provide a listing of clearances of hyperbaric chambers to date.

The basic framework governing the regulation of medical devices is established in the Medical Device Amendments to the Federal Food, Drug, and Cosmetic Act (the Act) and signed into law on May 28, 1976. These amendments gave FDA specific authority to regulate medical devices. These authorities were modified by several new laws including the Safe Medical Devices Act of 1990 (SMDA), the Food and Drug Administration Modernization Act of 1997 (FDAMA), the Medical Device User Fee and Modernization Act (MDUFMA) of 2002, the Food and Drug Administration Amendments Act (FDAAA) of 2007, and the 21st Century Cures Act.

A medical device is defined as ". . . an instrument, apparatus, implement, machine, contrivance, implant, in vitro reagent, or other similar or related article, including any component, part, or accessory, that is:

1. recognized in the official National Formulary, or the United States Pharmacopeia, or any supplement to them,
2. intended for use in the diagnosis of disease or other conditions, or in the cure, mitigation, treatment, or prevention of disease in man or other animals, or

3. intended to affect the structure or any function of the body of man or other animals, and which does not achieve its primary intended purposes through chemical action within or on the body of man or other animals, and which is not dependent upon being metabolized for the achievement of any of its principal intended purposes."[1]

From this definition, it is clear that many different types of products are medical devices. Examples include implantable defibrillators, ventilators, and of course, hyperbaric chambers. Anyone who engages in the manufacture, preparation, propagation, compounding, assembly, or processing of a device intended for human use that is a medical device is subject to the medical device regulations.

The regulatory class in which the device is placed by the agency governs the level of regulation or control necessary to ensure safety and effectiveness. The Act required the FDA to classify all medical devices intended for human use into three categories: Class I, general controls; Class II, special controls; and Class III, premarket approval. The three levels of control based on device class are as follows:[2]

Class I devices are those needing the lowest level of regulation and are subject to the general controls requirements. These include establishment (manufacturing site) registration, device listing, premarket notification [510(k)], and good manufacturing practices (GMP). Examples of Class I devices include nasal cannulas, laryngoscopes, manual sphygmomanometers, and scalpels. Most Class I devices are exempt from premarket notifications.

Class II devices are subject to special controls as well as general controls requirements. Special controls may include items such as labeling or a mandatory performance standard. A device is placed in Class II if the general controls by themselves are insufficient to provide reasonable assurance of the safety and effectiveness of the device but there is sufficient information to establish special controls to provide assurance, including the promulgation of performance standards, patient registries, development and dissemination of guidelines, recommendations, and other appropriate actions. Examples of Class II devices include hyperbaric chambers, ventilators, external open loop infusion pumps, and anesthetic gas machines.

Class III devices are devices for which general and special controls are not sufficient for ensuring safety and effectiveness. These devices are usually implants or life-sustaining devices. These devices cannot be marketed until a premarket approval application (PMA) is approved. A PMA includes more information than that typically found in a 510(k), including detailed information on the manufacturing of the device. Any subsequent changes to a Class III device must be reported in an annual report or a PMA supplement. Examples of Class III devices include implantable defibrillators, high frequency ventilators, and heart valves.

On November 2, 1979, FDA proposed classification rules for all anesthesiology and respiratory devices. After receipt and consideration of comments, a final regulation classifying these devices was published on July 16, 1982. Hyperbaric chambers were classified as Class II medical devices.

In 1990, Congress amended the Act. The Safe Medical Devices Act of 1990 (SMDA), which became effective on November 28, 1990, gave the FDA several new authorities and expanded and modified previous medical device requirements. New regulations that were introduced by SMDA and applicable to hyperbaric chambers include the following:

- Medical device user facilities (hospitals, nursing homes, ambulatory surgical facilities, and outpatient treatment and diagnostic facilities) are required to report incidents that reasonably suggest there is a probability that a medical device has caused or contributed to the death, serious illness, or serious injury of a patient. These reports are due as soon as possible but no later than 10 working days after the user facility becomes aware of the incident.
- Manufacturers, importers, and distributors are required to report to the FDA certain removals or corrections of a device. This includes removals and corrections to reduce a risk to health posed by the device or remedy a violation of the Act caused by the device that may present a risk to health.
- Good manufacturing practices includes design validation requirements.
- Provisions relating to 510(k)s include:
    - The manufacturer must obtain a substantial equivalence order before beginning commercial distribution of a device for which a premarket notification has been submitted.
    - FDA is allowed to make a determination of substantial equivalence to legally marketed predicate devices for which PMAs are not required, regardless of the date of introduction of the predicate device.
    - The premarket notification must include either a summary of the safety and effectiveness information upon which an equivalence determination could be based or a statement that safety and effectiveness information will be available to anyone upon request. FDA shall make 510(k) summaries available to the public within 30 days of a determination of substantial equivalence.
    - Class II has been redefined to include any device for which reasonable ensurance of safety and effectiveness can be obtained by application of special controls. Special controls may include such controls as performance standards, postmarket surveillance, and patient registries. The agency is currently working on the development of special controls for hyperbaric chambers with the help of the Medical Systems Subcommittee of *ASME-PVHO*.

The Act was amended by the Food and Drug Administration Modernization Act of 1997 (FDAMA). FDAMA contained provisions related to all products under FDA's jurisdiction. To view all modifications, visit website http://www.fda.gov/MedicalDevices/DeviceRegulationandGuidance/GuidanceDocuments/ucm094526.htm "Overview—FDA Modernization Act of 1997."[4] The following identifies some sections of the act that have been modified and affect hyperbaric chambers.

- Any determination of intended use of the device shall be based upon the proposed labeling submitted in the premarket notification. However, the director of the Office of Device Evaluation (ODE) may determine that there is a reasonable likelihood that the device will be used for an intended use not identified in the labeling that could cause harm. In such cases, the director will communicate FDA's concerns to the applicant in writing and require a statement in the labeling specifying limitations on uses of the device.
- The FDA cannot withhold a 510(k) decision for failure of a firm to comply with any provision of the Act unrelated to a substantial equivalence decision. This includes failure by the firm manufacturing the device to comply with GMPs, unless FDA finds that failure to comply with such regulations will potentially present a serious risk to human health.
- Manufacturers may disseminate written information concerning the safety, effectiveness, or benefit of a use not described in a device's approved labeling to health care practitioners, pharmacy benefit managers, health insurance issues, group health plans, or federal or state agencies provided certain requirements are satisfied. These requirements can be found at the website https://www.fda.gov/regulatory-information/search-fda-guidance-documents/overview-fda-modernization-act-1997-medical-device-provisions#401dissemination under Section 401—Dissemination of Information on New Uses.
- The FDA may, through publication in the Federal Register, recognize all or part of an appropriate standard established by a nationally or internationally recognized standards development organization.
- The FDA shall ensure that the Quality Systems Regulation conforms to the extent possible with all or part of internationally recognized standards defining systems.
- The FDA shall use the least burdensome approach to introduce devices into the marketplace.

Premarket Notification [510(k)]

At least 90 days before a device is intended for market, a firm must submit to FDA's Document Mail Center a premarket notification also called a 510(k) submission. The 510(k) submission must contain sufficient information demonstrating that a device is substantially equivalent to a predicate device. A predicate device is a device that was marketed prior to May 28, 1976, or has received a 510(k) clearance since. A premarket notification is also required for a product that has been or is being marketed by a firm when there is a significant change or modification, including intended use of the device, that may significantly affect the safety or effectiveness of the device. There is no application form for 510(k) submissions; however, a format can be found in 21 CFR 807.87.

The manufacturer must obtain a substantial equivalence order before beginning commercial distribution of a device for which a premarket notification has been submitted. For the purposes of determining substantial equivalence, the term substantially equivalent or substantial equivalence means, with respect to a device being compared to a predicate device, that the device has the same intended use as the predicate device and that the device has the same technological characteristics as the predicate device. Substantial equivalence also means that the device has the same intended use and different technological characteristics; the information submitted, including clinical data if necessary, demonstrates that the device is as safe and effective as a legally marketed device and does not raise new or different questions regarding safety and effectiveness from the predicate device.[3]

Hyperbaric chambers are classified with other anesthesiology and respiratory devices in the Code of Federal Regulations (21 CFR Part 868) as follows:

§868.5470 Hyperbaric Chamber

(a) *Identification.* A hyperbaric chamber is a device that is intended to increase the environmental oxygen pressure to promote the movement of oxygen from the environment to a patient's tissues by means of pressurization that is greater than atmospheric pressure. This device does not include topical oxygen chambers for extremities (§878.5650).

(b) Classification. Class II (performance standards)

Since hyperbaric chambers are classified as Class II devices, a premarket notification submission is required. The process is identical for both monoplace and multiplace chambers as well as accessories to hyperbaric chambers such as oxygen treatment hoods. There are specific items that should be included in the submission in order to demonstrate equivalence.

First, a device description should be provided that completely describes the features of the device, including the pressurization system, pressurization rates, depressurization rates, seating capacities, maximum pressure, built-in breathing systems, etc. Additionally, these features should be compared to a legally marketed predicate device. The descriptive information may also describe how the device conforms to *ASME-PVHO-1 Safety Standard for Pressure Vessels for Human Occupancy* and *NFPA 99 Standard for Health Care Facilities:* Chapter 20: Hyperbaric Facilities.

Performance testing should be supplied for the chamber and any components of the chamber. Examples of performance testing for chambers include pneumatic testing and deluge testing for multiplace chambers. Aspects of this testing are covered in *ASME-PVHO* and a declaration of conformity to *ASME-PVHO* may be supplied in lieu of the test results. Information demonstrating that the risks of the device have been mitigated to acceptable levels should be provided. This is typically done by providing information consistent with the principles described in ISO 14971: International Standard Organization, Medical Devices—Application of Risk Management to Medical Devices.

Labeling should be supplied within the submission. Labeling includes device manuals, instructions for use, labeling affixed directly to the device, and promotional literature. The device manual should include the indications for use, instructions for safe operation, cleaning instructions, and all appropriate cautions and warnings such as those affiliated with enriched oxygen atmospheres. Hyperbaric chambers are considered prescription devices under 21 CFR 801.109, and accordingly these devices should bear the prescription legend that states, "Caution: Federal law restricts this device to sale by or on the order of a physician." This label should be included on the device itself along with any manuals that accompany the device. Prescription devices are devices that adequate directions for use cannot be written. In the case of hyperbaric chambers, this would encompass the diagnosis of conditions for which hyperbarics would be suitable and the protocols for treatment.

If the chamber or chamber components are software controlled, software documentation should be supplied consistent with the level of concern for the software of the device. The agency currently has a software guidance document entitled, "Guidance for the Content of Premarket Submissions for Software Contained in Medical Devices," dated May 11, 2005. This guidance document may be obtained from the FDA at this link: https://www.fda.gov/regulatory-information/search-fda-guidance-documents/guidance-content-premarket-submissions-software-contained-medical-devices. This document outlines the documentation that should be supplied with computer-controlled medical devices. This guidance document identifies the information that should be supplied based on the level of concern for software of the device. There are three levels of concern: minor, moderate, and major. The level of concern is identified based on the consequences if there should be a software failure. For example, a hyperbaric chamber would be assigned a major level of concern for software that controls the pressurization and depressurization of chambers.

If the device includes electronic components, including microprocessors and oxygen analyzers, the electrical safety and electromagnetic compatibility of the device should be established. This will provide reasonable assurance that the device will not interfere with the safe operation of other medical devices in the vicinity such as ventilators, and devices such as cellular phones will not interfere with proper operation of the chamber or related accessories. The testing for these components that is typically conducted is in accordance with standards such as the IEC-60601 series of standards, as applicable.

The materials used in the chamber should be compatible with oxygen at the expected temperatures and working pressures. Documentation should be included that identifies the materials that are in contact with oxygen and an analysis that demonstrates that the materials are compatible with oxygen at the anticipated pressures and temperatures.

Human factors should be considered when designing hyperbaric chambers. The incorporation of human factors principles in the design of the console may help reduce or eliminate human errors that may impact patient safety. FDA has published guidance in this area entitled, "Applying Human Factors and Usability Engineering to Medical Devices," (2016), that is intended to assist industry in following appropriate human factors and usability engineering processes to maximize the likelihood that new medical devices will be safe and effective for the intended users, uses, and use environments.

Consensus Standards

At this writing, the agency has recognized both *NFPA 99:* Chapter 20: Hyperbaric Facilities and *ASME Pressure Vessel for Human Occupancy (PVHO).* A voluntary standard may be recognized in whole, in part, or not at all. Though the agency regularly updates its list of recognized voluntary standards to reflect changes in those standards (as in the case of *NFPA 99*'s relocation of hyperbaric facilities to Chapter 14), there may be some time lag before the most current version of a particular standard is formally recognized, though reviewers may be aware of updates to standards.

Therefore in lieu of providing data demonstrating the safety of the chamber, the manufacturer may provide a declaration of conformity to one or more of the recognized standards. A declaration of conformity includes the following information:

- Identifies the applicable recognized consensus standards
- Specifies, for each consensus standard, that all requirements were met, except for inapplicable requirements or deviations noted below
- Identifies for each consensus standard any way(s) in which the standard may have been adapted for application to the device under review, e.g., identifies which of an alternative series of tests were performed
- Identifies, for each consensus standard, any requirements that were not applicable to the device
- Specifies any deviations from each applicable standard that were applied (e.g., deviations from international standards which are necessary to meet U.S. infrastructure conventions such as the National Electrical Code ANSI/NFPA 70)
- Specifies what differences exist, if any, between the tested device and the device to be marketed, and justifies the use of test results in these areas of difference
- Provides the name and address of each laboratory or certification body that was involved in determining the conformance of the device with the applicable consensus standards and a reference to any accreditations of those organizations, if a test laboratory or certification body was employed

Each recognized standard includes an extent of recognition that identifies any portion of a standard that is not recognized or additional information that may need to be supplied. In the case of *ASME-PVHO*, the forms should be supplied in addition to a declaration of conformity. Furthermore, the Boiler and Pressure Vessel Inspector's Certificate should be supplied. More information regarding this topic, including the supplementary data sheets that include the extent of recognition may be found at https://www.accessdata.fda.gov/scripts/cdrh/cfdocs/cfStandards/search.cfm.

Indications for Use

All 510(k) submissions since January 1, 1996, are required to include an Indications for Use form. The indications for hyperbaric chambers currently recognized by the FDA include the following:[5]

1. Air or gas embolism
2. Carbon monoxide poisoning/carbon monoxide poisoning complicated by cyanide poisoning
3. Clostridial myositis and myonecrosis (gas gangrene)
4. Crush injuries, compartment syndrome, and other traumatic ischemias
5. Decompression sickness
6. Arterial insufficiencies
   a. Central retinal artery occlusions
   b. Selected problem wounds/diabetic ulcers (microvascular insufficiency)
7. Severe anemia
8. Intracranial abscesses
9. Necrotizing infections
10. Osteomyelitis (refractory)
11. Delayed radiation injury (soft tissue and bony necrosis)
12. Compromised grafts and flaps
13. Acute thermal burn injury
14. Idiopathic sudden sensorineural hearing loss

These indications are the same indications that are recognized by the Undersea and Hyperbaric Medical Society (UHMS). When the Medical Devices Classification panel made the original classification recommendation in 1978, a recommendation was also made to adopt the UHMS indications. As these are currently the only indications that are recognized by the agency, the promotion and advertising of hyperbaric chambers must be restricted to the above indications. FDA does not regulate the practice of medicine, accordingly, if a physician believes that the off-label use of a hyperbaric chamber is the best therapeutic option for a patient that is considered the practice of medicine and is not regulated by the agency. However, the device should not be promoted for that off-label use. If the device is promoted for off-label use, the compliance division of the agency may take action against those promoting the device. Complaints regarding the off-label promotion may be referred to the promotions and advertising group within CDRH.

Indications beyond the UHMS indications identified above would be considered new indications for hyperbaric oxygen. Accordingly, Center for Drug Evaluation and Research (CDER) would take the lead in the evaluation of the new indication. An investigational new drug (IND) application would need to be filed with CDER to obtain agency approval if the study is of significant risk. If the study is nonsignificant risk, then only Institutional Review Board approval is necessary.

Devices that are promoted for use in the hyperbaric environment should be specifically cleared for use in that environment if the hyperbaric environment may affect device performance. For example, if a manufacturer wishes to promote a ventilator for use in conjunction with hyperbaric chambers, then a 510(k) should be filed for the new intended use. The submission should include information demonstrating that the device operates as specified when used as intended.

Once a 510(k) has been cleared for marketing, the manufacturer may not indicate that the FDA has approved the device. Any representation that creates an impression of official approval of a device because of complying with the premarket regulations is misleading and constitutes misbranding.[6] The same is true for referencing establishment registration numbers.[7]

Additional Requirements

Manufacturers of medical devices are also subject to regulations such as establishment registration and device listing, quality system regulations, and medical device reporting. Manufacturers, US importers, re-labelers, and distributors of medical devices must register their facilities and list their products with FDA. Unless exempt under 510(g) of the FD&C Act, this is required within 30 days after beginning any of these activities: manufacture, preparation, propagation, compounding, assembly, or processing of a device intended for human use. Activities requiring registration include repackaging, relabeling, distributing of imported or domestic devices, and specifications development. Initial registration is made on the Initial Registration Form. For each registered facility, the devices that are manufactured or processed at that facility are to be listed as part of the device listing process. Additional information regarding registration and listing can be found at https://www.fda.gov/MedicalDevices/DeviceRegulationandGuidance/HowtoMarketYourDevice/RegistrationandListing/default.htm.

The GMPs regulations for medical devices were published in 1978. The regulations were not significantly changed until 1996, when the GMPs were replaced by the quality system regulation (QSR). These regulations can be found in 21 CFR 820. Most devices are subject to the QSR (GMPs). Quality system regulations focus on the methods used in and the facilities and controls used for the manufacture of medical devices. This regulation is very similar to the International Standard ISO 13485 Medical Devices, Quality Management Systems, and Requirements for Regulatory Purposes.

The QSR includes regulations that govern not only the manufacturing of medical devices like hyperbaric chambers but also the design of the device. Design controls require controlled procedures to address the following elements: design and development planning, design input, design output, design review, design verification, design validation, design transfer, design changes, and design history file. Design controls are intended to demonstrate the scientific validity of the design selected for the finished device and to demonstrate that when manufactured, the actual device meets all of its intended specifications and requirements. Design control documents are reviewed by field inspectors during a facility inspection. For manufacturers of hyperbaric chambers, the FDA will periodically inspect the manufacturing facilities to ensure compliance.

A postmarket requirement includes the reporting of device failures or adverse events, known as medical device reports (MDRs). Both manufacturers and medical device user facilities must submit MDRs. Manufacturers and medical device user facilities should submit a report when they receive or otherwise become aware of information that reasonably suggests that a device has or may have contributed to a death or serious injury. Manufacturers must report events which they have received or become aware of information that one of their marketed devices has malfunctioned and the device would be likely to cause or contribute to a death or serious injury if the malfunction were to recur.[8]

The United States has had a history of safe use with hyperbaric chambers. This is due in part to manufacturers' efforts to design safe devices and in part to the users' efforts to safely operate the device during use. With the explosive growth that the hyperbaric industry is experiencing, one hopes that the excellent record of safe hyperbaric use continues.

References

1. Federal Food, Drug, and Cosmetic Act, Section 201.[321](h), DHHS Publication. FDA 93-1051.
2. Federal Food, Drug, and Cosmetic Act, Section 513.[360c](a)(1), DHHS Publication. FDA 93-1051.
3. The Safe Medical Devices Act of 1990 and The Medical Device Amendments of 1992, HHS Publication. FDA 93-4243.
4. Food and Drug Administration Modernization Act of 1997.
5. Undersea and Hyperbaric Medical Society Hyperbaric Oxygen Therapy Committee Report; 2014.
6. 21 CFR 807.97, revised as of April 1,2018.
7. 21 CFR 807.39, revised as of April 1, 2018.
8. 21 CFR Part 803, revised as of April 1, 2018.

CHAPTER 3.6
Hyperbaric Therapy in Remote Locations: What Standards Are Acceptable?

Nicholas Bird, MD, MMM, FAAFP, UHM/FUHM

Introduction

This chapter focuses on the unique issues associated with remote hyperbaric oxygen treatment (HBO_2) as well as those factors that bear consideration when contemplating evacuation. Facilities in remote locations are geographically isolated or may have limited resources or expertise relative to specialty centers. This definition is quite broad but appropriately includes clinics and community hospitals whose care delivery may not meet standards associated with tertiary centers. Due to the current prevalence of remote diving activities and the loss of hyperbaric medicine centers with expertise in diving injuries, management of decompression illness is emphasized.

First Aid of Injured Divers

Emergency oxygen therapy is an integral first aid measure for injured divers.[1-2] High flow oxygen delivered under normobaric conditions enhances tissue oxygenation, promotes inert gas washout, and may enhance the efficacy of subsequent hyperbaric treatment.[3-5] Undersea and Hyperbaric Medical Society (UHMS) guidelines give emergency oxygen for decompression illness (DCI) an American Heart Association classification of 1C.[6,18] Research suggests that the use of emergency oxygen prior to HBO_2 slows DCI symptom progression and reduces the impact of treatment delays, especially when delays exceed six hours after surfacing from the incident dive.[5] Patients with DCI symptoms who receive pre-HBO_2 normobaric oxygen also appear more responsive to HBO_2.[5] The potential negative clinical impact of delays of more than six hours can be mitigated by the appropriate use of normobaric emergency oxygen.[7]

Dive accidents frequently occur in remote locations where oxygen supplies are limited. In these settings, rescuers face a dilemma between maximizing the fraction of inspired oxygen (FiO_2) and attempts to conserve supplies. The priority should always be maintenance of the highest FiO_2 possible, even if this reduces the overall treatment time.[1] Breathing near 100% O_2 optimizes the off-gassing gradient for dissolved inert gas and thus maximally expedites inert gas washout.

Oxygen supplies are optimally extended with the use of a demand valve (or manually triggered ventilator used as a demand valve). If continuous-flow delivery is required or the only method available, start at 10 liters-per-minute (Lpm) and increase in increments based on the needs of the diver, ensuring that the reservoir bag does not completely deflate with inspiration.[1]

Hydration efforts are commonly employed as adjunctive DCI therapy. Intravenous fluid (IVF) administration is the most expedient method of fluid replacement, but oral fluids are an acceptable alternative in the fully conscious patient.[5-6] Mechanisms supporting the adjunctive utilization of IVF include the following: dilutional reduction of inert gas concentrations; expedited transport of inert gas to the lungs; reduced blood sludging and improved intravascular volumes, which can support divers demonstrating signs of vascular compromise; third spacing; or shock.

Delays to Treatment

Logistical issues may delay hyperbaric treatment initiation. Use of emergency oxygen at maximal FiO_2 constitutes the best initial management of DCI and in some cases may represent a responsible alternative to HBO_2 in the face of risky or lengthy evacuations for mild disease. Data are limited regarding the clinical impact of treatment delays, but published reports and cumulative evidence support the conclusion that moderate delays in mild to moderate DCS have minimal impact on clinical outcomes.[5,7] Severe symptoms of DCS characterized by paralysis and urinary retention may persist or incompletely resolve, even when hyperbaric treatment is initiated without delay.[5]

Treatment

HBO_2 for suspected DCI should be initiated as soon as possible following symptom onset.[8] Evidence supports the prompt use of HBO_2, especially in cases of acute pulmonary and neurological DCI.[8] Latency periods (time following a dive prior to symptom onset) and rate of symptom progression, factor significantly in diagnostic and treatment considerations. Symptoms that occur within minutes or a few hours after surfacing are more likely to worsen and may progress rapidly.[8-9] In contrast, delayed symptom onset is frequently characterized by less severe symptoms that may or may not worsen and may resolve without recompression treatment.[6,8-10] Mild-moderate symptoms, especially when demonstrating neurological compromise, should not be ignored as they may suddenly worsen.[8]

DCI is treated with equal effectiveness in both monoplace and multiplace chambers.[7,11] Prompt treatment should not be delayed or evacuation initiated, based solely on the type of chamber available. As seen in Table 1, effective DCI treatment protocols are available for use in monoplace chambers and offer an operational alternative to the lengthier US Navy (USN) or US Air Force (USAF) Treatment Table 6 (Table 2 for USN

Table 1. Hart-Kindwall modified DCI Treatment Table for monoplace chambers.[12] Printed with permission.

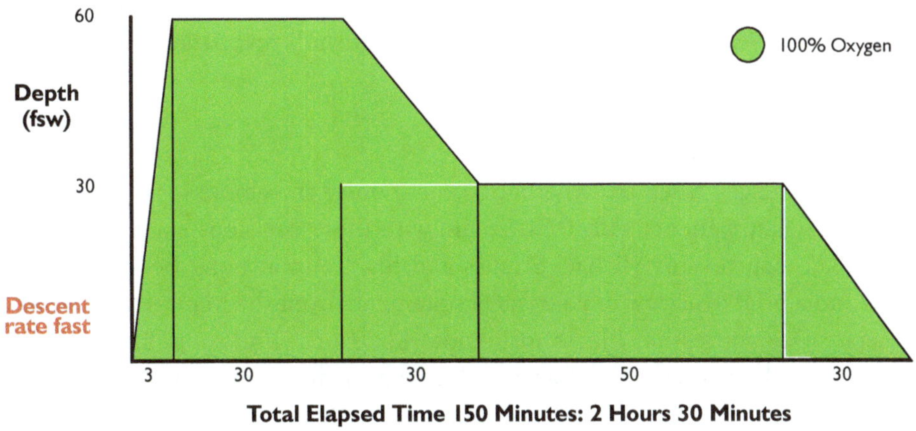

Treatment Table 6 and Appendix 1 for USAF Treatment Table 6).[8] Monoplace chambers equipped with air break capability can also perform a Treatment Table 6 and modified versions are commonly used to good effect (Table 1).[11-12,15]

Considerations Prior to Evacuation

The decision to evacuate a patient with suspected DCI should not necessarily preclude provision of an initial hyperbaric treatment. A common perception is that patients with DCI must only be treated initially with a Treatment Table 6 (TT6) and that both delays to treatment or ascents to altitude prior to HBO_2 are acceptable because of this perceived obligation. While the industry standard is indeed the use of a TT6 or its equivalent for DCI, it is entirely reasonable to optimize the time associated with evacuation preparation, which is frequently several hours. Early utilization of HBO_2 may serve to slow injury progression and reduce the risk of symptom and clinical exacerbation due to altitude exposure and expected time delays to the next hyperbaric treatment. If logistical factors limit the duration or frequency of treatment, but not the ability to provide safe recompression prior to evacuation, strongly consider the use of shorter treatment tables. Two treatment tables are discussed in this chapter but are not the only options available. (Equivalent tables are published and used in the United Kingdom Royal Navy Tables and the French have versions of the Comex tables.) If time prior to evacuation is limited and does not allow for completion of a USN or USAF TT6, then Tables 5 or 9 can be used with the intent to optimize inert gas washout, reduce the rate of disease progression, and optimize the patient's clinical status prior to evacuation.

Evacuation

Evacuation should be considered when there is a mismatch between patient status and local expertise, and available medical resources. Determining the need for evacuation is often highly subjective but should be guided by the present and trending pattern of the patient's medical condition. Considerations should include the impact of treatment delays, methods of travel, weather, time of day (planes may not be able to land at night), patient status, medical capabilities of evacuation aircraft and crew, patient comorbidities and overall clinical status.

Evacuation Decision Support

One of the challenges faced by hyperbaric practitioners in remote locations is when to treat or evacuate patients with DCI. To aid with these decisions, an algorithm has been included (courtesy of Michael Strauss and his group at Long Beach Memorial Hospital) and a brief overview of consensus statements from the Management of Mild or Moderate Decompression Illness in Remote Locations Workshop. The workshop was comprised of an international group of diving medicine experts who published proceedings to assist remote hyperbaric clinicians with the management of mild to moderate cases of decompression illness.[14,17]

Strauss et al. presented the following algorithm in 2010 to aid remote practitioners with evacuation decisions in patients with DCI.[13]

Table 2. Management and Transfer Algorithm

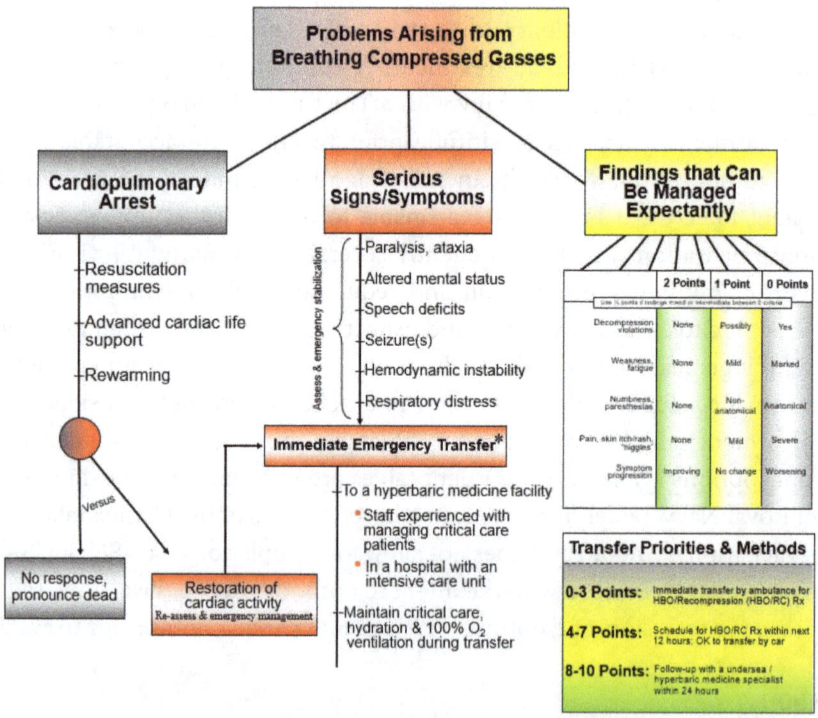

Printed with permission courtesy of Michael Strauss et al. from
An Algorithm for the Emergency Department Management and Transfer of Scuba Divers

Table 3. Summary of Consensus Statements[14]

- Mild DCI symptoms include limb pain, constitutional symptoms, skin rash, and non-dermatomal cutaneous sensory changes.
- Mild DCI symptoms in divers who have not received HBOT are unlikely to progress after 24 hours following the end of the incident dive, provided there is no further decompression stress or ascent to altitude.
- Treatment delays in cases of mild DCI symptoms are unlikely to result in a worsening of long-term outcomes (Level B evidence).
- Some patients with mild signs and symptoms of DCI can be treated adequately without recompression, although symptom resolution may take longer.
- Use of commercial airlines to evacuate selected divers with mild DCI symptoms may be appropriate to facilitate treatment or further evaluation following a surface interval of at least 24 hours. Mild DCI symptoms are unlikely to result in worsened long-term outcomes as a result of decompression in a pressurized cabin.

The complete document is downloadable on www.dan.org/research/.

Updated Consensus Guidelines for Prehospital DCI Management

The consensus summary above was published in 2004 and has been used as a guideline for medical management and evacuation decisions in cases of mild DCI.[14] In the years following its publication, further experience has been gained and clarification regarding particular aspects of the recommendations were provided in a follow-up consensus guideline for prehospital care in cases of DCI in 2018.[17] One of the essential concerns that occupied the latest publication related to the question of whether a thorough neurological examination performed by a qualified clinician was necessary to validate mild DCI characterized by the following: mild skin rash, lymphatic DCI, fatigue, some cutaneous sensory changes, limb pain, and the absence of significant neurological dysfunction.[17] The reason for this concern relates to the importance of a high quality medical assessment used to guide disposition (stay or evacuate) planning. Guideline authors provided a further refinement of the definition of mild DCI, a static or remitting symptom course for 24-hours after symptoms begin.

Technical Capacity

Requirements for safe chamber operation and maintenance are outlined in the *National Fire Protection Association's NFPA 99 Healthcare Facilities Code,* Chapter 14: Hyperbaric Facilities. *The American Society of Mechanical Engineers/Pressure Vessels for Human Occupancy (ASME PVHO)* provides standards for acceptable chamber construction for clinical use. These two organizations have established core industry standards for safe hyperbaric operations. Compliance with these two sets of standards is considered a foundation of all safe hyperbaric practices.

The essential technical capability necessary of any hyperbaric facility that treats injured divers is the capacity to perform a Treatment Table 6 or its equivalent. From a pressure perspective, this necessitates the ability to safely reach and sustain 2.8 atmospheres absolute (ATA).

Standard practice dictates that each facility have a backup gas supply to enable a complete Treatment Table 6 in the event of a power loss or other technical failure. For facilities not providing modified treatments tables (See Table 1), air break capacity and tender oxygen delivery are additional requirements. Multiplace centers must consider DCS risk associated with inside attendant duties and develop or acquire decompression and safety protocols to include oxygen-breathing systems.

Staff Training and Qualifications

Safe chamber operation necessitates sufficient foundational training followed by continuing education. The primary training required for work in the field of hyperbaric medicine is a UHMS-approved introductory course in hyperbaric medicine.[19] Guidelines for credentialing and privileging of hyperbaric providers were recently updated and published by the UHMS in 2018.[19] There are several UHMS-approved training programs in the United States. The UHMS has a complete list of available programs on their website (www.uhms.org). Additional training and educational opportunities exist beyond the primary course, which address the needs of particular career paths. For physicians interested in learning more about diving medicine, the UHMS Physicians Training in Diving Medicine Course and the Medical Examination of Divers Course provide opportunities for additional focused education in diving medicine. Further information is available at: www.uhms.org.

Summary

1. Hyperbaric oxygen therapy is the definitive treatment of DCI. Prompt recompression is associated with improved clinical outcomes in most cases. Treatment delays in mild-moderate symptoms are unlikely to worsen long-term outcomes.
2. In more severe cases of DCI, delays to treatment initiation of greater than six hours may be associated with slower or less complete recovery.[17]
3. Severe neurological DCS benefits from HBO_2, but many patients have residual symptoms despite minimal delays to treatment. Residual neurological or pain symptoms may persist after initial treatment and frequently benefit from additional HBO_2.
4. Providing the highest FiO_2 possible is the best first aid measure for suspected DCI and may protect against neurological symptom progression and may mitigate the potential clinical effects of delays in administering HBO_2.[13]
5. When available and when qualified medical personnel are on scene, use of intravenous fluids with nonglucose containing crystalloids, e.g., normal saline, is preferred.[17]

6. From a treatment mechanism perspective, all hyperbaric facilities can treat DCI with equal effectiveness with either a monoplace or multiplace chamber.
7. All hyperbaric facilities should maintain fundamental levels of staff training and technical standards. Guidelines for these are provided by the UHMS and include: *UHMS Guidelines for Hyperbaric Facility Operations 2nd Ed.* (2015), *Policies and Procedures Guidelines for Hyperbaric Facilities* (2017), and the *Hyperbaric Oxygen Therapy Indications 14th Ed.* (2019). Additional publications integral to safe administration of HBO_2 include the *NFPA 99* and *ASME PVHO.*
8. Decisions to treat versus evacuate are based on multiple factors that include the following: patient status, disease tempo (progression of symptoms), weather, travel distance, impact of treatment delays, time-of-day, available medical resources, and clinical expertise. Evacuation should be considered when patient treatment requirements or a patient's medical condition exceed local skill and technical capacity.
9. Consider providing an initial treatment with HBO_2 (Treatment Table 5 or 9) prior to evacuation if time does permit completion of a Treatment Table 6 or the facility is unable to provide a Treatment Table 6.
10. Decision support is available. Call DAN (+1-919-684-9111/+1-800-446-2671) or utilize some of the enclosed information to help guide treatment and evacuation decisions.
11. Hyperbaric treatment is the definitive treatment for DCI. However, it is important to rule out other potential causes of symptoms either before or after treatment(s) is initiated.

References

1. Divers Alert Network. Emergency Oxygen for Scuba Diving Injuries. 2011.
2. Markensen, D, et al. 2010 American Heart Association and American Red Cross Guidelines for First Aid. Circulation. 2010;122:S934-S946, doi:10.1161/CIRCULATIONAHA.110.971150.
3. Hyldegaard et al. *Undersea Biomed Res.* 1991;18:361-71.
4. Longphre et al. *Undersea Hyperb Med.* 2007;34:43-9.
5. Desola J, et al. Outcome of dysbaric disorders is not related to delay in treatment. Preliminary results of a multivariate analysis of 466 cases following a prospective study. Proceedings of the XXIII Annual Scientific Meeting of the European Underwater and Baromedical Society: EUBS 97, Bled, Slovenia.
6. Adjunctive therapy for decompression illness (DCI): Summary of UHMS guidelines; December 2002.
7. Stipp W. Time to treatment for decompression illness. Health and Safety Executive. 2007.
8. USN Dive Manual Revision 7. December 1, 2016.
9. Moon R. The natural progression of decompression illness and development of recompression procedures. *SPUMS J.* 2000;30(1):36-45.
10. Gempp E., Blatteau JE. Risk factors and treatment outcome in scuba divers with spinal cord decompression sickness. *J of Critical Care.* 2009;1-7.
11. Hart GB, Strauss MB, Lennon PA. The treatment of decompression sickness and air embolism in a monoplace chamber. *J Hyperbaric Med.* 1996;1:1-7.
12. Hart GB. Treatment of decompression illness and air embolism with hyperbaric oxygen. *Aerosp Med.* 1974;45:1190–1193.
13. Strauss MB, Miller SS, Lewis AJ, Alcock J, Kogen F, Aksenov IV. An algorithm for the emergency department management and transfer of scuba divers. Poster session presented at the Annual Scientific Meeting of the Undersea and Hyperbaric Medical Society. St. Petersburg Beach, FL. June 2010.
14. Mitchell SJ, Doolette DJ, Wacholz CJ, Vann RD (eds). Management of Mild or Marginal Decompression Illness in Remote Locations Workshop Proceedings. Durham, NC: Divers Alert Network. 2005.
15. Cianci PE; Green B; Slade JB, et al. [abstract] Delayed treatment of decompression illness with monoplace tables.
16. Denoble, Marroni, Vann. Annual Fatality Rates and Associated Risk Factors for Recreational Scuba Diving. DAN Fatality Workshop. Durham; April 2010.
17. Mitchell SJ, Bennett MH, Bryson P, Butler FK, Doolette DJ, Holm JR, Kot J, Lafere P. Prehospital management of decompression illness: expert review of key principals and controversies. Diving and Hyperbaric Medicine. 2018 March; 48(1):45-5.doi.10.28920/dhm48.1.45-55.
18. Applying Class of Recommendations and Level of Evidence to Clinical Strategies, Interventions, Treatments or Diagnostic Testing in Patient Care. (2015).

Retrieved October 25, 2018 from https://eccguidelines.heart.org/index.php/tables/applying-class-of-recommendations-and-level-of-evidence-to-clinical-strategies-interventions-treatments-or-diagnostic-testing-in-patient-care/.

19. UHMS Guidelines for Credentialing, Privileging and Supervision of Hyperbaric Oxygen Therapy in the U.S.A. (2018). Retrieved October 25, 2018 from https://www.uhms.org/images/PositionStatements/UHMS_Cred_and_Priv_Guide_Jan_31_2018.pdf.

Appendix

1. US Air Force Treatment Table 6 (*USN Dive Manual Revision 7,* 1 Dec 2016)

The US Air Force Treatment Table 6 is equivalent to the US Navy Treatment Table 6. The essential difference is that all of the oxygen periods and air breaks, with the exception of the ascent from 60 feet of seawater to 30 feet of seawater pressure, are consistently timed. This consistent pattern reduces the likelihood of operational errors.

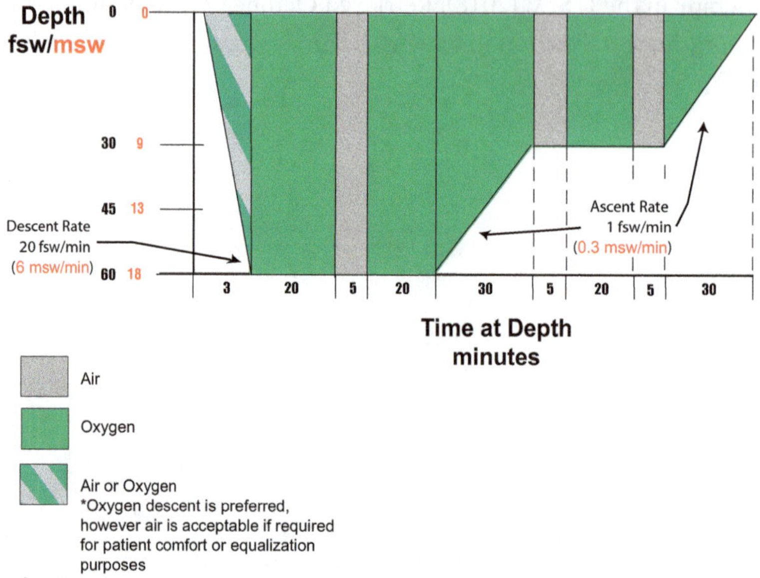

2. US Navy Treatment Table 5 (*USN Dive Manual Revision 7,* 1 Dec 2016)

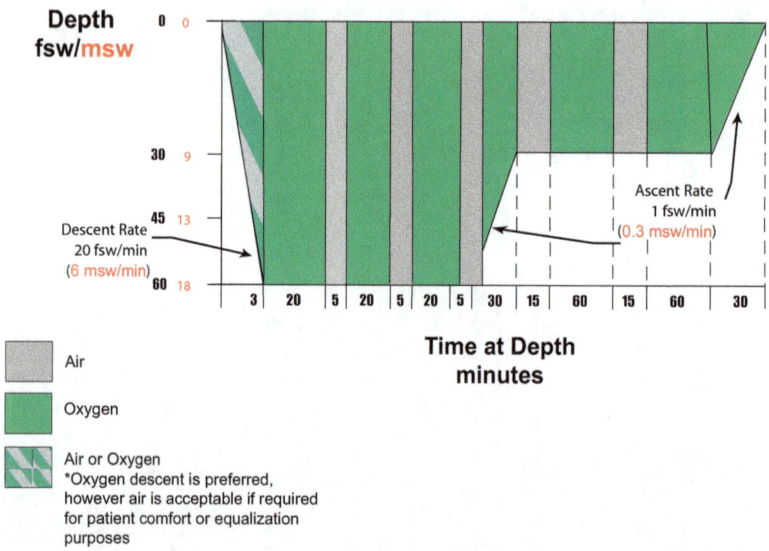

Treatment Table 5 may be used on a twice-daily basis for the treatment of residual DCI symptoms. As described above, Treatment Table 5 may be considered prior to evacuation if time or facility capacity does not safely allow for use of a Treatment Table 6.

3. **US Navy Treatment Table 9** (*USN Dive Manual Revision 7*, 1 Dec 2016)

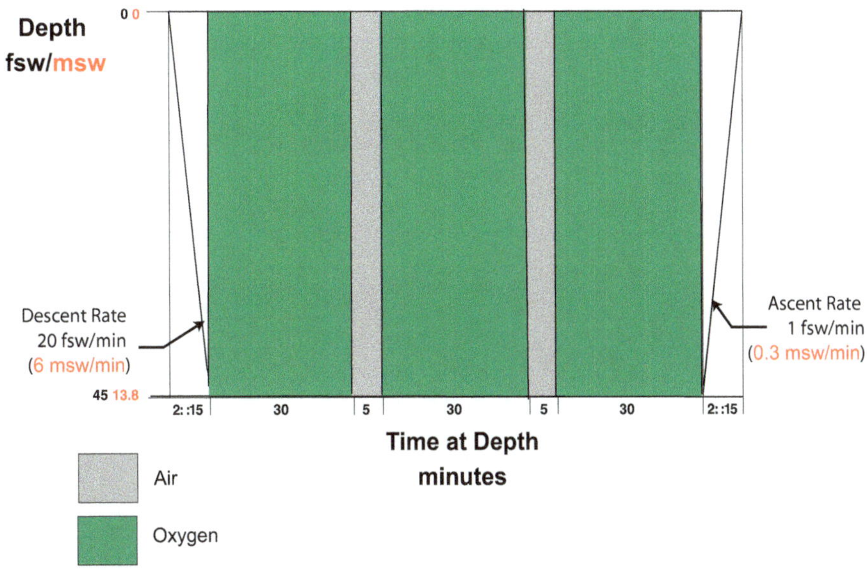

Treatment Table 9 is most frequently used for standard wound care treatments, but twice-daily treatment protocols may be used for the treatment of residual DCI symptoms.

CHAPTER 3.7
The Role of Quality Assurance in the Design and Fabrication of Hyperbaric Oxygen Chambers Intended for Clinical Use

Deepak Talati, BSME, MSIE and Greg Godfrey, BS, MBA, RAC, CQE, CQA

Introduction

Quality assurance is continually playing an increasing role in the fabrication of pressure vessels in the United States and throughout the world. The role of quality assurance is to ensure compliance with all applicable standards and manufacturing requirements involved with the design, fabrication, and installation of the hyperbaric chamber. The standards specifying quality assurance requirements for hyperbaric chambers have diverse origins and goals. It is the intent of this chapter to describe, in a general manner, the quality assurance requirements for the fabrication of hyperbaric chambers and the relevant standards from which they originate. It is not the intent of this chapter to describe the specific product standards governing the design or manufacture of the hyperbaric chamber.

History of Quality Assurance Standards

Customers and users have had concerns regarding product quality since humans began manufacturing products for commercial distribution. The quality of the product or service was generally at the whim of the person providing the service or producing the product, leaving the customer with no assurance the service provided would meet their expectations or that the product would work as intended.

Product standards were developed over the last hundred years to specify minimum requirements products must meet to be considered acceptable. This was the beginning of quality control, as there was now a means to specify and determine the quality of a product. These standards were then incorporated into purchasing contracts and national standards as customers and users began specifying the quality expectations of the product they were purchasing.

The development and acceptance of product standards had a direct effect on improving the quality of products and services. Unfortunately, there was considerable variability, as there were no controls in the quality of the products produced to these standards resulting in unacceptable product reaching the customers. It became evident that something more was needed to ensure the products received would meet the specified product standards and perform as they were intended. During World War II (WWII), munitions and equipment sent to the field experienced high levels of defects. Bombs wouldn't explode, rifles would jam, and bullets wouldn't be ejected. This was of great disappointment to the customers whose lives depended on the products working correctly. The United States Department of Defense began specifying certain quality system requirements be adopted by its suppliers to reduce the amount of faulty product reaching the battle field. It was realized that the manufacturing activities needed to be controlled to reduce the variability in quality of outgoing products. This was the beginning of the quality assurance movement. Following WWII, quality assurance standards were developed and imposed on suppliers by the purchasers of many types of products. Many countries and industries developed similar standards with the intent of ensuring routine product quality, especially where public safety was concerned. Some of the more notable industries included aerospace, medical products, automotive, nuclear, and defense contracting.

Industry Standards

The American Society of Mechanical Engineers (ASME) established the Boiler and Pressure Vessel Committee to develop rules for the construction of steam boilers and other pressure vessels in 1911. These rules were published as *ASME Boiler and Pressure Vessel Code (BPVC)*[1] with specific rules for construction of pressure vessels listed in Section VIII.

The *ASME PVHO-1 Safety Standard for Pressure Vessels for Human Occupancy*[2] is a branch of *ASME* Section VIII of the *ASME BPVC* and was established in 1974 to cover important considerations such as acrylic viewport windows, not covered in *ASME* Section VIII. Requirements for a quality assurance program were added to the *ASME PVHO-1 Safety Standard* in 1984.

In 1946, the National Board of Boilers and Pressure Vessel inspectors published *National Board Inspection Code (NBIC)*[3] establishing rules for inspection and repairs to boilers and pressure vessels. The main purpose was to provide assurance that pressure retaining components were constructed in accordance with the *ASME BPVC* and that they were inspected by a qualified national board commissioned inspector. The *NBIC* was restructured in 2017 into four parts: installation, inspection, repairs, and alterations and pressure relief devices.

The manufacturer or assembler's quality control system must be audited and certified by ASME to the requirements stated in Section VIII of the code. The manufacturer or assembler must also contract with an ASME-authorized third-party inspection agency, referred to as the authorized inspection agency (AIA), to inspect the hyperbaric chambers against the requirements of the code and to the fabricator's design and manufacturing specifications implementing the code.

Hyperbaric chambers installed in the United States are fabricated, tested, and stamped in compliance with the requirements of the *ASME Boiler and Pressure Vessel Code* and *ASME Pressure Vessels for Human Occupancy PVHO-1 Safety Standard.* Registration of pressure vessels with a national board number is required and can be completed with the manufacturer submitting an original manufacturer's data report to the national board for permanent retention. The data report is certified by both the manufacturer and the national board commissioned inspector. Additionally, pressure vessels for human occupancy intended for use in health care facilities shall comply with requirements of *NFPA 99, Health Care Facilities Code,* Chapter 14: Hyperbaric Facilities[4] and local city/ state jurisdictional requirements.

At present, other than self-certification and verification to the requirements of the *ASME PVHO-1 Safety Standard,* there are no requirements for a third-party inspection agency or system certification. The manufacturer or assembler must verify and record fabrication activities and testing as required by *ASME PVHO-1 Safety Standard and PVHO-2 Safety Standard for Pressure Vessels for Human Occupancy, In-Service Guidelines.*[5]

ASME Quality System Requirements

ASME Section VIII, Division 1 BPVC

The *ASME* Section VIII, Division 1 BPVC quality system that applies to the manufacturer or assembler of pressure vessels is found in the *ASME Boiler and Pressure Vessel Code, Section VIII, Mandatory Appendix 10, Quality Control System.* The manufacturer or assembler is required to implement and maintain a quality control system, which can show objective evidence that all code requirements including material, design, fabrication, test, and inspection by the authorized inspector of pressure vessels and components are met. It also provides a guide to some of the features required to be covered in the written description of the *Quality Control System* manual.

ASME PVHO-1 Safety Standard

The *ASME PVHO-1 Safety Standard* requires PVHOs to be designed, fabricated, tested, marked, and stamped in accordance with the requirements of *ASME PVHO-1 and ASME BPV* code Section VIII, unless otherwise permitted within the applicable standards. In-service requirements for PVHOs are found in *ASME PVHO-2, Safety Standard for Pressure Vessels for Human Occupancy, In-Service Guidelines.*

The quality assurance requirements for implementing and maintaining a quality assurance program for PVHO Manufacturers and Acrylic Window Fabricators can be found in Section 3 of the *Safety Standard.* Specific quality assurance requirements relating fabrication of viewport which includes window, flange, retaining rings, and seals are stated in fabrication and inspection subsections of Section 2, viewports section.

The PVHO Manufacturers and Acrylic Window Fabricators are responsible for implementing and maintaining the quality requirements as described in ISO 9001 Quality Management Systems[6] or ISO 13485, Medical Devices—Quality Management Systems,[7] whichever is applicable. They are also required to certify compliance with PVHO-1 Safety Standard by furnishing the purchaser with the appropriate PVHO-1 forms and marking the PVHO in accordance with the requirements stated in the standard.

The requirements for establishing and maintaining quality assurance programs to control the quality of work performed by the repairers of severely damaged acrylic windows can be found in Mandatory Appendix III, Quality Assurance program for repair of severely damaged windows, of *ASME PVHO-2, In-Service Guidelines.*

Medical Device Regulatory Requirements

United States Food and Drug Administration (FDA)

In 1976, the United States Congress amended the Food, Drug & Cosmetic Act to extend regulatory coverage by the United States Food and Drug Administration (FDA) to medical devices. Hyperbaric chambers are classified as Class II medical devices under the United States Code of Federal Regulations (CFR), Title 21, Part 868 Anesthesiology Devices, requiring compliance with CFR Title 21, Part 820, Quality System Regulation.[8]

In 1990, FDA undertook the start of the revision of the Current Good Manufacturing Practice (CGMP) regulation to add the design controls authorized by the Safe Medical Devices Act. Also, the FDA believed that it would be beneficial to the public and the medical device industry for the CGMP regulation to be consistent, to the extent possible, with the requirements for quality systems contained in applicable international standards, primarily the International Organization for Standards. After an extensive effort, the part 820 revision was published on October 7, 1996 and went into effect June 1, 1997.

A quality system is a necessary component of any medical device commercialization effort. Medical device manufacturers seeking regulatory clearance or approval in the United States, 21 CFR Part 820 of US Code of Federal Regulations, must meet quality system requirements (QSR) to bring their products to market.

In order to achieve FDA QSR compliance, you must implement a quality system covering the design, manufacture, packaging, labeling, storage, and delivery of your medical device. Quality system requirements of 21 CFR Part 820 explain your obligations in the following areas:

- Management Responsibility
- Quality Audit
- Personnel
- Design Controls
- Document Controls
- Purchasing Controls

- Identification and Traceability
- Production and Process Controls
- Acceptance Activities
- Nonconforming Product
- Corrective and Preventive Action
- Labeling and Packaging Control
- Handling, Storage, Distribution, and Installation
- Records
- Servicing
- Statistical Techniques

Europe Economic Union

CE Marking

The letters "CE" are the abbreviation of French phrase Conformité Européenne, which means European conformity. The term initially used was CE mark and it was later replaced by CE marking in 1993.

Before a medical device can be launched in the European Economic Area (EEA), it must receive CE marking. The CE marking confirms that the medical device meets certain essential requirements of the European General Medical Devices Directives (i.e., that it is fit and safe for the intended purpose). Certain directives include options for the responsible organizations to provide a declaration of conformity stating that the product meets the requirements of the applicable directives. Other directives pertaining to products affecting health and/or safety such as hyperbaric chambers require a specific certificate from the notified body. CE marking also shows that the medical device can be freely marketed anywhere in the EEA without further control.

CE marking is mandatory for medical devices sold in the EEA, even if the medical device was manufactured outside the EEA. It is the manufacturer's sole responsibility to obtain and place the CE mark on the product. If the product is imported from outside the EEA, then this responsibility falls to the importer within the community.

EU Medical Device Regulation (MDR) 2017/745

Effective June 14, 1998, all medical devices and their accessories intended for market in the European Economic Union must comply with the requirements of Council Directive 93/42/EEC of June 14, 1993.

Medical device manufacturers will soon be confronted with major changes in the EU's decades-old regulatory framework which governs market access to the European Union (EU). The EU Medical Device Regulation will replace the EU's current Medical Device Directive (93/42/EEC) and the EU's directive on active implantable medical devices (90/385/EEC).

The EU Medical Device Regulation (2017/745)[9] was officially published on May 5, 2017, and came into force on May 25, 2017. Manufacturers of currently approved medical devices will have a transition time of three years until May 26, 2020, to meet the requirements of the MDR. For some manufacturers, the new MDR provides an additional time after the date of application allowing them to place new products for a maximum of four (4) more years to May 26, 2024. Additional requirements will apply for this extended transition period.

The MDR differs in several important ways from the EU's current directives for medical devices and active implantable medical devices. Hyperbaric chambers are classified as Class IIb medical devices under Rule 12 of the MDR regulation and some of the significant changes in the regulation include the following:

- **Product scope expansion:** The definition of medical devices and active implantable medical devices covered under the MDR will be significantly expanded to include devices that may not have a medical intended purpose, such as colored contact lenses and cosmetic implant devices and materials. Also included in the scope of the regulation are devices designed for the purpose of prediction and prognosis of a disease or other health condition.
- **Identification of a qualified person:** Device manufacturers will be required to identify at least one person within their organization who is ultimately responsible for all aspects of compliance with the requirements of the new MDR. The organization must document the specific qualifications of this individual relative to the required tasks.
- **Implementation of unique device identification:** The MDR mandates the use of unique device identification (UDI) mechanisms. This requirement is expected to increase the ability of manufacturers and authorities to trace specific devices through the supply chain and to facilitate the prompt and efficient recall of medical devices that have been found to present a safety risk. In addition, the European Databank on Medical Devices (Eudamed) is expected to be expanded to provide more efficient access to information on approved medical devices.
- **Rigorous post-market oversight:** The MDR will grant notified bodies increased postmarket surveillance authority. Unannounced audits, along with product sample checks and product testing, will strengthen the EU's enforcement regime and help to reduce risks from unsafe devices. Annual safety and performance reporting by device manufacturers will also be required in many cases.
- **Specifications:** The MDR plans to allow the EU Commission or appointed expert panels to publish common specifications which shall then be taken into account by manufacturers as well as notified bodies. These common specifications shall exist in parallel to the Harmonized Standards and the State of the Art.

- **Reclassification of devices according to risk, contact duration and invasiveness:** The MDR will require device manufacturers to review the updated classification rules and update their technical documentation accordingly by considering the fact that Class III and implantable devices will have higher clinical requirements and a regular scrutiny process.
- **Systematic clinical evaluation:** Manufacturer will need to re-prepare their clinical evaluation by considering the new wording of the regulation on when an equivalence approach and under which circumstances it is possible to justify not conducting a clinical investigation.
- **No grandfathering provisions:** Under the MDR, all currently approved devices must be recertified in accordance with the new requirements. Exemptions are under negotiation at the time of this writing.

EU Pressure Equipment Directive (PED) 2014/68/EU

The Pressure Equipment Directive (PED) 2014/68/EU (formerly 97/23/EC)[10] of the EU sets out the standards for the design and fabrication of pressure equipment (steam boilers, pressure vessels, hyperbaric chambers, piping, safety valves, and other components and assemblies subject to pressure loading) generally over 0.26 gallons or one liter in volume and having a maximum pressure more than 7.25 PSIG or 0.5 bar gauge. It also sets the administrative procedures requirements for the conformity assessment of pressure equipment for the free placing on the European market without local legislative barriers. It has been mandatory throughout the EU since May 30, 2002, with 2014 revision fully effective as of July 19, 2016. This is enacted in the UK as the Pressure Equipment Regulations (PER). The set of standards and regulations regarding pressure vessels and boilers safety is also very close to the US standards defined by the American Society of Mechanical Engineers (ASME).

Rest of World

There are many different requirements throughout the rest of the world for compliance to quality assurance systems covering the design and manufacture of medical devices. Many countries accept compliance with U.S. FDA regulations or compliance with the European Medical Device Directive for the import of medical devices. The number of government agencies requiring compliance and certification to a quality assurance standard for registering medical devices in their countries is increasing every year. The most widely accepted quality assurance standard is ISO 13485:2016 Medical Devices Quality Management System Standard.

Quality Management System (QMS) (ISO 13485:2016)

ISO 13485:2016 – Medical Devices Quality Management Systems Requirements for regulatory purposes specify requirements for a quality management system where an organization needs to demonstrate its ability to provide medical devices and related services that consistently meet customer and applicable regulatory requirements. Such organizations can be involved in one or more stages of the life cycle, including design and development, production, storage and distribution, installation or servicing of a medical device, and design and development or provision of associated activities (e.g., technical support). ISO 13485:2016 can also be used by suppliers or external parties that provide product, including quality management system-related services to such organizations.

Requirements of ISO 13485:2016 are applicable to organizations regardless of size and type, except where explicitly stated. Wherever requirements are specified as applying to medical devices, the requirements apply equally to associated services as supplied by the organization.

The processes required by ISO 13485:2016 that are applicable to the organization, but performed by another organization (supplier/contractor), are the responsibility of the organization and are accounted for in the organization's quality management system by monitoring, maintaining, and controlling the processes performed by those parties.

If applicable regulatory requirements permit exclusions of design and development controls, this can be used as a justification for their exclusion from the quality management system. These regulatory requirements can provide alternative approaches that are to be addressed in the quality management system. It is the responsibility of the organization to ensure that claims of conformity to ISO 13485:2016 reflect any exclusion of design and development controls.

If an ISO 13485 requirement is not applicable to the activities performed by an organization, it may be excluded from the organization's QMS. However, the organization needs to document the justification for excluding it from their quality management system.

Quality Assurance System Benefits

Customer Satisfaction

Many benefits result from having an established comprehensive quality system. The most important benefit is customer satisfaction. It is the customers purchasing the medical device who will make positive or negative comments based on their experience to others who may be considering purchase of the same device. In addition, many purchasers of capital equipment require the submittal of references prior to signing a purchase agreement.

Perceived product quality also provides a competitive advantage in today's market.[11] Quality is generally associated with cost-effectiveness and product safety, key issues in the clinical environment. High quality will continue to be a competitive advantage until the quality of all suppliers is considered equal.

Contract Compliance

A comprehensive quality assurance system will ensure that specific customer and contractual requirements, if required, are addressed in the design and manufacture of the chamber. Failure to meet contract requirements not only results in customer dissatisfaction but can also be considered breach of contract.[12] This issue takes on more importance in the manufacture of multiplace chambers versus monoplace chambers. Multiplace chambers are built to detailed customer specifications where monoplace chambers are usually built to the manufacturer's specifications. A product which fails to meet its intended purpose may be considered as a breach of contract, resulting in additional expenses to the manufacturer.

Reduced Quality Problems

The level of product quality will vary from one finished unit to the next. Significant levels of variability result in increased quality problems, reduced reliability, increased costs, and customer dissatisfaction. A good quality assurance system will provide the necessary process control to reduce the variability of outgoing products in addition to eliminating the causes of quality control problems. The quality system also establishes the baseline for continuous improvement efforts, including product and process cost reduction activities.[13]

Quality Costs

Poor quality associated with product design and manufacture leads to considerable costs to the manufacturer and to the customer. The manufacturer time spent addressing process quality problems is calculated in person-hours spent addressing the problem and lost opportunity costs in person-hours that should have been spent doing value added activities. Continuous improvement through corrective and preventive action activities will reduce the amount of scrap and rework generated through nonconforming product. A comprehensive quality assurance system will continue to reduce the number of quality problems over time, resulting in an improved bottom line for the manufacturer.[14]

Improved outgoing product quality also reduces the amount of warranty-related activities which occur. A product that does not perform as intended or specified can be considered a violation of an implied warranty or capability, possibly resulting in extensive warranty and/or legal costs to the manufacturer.[15]

Product Liability Protection

Manufacturers in the United States have significant liability exposure associated with the use of their products. Every ethical device manufacturer has a primary goal of ensuring patient and user safety. Manufacturers are required to maintain a risk-based quality assurance system to ensure the design and manufacturing processes result in safe and efficacious products. This will not only help ensure their products are safe to use but will also help avoid costs associated with product liability lawsuits and subsequent recalls or corrective actions. In addition, having a sound quality assurance/safety system may provide the manufacturer some limited protection relating to negligence claims in addition to possible avoidance of criminal charges.[16]

Future Directions

The International Medical Device Regulators Forum (IMDRF) recognizes that a global approach to auditing and monitoring the manufacturing of medical devices could improve their safety and oversight on an international scale. At its inaugural meeting in Singapore in 2012, the IMDRF identified a work group to develop specific documents for advancing a medical device single audit program (MDSAP).

The MDSAP allows an MDSAP-recognized auditing organization to conduct a single regulatory audit of a medical device manufacturer that satisfies the relevant requirements of the regulatory authorities participating in the program. These requirements are in addition to the QMS requirements stated in ISO 13485.

International partners that are participating in the MDSAP include the following:

- **Australia:** The Therapeutics Goods Administration (TGA) uses the MDSAP audit report as part of the evidence that is assessed for compliance with medical device market authorization requirements unless the medical device is otherwise excluded or exempt from these requirements or if current policies restrict the use of MDSAP audit reports.
- **Brazil:** The Brazilian National Health Surveillance Agency (ANVISA) utilizes the outcomes of the program, including the reports, to constitute an important input on ANVISA's premarket and postmarket assessment procedures, providing, when applicable, key information that is expected to support regulatory technical evaluation on these issues.
- **Canada:** Health Canada HC is using MDSAP audit as part of their Canadian Medical Device Conformity Assessment System (CMDCAS) certification program effective January 1, 2019. The MDSAP is now the mechanism to achieve regulatory compliance for quality management system requirements in Canada.
- **United States:** U.S. Food and Drug Administration's Center for Devices and Radiological Health FDA will accept the MDSAP audit reports as a substitute for FDA routine inspections. Inspections conducted for cause or compliance follow-up by FDA will not be affected by this program. Moreover, this MDSAP would not apply to any necessary pre-approval or post-approval inspections for premarket approval (PMA) applications or to decisions under section 513(f)(5) of the Act (21 U.S.C. 360c(f)(5)) concerning the classification of a device.
- **Japan:** The Ministry of Health, Labour and Welfare (MHLW) and Pharmaceutical and Medical Devices Agency (PMDA) will utilize these audit reports in both premarket and periodical postmarket audit under regulations in Japan. Japan officially joined the pilot in June 2015 and began accepting MDSAP audit reports in June 2016.

Based on its evaluation of the MDSAP Final Pilot Report, the MDSAP Regulatory Authority Council (the international MDSAP governing body) determined that the MDSAP pilot had satisfactorily demonstrated the viability of the Medical Device Single Audit Program.

As of the date of this publication, only Canada has adopted MDSAP. Other participating countries may or may not require MDSAP compliance from countries importing their devices.

FDA will continue to accept MDSAP audit reports as a substitute for routine agency inspections. Firms with activities related to the electronic product radiation control (EPRC) provisions of the Act will continue to be subject to FDA inspections for the EPRC activities.

References

1. ASME. American Society of Mechanical Engineers Boiler and Pressure Vessel Code Section VIII – Rules for Construction of Pressure Vessels Division 1, Appendix 10. ASME; 2019.
2. ASME. American Society of Mechanical Engineers Safety Standard for Pressure Vessels for Human Occupancy PVHO-1. ASME; 2016.
3. National Board Inspection Code (NBIC). National Board of Boiler and Pressure Vessel Inspectors; 2017.
4. NFPA. NFPA 99 Health Care Facilities Code. National Fire Protection Association; 2018.
5. ASME. American Society of Mechanical Engineers Safety Standard for Pressure Vessels for Human Occupancy In-Service Guidelines PVHO-2. ASME; 2016.
6. ISO 9001:2015 Quality Management Systems – Requirements. International Organization for Standardization; 2015.
7. ISO 13485:2016 Medical Devices – Quality Management Systems – Requirements for Regulatory Purposes. International Organization for Standardization; 2016.
8. United States Code of Federal Regulations, Title 21, Part 820 Quality System Requirement. U.S. Government Printing Office; April 1, 2018.
9. Regulation (EU) 2017/745 of the European Parliament and of the Council of 5 April 2017 on Medical Devices. Amending Directive 2001/83/EC, Regulation (EC) No 178/2002, and Regulation (EC) No 1223/2009. Repealing Council Directives 90/385/EEC and 93/42/EEC.
10. Pressure Equipment Directive PED2014/68/ EUGuidelinesENv5.2.
11. Atkinson H, Hamburg J, Ittner C. Linking Quality to Profits. American Society for Quality Control Quality Press; 1994.
12. Welch C, Geissler P. Bringing Total Quality to Sales. American Society for Quality Control Quality Press; 1992.

13. Pyzdek T, Keller P. Quality Engineering Handbook. Marcel Dekker, Inc., 2003.
14. Campanella J, Hagan J. Principles of Quality Costs. American Society for Quality Control Quality Press; 1990.
15. Goestsch D, Davis S. Total Quality Handbook. Prentice Hall; 2001.
16. Kolb J, Ross S. Product Safety and Liability. McGraw-Hill Book Company;1980.

CHAPTER 4
Hyperbaric Chamber Systems

CHAPTER 4.1
Pressurization Systems

Michael W. Allen

General

Pressurization systems are a critical element in any hyperbaric system; they are the link between the source of gas and the point at which it enters the chamber(s). In a clinical hyperbaric facility, the pressurization gas can be air, oxygen, or both depending on chamber type and facility operating policies (i.e., Do they use air breaks?).

This chapter is written from the perspective of you as a system user rather than system designer. The objective is to provide practical information on various aspects of pressurization systems that will be helpful to you on a day-to-day basis. It is recommended that you go beyond the basic information provided here and become familiar with Chapter 5: Gas and Vacuum Systems and Chapter 14: Hyperbaric Facilities chapters in *NFPA 99 Health Care Facilities Code.*[1] *NFPA 99* is the standard which governs the design, construction, and utilization of hyperbaric systems in U.S. health care facilities; it is also used by authorities having jurisdiction (AHJ) such as federal, state, and municipal regulatory agencies and third-party accreditation bodies in their assessment of your operation. Keep a copy of the latest edition of *NFPA 99* in your facility technical library. It will complement this chapter and serve as a ready reference. Become familiar with the relevant sections to help you spot compliance problems with your equipment and be a source of reference in the event your facility is inspected.

Unless otherwise specified in *NFPA 99*, piping systems dedicated to clinical hyperbaric chambers are required to comply with *American Society of Mechanical Engineers (ASME) Safety Standard for Pressure Vessels for Human Occupancy (PVHO-1).*[2] The pressurization system is a subsystem critical to the overall performance of the equipment and must be capable of meeting the performance requirements established for any normal and emergency condition. To comply with PVHO-1, system performance criteria must be clearly laid down in a document known as a *User's Design Specification (UDS).* When it is completed and agreed upon, the *UDS* becomes the road map for the designer. I recommend you also acquire a copy of *ASME PVHO-2 Safety Standard for Pressure Vessels for Human Occupancy: In Service Guidelines,*[3] which provides valuable guidance on the care and maintenance of your equipment. It is recommended that you acquire a copy of each standard for your facility technical library and familiarize yourself with the contents.

In the case of multiplace chambers, which are built to comply with a user's particular requirements, the criteria will be specified in the contract issued to the system supplier. For monoplace chambers, which are normally production units purchased "off-the-shelf," they will generally be listed in the manufacturer's literature. In each case you should also find a detailed description of the chamber performance criteria in the documentation package provided with the equipment. A copy of this should be held onsite.

As a minimum, the pressurization system must meet the following functional requirements in order for the chamber to perform in accordance with specification:

- Have the flow capacity to pressurize the chamber at its maximum specified pressurization rate throughout the rated pressure range.
- Be capable of pressurizing the chamber to its maximum allowable design pressure.
- Have the flow capacity to allow the chamber to be ventilated in accordance with the specified performance criteria or, as a minimum, the requirements of the edition of *NFPA 99 Health Care Facilities* in force at the time of construction.
- Be capable of providing gas, which meets or exceeds the purity standards laid down in the edition of *NFPA 99* in force at the time of construction.
- Have the capacity to support the chamber(s) under all operating and emergency conditions.

The pressurization system designer will develop the design around these basic requirements, so it is very important that chamber specifications are clearly stated and detailed in the planning stages of the facility.

Supply Pressure

One of the biggest problems associated with chamber pressurization systems is pressure drop. It is one thing to have a given pressure showing on a gauge at your chamber control panel when there is no flow into the chamber, it is quite another to watch that pressure drop away as gas flow is introduced to the chamber. This situation is the result of one or both of these design related factors:

1. The gas source is not capable of meeting all volumetric demands of the chamber(s) while maintaining an acceptable minimum supply pressure.
2. Every valve, pressure regulator, check valve, elbow, and linear foot of pipe in a given pipe run will present a disturbance to flow. If the designer has not adequately allowed for this in his or her calculations, it will be seen as an excessive reduction in pressure and flow between the source and the final outlet at the chamber.

The pressurization system must be capable of maintaining the minimum acceptable supply pressure and volume of gas at the chamber inlet in order to maintain the maximum rates of pressurization and/or ventilation throughout the operating range of the chamber. We will look at these technical issues as they affect the design and construction of pressurization systems and relate to the two types of chambers utilized in hospital-based hyperbaric facilities.

Multiplace Systems – Human, Multiple Occupancy Chambers

Clinical multiplace chambers are pressurized with air. This is normally done using dedicated air compressors, which are usually located in a self-contained machinery space immediately adjacent to or close by the chamber room. Such spaces should be isolated from the chamber room for protection in the event of fire but easily accessible in the event of an emergency. *NFPA 99* provides clear requirements for fire-resistant construction to be used in buildings that house hyperbaric chambers.

The technical requirements for pressurization systems in a facility providing nonacute care, i.e., where a system shutdown will not put patients in the chamber directly into a life-threatening situation, are less complex than those required for an acute-care operation and must comply only with the requirements of *NFPA 99* in force at the time of construction.

An example of an acute-care situation would be a diver being treated for decompression sickness. A system shutdown would present a significant threat to that individual if adequate redundancy and other support were not immediately available to maintain system integrity, at least for the duration necessary to permit completion of the treatment. This is a flag to point out that clear specifications can only be established when there is an equally clear view of the type of patients to be treated.

Bear in mind that regardless of the year of construction, any modifications or upgrades must comply with the current edition of the code(s) and any applicable state or local ordinances. Thus, it is important to recognize that upgrading any program, from a nonacute care to an acute-care operation will involve more than just a single decision point; there will be a series of technical consequences and associated costs to be taken into account.

Air supplied from compressors for compression and ventilation in stand-alone chamber systems must comply with the *NFPA 99* in force at the time of installation. The 2018 edition states that air supplied exclusively to Class A and B chamber systems must, as a minimum, meet the requirements of Compressed Gas Association (CGA) Standard ANSI/CGA G-7.1-1997 Grade E, normally referred to as CGA Grade E.[4] *NFPA 99* also places an additional restriction on the presence of permanent particulates, which are limited to ≤ 1mg/m^3 @ 1 micron or larger. Permanent particulates, also known as particulates or particle pollution, are terms used to describe the various-sized bits of solid and semisolid matter, such as dust, smoke, pollen, and bacteria and viruses found in the atmosphere. Really fine particles can remain suspended almost indefinitely and travel for miles driven by the wind until they come into contact with a surface or are washed out of the air by rain or snow. Most of the particulates we inhale are filtered out in our nasal passages but really fine ones can pass through and get trapped in the lungs. These trapped particles can lead to health problems. Class A and B chamber systems that take pressurization air from, or supply it to, a hospital central medical air system must comply with the higher CGA Grade N, which is the grade called out by the U.S. Pharmacopeia (USP) for medical air. Likewise, when breathing air for Class A and B chambers is supplied from cylinders, it must comply with CGA Grade N.

Compressor Selection

NFPA 99 requires that there be at least two compressors serving the hyperbaric system. Compressor capacity (pressure and volume output) should be such that flow rates commensurate with the chamber performance specification can be maintained with only one compressor operational. Power to each compressor must be supplied through separate electrical branch circuits to help protect against shutdown due to a power failure within the facility.

The compressor set will be configured to work on an automatic lead-lag system, which means the running time for each compressor is monitored to ensure the workload is evenly spread and no one compressor gets more running hours just because it's on/off switch happens to be closest to the operator. This ensures wear and tear is even and helps reduce overall maintenance costs.

The designer will select the operating pressure of the compressor(s) based on the performance specification of the chamber. The choice can be loosely divided into three categories based on output pressure:

- Low pressure (LP) with an output range of 100-125 pounds per square inch (PSI)
- Medium pressure which has an output range of 125-500 PSI
- High pressure (HP) where the output range is over 125 PSI or over 500 PSI, depending on the system

Unless they were originally designed for deep-diving research, most hospital-based multiplace chambers have a maximum operating pressure of 6 atmospheres absolute (ATA) and generally run at not more than 3 ATA during day-to-day operations treating clinical patients. On this basis, the most likely selection is going to be low or medium pressure compressors with output based on the total volumetric requirement necessary to meet the performance specification of the hyperbaric system.

For the purpose of this discussion, which stresses safety, there are three basic types of compressor that meet the requirements of *NFPA 99.*

- **Oil-less compressors** have no oil in the crankcase. They use sealed bearings and piston rings made from a self-lubricating material such as Teflon®, which seals the cylinder bore and reduces friction. A filtration system should be used to remove moisture and any particulate matter.

- **Oil-free compressors** have oil in the crankcase but the term is misleading. The oil is sealed off so that it cannot contaminate the compression chamber until the seals eventually wear or break. A filtration system should be used to remove moisture and any particulate matter.
- **Oil-lubricated compressors** are permitted as long as they incorporate an air filtration package on the downstream side rated to deliver the required air purity at the maximum pressure and flow rates necessary to meet the performance requirements of the chamber(s).

Air Intake

The pressurization system really starts at the mouth of the air intake, which is routing atmospheric air being drawn in to the compressor(s) and must be open to the outside of the building. The air intake functions at ambient atmospheric pressure; therefore, it is critical that the size of the ducting is adequate to ensure an unrestricted supply of fresh air can be drawn into the compressor(s) at all times. Any restriction will severely compromise the effectiveness of the pressurization system and could damage the compressors.

The positioning of the main air intake must be considered very carefully, and each location will have its own set of circumstances to be taken into account. The distances given below are those cited in *NFPA 99* and are considered by this author to be minimums. An increase in any of these parameters will help to improve the quality of air taken into the system. To minimize the risk of pulling in contaminated air, the mouth of the intake needs to be located at least 20 feet (6 meters) above ground level, not less than 10 feet (3 meters) from any window, door, or other building openings, and at least 25 feet (7.6 meters) from ventilation system exhausts, plumbing (particularly toilet) vents, fuel storage vents, combustion engine exhausts, discharge vents for waste anesthetic gases, and any other areas where inadequate ventilation might allow vehicle exhaust or other noxious fumes to accumulate.

We also need to avoid the exhaust outlet from our own chamber oxygen breathing system. Ideally the intake should terminate above the roofline where a continuous supply of fresh air is almost guaranteed. A dry filter screen should be located in the mouth of the intake to take out small airborne debris, flying insects, etc. The opening of the intake should be finished in a "swan-neck" configuration, which means the mouth of the intake should be turned through 90 degrees to face down and finished high enough above any flat surface to prevent water ingress. Finally, a protective cover made of non-corroding material should be fitted to the opening and have a mesh small enough to prevent animals, such as birds and vermin, taking up residence but large enough to prevent clogging and restriction of air flow. The cover should be both firmly fixed and flexible enough to absorb contact with flying debris, made with material that will not disintegrate and damage the filter screen, and migrate to the compressor inlet(s) with the consequent risk of damage. Clearly the air intake inlet is something that needs to be included in a regular inspection and maintenance schedule, so access for inspection must be considered in deciding the final location. Ensure the intake is clearly marked with a sign indicating what it is and that it should be kept clear. The conduct of any work around the intake area should be included in the facility "hot work" permitting system so that activities such as welding or the laying of new roof felt are undertaken when the system is shut down, and proper precautions to prevent contamination are taken.

Aftercoolers, Driers, and Filtration

When gases are compressed, they get hot. Incorporating aftercoolers and driers into the pressurization circuit provides the means to reduce the gas temperature and water condensate in the air stream before it enters the storage receiver. These will be acquired from the compressor manufacturer to ensure compatibility and sized to handle the maximum pressure and flow output from the compressor(s). They can be set up as single units per compressor or connected into duplex or multiplex sets that serve multiple compressors. Regardless of how it is done, there should be in-line valves to isolate and bypass each part of the system for repair or maintenance without shutting down the supply of compressed air to the storage receiver.

In-Line Filtration

An in-line filtration set will be required and should be located upstream of the aftercooler/drier assembly. The range and type of filters to be included will be dependent on the type of compressors and ambient air quality at the location. Whatever filters are needed, they must all be rated to process the maximum flow requirements at the maximum design pressure. As a minimum, the filter set must be appropriate for the conditions of the intake air, i.e., it should catalyze or absorb any carbon monoxide (CO), remove at least 98% of particulate matter of one micron or bigger, have a coalescing filter(s) to trap, and remove moisture and a charcoal filter(s) to remove odors from fumes brought in through the air intake. Each filter should be fitted with a watchdog monitor to give clear indication when it needs to be cleaned or replaced. Ideally this information will be relayed to the chamber operator by means of a remote condition indicator panel located on or adjacent to the chamber control console. The filtration set(s) should be included in the regular inspection and maintenance schedule to ensure proper performance.

Incorporating the filtration necessary to properly process and remove contaminants from the compressed air before it enters the chamber is a very important element in the design of the pressurization system. Just two examples should serve to make the case. It is common knowledge within the hyperbaric community that many people are treated for carbon monoxide poisoning every year; it can be a lifesaving intervention. CO is a very poisonous gas even at low levels; it is not uncommon in any large town or city to read high levels of CO in atmospheric air samples taken at busy traffic junctions or a street. CO levels as low as 150 parts per million in your sample could produce symptoms in as little as 10 minutes at atmospheric pressure.[5] If we take contaminated air and compress it, there is a real risk the result could be toxic if not actually lethal for the chamber occupants. Similarly, moisture and particulates in the pressurization air will react with piping and the metallic parts in valves and regulators setting up corrosion and/or erosion, which over time may cause them to fail in service. Potentially this could lead to the development of a hazardous situation; at the very least it is going to cost money for repair and maintenance.

Air Receivers

The chamber(s) should never be pressurized directly from the compressors. It is important that there is an in-line air receiver with an allowable working pressure equal to or greater than the output pressure of the compressor(s). The receiver must be built in accordance with a recognized standard. In the United States, *NFPA 99* mandates this will be the *ASME Boiler and Pressure Vessel Code (ASME-BPVC),* Section VIII, Unfired Pressure Vessels.[6] It should be manufactured using corrosion-resistant material or have been treated to be corrosion resistant. You will find a plate giving manufacturing details. Take a clear photograph or rubbing of the plate, and keep it with your other system records. There is no set size for air receivers relative to the chamber it is connected to; this is left to the designer. As a minimum it should have sufficient capacity. When the high-low pressure sensors controlling compressors are correctly set, there is enough volume capacity to prevent short-cycling. Short-cycling is the rapid on-off cycling of a compressor that occurs when pressure sensors are not set correctly or the receiver storage capacity is too small relative to the size of the compressors.

The air receiver will be used to store output from the compressors and is important because of the following:

- It allows large volumes of air to be stored at the output pressure of the compressors, which will be several times the maximum working pressure of your chamber(s).
- Dependent upon the volume of the receiver, this will provide a substantial reservoir of air ready to use.
- It helps reduce the total workload on the compressors by buffering air consumption.
- It ensures the source air for the chamber is at or near ambient temperature when it is supplied to the chamber and helps keep the overall increase in chamber atmospheric temperature during pressurization to more comfortable levels.

The receiver(s) should have separate inlet and outlet ports, each fitted with an isolation valve. An in-line check valve should be located on the supply side before the isolation valve to prevent back pressure on the compressors when they are in the shutdown mode. A bypass system should be set up on the inlet side to allow one or more compressors to be offline for service or maintenance while the system remains operational.

A pressure gauge should be located in a place that is easy to see, ideally at eye level. This is a standard pressure reading so the gauge should be calibrated in pounds per square inch (PSI) unless you are located in a metric country, in which case it will be in kilograms per square centimeter (kg/cm^2) or perhaps kilopascals (kPa). Whichever it is, make sure all gauge readings throughout the pressurization system are consistently imperial or metric to avoid confusion.

For operational safety and common sense, the receiver must be fitted with an approved pressure relief valve (PRV). This is also a code requirement under *NFPA 99* and, as with the receiver itself, the PRV must meet the requirements of the applicable sections of *ASME BPVC* Section VIII. A shutoff valve should be located between the relief valve and the receiver and set in the open position with a frangible tie-seal. An open-ended line should be fitted to the PRV outlet and directed to ensure any pressure vented is routed safely away from personnel who might be close. An automatic drain should be located at the lowest point of the receiver to allow any moisture buildup to be vented. A manual valve fitted in a "T" configuration should be located between the receiver and the auto-drain to allow manual operation. This should be set in the normally closed position and secured with a frangible tie-seal. An open-ended line should be connected to the receiver drain so that any liquids released are routed to a floor drain. There should be an inspection hatch and cover intended to permit periodic visual inspection of the receiver. It is important that the receiver is oriented to give access to this hatch.

System Integration

Starting with the air intake and ending at the final in-line valve mounted on the chamber, each element of the pressurization system is conjoined to form a single operating unit capable of delivering pressurization gas to the chamber. There are many ways in which this can be done, but there are some common issues which must be addressed to ensure the system is safe to operate.

Equipment Mounting

All floor-mounted equipment, particularly rotating machinery such as compressors, should be set on vibration mounts. Final connections between the piping and any active machinery should be made using flexible couplings to help reduce and protect against failure due to vibration during normal operation and provide better resistance to damage due to natural phenomena such as earthquakes. ***Note:*** In certain locations there may be additional building code requirements in place to allow for seismic activity. The facility engineering department should be able to advise you on this.

Climactic Conditions

Apart from the general comfort of individuals in the area, ambient climactic conditions such as heat, cold, and humidity will have an impact on the effort necessary to process the pressurization air and control conditions within the chamber itself. For example, the machinery room air conditioning will need to be capable of dealing with both local environmental conditions, the heat generated by the machinery in operation, and the aftercooler-drier system. For example, the aftercooler-drier system will have to process the compressed air but do it in the ambient conditions of the hyperbaric facility machinery room. Equipment located in a machinery room where the environment is well-controlled will have less work to do than the same equipment in an uncontrolled space.

Interconnecting Pipework

The interconnecting pipes are the arteries of the multiplace pressurization system and critical to its operation. In a self-contained system, it is necessary to comply with the hyperbaric facilities chapter of *NFPA 99* in force at the time of construction. If the chamber(s) take air from the hospital central air distribution system, then the requirements become significantly more stringent and must meet the standards for hospital medical gas piping. For many years, systems have been built with the piping in plain view, but it is becoming more common to "box" it in so it cannot be seen by patients. However your system is configured, the piping must still be easily accessible and properly supported and labeled.

Piping Support

All piping from the machinery room to the final valve on the chamber(s) must be adequately supported to ensure it is secure and safe to use in its intended service. The information below is summarized from *NFPA 99* and supplemented by many years practical experience.

- Any floor level piping must be protected from impact from gurneys and wheelchairs etc., which are a fact of life in a medical hyperbaric facility.
- Any piping below floor level should be located in a chase with easily removed covers to facilitate routine inspection and maintenance.
- Any piping going from floor to ceiling (aka risers) that is exposed, whether servicing the hyperbaric facility or simply passing through the space, should be protected particularly up to the maximum height of your wheeled equipment.

Look around your facility. Pipework you can strike with any of your wheeled equipment should be given additional protection.

All pipework, whether vertical or horizontal, overhead or below floor level, should be anchored to the structure of the building itself. Support is provided using hangers sized to hold the pipe securely, reduce movement, and act as a vibration damper. The distance between hangers is dependent upon the size of the pipe. The terms pipe and tube are used in relation to piping, but they are practically interchangeable. However, tube is manufactured to tighter engineering tolerances than pipe. Pipe is sized using the nominal pipe size (NPS) system in which the internal diameter (I.D.) is stated but the outside diameter may change based on intended service (pressure), which will define the wall thickness (schedule) of the pipe. Tubing sizes are always based on the actual outside diameter, meaning that the actual inside diameter (bore) of the tube is reduced by the wall thickness. When it comes to setting support hangars, the spacing does not change between pipe and tube. The required distances will be laid down by the local jurisdiction and reflect local conditions. In other countries, these may differ from those given in Table 1, which was assembled for guidance purposes using the values given in *NFPA 99*. Always confirm the distances with your local jurisdiction.

Table 1. Maximum Pipe Support Spacing. Created using values given in Table 5.1.10.11.4.6, *NFPA 99 2018*, Chapter 5: Gas and Vacuum Systems.[1] Based on *MSS SP-58, Pipe Hangers and Supports: Materials, Design, Manufacture, Selection, Applications, and Installation.*[7]

Tube/Pipe Size - O.D. in(mm)	Hanger Spacing – feet (mm)
3/8" (13.72)	5 (1520)
1/2" (17.15)	6 (1830
5/8" (21.34)	6 (1830)
7/8" (26.67)	7 (2130)
1-1/8" (33.40)	8 (2440)
1-3/8" (42.16)	9 (2740)
1-5/8" (48.26) and up	10 (3050)
Vertical risers, all sizes, not to exceed . . .	15 (4570)

Labeling

When you are working on a piping system for any reason, there is almost nothing worse than trying to trace a given pipe around a room, through wall penetrations, and up and down floors when you have no way to be sure which pipe it is, what is in it, and the direction of flow. Clearly marked pipework throughout the system is not only helpful for inspection and maintenance, it improves safety by enabling rapid recognition of a given pipe in an emergency, and, if that is not enough, it is mandated by *NFPA 99*. If your facility has suspended ceilings, it is recommended you add markings on the wall or a ceiling panel to clearly show the location of any thru-wall penetrations and riser floor penetrations that are hidden above the ceiling line so you know which panels to lift to get at the piping quickly in the event of an emergency.

All system pipework should be clearly marked for content, pressure, and direction of flow using stencils or adhesive markers/tape. These requirements have been substantially unchanged for many years. Any inspection of your facility will be conducted using the locally accepted standard. It is recommended all piping be brought into compliance with the current edition, whichever standard you are required to comply with. In the United States, this will be *NFPA 99*. Table 2, System Identification Markings, which is based on the values found in Table 5.1.11, *NFPA 99:* Chapter 5: Gas and Vacuum Systems, 2018. The required colors will be laid down by the local jurisdiction and may differ from those given in Table 2. Always confirm the color markings with your local jurisdiction.

Only those markings relevant to pressurization systems have been extracted from each listing. Make sure to post a notice in a prominent position clearly describing the markings used complete with symbols and color codes. Helium and medical vacuum (med vac) are included to ensure facilities treating divers or with a medical vacuum system installed can mark the relevant pipework appropriately.

Table 2. Pressurization System Markings for Hospital Medical Air and Gas Systems Based on Data Given in Table 5.1.11 Standard Designation Colors and Operating Pressures for Gas and Vacuum Systems, *NFPA 99*.[1]

Gas Service	Abbreviated Name	Colors (Background/text)	Standard Gauge Pressure- PSI(kPa)
Medical Air	Med Air	Yellow/Black	50-55 (345-380)
Oxygen	02	Green/White or White/Green	50-55 (345-380)
Helium	He	Brown/White	50-55 (345-380)
Medical-surgical vacuum	Med Vac	White/Black	380mm-760mm (15in. to 30in.) HgV

All piping should be marked with one-inch-wide bands of paint or adhesive tape located at each bend or intersection, immediately adjacent to each side of an obstruction, such as a wall or floor penetration, and at least once on every floor of a building any piping riser passes through. There should be a minimum of three bands where piping is crossing a large area, such as a room. In addition to the color bands, pipes should be marked with the name or symbol of the contents and arrows indicating direction of flow. Ready-made colored tapes, many with names and arrows, are available online or from local safety product suppliers who will most likely already be known to your facility maintenance and purchasing departments.

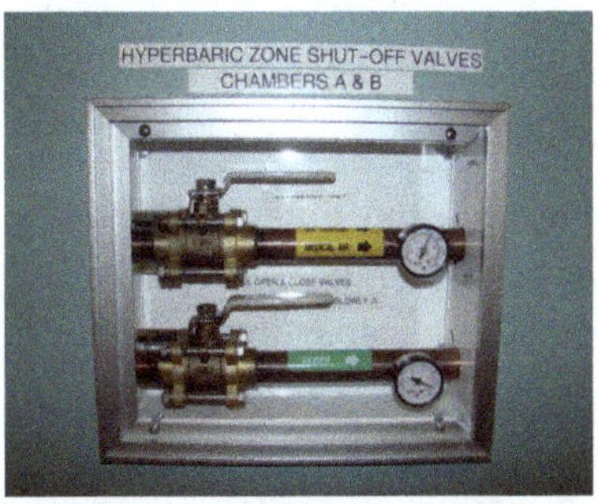

Figure 1. Piping marked for service with off-the-shelf adhesive tape.
Photo courtesy of CentraState Hospital and Medical Center, Freehold, New Jersey.

Where piping has been painted, a background color should be applied first to ensure the markings contrast well and can be easily seen. *NFPA 99* does not specify flow direction markings, but it is good practice and will be helpful for any personnel working on the system. ***Note:*** Piping used for medical air and gas service should not be painted except as required to apply the identification markings.

Chamber Control Panel

The chamber control panel is the brains of the pressurization system; for safety and efficiency, everything directly related to chamber function should be controlled and/or monitored from this location. There are many ways to control the chamber. It may be with large bore control valves big enough to pass the full flow of air through the console. It could be with small-bore pilot valves using instrument air to operate valves and regulators located remotely on the chamber or elsewhere on the system. It is increasingly common to utilize computer-based control systems and "fly by wire" technology. However it is done, there are certain things related specifically to the pressurization system that should, as a minimum, be located on the chamber control console to ensure the operator has all of the information necessary to operate the system safely. In this author's opinion these are as follows:

- A supply pressure gauge for each source of gas on line to the system. This will be a standard pressure gauge, i.e., it will read zero (0) at atmospheric pressure (ATA).
- A separate absolute pressure gauge for each compartment that can be independently pressurized in the chamber. Remember, we read chamber pressure in absolute terms and these gauges should be calibrated accordingly, i.e., an absolute pressure gauge will read one (1) ATA. Gauges on medical chambers are most commonly calibrated in ATA or Bar/kPa in countries that are metricated, which generally ties in well with the way treatment protocols are written. There will be an alternative reading shown on the gauge; this should also be expressed in absolute terms.
- A condition indicator panel showing the status of machinery supporting the system, such as the compressor(s) running or on standby in response to the demand for air. This should be fitted with an audio-visual alert/alarm system as appropriate to alert the operator in the event of a failure.
- A condition monitoring panel indicating important and potentially rapidly changing information such as air quality, CO levels in compressor intakes, and status of the filtration system. This should be fitted with an audio-visual alert/alarm system as appropriate.

Air Sampling

Regardless of compressor type or filtration package used, samples of air should be drawn and tested at least once every six months and on completion of any major repair or modification. You can send the sample to a registered test lab and get a report that will list findings. Be sure to tell the lab what CGA standard they must test to. If you are unsure, a qualified lab will be able to advise you. Alternatively, you can draw the sample and test it yourself using one of a number of colorimetric tube testing systems that are commercially available. Measurements are made by passing sample air through a detector tube filled with a high purity reagent, which reacts to the specific component being measured. The presence of the component causes the reagent to stain in direct proportion to its level in the sample and you can read the result on the tube, which will be calibrated accordingly. If you send your sample to a lab, you will get a signed report listing the tested parameters on their letterhead. If you do your own testing, I recommend you create a check sheet to record the results. As a minimum, record the result for each parameter tested; identify the grade you are testing to and the acceptable level of each substance in that grade; test date, details of the tube kit you used; and get two original signatures, one of which should be the hyperbaric safety officer/director to verify the result. Keep these reports on file. They are important in the event you get audited or wish to go for facility accreditation at some time.

Monoplace Systems – Human, Single Occupancy

Hospital-based monoplace chambers are most commonly pressurized with 100% oxygen. The typical monoplace pressurization system, therefore, starts at the bulk liquid oxygen (LOX) storage system which may or may not be dedicated to the hyperbaric facility. Monoplace chambers located in a hospital and pressurized with air will be subject to the same requirements as those described above for multiplace chambers. For the purpose of this chapter, we assume that the method of pressurization is 100% oxygen. The system must comply with the relevant sections of *NFPA 99* in force at the time of construction. As indicated above, changes, modifications and/or additions must be made in compliance with the current edition of the code.

It is highly unusual to see a monoplace hyperbaric facility with less than two chambers. Many organizations will start with two chambers but plan for expansion by installing piping capable of supporting four or more. It is worth noting that in all but a very large hospital, even a two-chamber hyperbaric operation is likely to consume more oxygen than all of the other consumers put together on a daily basis.

Bulk Liquid Oxygen (LOX) System

This is not a discussion about liquid storage systems, so the information is limited to what will help you better understand where your gas that pressurizes your chambers comes from and how it is managed. An onsite liquid storage system normally consists of a storage tank with fill valves and status telemetry system, a vaporizer, and a control manifold to regulate delivery into the distribution system. The liquid is delivered to site in trucks and then transferred into the storage tank. Storage tanks range in size from 500 gallons to as big as 11,000 gallons. In my experience the most common size of bulk tank used at hospital sites is 6,000 gallons. Smaller volume users or those in locations such as inner cities, where space for bulk gas storage is limited, may opt to use micro-bulk or portable LOX tanks. A full range of storage systems are offered by all of the major suppliers.

The vaporizer receives liquid from the tank and warms it; the liquid turns to gas which can then be fed into the control manifold and out to the distribution system. The most widely employed type of vaporizer, and the one you will see at your hospital, takes heat from ambient air to do the warming. They are basically manifolds of finned tubes joined together so that the liquid entering the system gets warmed and enters its gas phase. The fins are thin plates fixed to the outside circumference of the pipe, which significantly increases the surface area available for heat exchange relative to the nominal surface area of a similar pipe without fins. Vaporizers are built up in sections known as "arrays," with each additional array increasing the amount of liquid oxygen the vaporizer will process. The nominal performance of a vaporizer is based on eight-hour cycles after which icing tends to occur and may reduce its efficiency. When you see a vaporizer covered in ice, this is an indication the unit has been running continuously for too long without a shutdown or that demand is exceeding vaporizer capacity and additional array(s) should be added.

Control Manifold

The typical control manifold is made up of shutoff valves, check valves, strainers, regulators, and gauges and controls the pressure of the oxygen delivered to the hospital's distribution system. It also helps to prevent excessively cold gas or even liquid being carried over into the circuit, which could damage the system and result in a hazardous situation. In the United States, onsite hospital oxygen bulk oxygen storage systems are regulated by code to supply gas at a pressure of 50-55 PSIG; this is then delivered by means of a central distribution system to all operating rooms and patient areas of the hospital.

Consumption

The original LOX tank will have been sized based on total estimated consumptions for the hospital and minimizing the number of deliveries that need to be made to service the demand. Following the initial installation of the LOX system, the most expensive part of maintaining the oxygen supply is trucking the liquid to site.

It is critical that gas is supplied at a pressure and flow that will ensure chamber performance specifications can be met. This can have both a technical and economic impact. If the chambers selected for the program require a supply pressure higher than the standard 50-55 PSI as permitted in the code, then a second regulator set at a higher pressure, say 70-80 PSI, with its own vaporizer and control system serving a separate piping system dedicated to the hyperbaric chambers, will be required. Because of the pressure difference, this must be isolated from the main hospital system.

It may be that adding hyperbaric chambers will put such a demand on the system that the existing storage tank is too small to serve all users without an excessive increase in the number of deliveries. This will cause a significant escalation in the unit cost of oxygen. It is not unusual to find it is more economical to install a second LOX storage tank dedicated to the hyperbaric program. As indicated previously, if this is to work at the higher supply pressure, it will need to have a dedicated piping system and be isolated from the main hospital distribution system. Figure 2 below shows a typical two-tank bulk setup.

To put this into perspective and by way of an example, we can do some calculations

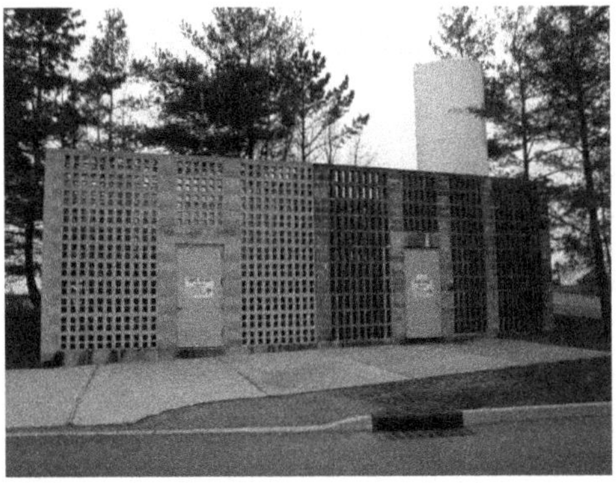

Figure 2. Typical two-tank setup. The large 6,000 gallon tank on the right is serving the hospital, while the smaller 3,000 gallon tank on the left is dedicated to the hyperbaric unit. They are protected by separate retaining walls with open-mesh blocks to ensure the area(s) ventilate freely.

NOTE: Each access door is marked with a warning sign. There is easy access from the road to facilitate parking for the tanker truck and provide a spill pad. Surrounding trees are cut back to avoid overhanging the area.

Photo courtesy of CentraState Hospital and Medical Center, Freehold, New Jersey.

to estimate the daily consumption of a two-chamber monoplace operation conducting eight treatments during a normal eight-hour working day. The gas flow rate through a monoplace chamber is adjustable. Patient comfort in a typical monoplace chamber is achieved by adjusting the flow rate and using the mass flow of gas to influence the temperature inside the chamber. Flow rate is generally referred to in standard liters (volume measured at atmospheric pressure) and ranges between 100-400 standard liters per minute (slpm). If we assume the average of flow rate is 250 slpm throughout a treatment, we do eight treatments per day, and the average treatment time is 110 minutes, we should end up with a reasonably accurate daily consumption.

- Conversion factor for standard liters (L) to standard cubic feet (ft^3) - 1 liter = 0.035315 ft^3
- Total gaseous consumption per treatment is 250 slpm x 110 mins = 27,500 standard liters or 972 ft^3
- Total gaseous consumption per day is 27,500 x 8 = 220,000 standard liters or 7,776 ft^3
- Conversion factor for gaseous oxygen (liters) to liquid (U.S. gallons) - 1 U.S. gallon = 115.1 ft^3
- Total estimated daily consumption – 7,776/115.1 = 67.56 or 68 U.S. gallons

Such a consumption rate will significantly change the refill rate of any existing storage system it is attached to, which is why the best solution is normally the dedicated tank.

To ensure continuity of supply, a delivery will be scheduled when the telemetry system signals the tank is down to a preset minimum volume of liquid remaining. This will not be less than 15 - 20% of total volume, or 450 - 600 gallons in the case of a 3,000 gallon tank to ensure that even if a delivery is delayed by a few days, the system remains operational. Based on our example consumption rate, a 3,000 gallon tank will have a usable volume of 2,400 gallons and trigger a refill approximately every 35 days (2,400/68 = 35.29).

If you have chambers that are capable of operating with gas supplied at the standard 50-55 PSI pressure range, then it is possible the hyperbaric program could be serviced by the existing system without significant modification. This will be a more economic approach assuming the following:

- A point from which to pick up the oxygen supply from the central distribution system is within a reasonable distance from the hyperbaric facility.
- The piping system is capable of flowing gas to all consumers in the circuit without an unacceptable pressure drop, i.e., if low-pressure oxygen alarms go off in the hospital every time you pressurize your chamber(s), the system is inadequate.
- The additional demand on the existing storage tank does not impact deliveries beyond that which is economically acceptable.

As indicated above, we can easily estimate the impact of increased consumption on the system. Similarly, the designer can calculate the impact of the increased demand on the actual piping system. Can it support the additional flow without unacceptable pressure drop(s) in all circuits affected? Because of the potential cost impact, it is also helpful to confirm the calculations by conducting a flow-study. This is done by setting up gauges to measure pressure variations in different parts of the system. Noncritical and critical zones such as the emergency room and ICU should be measured for pressure drop. Flow rates are introduced to the system to simulate variations in demand encountered at different phases of a treatment. The highest demand will occur at the commencement of compression with gas flowing at the maximum compression rate of the chamber(s) to be installed. One test should simulate all chambers being compressed to the maximum pressure with oxygen flow set at the highest operational flow rate. Monitoring the actual pressure drop at the selected locations will provide a picture of how the system is going to perform under actual working conditions. If this flow study is to have real value, it must be done during the initial engineering assessment that will be carried out by the hospital engineering team and their gas system contractors.

Piping System

By code the medical grade oxygen and air supplied to monoplace chambers through a hospital central distribution system, or a separate dedicated piping system, must be compliant with the relevant sections of *NFPA 99* in force at the time of construction. Whether the pipework is a dedicated line or connected to the main hospital distribution system, it should be sized to carry the projected worst case volume at the required pressure in the dynamic flow condition. The piping system protection and support requirements outlined in the Multiplace Systems section of this chapter also apply here.

Oxygen

As we discussed previously with multiplace chambers, pressure drop is usually the major problem associated with your pressurization system. This is particularly true in high-flow, low-pressure systems and will impact the way in which you can pressurize your chambers and manage your patient load. There are several manufacturers marketing monoplace chambers to the medical market. These chambers consume between 100 and 400 slpm of oxygen in order to maintain pressure, ventilation, and optimize patient comfort. The chambers which have mechanical-pneumatic systems tend to have flow-rates that vary from 240 – 400 slpm, whereas the current computer-based systems can maintain control with flows as low as 100 lpm. Chambers with mechanical-pneumatic control systems also tend to require higher supply pressures to compensate for losses occurring in the control system itself. In every case, the gas system designer needs to plan and provide for the worst case pressure and flow condition.

Running medical grade piping in a hospital is expensive, so it is prudent to make sure there is redundant capacity built into the system feeding the hyperbaric program. This is important for the oxygen piping which, of course, moves the therapeutic gas we supply to our patients. The additional materials and minor increase in labor costs for building in redundant capacity (oversized piping and additional pipe drops that are terminated at a known location inside a wall) during initial construction versus sizing it to just meet current demand is minuscule compared to the disruption and cost of carrying out upgrade work to support additional chambers later. The other major advantage of oversizing the pipework is that it minimizes pressure drop by acting as a reservoir to help buffer variations in demand. Wherever possible, this oversized piping should be run all the way through to the gas control panel(s) serving the chamber(s). As previously noted, any new construction or additions to an existing system must be compliant with the current code, which, at the time of writing, is *NFPA 99* 2018 edition.

Air

There is no current code requirement that mandates air must be available for a monoplace facility to be compliant. Not all hyperbaric operations have air on line to the chambers. This is often the case with facilities that have been open for a number of years. Most treatment protocols used today have "air breaks" built into them to mitigate the onset of oxygen seizure. It is becoming rare to find a new facility that does not have air readily available to the chambers.

In a typical monoplace operation, the demand for air is low and generally only used for providing air breaks. Based on the operational procedures established in your facility, air may also be used to replace oxygen as a step in the management of an oxygen seizure should one occur during treatment.

If medical air is not readily available from the central distribution system, an alternative and less expensive option than piping it in is to use high-pressure cylinders brought together in a manifold connected to an automatic switchover panel. The outlet from this panel is then fed to the chamber room. This assembly must be housed in a purpose-built "closet" space protected and secured by a set of lockable double doors which will open to give full access for cylinder handling (Figure 3). For efficiency this should be located as close as possible to the chamber room. In my experience, two sets of three "J" cylinders in a manifold with one set on each side of an automatic switchover box is very effective (Figure 4). The switchover panel contains a pressure regulator to control on-line pressure to the chambers. It will switch manifolds when the set minimum pressure is reached to ensure on-line pressure is always adequate. Status is displayed on the central condition indicator panel (Figure 5). When used just for air breaks during a normal eight-hour working day, each triple-cylinder manifold will support a two-chamber operation for approximately six to seven days before switching.

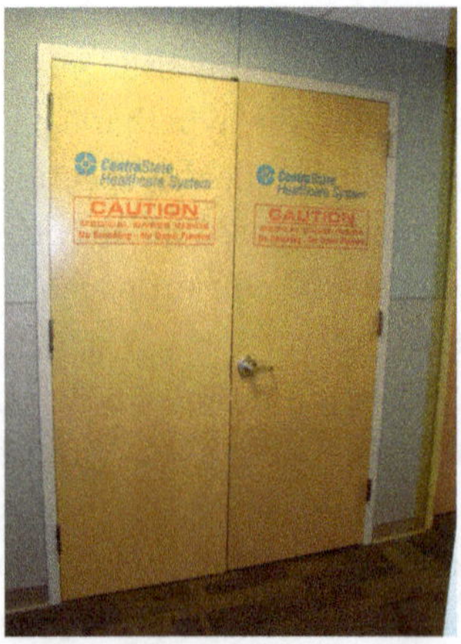

Figure 3. Typical air supply closet. The door to the chamber room can be seen on the extreme right. Note: The warning sign is posted at eye level to ensure it is clearly seen. Photo courtesy of CentraState Hospital and Medical Center.

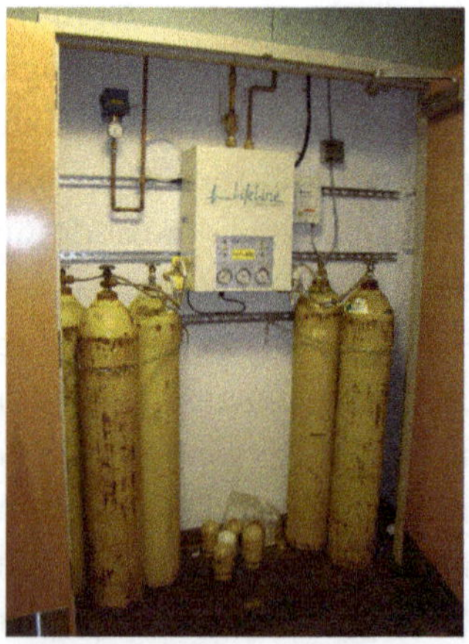

Figure 4. Triple-cylinder manifolds on either side of the automatic switchover box. Note: The cylinders are secured to the wall by a rack and chains. Photo courtesy of CentraState Hospital and Medical Center.

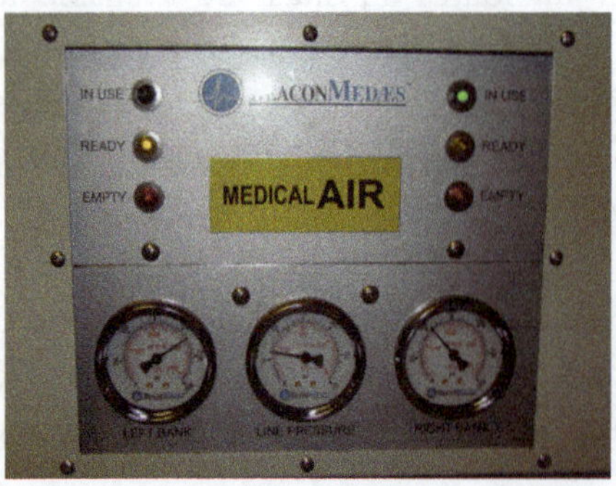

Figure 5. Condition Indicator Panel. The indicator LEDs show which manifold is in-use and which is ready. The left and right gauges show manifold pressure. On-line pressure is displayed on the center gauge. Photo courtesy of CentraState Hospital and Medical Center.

Zone Valve Box

Both air and oxygen must run through a "zone valve" box (Figure 6) before they enter the chamber space. A zone valve is an in-line quarter-turn valve, which allows the gas supply into a given space to be shut off. This is for safety purposes like in the case of fire or maintenance in the protected zone. Gauges are located in-line to show the pressure at the valve. You will find zone valves throughout the hospital; they are located so that given areas can be isolated selectively without shutting down the whole system. They are always located in open areas such as a corridor, which guarantees easy access and makes them highly visible.

Zone valves are mounted in a box recessed into a wall about five feet above the floor so that they are approximately at eye level and can be actuated by an average person without bending. The box has a clear plastic cover that must be removed to access the valve handles. They must be located as close as possible to an access point, such as the main door into the chamber room, and always outside of the zone it is protecting. While a zone valve may protect several rooms/areas on a single floor, it cannot be used to protect zone(s) on floors above or below its location. Sometimes there may be several zone valves in close proximity; each one must be clearly marked to show which area(s) it protects. The hyperbaric chambers normally warrant a dedicated zone valve box.

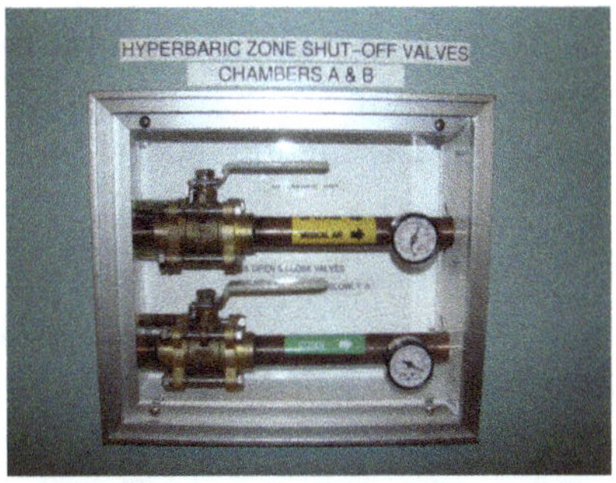

Figure 6. Zone valve box with protective cover removed showing the shutoff valves in normal operating position. Note the clear identification above the box and on the piping. The analog supply pressure gauges on each line can be seen through the clear window in the protective cover. Photo courtesy of CentraState Hospital and Medical Center.

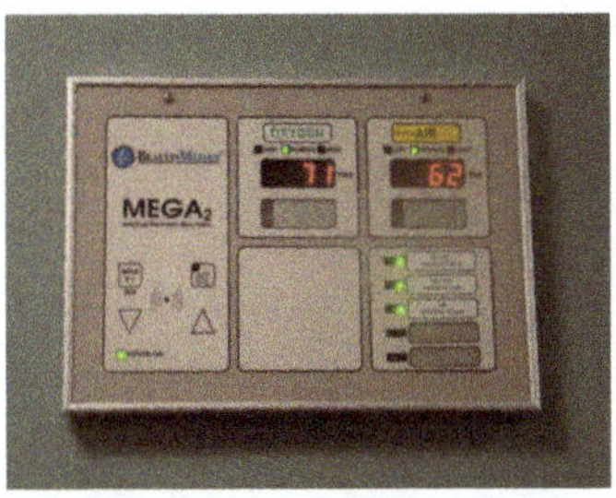

Figure 7. Typical alarm panel showing the supply pressure for oxygen and air on line to the chamber room. Photo courtesy of CentraState Hospital and Medical Center.

Alarm Panel

An alarm panel (Figure 7) is required, which displays the status of the gas supply to the chamber room. This will have a digital display of the pressure in each circuit. It will have an audio visual system, which changes color and sounds an alarm in the event supply pressure moves outside the preset parameters. Figure 8 shows a typical alarm panel and zone valve set up adjacent to the chamber room door.

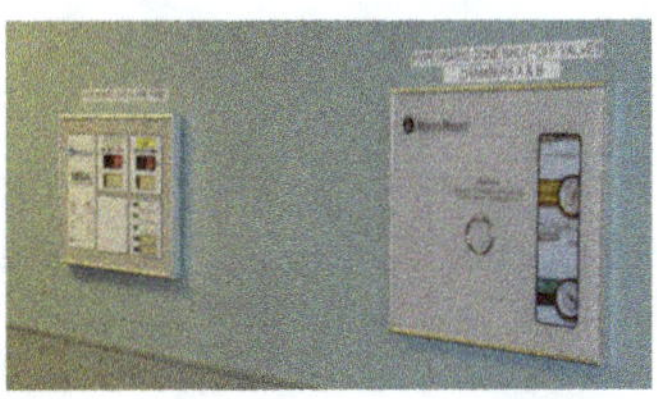

Figure 8. Typical setup showing from left to right, the alarm status panel and the zone valve with its protective cover in place. Photo courtesy of CentraState Hospital and Medical Center.

Chamber Gas Control Panel

In the case of monoplace chambers, the final point of monitoring and control before the gas arrives at the chamber is generally a wall-mounted panel that allows oxygen and air to be switched during a treatment for the administration of air breaks and for the gas supply to the chamber to be switched off in the event of an emergency. There are many variations of such panels; each manufacturer offers their own panel design as an optional extra. Some service providers have very specific requirements and make their own panels. These panels should be located between each pair of chambers so that they can be easily reached by the chamber operator. Whatever approach is used, there should be at least a separate in-line shutoff valve and pressure gauge indicating the pressure of incoming gas for each chamber. If air is available, there will also be a three-way valve which will allow the operator to switch the gas online to the chamber from oxygen to air and back by changing the direction of the valve handle.

Conclusion

Our experience in designing and building pressurization systems that will support hyperbaric chambers and ensure and safeguard the purity of the gases they carry has evolved over many years. Regardless of which type of hyperbaric chamber(s) you have or will become involved with, there are clear code requirements based on good engineering practice and bolstered by many thousands of man-years of practical experience across the industry. Today, when a designer is given clear performance requirements and follows applicable codes and standards, the result will be a compliant system which performs in accordance with the user's design specification in all normal and emergency conditions. I have no doubt that as we gain more experience, the hyperbaric equipment we rely on to provide care for our patients will continue to become safer and more reliable.

Acknowledgments

Special thanks to CentraState Medical Center, Freehold, New Jersey, for permission to use the photographs of their facility.

References

1. National Fire Protection Association. NFPA 99 Health Care Facilities Code, 2018 Edition. Quincy, MA: National Fire Protection Association; 2018.
2. ASME PVHO-1 Safety Standard for Pressure Vessels for Human Occupancy. New York, New York: American Society of Mechanical Engineers; 2016.
3. ASME PVHO-2 Safety Standard for Pressure Vessels for Human Occupancy: In Service Guidelines. New York, New York: American Society of Mechanical Engineers; 2016.
4. CGA G-7.1-2018: Commodity Specification for Air – 7th Edition. Chantilly, VA: Compressed Gas Association; 2018.
5. Weaver LK. Carbon Monoxide Poisoning. In Weaver LK (ed) Hyperbaric Oxygen Therapy Indications, 13th Edition. North Palm Beach, FL: Best Publishing Company; 2014:47-64.
6. ASME Boiler and Pressure Vessel Code, Section VIII, Rules for Construction of Pressure Vessels, Division 1. New York, NY: American Society of Mechanical Engineers; 2015.
7. MSS SP-58- Pipe Hangers and Supports — Materials, Design, Manufacture, Selection, Application and Installation. Veinna, VA: Manufacturer's Standardization Society of the Valve and Fittings Industry, Inc.; 2009.

CHAPTER 4.2
Piping Systems

Stephen D. Reimers, PE and Ramesh K. Dixit, PE

Introduction

The functional capabilities of a hyperbaric facility are heavily influenced and often controlled by the piping systems that provide its necessary services. Consequently, decisions regarding piping issues usually have a substantial and sometimes unexpected impact on the facility as a whole. This chapter deals with current code requirements and selected other topics that influence the design and construction of hyperbaric facility piping systems.

Effective Editions of Applicable Codes and Standards

The very first requirement is determining what codes and standards apply. This may seem straightforward. Often it is not. Codes and standards are living documents periodically updated by the organizations that manage them. Each code or standard has an approximate timetable for publishing new editions and/or addenda to existing editions. In addition to determining which codes and standards are applicable to a given facility, it is also necessary to know which editions are the governing ones. The economic penalties for getting this portion of the job wrong can be substantial.

For standards where compliance is voluntary, there are no hard and fast rules regarding which edition of a particular code or standard is the governing one. Generally accepted conventions are as follows:

- New editions and revisions for voluntary codes and standards become applicable to new construction projects six months after their publication date.
- The edition of the codes and standards applicable at the time a device/facility was built remains applicable throughout the life of the device/facility. The only exceptions are situations where something permitted in a code or standard is later found to be obviously hazardous. As one might expect, such an occurrence is very rare.
- If modifications/upgrades are performed, they can be done either to the original construction code/standard or the edition being adopted by the city or state

at the time of the work. Usually, major modifications to the existing structures and equipment may be needed using the version of code or standard currently adopted by the authority having jurisdiction (AHJ).

For codes and standards subject to adoption and enforcement by local jurisdictions, such as *NFPA 99 (Health Care Facilities Code), NFPA 55 (Compressed Gases and Cryogenic Fluids Code)* and the building code (uniform building code, etc.), the situation is different. For these codes the situations generally encountered are as follow:

- When governing bodies (legislatures, city councils, etc.) adopt a certain code or standard for their jurisdiction, they have a need to know precisely what they are adopting. Instead of adopting a code or standard as a living document subject to alteration by bodies over which they have no control, they adopt a specific edition. The codes and standards applicable to new construction projects within the affected jurisdiction are the specific editions of those documents adopted by the local governing body. The local governing body is referred to in code language as the "authority having jurisdiction." As newer editions of codes and standards become available, adoption of them usually requires another separate action by the AHJ. The *edition officially adopted and therefore enforced is often several editions behind the last one available.* For example, at the time this chapter was updated (2019), the edition of *NFPA 99* that is officially adopted and enforced by the city of New York is the 2012 edition.
- Major modifications to existing structures and equipment may be required according to the the edition currently adopted instead of the one under which a device/facility was originally built. Repairs and minor modifications can usually be done under the original construction rules. Consumers in some situations may be compelled to use new relevant codes in the event the previous code is superseded by the new one. One such relevant code is *NFPA 50 (Standard for Bulk Oxygen Systems at Consumer Sites),* which has been withdrawn in 2004 and incorporated into *NFPA 55.*

The technical and financial implications of accurately determining which edition of each applicable code is being enforced can be substantial. This is especially true for hyperbaric facilities since the codes for them are still maturing and the economic and technical impact of changes from one edition to the next are significant. It should also be understood that determining which edition is the one being enforced is not always easy. One should be persistent. Sometimes several inquiries are required before the correct answers become clear. The best contact point for inquiries regarding the fire code in a large city is usually the plan review department. In smaller jurisdictions, it is often the fire marshal's office. For inquiries regarding applicable pressure vessel regulations in the United States and Canada, usually the best initial point of contact is The National Board of Boiler and Pressure Vessel Inspectors. (https://www.nationalboard.org)

Multiplace Facilities

Where the Rules Come From: The "Major Players"

The two current principal hyperbaric facility codes are *NFPA 99: Health Care Facilities Code, 2018 edition,* Chapter 14: Hyperbaric Facilities and Chapter 5: Gas and Vacuum Systems and *ASME PVHO-1: Safety Standard for Pressure Vessels for Human Occupancy, 2016 edition.*

Figure 1 illustrates the boundaries of the applications of those codes and the other codes and standards known to apply to multiplace facilities.

With respect to piping systems, Chapter 14 (para 14.2.1.3)[2] gives performance requirements for the fire suppression system and requires construction of the piping systems in accordance with rules listed in the Piping Systems section of *PVHO-1* standard. Although *PVHO-1* has an entire section dedicated to piping, it does not give overall system performance requirements. That part is left up to the builder and/or purchaser as defined in a document known as the *User's Design Specification.* Rather, *PVHO-1* provides a coherent set of do's and don't's that experience has shown produce safe and reliable piping systems. *PVHO-1* piping rules also include prohibitions against several design details found to encourage operational errors.

For hyperbaric facilities part of a hospital or other large health care facilities, the boundaries between the application of the principal hyperbaric codes described above and the codes applicable elsewhere in the institution are sometimes intricate and always important.

Similar to Chapter 5, application of Chapter 14 requirements is also divided into four categories. The difference between various categories is the nature of risk associated with hyperbaric care being provided in the hyperbaric facility. Category 1 thru 4 hyperbaric care are described as follows in Chapter 14:[2]

- **Category 1 Hyperbaric Care:** Where interruption or failure of medical gas supply or electrical service are likely to cause major injury or death of patients, staff, or visitors, the medical gas system and electrical service are considered to be Category 1.
- **Category 2 Hyperbaric Care:** Where interruption or failure of medical gas supply or electrical service are likely to cause minor injury or death of patients, staff, or visitors, the medical gas system and electrical service are considered to be Category 2.
- **Category 3 Hyperbaric Care:** Where interruption or failure of medical gas supply or electrical service are not likely to cause injury to patients, staff, or visitors, the medical gas system and electrical service are considered to be Category 3.
- **Category 4 Hyperbaric Care:** Category 4 is reserved for future use per 2018 edition of *NFPA 99.*

Chapter 14 also provides classification of the chambers based on their occupancy.[2]

- Class A: Human, multiplace occupancy (multiplace)
- Class B: Human, single occupancy (monoplace)
- Class C: Animal, no human occupancy

Chapter 14 is divided into three major sections. Section 14.1 provides scope and general requirements of hyperbaric facilities. Section 14.2 provides requirements for construction and equipment for hyperbaric facilities. Section 14.3 addresses administration and maintenance.

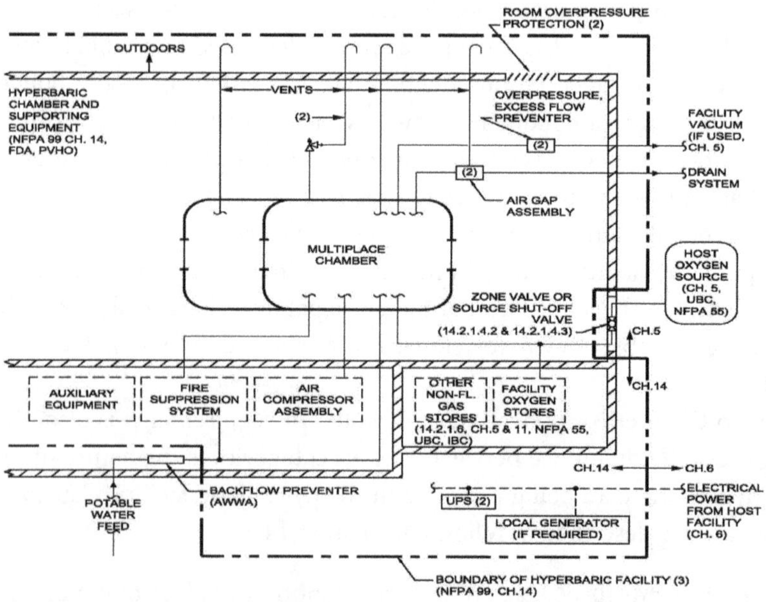

Figure 1. Codes and standards application to multiplace facilities. Diagram courtesy of authors.

Notes:

1. Requirements for the oxygen storage and handling within the hyperbaric facility must meet Chapter 5 and/or NFPA 55 storage requirements also apply where invoked by Chapter 5.
2. This is not currently a code requirement but recommended.
3. Primary standards only are shown. Additional standards that apply to varying degrees include *NFPA 70, NFPA 250,* and *NFPA 101*. Other standards may also apply depending on the jurisdictional requirements.
4. Abbreviations:

AWWA	American Water Works Association	IPC	International Plumbing Code
UBC	Uniform Building Code	CGA	Compressed Gas Association

5. Paragraph and chapter designations refer to ***NFPA 99, 2018 edition.***

Where the Rules Come From: "Satellite Players"[1]

Chapter 5 rules are intended for piping that is embedded in walls, ceilings, and other hard-to-reach places. It is much more restrictive than Chapter 14 with respect to joining techniques and selection of materials. Building a workable hyperbaric facility to Chapter 5 rules would be somewhere between difficult and impossible. However, many hyperbaric facilities are supplied with air and oxygen from host institution piping systems that fall under Chapter 5 rules. It is essential to clearly establish where the applicability of Chapter 5 rules ends and the applicability of Chapter 14 picks up. A simple way is to declare the hyperbaric facility a "zone" supported by the Chapter 5 system. The feed from the Chapter 5 system is then terminated with a zone valve under Chapter 5 rules, and Chapter 14 rules are considered to apply downstream from the zone valve.

In Chapter 5, requirements for medical gas and vacuum systems (MGVS) are categorized on the basis of the level of risk to patients from a failure of the supply system. A Category 1 MGVS is intended to be most reliable and redundant of the three risk categories. In a similar fashion, Chapter 14 dictates the requirements for Category 1-4 hyperbaric care.

Requirements for gas and vacuum systems in Chapter 5 for *NFPA 99* have been organized by Category 1 (Section 5.1), Category 2 (Section 5.2), and Category 3 (Section 5.3). Chapter 5 is organized conveniently for the user and similar requirements in the above three categories are numbered in parallel. For instance, requirements of labeling are numbered 5.X.11. These labeling criteria can be found under 5.1.11 for Category 1, 5.2.11 for Category 2, and 5.3.11 for Category 3. Applicable categories can be determined by using the risk category procedures described in Chapter 4. Commentary Table 5.1 Quick Locator of Category 1, Category 2, and Category 3 Systems Requirements from Chapter 5 of *NFPA 99* also summarizes these in a tabular form.[5]

Chapter 14 of *NFPA 99* contains references to certain Chapter 5 requirements, primarily to the Chapter 5 provisions regarding the storage and handling of nonflammable medical gases. However, the generally accepted understanding is that Chapter 5 requirements apply to hyperbaric facilities only where specifically cited by Chapter 14.

With respect to the storage of nonflammable medical gases stored within the hyperbaric facility, Chapter 14 (para. 14.2.1.6)[2] requires that such gases be housed in accordance with Chapter 5 and Chapter 11 rules. Chapter 5 (para 5.1.3.3.1.6)[1] requires that cryogenic central supply systems to comply with *NFPA 55*. Table 6.3.1.1 of *NFPA 55* provides the cryogenic oxygen storage limits for within the hyperbaric facility.[3] Cryogenic oxygen storage above 180 gal (681 L) is not permitted inside a structure per *NFPA 55* storage limits.

The Chapter 14 reference to Chapter 5 requirements for the storage of medical gases stored within the hyperbaric facility is located in the Chapter 14 (section 14.2.1.6 Storage and Handling of Medical Gases.)[2] In that location it is easily overlooked but should be followed. Also, many building codes contain limitations on the amount of gas that can be stored inside a structure. Those limitations are often more severe than the limitations imposed by the fire code. See the section Effects of Building Codes in this chapter.

There are often times when it would seem logical to use the hyperbaric facility air and oxygen resources to support other consumers within the same health care institution. This situation, however, requires careful planning. As soon as the hyperbaric air or oxygen resources are used to provide support to nonhyperbaric consumers, those resources become subject to Chapter 5 rules. Chapter 5 rules are designed for air and oxygen services that must be extremely reliable, operate unattended for long periods of time, and be maintainable without significant disruption of service. The Chapter 5 rules for redundancy and supervision are much more comprehensive than Chapter 14 rules for the same services. For facilities where the nonhyperbaric oxygen demand is small, the cost of upgrading a hyperbaric facility oxygen service to comply fully with Chapter 5 rules is often manageable. However, the cost of upgrading a hyperbaric air plant to comply fully with Chapter 5 rules is usually sufficient to convince facility planners that a better approach is to keep the two services separate.

Many multiplace facilities are equipped with a medical suction capability and a capability to discharge exhaled oxygen outside the facility. At pressures in excess of 1.5 atmosphere absolute (ATA), the differential between chamber pressure and outside atmospheric pressure is normally sufficient to power the service. However, if it is desired to have medical suction and/or overboard dump services that function in the region between 1.5 ATA and 1.0 ATA, it is usually necessary to provide an auxiliary vacuum source. Medical vacuum systems (Chapter 5 rules) can be used for this function. However, if this is to be done, the connection should be done in such a way that misoperation of the hyperbaric controls cannot result in overpowering the vacuum system. Most facilities that have installed auxiliary vacuum sources have elected to keep them completely separate from the host institution's medical vacuum system.

Electrical Codes for Oxygen Storage Rooms

With respect to the electrical requirements for an oxygen storage room, *NFPA 99*, Section 5.1.3.3.2(8)[1] clearly states that the location is an "ordinary location" under the rules of *NFPA 70 National Electrical Code* with the limitation that all electrical devices be located at least five feet above the finished floor level to avoid physical damage (presumably from impacts from moving cylinders).

Effects of Building Codes

In many sites, the Chapter 5 rules for the storage of oxygen and other nonflammable medical gases are not the only ones that apply. Many building codes also have rules regarding the storage of pressurized gases within the building envelope. Similar to Chapter 5 and Chapter 14, the fire code rules are also based on risk. Building code rules are generally based on occupancy. *Building code restrictions on the amounts of medical gases that can be stored inside a structure are often substantially more restrictive than the corresponding restrictions in* NFPA 99 *or* NFPA 55. Many building codes limit the amount of oxygen that can be stored inside a structure without changing the classification of the entire structure to hazardous occupancy to 3,000 to 5,000 scf, depending on the circumstances of the installation. Hazardous occupancy ratings involve so many requirements that such occupancies are often referred to as "occupancies from hell." When such building code limitations are encountered, it is best to design the hyperbaric service oxygen storage to stay within the amounts permitted for a nonhazardous building occupancy rating.

When designing the hyperbaric facility equipment and piping, it is important to know what building code is used by the local jurisdiction and what edition of that code they are enforcing. In most locations, a medical office is considered by the building code as a normal business occupancy. The presence of hyperbaric chambers does not normally affect the occupancy classification under the building code. As stated in the above paragraph, storage of large amounts of oxygen inside a structure can affect the occupancy classification and force it into an "H" class (hazardous use) occupancy.

Potable Water Codes

Normal fire main water is generally dirty, and inadvertent discharges of hyperbaric chamber fire suppression systems do sometimes occur. It is also essential that the systems be tested periodically at full flow. It is desirable for the water in the fire suppression system to be clean. Often the simplest way to have clean water is to supply the hyperbaric chamber fire suppression system from the local potable water system. This also opens up the possibility of using the chamber fire suppression system as an inexpensive source of potable water in the chamber. This practice is generally permissible but with a proviso. Whenever a public water system is connected to a consumer where the downstream pressure may exceed the pressure in the water system, an approved backflow preventer must be installed at the connection point. Such devices are readily available from many plumbing supply houses.

Selected Other Issues

Sanitary Drain Connections

Larger multiplace facilities sometimes include a sink and/or toilet inside one or more chambers. These devices have drains that must be connected to the local sanitary drain. Applicable codes in this situation are obscure, if there are any at all. However, this connection must be made with care lest misoperation of the controls result in pressurization of the sanitary drain. With a poor design and a little bad luck, it is possible to turn nearby toilets into fountains. This situation can be avoided by adding an air gap or properly vented interface tank between the hyperbaric piping and the local sanitary drain.

Chamber Exhausts

The normal exhaust from a chamber is required by Chapter 14 to be piped to a location outside the building well clear of intakes and other building openings. This can sometimes require a long run of pipe. Multiplace chambers usually are also multi-compartment chambers with each compartment fitted with controls to permit it to be operated independently of the others. In locations where long exhaust lines are required, there is a strong temptation to combine the lines from individual compartments into a common line for the run to the building exterior. This can lead to some embarrassing consequences.

Most clinical chambers relay on some level of constant ventilation to keep the atmosphere in the chamber fresh and uniformly "stirred." This results in a small but constant exhaust flow from each chamber any time it is under pressure. The pressure buildup at the chamber end of the exhaust line from the accumulated effect of these small flows can often reach 1 PSIG (pounds per inch [gauge]) or more. Suppose now that it is desired to bring one compartment to surface pressure while this is happening. The compartment will depressurize to the point where its pressure equals the pressure at the chamber end of the exhaust line and no further. The usual result is that the compartment door to the exterior cannot now be opened. A 1 PSIG differential over a 30-inch diameter door, for example, results in a total force on the door of 707 lbs, enough to prevent even the most muscle-bound chamber attendant from opening the door, assuming the door opens inward against pressure as most do. This is also enough pressure on an outward opening door to cause it to open with great velocity if the operator should somehow succeed in releasing the door restraints. Most outward opening doors have interlocks to prevent this from occurring, but not all do.

What is the solution to this situation? One solution that can always be done is to temporarily stop the exhaust flow from all other compartments whenever one compartment is brought to surface pressure. A much more satisfying solution is to route the exhaust from each chamber to the building exterior in a separate line. Each individual compartment can then be returned to surface pressure independently of what is happening in the others.

There are code requirements that address how fast a monoplace or multiplace chamber should be evacuated under emergency conditions. Chapter 14 (section 14.2.5.2)[2] requires that Class B (monoplace chambers) are capable of depressurizing from 3 ATA to door open in less than 2 minutes. Most monoplace chambers have an "emergency dump" valve that will permit them to be depressurized from 3 ATA to surface pressure in about one minute. Emergency depressurization requirement for multiplace chambers from 3 ATA to surface is less than 6 minutes per Chapter 14 (section 14.2.5.1.)[2] However, there is no specific requirement for multiplace chambers to have an emergency depressurization valve. These valves are rarely found on multiplace chambers. The ability to evacuate a chamber quickly should the need arise is a significant safety consideration. It needs to be carefully addressed during the facility planning stages as its presence or absence can significantly affect emergency response plans. Chambers that take a long time to depressurize to surface pressure can also be annoying to personnel and wasteful of time resources.

Room Barotrauma

Some years ago, an altitude chamber operator was demonstrating the operation of the emergency resurface valve on his altitude chamber to a guest. This valve admitted outside room air into the chamber at a high rate to cause it to quickly return to surface pressure from high altitude. When the operator opened the chamber door, he found the ceiling of his laboratory on the floor.

The potential for the same event to occur, but in the opposite direction, exists for many hyperbaric chambers, especially large chambers located in small rooms. During any installation, the possible effects of a major loss of chamber pressure integrity on the room housing the chamber should be considered. A sudden rise in room pressure of less than 1 PSIG is generally sufficient to do significant damage, such as blowing the walls out. Most rooms have sufficient exhaust capability to handle normal chamber gas discharges. However, the sudden opening of a main chamber relief valve or a failure of a major door seal in a small, tightly sealed room could have spectacular consequences. To avoid such possibilities, the exhausts from all major relief valves should be piped outdoors and the exhaust capability of the room should be checked against the credible sources of gas discharge into the room. If more exhaust capability is indicated, it can usually be easily added by installing a bank of gravity louvers somewhere on an available exterior wall.

Monoplace Facilities

Applicable Codes and Their Boundaries of Application

Figures 2 illustrates the boundaries of application of the applicable codes and standards to an oxygen ventilation monoplace chamber facility. Figure 3 shows their application to air ventilation monoplace facilities.

In general, the codes and standards that apply to multiplace chambers apply to monoplace chambers as well. However, there are some important differences in requirements.

The Impact of Piping System Design on the Requirements for the Space Housing a Monoplace Hyperbaric Facility

Chapter 14 requires sprinkler protection and a two-hour-rated fire perimeter around permanently installed multiplace chamber (Class A) facilities. However, per 14.2.1.1.2,[2] monoplace chambers (Class B) and animal research chambers (Class C) are not required to be protected by two-hour fire resistant-rated construction.

In recent revisions made to *NFPA 99* standard, Chapter 14 (para 14.2.1.2)[2] now permits using a clean agent fire protection system designed to *NFPA 2001* requirements or

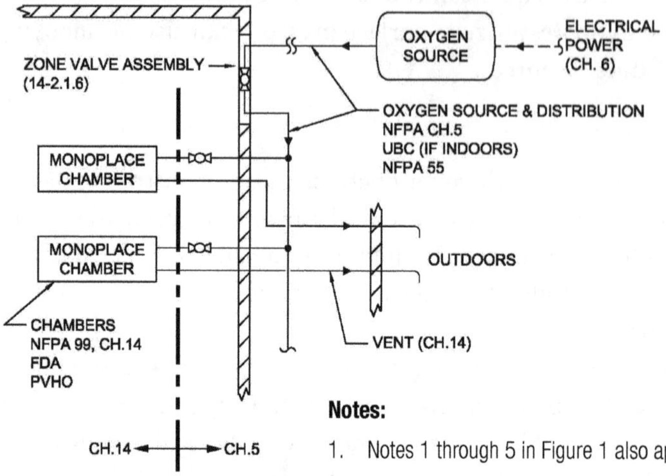

Notes:

1. Notes 1 through 5 in Figure 1 also apply.

Figure 2. Codes and standards application to a typical oxygen ventilation monoplace chamber facility. Diagram courtesy of authors.

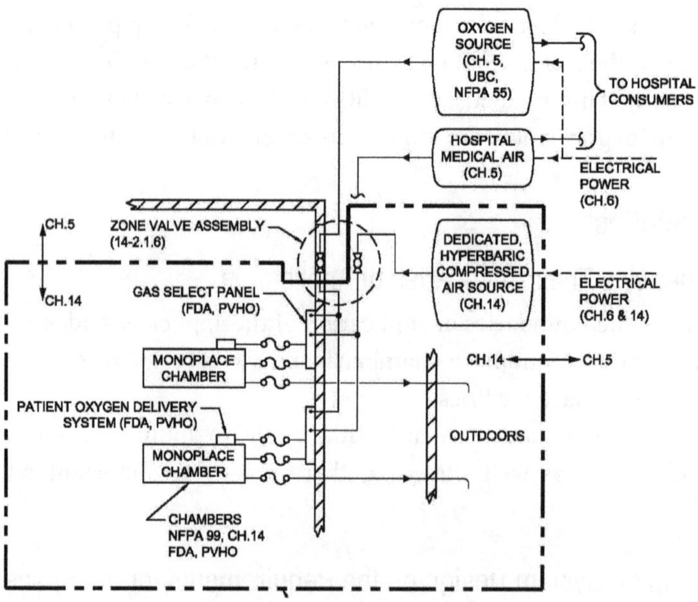

Figure 3. Codes and standards application to a typical air ventilation monoplace chamber facility. Diagram courtesy of authors.

Notes:

1. For most sites, the oxygen source will need to meet the requirement for Category 1 piped systems under Chapter 5 rules. Smaller sites sometimes can be installed under the rules for Category 3 piped gas systems.
2. Notes 1 through 5 in Figure 1 also apply.

automatic wet pipe sprinkler system meeting the requirements of *NFPA 13* and water mist system meeting the requirements of *NFPA 750* for facilities housing Class A, Class B, or Class C chamber and ancillary equipment.

Conclusion

Design and construction of the piping systems for hyperbaric facilities is an art form that requires not only the basic knowledge of engineering principles and construction materials but also the adequate knowledge of applicable codes and safety standards. Application of these codes and standards varies by state and from one jurisdiction to another within the same state. Depending on which code is applied for construction of your facility will not only affect its financial obligation but the overall safety of the facility and quality of patient care. It is highly recommended that one should thoroughly study and understand the applicable patient safety, design, and construction codes and standards along with associated financial obligations of a hyperbaric care facility.

References

1. National Fire and Protection Association. Chapter 5: gas and vacuum systems. NFPA 99 Health Care Facilities Code, 2018 edition. Quincy, MA: National Fire Protection Association; 2018;99-28 to 99-69.
2. National Fire and Protection Association. Chapter 14: hyperbaric facilities. NFPA 99 Health Care Facilities Code, 2018 edition. Quincy, MA: National Fire Protection Association; 2018;99-108 to 99-121.
3. National Fire Protection Association. NFPA 55 Compressed Gases and Cryogenic Fluids Code, 2016 edition. Quincy, MA: National Fire Protection Association; 2016.
4. American Society of Mechanical Engineers. ASME PVHO-1-2016 Safety Standard for Pressure Vessels for Human Occupancy, 2016 edition. NY: The American Society of Mechanical Engineers; 2016.
5. Hart, JR, Rubadou, CB. NFPA 99 Health Care Facilities Code Handbook, 2018 edition. Quincy, MA: National Fire Protection Association; 2018;84.

CHAPTER 4.3
Breathing Gas Systems

Glenn J. Butler, Mark Chipps, and Regina Sonnenrein

Introduction

The primary safety considerations in hyperbaric medicine are the ability to provide a safe environment that minimizes the inherent danger of fire and explosions and to provide the patient under pressure with a physiologically appropriate gas. Most modern clinical hyperbaric breathing gas system designs come from the historically hazardous environments of commercial diving, aerospace, and mine, tunnel, and caisson work in hypoxic/toxic atmospheres.

It is worthwhile to go back to the beginning of breathing gas system (BGS) design philosophy and review individual materials and components for a deeper understanding of BGS design and safer operational use. While most BGS have been designed to help prevent operator misuse, it is essential to remember that through operator error or mechanical design, every BGS has the ability to provide the patient a physiologically inappropriate gas—or none at all.

Today, most clinical hyperbaric personnel work with hyperbaric chambers and breathing system equipment that they have not designed or constructed. Many hyperbaric chamber operations staff have a limited understanding of "how" a system functions, and therefore, rely on the manufacturer for training or service work. It is important to receive formal training for the safe operation of hyperbaric equipment; it is just as important that hyperbaric personnel have an appreciation of chamber and breathing system hardware component functions, limitations, and materials and why these systems have been designed in a specific manner. Such knowledge is a matter of life and death for the patient and also for the personnel operating hyperbaric chambers.

The use of oxygen is the primary design and materials consideration in any breathing system. A critical concept is that almost everything will burn (oxidize) to some degree when heated to a sufficiently high temperature in the presence of oxygen, which is a strong oxidizer. A good example of this is an oxyacetylene cutting torch, with which steel a foot thick may be cut (actually burned) by heating the steel to temperatures over

600°C (1100°F) and blowing a stream of oxygen onto it.

Every day, oxygen (O_2) and high-oxygen mixtures are used safely in the welding, diving, and aviation industries, and in medical applications. These industries have learned that the key to oxygen safety is the use of specially prepared and compatible equipment by trained personnel following specific procedures. These principles and philosophies and how they can be applied to the use of oxygen-enriched breathing mixtures are covered in this chapter.

Note: Oxygen safety is a matter of degree. All breathing systems must be designed for oxygen service.

The NFPA-99 Code[1]

For some years, the U.S. National Fire Protection Association (NFPA) has published a standard regarding fire safety for hyperbaric facilities.[1] It is a constantly evolving code thanks to the input of various experts and contributors, with the goal of producing a practical and up-to-date guideline.

Hyperbaric Chamber Fire Safety

Special precautions during hyperbaric operations are needed to ensure fire-free safety, especially since clinical treatment chambers utilize 100% oxygen and oxygen breathing gas mixtures; their design may make quick escape of occupants impossible. Specific details are beyond this chapter's scope, but a great deal about oxygen safety and safe handling of enriched mixtures is to be learned from the principles involved in chamber fire safety.

Oxidizer

Oxygen Use in Hyperbaric Chambers

Hyperbaric chambers are basically of two types, a large, steel chamber that takes several patients at one time (multiplace—Class A) and smaller single-person (monoplace—Class B) chambers usually made of acrylic plastic and filled with oxygen.

The Fire Triangle—oxidizer, fuel, and ignition—applies to all hyperbaric chamber and facility designs, and all three legs of the triangle are involved in the system.

Oxygen in Multiplace Chambers

Multiplace chambers are compressed on air, and a major component of chamber fire safety is to maintain the oxygen content in the chamber atmosphere at 21%. Oxygen breathed by patients as part of their treatment is not normally released into the chamber. An outside chamber, or "overboard" oxygen exhaust system is utilized with a mask or continuous flow hood system to release the gas outside the chamber. This exhaust system compensates for the difference in pressure between the inside and outside of the chamber and protects the patient from a mask suction injury by maintaining about a 1 atmosphere negative differential to exhaust exhalation gases outside the chamber regardless of the actual pressure inside the chamber.

Even with these precautions, there can be some oxygen leakage into the chamber. Therefore, the atmosphere in a multiplace chamber is continuously monitored by an oxygen analyzer, which alarms at the level of 23.5% oxygen. Controlling ventilation takes a large volume of air.

While 21% oxygen atmospheric air will support combustion, the same 21% oxygen air compressed into a multiplace chamber at 3 atmospheres may facilitate rapid combustion and flame propagation because there are more oxygen molecules available to the combustion process, and the increased density promotes conduction and flame spread.

Burning rate is a complex combination of partial pressure of oxygen (PPO_2), chamber pressure, and inert gas background. It is possible to have atmospheres that will not support combustion but that are safe to breathe. Per the *US Navy Diving Manual*, for hyperbaric applications this is called the zone of no combustion.[16]

Oxygen in Monoplace Chambers

Monoplace chambers, with few exceptions, are compressed with oxygen, with the flow of oxygen used to provide ventilation for control of carbon dioxide, moisture, and temperature. The patient does not have to wear a mask in this oxygen environment. In air-ventilated monoplace chambers, oxygen needs to be delivered by a tight-fitting mask, oxygen hood, or another device.

Fuel

Items that can burn are kept to a minimum in the chamber. Materials normally considered fire resistant may burn in oxygen-enriched environments. Items safe for hyperbaric chamber environments are available for wiring insulation, clothing, and other applications.

There are a wide range of fuels that can be introduced into the hyperbaric environment.[1-2]

- Bedding
- Linens
- Clothing
- Patient monitoring devices
- Human body, particularly hair
- Refreshment containers
- Flammable vapors
- Lint/dust

In some multiplace chambers, reading materials are not allowed or kept to a minimum.[1] Clothing and bedding in some facilities are made of special oxygen-compatible polymers. Mattresses and cushions are covered with oxygen compatible materials or made of flame-resistant matter.

Some experts feel cotton clothing and bedding is better than polyester blends, since cotton is less prone to static discharge and absorbs more moisture. However, cotton fiber dust is an excellent fuel; any chamber interior and exhaust should be thoroughly cleaned during regular maintenance.

Ignition

Monoplace chamber fires have been caused in most cases by items taken into the chamber by the patients, such as hand warmers, smoking materials, or sparking toys. Ancillary medical equipment like cardiac monitors or intravenous fluid pumps are positioned on the outside of the chamber for safety.

The main source of ignition in multiplace chambers comes from electrical power, like patient monitors, medical equipment, or entertainment systems. These can be used safely if properly insulated, enclosed in metal, and/or blanketed in inert gas such as nitrogen, and switching power on and off is normally done externally.

Masks, Fire Extinguishing, and Escape

Emergency breathing masks that deliver life-sustaining gas are essential in case of fire inside a multiplace chamber. Ultraviolet (UV) fire detection devices alert the chamber personnel or trigger a water deluge system, which together with a hand-directed hose, is the best available countermeasure in case of a fire. Power must be turned off and emergency lights on, if needed. Lockout hatches are designed to allow occupants to escape from one lock to another (Figure 1).

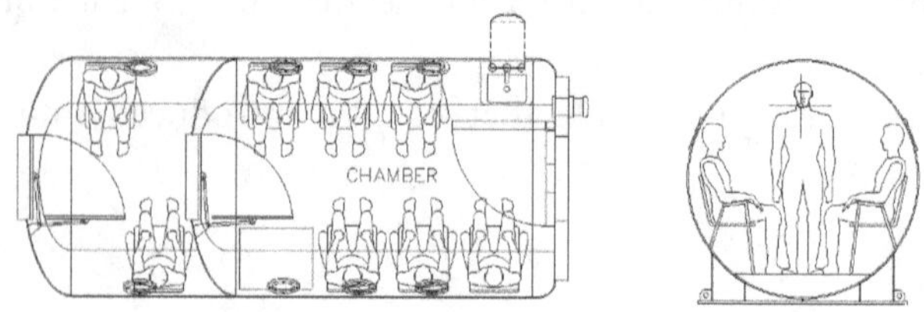

Figure 1. Multiplace chamber. Image courtesy of Reimers Systems.

Fire and Pressure

Almost all breathing gas systems fires occur with high-oxygen mixtures during rapid transitions from low to high pressure, and/or high velocities in the presence of particulates or oil contamination. As oxygen pressure and therefore the number of molecules increases in the presence of a fuel, the temperature necessary to initiate combustion of the fuel—the auto-ignition point—decreases dramatically, making it easier to start a fire.[3-4] In 3,000 PSIG oxygen systems, for example, the auto-ignition point of a given valve seat material may be only a fraction of the temperature required to set the material on fire in atmospheric air, if indeed it will burn in air at all.

Many materials that will not readily burn in high-pressure air conditions, even at very high temperatures, may explode in the presence of high-pressure oxygen. The selection and use of the materials most resistant to auto-ignition in high-pressure oxygen is critical to preparing equipment for oxygen-rich service safety.

Remember: Always work with oxygen at lowest possible pressure.

Design Principles for Oxygen Systems

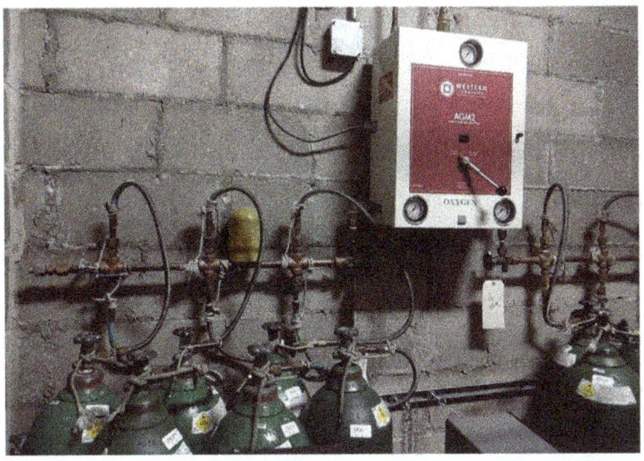

Figure 2. Photo courtesy of Life Support Technologies Group.

Avoid Adiabatic Heating by Compression

A common source of high temperatures in gas systems is heating caused by rapid compression of the gas within the pressure compartments and piping system, a phenomenon known as dieseling.[4] This is the same process that occurs in diesel engines. Rapid compression of a manifold with a working pressure of 3,000 PSIG (200 bars) can produce momentary gas temperatures in excess of 900°C (1,600°F), a value in excess of the 200 to 315°C (400 to 600°F) auto-ignition temperatures of ordinary lubricants. Fast-moving gas heats up; a cylinder valve can generate temperatures to 1,400°F.

Do not use ball valves in high-pressure (HP) oxygen systems. Only globe valves should be used in HP systems. Ball valves may be located downstream, where pressure does not exceed 125 PSI. The ball valve should NEVER be operated to quickly release 02 pressure into a volume container, such as a chamber or a pipe system.[1]

Maintain Low Velocity of Gas

Minimizing gas velocities is an effective method of preventing fires in a high-pressure gas mixing system. A rapidly opened cylinder gas valve outlet can create high gas velocities, which in turn may produce high adiabatic temperatures, causing materials to reach auto-ignition temperatures; high gas velocities can also carry particles, which can produce ignition by particle impingement or friction. Even a small steel particle has substantial energy on impact. Another source of high temperatures in gas systems is caused by the localized friction which occurs as gas moves through valves and orifices at sonic or near-sonic velocities.

Always work at the minimum velocities, pressures, and rates of compression that are both possible and practical.

Reduce Impingement by Limiting Foreign Matter in the System

Particle impact is a likely cause of auto-ignition in larger storage and manifold systems.[4-5] High gas velocities can pick up and carry metal particles and other debris downstream at hundreds of feet per second, and this can cause sparking and very high localized temperatures as the particles hit bumps and bends in the piping. Sharp turns are not recommended.

Most systems contain filtration to prevent the contamination of the system by connection to contaminated supply sources. One such source of continuing contamination is from the connectors of gas cylinders which may collect various particulate matter. Particle filters should be located at gas cylinder connections and prior to critical components in the system. (Blow out cylinder valve first.)

Another source of contamination is oil mist or entrained hydrocarbons from air pumped by oil-lubricated compressors. Compressed Gas Association (CGA) grade D or E air, while safe to breathe is not compatible for mixing with oxygen.

Use Oxygen-Compatible Materials

Fuel is found as contaminants in the system and in the materials of the system itself. Some fires that have burned system components appear to have been started by some contamination in the system. Minimizing fuel in the form of contaminants is accomplished by care during manufacture, cleaning before use, and strict control when the system is opened.

Selection of Valves

Valves are key players in a safe oxygen manifold. Valves that would allow rapid compression with the accompanying heat buildup are bad news. Cylinder valves can be misused. Relief and check valves have their place.

Ball vs. Globe Valves

Only rotating stem type valves or globe valve patterns should be used in high-pressure oxygen circuits. Ball valves can be used as shutoff valves and are ideal for rapid shutoff applications. Use slow-opening, bubble-tight valves for isolation. Proportional flow or metering valves are best to control flow, with minimal pressure across the valve. Tight shut-off is not the main goal in a metering valve; use them in conjunction with an isolating valve and/or a regulator to control pressure.

Regulators as Valves

Regulators act as pressure reducing valves, for example to control the pressure when transferring gas at cylinder pressure.

Check Valves

Check valves ensure correct procedural use of a system. They prevent reverse flow in a manifold, especially when cascading from cylinders, to prevent backflow and reduce chance of a seat sticking and holding a cylinder closed.

Cylinder Valves

Cylinder valves should be either fully open or fully closed and should not be used to throttle flow.

Safety and Relief Valves

The primary use of relief valves is for overpressure protection. Rate all components for full pressure + 10% (minimum).[15] Pressure protect each section of the system, including gauges. Use resealing type relief valves; total loss of gas due to overpressure is not only wasteful, it can cause a fire or' allow one to spread. Cylinder rupture disks do not substitute for relief valves. Be sure to vent oxygen relief valves in a safe area, and ensure that reaction forces do not do damage.

Material and Lubricant Compatibility with Oxygen

1. Presence of Flammable Materials

When materials are exposed to oxygen or oxygen-enriched atmospheres, their compatibility from a flammability point of view must be considered. By compatible, we mean that the material will not burn easily in oxygen. Materials that have already reacted with oxygen (oxides) cannot participate in a combustion process. Hence, one way to control propagation is to prevent it entirely. This would be equivalent to removing the fuel leg of the fire triangle. Unfortunately, this more conservative approach is usually not practical.

The most likely source of fuel in compressed air or enriched air systems is liquid oil. This oil contamination may be the result of improperly cleaned parts attached to the system or compressor lubrication oil which has been allowed to accumulate in the system.

While the amount of oil necessary to support the combustion process are dependent on many factors, some of the lubricating oils that are recommended by manufactures and selected for their low-toxicity properties for use in high-pressure breathing gas compressors will ignite spontaneously if heated to their 150°C to 230°C (300°F to 450°F) auto-ignition temperature in the presence of oxygen.[5]

The amount of condensed hydrocarbon-based oil necessary to allow sustained combustion in a high-pressure air system has been established experimentally at values as low as 20 milligrams of condensed oil per square foot (0.093 m^2) of internal piping area, under certain conditions.[6] The exact amount of contamination one might expect is proportional to the amount of air pumped by the compressor, adjusted for the quality and frequency of the filters and the maintenance of the compressor.

Other potential fuels may include component soft goods such as valve seats, regulator diaphragms, O-rings, and thread-sealing tape that comes into direct contact with the gas streams. As a general guideline, components designed and cleaned for oxygen service are acceptable for high-pressure enriched air systems.

To minimize risk, lubricants used in gas exposed components such as valve stem threads should be rated for oxygen service. Ignition has occurred with silicone greases used in high-pressure air systems. There is a popular misconception that silicones are not flammable, but any silicones used in the system should be replaced with a more oxygen-compatible lubricant.

2. Oxygen Compatibility

Oxygen compatibility is the ability of a substance to coexist with both oxygen and a potential source of ignition within the acceptable risk parameter of the user, at an expected pressure and temperature. [10]

This is very important when using oxygen-enriched air at high pressure. Oxygen is not a flammable gas or vapor such as acetylene or ether, but it is a strong oxidizing agent and will combine chemically with compounds and fuels, causing an exothermic chemical reaction. Other oxidants are chlorine and nitrous oxide. The rate at which this chemical reaction or oxidation takes place is very important; it may be slow or fast.

The following are some materials considered compatible for oxygen service:

- Teflon and Kel-F: Proprietary polymers used for valve seats, tubing, and linings, etc., may be metal or glass-filled or reinforced. These have excellent high-temperature resistance to slow oxidation and to burning in high oxygen but are not usable in some "dynamic" applications.
- Hypalon, Viton-A, Fluorel: High-temperature oxygen applications such as compressors, etc.
- Viton-A shows good resistance to the oxygen-compatible lubricants that contain chlorine.
- Buna-N and neoprene: Low-temperature O-rings and diaphragms (may be fabric reinforced). The least oxygen compatible in this list.

All these materials have minimal chemical interaction with strong oxidizers, but they all will burn rapidly in oxygen if heated to their ignition temperature of 400-500° F. Proper cleaning is important to prevent initial combustion.

Some components of an oxygen system (valves, regulators) require lubrication for proper operation. Special lubricants are required for oxygen service. Perfluorinated polyether-based oils with fluorotelomer thickeners are the most inert and probably the best. Perfluoroalkyl products work well, but they tend to lose some of their lubrication qualities at low temperatures. Perfluorinated polyether-based oils have good low-temperature characteristics and are comparatively low-priced. These materials are compatible with most common elastomers and are superior to ordinary and/or silicone-based lubricants, which should not be used on oxygen or enriched air systems.

- Fluorolube, a chlorofluorocarbon by Hooker, is oxygen compatible, but it is not compatible with aluminum and is not as well tolerated by Buna-N. Chlorine in this compound reacts with aluminum.
- Krytox, a perfluoroalkyl polyether by DuPont, is oxygen tolerant, but is not as good a lubricant at low temperatures as the perfluorinated polyethers.
- Christo-Lube MCO-ll1, a line of perfluorinated polyether-based oils by Lubrication Technology, Inc., has good low-temperature lubricant qualities and is oxygen compatible. This company also makes Scubalube, which is also good.
- Braycote by Castrol is another perfluoroalkyl polyether oxygen-compatible lubricant. It is used extensively by National Aeronautics and Space Administration (NASA).
- Mollycote(R) 111 Compound, a silicone grease by Dow Corning, is not recommended for oxygen service above 100 PSIG.
- Silicone greases are improperly regarded by some as oxygen safe. They are better than ordinary grease but they are NOT suitable for high-pressure oxygen service. The better quality lubricants are slightly more expensive, but where oxygen compatibility is needed, they are well worth it.

Cleaning for Oxygen Service

The Practice of Oxygen Cleaning

The Compressed Gas Association (CGA) in the pamphlet, "Cleaning Equipment for Oxygen Service," (CGA 0-4.1, 1985)[8] and the American Society of Testing and Materials (ASTM G-93, 1992)[9] recommend that all system components having either direct contact with oxygen or the indirect possibility (i.e., not normally in contact with oxygen, but which might be as a result of a reasonably foreseeable malfunction) be constructed of oxygen compatible materials and cleaned to oxygen-service standards. The same recommendation applies to enriched air mixtures, especially those above about 40 or 50% oxygen by volume.

Gas Handling Hardware

A breathing gas system (BGS) for making and/or handling oxygen and special gas mixes should be designed for oxygen service, using materials approved for use in oxygen and of an inherent design that limits rates of flow and compression effecting gas temperatures.

1. High- and Low-Pressure Oxygen Systems

Compressors and gas handling systems can be loosely divided according to pressure:

- Low pressure (LP) is up to 125 PSI.

- Medium pressure is 125-500 PSI.
- High pressure (HP) is over 500 PSI.

2. Materials for Oxygen Systems

Candidate materials include common metals and some not well known in other applications.

- Brass, bronze, copper alloy are the most commonly used materials for handling oxygen. Heavy-walled, annealed copper (6x9 mm; 6 mm ID, 9 mm OD) is common for pigtails. These materials are often connected by silver brazing.
- Stainless steel seamless tubing and fittings:
  - 304 and 316 alloys have high nickel concentration and are more spark resistant.
  - Most tubing is designed to be cold bent[10] and tubing is most often used with compression and flare type fitting systems at high pressures.
- Monel. For many years the U.S. Navy (USN) would only allow monel (a nickel-copper alloy) to be used in its oxygen systems. It is the most resistant to impact and auto-ignition. Monel was believed by many to be unnecessarily expensive. Now the USN allows 300 series stainless steel (>20% Ni-Cr) and brass to be used for pressures up to 3000 PSI. Tubing, piping, and most types of fittings are available in Monel.
- Tungum tubing is often used in Europe. Tungum is a very hard copper-nickel alloy; when used with compression fittings it requires stainless steel fittings and ferrules to bind or swage the pipe.
- Hasteloy and Inconel are proprietary nickel and copper alloys which are acceptable for oxygen service.
- Aluminum, 600 series, is used for aircraft oxygen systems. Aluminum is not very oxygen compatible and ignites at lower temperatures and burns more rapidly than other materials listed. However its low weight advantage in aircraft predominates.
- Galvanized and carbon steel are used to carry oxygen in air reduction and chemical plants for medium pressure, large volume service. Not used for high-pressure oxygen systems. Note: An oxy-acetylene cutting torch burns steel.

Fittings and Connectors

1. Overview of Fittings

The basic function of fittings is to provide the transition between the piping material or tubing and the components of pressure control, regulation, and/or shutoff used to control the gas or liquid medium in the piping system. This transition implies adaption from the types of connection used on the different components. As an example, a fitting transition may provide a compression connection to the tubing on one side and an U.S. National Pipe Thread (NPT) connection to a regulator component on the other. The term "fitting" implies this adaption.

Fittings are made of all the materials used for piping or components like copper or galvanized steel. Fittings for high-pressure oxygen systems, however, are designed with high-pressure stainless steel, copper, or brass, or monel materials as being most compatible.

2. Types of Fittings (not all-inclusive)

- Threaded, tapered, pipe connections
- Threaded, parallel threads with gaskets
- Soldered socket or welded joints
- JIC 37.5° and 45° flare fittings; also known as AN (army-navy) fittings
- Compression fittings:
  - Swagelok two ferrule
  - Gyrolok two ferrule
  - A-10k two ferrule Parker
  - CPI single ferrule Parker
- Zero clearance, flat, flanged-type with O-ring seal
- Nut and nipple, as used on gas cylinders

3. Tapered Thread Connections

Tapered fittings are designed to develop both their mechanical strength and gas pressure seal on the threads themselves using a thread filler and lubricating material such as polytetrafluoroethylene tape (PTFE). The disadvantage is the need for at least a five-thread engagement for full pressure rating. In order to tighten a fitting elbow sufficiently, the elbow can end up pointing in a less desirable direction. It is important to ensure similar but different pipe patterns, like BSP and ISO, are not cross-threaded.

Assembling NPT pipe and fittings: Higher pressure NPT fittings are often provided with hexagonal shapes or flat spots for applying a wrench, and some high quality nipples are machined from hexagonal stock material, threaded at both ends, and drilled out in the center. Most high-pressure NPT piping systems, such as manifolds for gas, are available precleaned and packaged for high-pressure oxygen service.

Selecting sealants for NPT connections: The best overall material for tapered thread sealing is PTFE (Teflon) tape. It is clean and easy to use, but requires some training in order to place it on the fitting and to tighten the joint properly. PTFE is extremely inert, oxygen compatible, and is acting as an excellent lubricant to permit the tapered fittings to tighten together smoothly and to provide a material to fill the space between the threads.

4. Parallel Threaded Connectors

Several straight or parallel thread system designs are available to minimize limitations of tapered fittings. SAE and BSPP thread systems use the parallel threads and O-rings or gaskets to provide the mechanical connection and pressure rating. This design permits unlimited orientation over a full 360°area while remaining gas tight.

5. Soldered, Brazed, and Welded Socket Connections

This method of piping connection is the most widely used in HP oxygen manifolds. Higher pressure systems designed for gas, and in particular enriched air or high oxygen mixtures, use a silver brazing technique with an oxygen-compatible water-based compound as the flux. A silver-based alloy containing up to 50% silver is used to braze or silver solder the connection. Silver-soldered sweat fittings are the most often used in factory-assembled high-pressure gas and oxygen manifolds.

Socket weld fittings: Socket weld fittings are basically the same design as sweat solder fittings and are assembled in the same manner and welded. They cannot readily be disassembled.

Joint Industrial Council (JIC) 37° flare fittings or AN fittings: The flare fitting design uses a tapered nut and male bullnose fitting with a 37° sealing face. The tubing end is flared outward to match this 37° male flare (thus the tube becomes the female component), and the nut and following collar presses the back of this flare against the fitting face, forming a seal.

6. Compression Fittings

Compression fittings for tubing form a seal by a ferrule being compressed into the tubing wall by a threaded nut (Figure 3). Joints may be loosened and retightened, but ferrules cannot be reused, and the nut is captive once sealed. (Tubing has to be cut to do a new joint.) This compression of the tubing allows for extremely high pressures without blowing the tubing out of

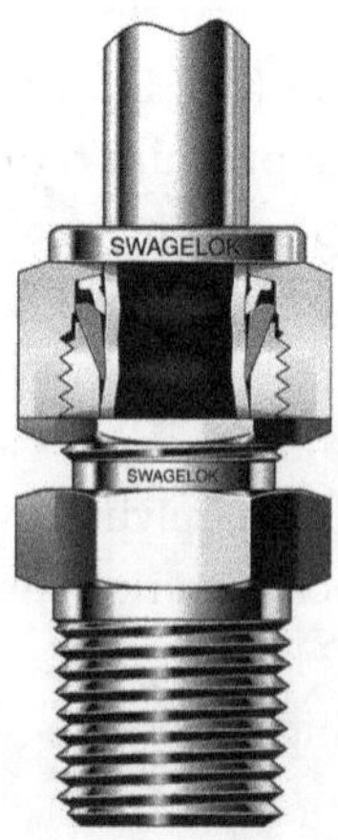

Figure 3. Example of a typical ferrule compression fitting. This system provides both a gas tight seal and mechanical strength at the tubing and ferrule connection. Photo courtesy of Swagelok Company, Solon, OH.

the compression fittings, consistent with the strength of the materials. The gas seal in this compression fitting detail is metal-to-metal and requires that tubing be free from scratches, saw marks, and other defects on the outside surface.

Tubing for compression fittings: The key to the proper and safe use of compression fittings is that the tubing must always be softer than the compression fitting material, specifically the ferrule. Compression fittings are designed to be used either with fully annealed soft copper (refrigeration) tubing in rolls or rigid tubing lengths designed to conform to ASTM-A269 or A213 specifications.[11,13] It references tubing which may be bent while cold and is designed for compression and flare applications. Most high-pressure compression fittings such as Swagelok, Gyro-lok, or Parker brand fittings are designed to be used with the ASTM-269 specification[10] (can be bent cold). Light gases such as helium can escape through even the most minute leak path. A compression fitting nut should be tightened 1½ turns beyond hand tight to properly swage the fitting.

7. Zero Clearance O-Ring Flanged Fittings

Q-ring sealed zero clearance fittings have zero insertion depth and universal orientation. They are often used in relief valves or regulators that must be removed and serviced. The flanged O-ring face fittings are adaptable to NPT, silver solder, socket weld, and welded interface attachment to piping and tubing.

8. Gas Cylinder Connectors; Nut and Nipple

The US-based CGA and other equivalent international organizations have designed a series of noninterchangeable gas cylinder connections. The connections for each gas group, such as inert gases, mixtures, oxygen, nitrous oxide, etc., are each dimensionally unique and are intended to prevent an inadvertent cross-connection of gas supply which may cause a hazardous or life-threatening condition.

With few exceptions, cylinder connectors are designed to seal metal to metal. Carbon dioxide, phosgene, and a few other gases utilize washer inserts.

Sealing tapes or sealants are not necessary to make cylinder connections leak tight and might have the opposite effect. The inside of cylinder valve connections quickly collects contaminants ranging from insect nests to diesel smoke residue. Always ensure that the valve orifice is clear before connection. Purge the cylinder valve before connecting to it.

9. Cylinder Valves

Types of cylinder valves: Cylinder valves (Figure 4) are designed to be reliable, have gas-tight shutoff, and to fail safely using an integral rupture disk in the event of over pressurization. One of the two basic types of cylinder valve designs is the nonrising stem design, utilizing a spinning handle linked to a shaft by a keyway. Turning the handle turns the shaft, which turns the valve seat, which is threaded. It is difficult to tell if this type of valve is open or closed, except to test it by closing (clockwise) and/or attempting to open counterclockwise.

The second design uses a metal diaphragm instead of stem packing glands to eliminate leakage. More costly and designed for toxic or flammable gases, the stem of this type valve is isolated from the gas by thin metal diaphragms. Clockwise turning exerts pressure on the diaphragm, which pushes the valve assembly onto the seat and shuts off gas flow. Counterclockwise turning releases pressure from the diaphragms and allows gas to escape. The nonrotating internal stem minimizes wear of the seat assembly seal and the seat as compared to the other valve design.

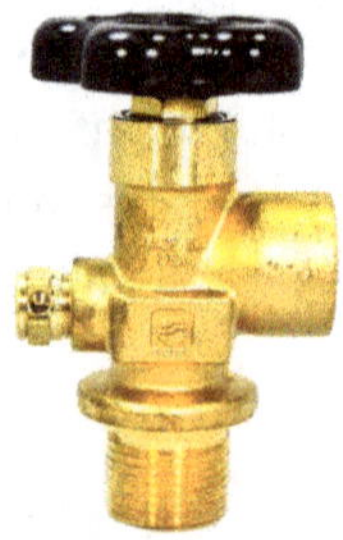

Figure 4. Example of a high-pressure gas cylinder shutoff valve. All cylinder valves are required to incorporate a rupture disc to prevent overpressurization of the cylinder. This design features a nonreaction rupture disc and rotating soft stem seat.
Photo courtesy of Sherwood Scuba.

Cylinder valve connector uniqueness: In the United States, cylinder valve connections are specifically designed by CGA to be dissimilar, to prevent the wrong regulator from connecting to the wrong cylinder or type of gas, or the wrong type of gas being delivered to a specific service. Medical breathing gas cylinders cannot be connected to a nitrogen connection used for operating room tools nor can a nitrogen cylinder be connected to a medical oxygen manifold allowing nitrogen to be delivered to the anesthesia machine and breathed by a patient.

Medical oxygen cylinders rated to 3,000 PSI (200 bars) use the CGA 540 connection,[12] a right-handled female nut on the regulator, and male parallel thread on the cylinder. Inert gas (nitrogen, helium, argon) cylinders use a CGA 580 connection,[15] which is female on the cylinder.

Using cylinder valves to control flow: Gas cylinder valves are not designed to control flow; they function best as on-off valves. They should be opened or closed by finger strength only. If wrenches or tools are needed to open or close cylinder valves, there is something mechanically wrong with that valve and it should be taken out of service until the problem can be identified.

Cylinder valve seat can stay in place: Cylinder valves can cause a specific problem when used in cascade gas mixing manifolds, since they are designed to keep gas in, not out. If a valve is opened when there is pressure on the outside, the seat may stay in place and not open; it can wreak havoc with mixing. Use a valve independent of the cylinder valves for control and have the cylinder valves either be fully open or fully closed.

Regulators for Pressure Control

Gas pressure regulation devices are designed to control supply and discharge pressure differentials for specific applications:

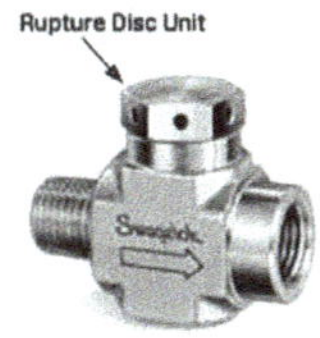

Figure 5. Rupture disk. PHoto courtesy of Swagelok Company.

1. Types of Regulators

- Hand-operated cylinder regulators
- Low-pressure line regulators
- Dome-loaded regulators
- Back-pressure regulators
- Tracking and self-relieving regulators
- Balanced and unbalanced regulators

Cylinder and low-pressure line regulators: These are for use with high-pressure cylinders and are usually hand-loaded (adjusted) or have a fixed spring pressure and delivery pressure. A special type of cylinder regulator allows the full pressure of the supply tank to be discharged under control (Figure 6).

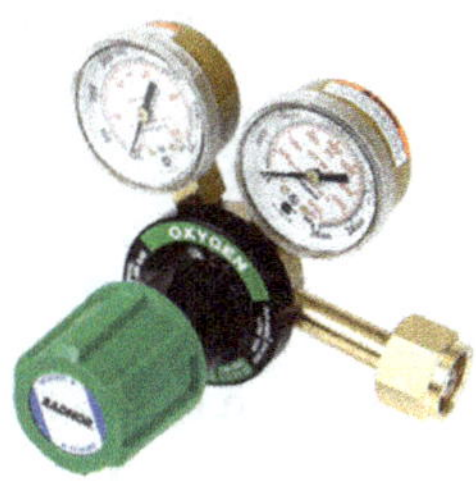

Figure 6. Regulators. Typical single-stage, high-pressure cylinder regulator. Photo courtesy of Airgas.

Dome-loaded regulators: Similar to other high-pressure hand-loaded regulators but use gas or fluid pressure on a diaphragm to load the regulator control valve instead of spring tension developed by hand. They may be remotely controlled, so dome-loaded regulators are often used where large volumes of gas and large diameter piping may be routed directly from the supply source to the point of gas utilization.

Back-pressure regulators: These regulators are often used in multiplace chambers for the oxygen mask overboard-dump system. As the patient exhales into the system, the pressure is increased slightly, causing the regulator to release gas and maintain the set pressure. Back-pressure units are considered tracking regulators.

Balanced and unbalanced regulators: Simple, unbalanced regulators begin to lose their discharge pressure stability as the inlet pressure begins to drop off and may open completely with a rush of gas as the last of the gas in the cylinder is used. Balanced regulators have internal pressure connections that provide feedback pressure to balance it with the inlet valve and compensate for depleting inlet pressure (Figure 7).

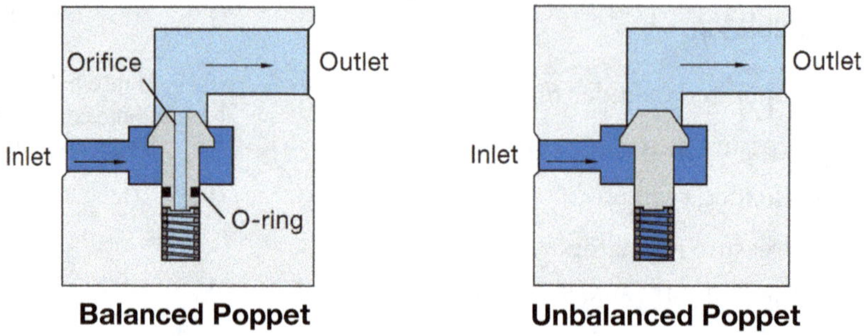

Figure 7. Balanced and unbalanced regulators. Right: Highly simplified schematic of a standard unbalanced regulator. This design is not entirely independent of inlet pressure. As inlet pressure falls, the outlet pressure rises typically 0.5 PSI per 100 PSI drop in inlet pressure. Left: The balanced regulator design partially compensates for decaying inlet pressure by balancing the poppet valve forces. Images courtesy of Swagelok Company.

Self-relieving regulators: This design feature is offered as an option with most conventional regulators. It permits downstream gas pressure to be vented from the regulator when this pressure exceeds the regulator set point. The self-relieving or downstream-vented regulator is designed to exhaust to the atmosphere any downstream gas pressure in excess of the set point. This may be used to control discharge pressure as an integral relief valve.

2. Regulator Pressure Stages

Regulators are designed to reduce supply pressure to discharge pressure in one, two, or even three steps or stages. In single-stage regulators, this pressure control occurs in one pressure drop. A two-stage regulator will drop the inlet to an intermediate pressure, which will then feed a second stage. Due to a smaller pressure drop, a two-stage regulator tends to have a more stable discharge pressure over the full range of output supply pressures.

Gauges

Gauges are an essential part of safety and control of gas systems. Gauges sense pressure and indicate and display that pressure. There are two main types of detectors, and two main types of display. Detectors include Bourdon tubes and strain gauges. Displays include the familiar analog faces with rotating needle indicators and a wide variety of digital readouts.

Readings of pressure are expressed in absolute and gauge terms. Absolute pressures are referenced to a zero pressure vacuum, while gauge pressures are referenced to the ambient atmospheric pressure. In any case, gauge pressures are differential pressures.

Types of Pressure Sensor

The simplest sensing device and yet the most elegant is the Bourdon tube. It consists of a flattened hollow tube that is curved into a "C" shape or spiral. One end is anchored, the other is attached to an indicator needle, linkage, or gear mechanism, which connects to the dial face, either analog or digital.

Accuracy Requirements for Gauges Used for Mixing

Accuracy vs. precision: Accuracy refers to the correctness of a reading and how close it is to giving the true value. Precision refers to how closely the value may be read to how many decimal places. High precision does not necessarily imply high accuracy.

Concept of a master gauge: Where mixing is done by partial pressure, the accuracy of the mix depends strongly on the accuracy of the gauge used for measuring the pressures. For best results from mixing, it is necessary to use a high-quality gauge that provides both accurate and linear readings, and that the gauge can be read with sufficient precision for the type of mixing being done. This is a master gauge.

Gauges can be ordered from the manufacturer to selected, and calibrated to, various specifications, which may be etched on the face. They should be purchased factory-cleaned for oxygen service. Protect gauges from weather, dust, and shock. Sudden shock to a gauge, such as dropping it may dramatically affect accuracy. Test (master) gauges should be protected from being dropped and maintained in a cushioned box if portable.

To prevent rapid pressure fluctuations and promote a smooth, mechanical transition of the pressure sensor, snubbers or filters can add safety. Snubbers also prevent contamination from entering the pressure-sensing Bourdon tube or crystal and also serve as flame arresters in oxygen systems.

Compressors for Breathing Gas Systems

High-pressure breathing air compressors may be divided into three basic design categories:

- Oil-lubricated
- Oil-free
- Oil-less

Oil-free and oil-less compressors can be grouped together and compared with oil-lubricated compressors. Oil-lubricated compressor designs are generally less expensive to purchase and maintain but need filtration and frequent preventive and interval maintenance.

Oil-free and oil-less compressors are initially more expensive to purchase, but eliminate both oil contaminants and the possibility of producing carbon monoxide during the compression process.

Compressors are used to fill larger air receivers for storage in multiplace facilities or for smaller cascade systems of air cylinders, where commercial delivery is not desired or feasible.

Industrial Gas Cylinders

Ownership

While scuba tanks are generally owned by the individual user, large industrial gas U.S. Department of Transportation (DOT) cylinders are usually owned by the gas supplier/distributor and leased to the health care facility operating it.

DOT

In the United States, standards for portable cylinder design and testing is set by DOT, and they require frequent inspection. Large ASME storage tanks, once in place, are designed not to require periodic inspection or hydro-testing due to their size.[16]

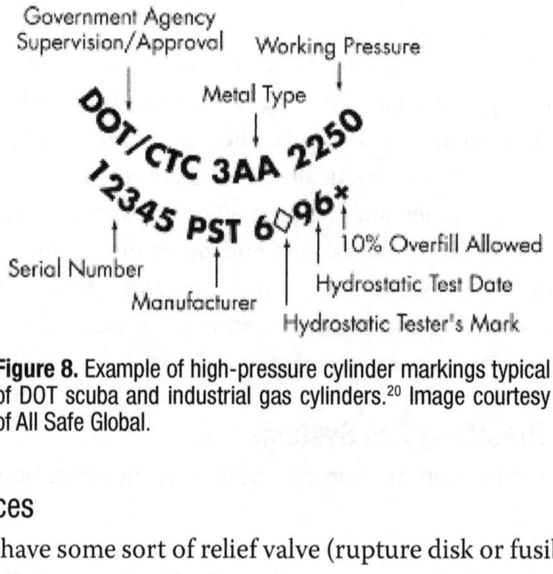

Figure 8. Example of high-pressure cylinder markings typical of DOT scuba and industrial gas cylinders.[20] Image courtesy of All Safe Global.

Safety Relief Devices

Pressure vessels all have some sort of relief valve (rupture disk or fusible plug) to release pressure in a controlled way. For cylinders, these are specifically to prevent catastrophic failure and explosion of tanks in the event of fire.

Large Receivers (Compressed Gas Storage Tanks)

ASME-coded (American Society of Mechanical Engineers) pressure vessels are used in clinical installations. Large tubes (usually arranged horizontally in racks), once in place, do not need periodic hydrostatic testing but do need annual inspection. They are overdesigned, extra thick, and inspected carefully in manufacture.

Storage of Cylinders

- Oxygen breathing gas mixtures in high-pressure cylinders should be stored in a well-ventilated area and out of direct sunlight. Some rules call for special rooms for oxygen with detectors or storage outdoors.
- Oxygen cryogenic dewars should be stored out of direct sun and in a ventilated area, since they bleed off 1 to 5% gas per day. Additional insulation such as space blankets may be indicated in warm climates.
- Inert gases and mixes have special requirements, especially for gases heavier than air that can collect in low spots. Storage should be in a well-ventilated area out of direct sunlight.

Cylinders stored vertically must be secured to walls or racks, which minimizes risks of damaging valves, regulators, and whips attached to them.

Liquid Oxygen (LOX)

1. Properties of Liquid Oxygen

In light of the safety considerations for gaseous oxygen, there are some special considerations for the safe use of LOX.

At cryogenic temperatures, below -297°F (-183°C), oxygen is a transparent pale blue liquid that is slightly heavier than water. Liquid oxygen has an expansion to gas ratio of 860:1, which means that one liter of oxygen will expand to become 860 liters of gaseous oxygen at standard temperature and pressure. Liquid oxygen is stored in a multiwalled, vacuum-insulated container. The container is maintained at a pressure of 230 PSI (15 bars). Although the containers are well insulated, the liquid still boils off at a rate of about 1% per day. This boil-off can cause significant pressure if the gas is not allowed to escape. Although the liquid vaporizes continuously at a low rate, if large quantities of gas are needed, in order to convert this liquid to gaseous form, it is necessary to warm it. This is done with a vaporizer, a finned heat exchanger that uses ambient outside air temperature to warm the liquid. The liquid flows into the vaporizer, picks up heat, vaporizes into a gas, and exits the vaporizer at roughly ambient outside temperature.

Liquefied compressed gases are stored at pressures less than those for nonliquefied gases. Storage pressures are usually well above those of final use pressures, and therefore pressure relief regulators and pressure relief devices are used.

2. Liquid Oxygen Safety

Some basic rules regarding LOX, some of which are applicable to all cryogenic liquids, are as follows:

- LOX is an extremely cold liquid that can freeze tissue on contact and cause skin that touches a cold pipe to stick to that pipe. This extreme cold causes embrittlement of carbon steel, plastics, rubber, and other materials.

- Extreme pressure can occur from rapid vaporization of the refrigerated liquid if it is subjected to rising temperatures from leakage of heat into the cryogenic container or system or if the LOX escapes from the cryogenically insulated container and vaporizer system.
- Fire and/or explosion can occur in escaping liquid oxygen, which, while itself not a flammable gas, can combine with organic materials such as asphalt to create an explosion.
- Liquid oxygen containers, piping, and equipment must be properly cleaned for oxygen service. They must be kept clean and free of grease, oil, or other hydrocarbon materials which can combine with oxygen with and explode. The system and procedures should be designed to prevent liquid oxygen from coming in contact with any organic materials or flammable substances of any kind.

Gas Analyzers and Gas Analysis

The majority of clinical monoplace and multiplace chamber facilities are operating from hospital liquid bulk oxygen tanks, with medical grade air for air breaks piped into a switchover panel.

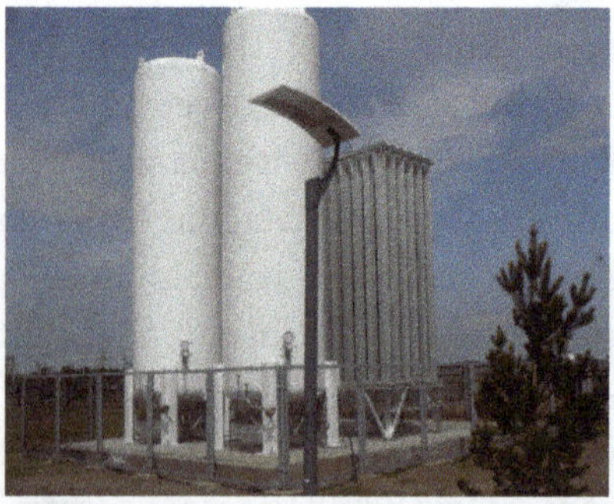

Figure 9. Photo courtesy of Life Support Technologies Group.

Most *NFPA-99* compliant multiplace hyperbaric chambers have fixed oxygen as well as infrared carbon dioxide gas analysis systems with dedicated calibration and sampling circuits for each chamber compartment. In some multiplace facilities, helium may be analyzed as well.

Oxygen analyzers work on chemical, electrochemical, or magnetic principles. All are reliable, but ease of operation and response time may vary.

All of the above safety measures and analyses are established in order to facilitate patient safety and comfort, while delivering the appropriate breathing gas for best treatment outcome.

Patient Oxygen Delivery Systems

Hood System

The most common way to deliver treatment gases to patients in a multiplace chamber is through the use of a hood system/tent. Hoods are versatile and can be used for multiple treatments. The system consists of the hood (clear vinyl with a visor and hard plastic ring) and a neck seal/neck dam. Other respiratory items are used to supply and exhaust treatment gases, e.g., corrugated tubing, in-line filters or noise dampeners, T-pieces, check valves, Y-Pieces, etc. There are several ways to set up the semiclosed circuit system.

Neck seals consist of a rigid plastic outer ring (connecting to the hood via an O-ring seal) and a softer material that is cut to fit snugly on the patient's neck or torso for pediatric patients. Tape-on vinyl neck seals have been used with patients who have asymmetrical anatomy of the neck and with tracheotomy patients. Ports to connect the gas supply and exhaust tubing are located on the rigid portion of the neck ring.

Special Considerations

a) The majority of hood systems, as shipped from the manufacturer, do not include an anti-asphyxiation mechanism, and a vacuum breaker must be in place prior to patient use. A respiratory check valve or series of respiratory check valves, located on the exhaust line, are normally used to serve this purpose. If the supply is interrupted, the hood will begin to deflate and at a certain point, the check valves will open with patient inspiration, allowing them to breathe chamber atmosphere. One manufacturer uses a reference hose on the hood exhaust side, which is open to chamber atmosphere.

b) Hood systems are multiple use devices and infection control must be taken into account. Some manufacturers approve their hoods but not neck seals for multipatient use; in these cases it is imperative that proper disinfecting procedures are followed.

c) Multiple factors need to be evaluated when choosing the proper flow rate for hood systems. These include hood volume, patient size, respiratory rate, sitting vs. standing, as well as other factors. For some time now, the customary flow rate used has been 28-30 actual liters per minute.[14] This rate will keep humidity and CO_2 at comfortable levels. Although it is acceptable for most cases, the flow may need to be increased for larger patients and decreased for pediatric patients.

Freeflow, Nonrebreather Masks

This section does not refer to demand regulator masks.

Mask systems are used in monoplace chambers to give air breaks and in multiplace chambers for patients who cannot tolerate an oxygen hood, have anatomical malformations of the neck, or by preference of the patient or facility. Some units use anesthesia masks, but there are manufacturers who use units specifically designed for this application.

Special Considerations

a) There is very little dead space when compared to hoods, so special system features must be in place to protect the patient from loss of gas flow and more importantly, over-exhaust that can lead to a suction injury. Optimally, the circuit should have one 3-liter respiratory bag on the supply and exhaust side. This will increase the dead space and compensate for a patient who increases or decreases his or her respiratory rate. A series of respiratory check valves should be put in-line on the exhaust side as secondary protection against suction injuries.

b) Typical, Y-type connector, with check valves, is connected directly to the mask. This prevents inspiration of exhaled gas, ensuring the patient receives the appropriate dosage of the treatment gas.

c) The mask must fit snug against the patient's face to ensure a complete seal. A head net or strap will provide four points of connection to the mask, and each can be adjusted to securely fit the system to the patient's face.

d) Infection control and cleaning of this system is very important. The mask should be cleaned per manufacturer instructions, and some can be sterilized for multiple patient use. It is good policy to entirely replace the exhaust side of the mask on a routine basis to prevent bacteria growth and lung discharge accumulation in the 3-liter bag. Having the infection control department involved with the decision process is useful, but typically units will replace the exhaust at the end of each week.

e) Gas flow to the patient is, again, dependent on the patient size, respiratory rate, and other factors. As a standard, keeping each 3 liter bag, ¾ full usually suffices. Make small adjustments for patient comfort.

Demand Regulator Breathing Mask

Typically referred to as BIBS masks, (built-in breathing system), this delivery system is commonly used for multiplace staff oxygen decompression. It also serves as a lifeline of clean gas in the event of a fire or contaminated atmosphere. Some facilities use BIBS masks to treat injured divers, but it's not necessarily the best delivery method for patient use in the clinical environment. A complete system with mask, regulator, hoses, and connectors average in price from $1,000 and up.

Special Considerations

a) Facilities utilizing oxygen from a LOX system normally maintain a line pressure near 50 PSI. This is not enough pressure for BIBS masks to function normally when under pressure in the chamber. A demand regulator of this type ordinarily needs a line pressure of 50 PSI above chamber pressure. A high-pressure oxygen manifold system would fulfill this need. The manifold can regulate down the HP oxygen to a line pressure of 100 PSI, and this would act as a dedicated supply to the inside tender.

b) Most units have masks for each of their staff members. They should be cleaned per manufacturer recommendations. The regulators should also be part of a regular maintenance program and cleaned on a schedule recommended by the manufacturer. The regulator is sensitive and can freeflow or malfunction if foreign object debris (FOD) gets into the valves. One piece commonly overlooked is the quick-disconnect on the T-piece/mask interface. This is located directly in front of the tender's mouth when decompressing on BIBS and is a hot-spot for germ transfer.

c) The O-ring at the mask/regulator connection, as well as the regulator diaphragms, should be lightly lubed with oxygen safe grease. This will allow ease of mask connection and keep the components from drying.

Tracheal Cuff

The system design for a trach set is very similar to the mask. However, there needs to be added caution due to the limited area of dead space. Different connections to the trach can be used, but the two most common are using a trach shield or a respiratory T-piece connected directly to the patient. A trach shield can be uncomfortable and also leak treatment gas. The T-piece provides a snug fit directly on the trach itself, but the tender needs to be vigilant when connecting and removing the piece.

Special Considerations

a) Check valves are on either side of the T-piece to prevent inspiration of exhaled gas, ensuring the patient receives the appropriate dosage of the treatment gas.

b) Similar to a mask system, infection control and cleaning is very important. It is good policy to entirely replace the exhaust side of the mask on a routine basis to prevent bacteria growth and lung discharge accumulation in the 3-liter bag. Having the infection control department involved with the decision process is useful, but typically units will replace the exhaust at the end of each week.

c) Gas flow to the patient depends on the patient size, respiratory rate, and other factors. As a standard, keeping each 3-liter bag ¾ full usually suffices. Make small adjustments for patient comfort.

Ventilators

The majority of patients who are treated in hyperbaric units are stable, alert, and oriented and not dependent on life-saving equipment. However, there are few ICU patients who require ventilator support for respiratory failure who also need hyperbaric oxygen therapy. As with all the equipment used in conjunction with hyperbaric chambers, the specifications and regulations for a ventilator is no exception. Rigorous testing for safety is required prior to the use of a ventilator, either with a monoplace chamber or within a multiplace chamber. Patients requiring life-support equipment should always be under the constant surveillance of competent medical practitioners.

Over the years, a variety of ventilators have been modified for hyperbaric use. The first purpose-built hyperbaric vent was the Sechrist 500A pressure cycle vent, but this unit is discontinued. Other ventilators used under hyperbaric conditions include Siemens Servo 900C (although this was not a purpose-built ventilator for hyperbaric applications), Bird models, the Eagle Impact transport ventilator, and the Monaghan 225, but presently, the Atlantis is the only ventilator available on the market that is designed, built, and FDA 510(k)-cleared for the specific purpose of ventilating in a hyperbaric environment. When the Atlantis ventilator is used in both monoplace and multiplace hyperbaric chambers, the chambers are pressurized up to 6 atmospheres absolute (ATA).

Before the Atlantis received 510(k) clearance and was available on the market, hyperbaric practitioners and manufacturers were forced to modify existing ventilators for use with hyperbaric chambers. The use of a non-FDA-cleared ventilator creates several medical and legal issues for hyperbaric practitioners and administrators, such as performance reliability, insurance carrier notification requirements, trouble complying with accreditation standards, and the obligation to meet enhanced standards for informed patient consent.

When used in a monoplace setting, the control module is located outside the hyperbaric chamber and is connected to the chamber via a pass-through fitting located in the chamber door or bulkhead. The patient breathing circuit is located inside the chamber, where the tidal volume hose and exhalation valve driveline tubes are attached to the inner portion of the chamber door, using the same pass-through fittings. In a multiplace setting, the entire ventilator is permitted inside the chamber.

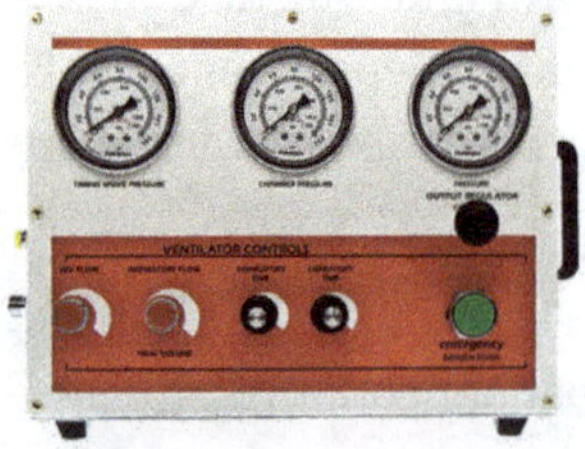

Figure 10. Atlantis BaroVent. Photo courtesy of Providence Global Medical, Holladay, UT.

Other ventilators would have the pneumatic component brought inside the chamber and electrical component outside and communicated via pass-throughs on the chamber hull.

Conclusion

Modern hyperbaric chamber breathing gas systems for clinical and diving applications are designed, manufactured, and installed with safety in mind. They include materials, features, and components specifically tested for oxygen compatibility and hyperbaric environments. Overall safety, however, still depends on a well-trained and educated operator or team with a thorough understanding of the BGS at their facility, following established procedures for safe operations.

References

1. NFPA. NFPA 99: Standard for Health Care Facilities, 2018 Edition. Quincy, MA: National Fire Protection Assn; 2018.
2. ASTM. ASTM G 72-01. Standard test method for autogenous ignition temperature of liquids and solids in a high-pressure oxygen-enriched environment. Philadelphia: American Society for Testing and Materials; 2001.
3. Barthelemy H, Vangard G. Ignition of PTFE-lined hoses in high-pressure oxygen systems: test results and considerations for safe design and use. In: Schroll DW, ed. Flammability and sensitivity of materials in oxygen-enriched atmospheres. Volume III, ASTM STP 986. Philadelphia, Penn: American Society for Testing and Materials; 1988:289-304.
4. Benz FJ, Williams RE, Armstrong D. Ignition of metals and alloys by high-velocity particles. In: Benning MA, ed. Flammability and sensitivity of materials in oxygen-enriched atmospheres. ASTM STP 910. Philadelphia, Penn: American Society for Testing and Materials. 1986:16-37.
5. Moffett GE, Pedley Md, Schmidt N, Williams RE, Hirsch D, Benz FJ. Ignition of non-metallic materials by impact of high-pressure gaseous oxygen. In: Schroll DW, ed. Flammability and sensitivity of materials in oxygen-enriched atmospheres. Volume III, ASTM STP 986. Philadelphia, Penn: American Society for Testing and Materials; 1988:218-232.
6. Werley BL. Oil film hazards in oxygen systems. In: Werley BL, ed. Flammability and sensitivity of materials in oxygen-enriched atmospheres. ASTM STP 812. Philadelphia, Penn: American Society for Testing and Materials; 1983:108-125.
7. Werley BL, ed. Fire hazards in oxygen systems. ASTM Committee G4.05 standards technology training coursebook. Philadelphia, Penn: American Society for Testing and Materials; 1990.

8. CGA. Cleaning equipment for oxygen service. Pamphlet CGA G-4.1-1985. Arlington, VA: Compressed Gas Association; 1985.
9. ASTM. ASTM G93, Standard guide for evaluating metals for oxygen service. Philadelphia, Penn: American Society for Testing and Materials; 1992.
10. ASTM. ASTM A269/A269M-15a, Standard specification for seamless and welded austenitic stainless-steel tubing for general service. ASTM International, West Conshohocken, PA; 2015.
11. ASTM. ASTM A213/A213M-18b, Standard specification for seamless ferritic and austenitic alloy-steel boiler, superheater, and heat-exchanger tubes. ASTM International: West Conshohocken, PA; 2018.
12. CGA. Handbook of Compressed Gases. Arlington, VA: Compressed Gas Association; 2013.
13. CGA. Standard color marking of compressed gas containers intended for medical use. Arlington, VA: Compressed Gas Association; 1988.
14. Reimers, SD. Flow dynamics of patient hoods. Reprinted from Proceedings of XIV Int'l Congress of Hyperbaric Medicine, 2002. Reimers Systems, Inc., Springfield, Virginia; 2002.
15. ASME. ASME PTC 25. Pressure Relief Devices, API 527. NY, NY:ASME. 2014.
16. US Navy. US Navy Diving Manual. 1991. Chapter 15: 15-17.
17. U.S. Department of Transportation. Washington, DC.

Bibliography

1. Butler GJ, Crowley WF, Rugh S, Desautels DA, Sullivan N. 1993 Apr. Accident risk assessment and safety training programs for clinical hyperbaric facilities. Presented at Gulf Coast Chapter, Undersea Hyperbaric Medical Society, Fort Lauderdale, FL.
2. Hamilton RW, chairman. 1992 Jan. Workshop findings: Evaluating enriched air ("nitrox") diving technology. Scuba Diving Resource Group: Boulder, CO.
3. NFPA 53: Recommended Practice on Materials, Equipment, and Systems Used in Oxygen-Enriched Atmospheres. Quincy, MA: National Fire Protection Association; 2016.
4. McFall G. NOAA Diving Manual. Sixth edition. North Palm Beach, FLA: Best Publishing Company. 2017.
5. Commercial Diving Operations, 29 CFR 1910, Subpart T. Washington: U.S. *Dept.* of Labor, Occupational Safety and Health Administration; 2011.
6. Overland T. Discussion by Mr. Terry Overland. In: Hamilton RW, Hulbert AW, Crosson OJ, eds. Harbor Branch workshop on enriched air nitrox diving. Technical Report 89-1. NOAA Office of Undersea Research: Rockville, MD; 1989.
7. Rollins JP, ed. Compressed air and gas handbook. Fifth edition. Englewood Cliffs, NJ: Prentice Hall PTR; 1989.

8. Schoenman L, Stoltzfus J, Kazaroff L. Friction-induced ignition of metals in high-pressure oxygen. In: Schroll DW, ed. Flammability and sensitivity of materials in oxygen-enriched atmospheres. Volume III. ASTM STP 986. Philadelphia, Penn: American Society for Testing and Materials; 1988:105-133.
9. Slack DS, Gault WS. Compressor-produced gas contaminants. In: Proceedings 1976 Divers' Gas Purity Symposium. Rept 7-76. Columbus,OH: Battelle Columbus Laboratories; 1976.
10. Sullivan GD. Evaluation of Bauer high pressure breathing air P-2 purification system. NEDU Report 10-91. Panama City, FL: Navy Experimental Diving Unit; 1991. AD A243535.
11. US Navy Department. US Navy Diving Manual. NAVSEA 0994-LP-001-9020. Volume 2, Revision 3. Washington DC: Navy Department; 1991.
12. Vann RD. Physiology of nitrox diving. In: Hamilton RW, Hulbert A W, Crosson OJ, eds. Harbor Branch workshop on enriched air nitrox diving. Technical Report 89-1. Rockville, MD: NOAA Undersea Research Program; 1989.
13. Wells JM. Nitrox diving within NOAA: History, applications and future. In: Hamilton RW, Hulbert A W, Crosson DJ, eds. Harbor Branch workshop on enriched air nitrox diving. Technical Report 89-1. Rockville, MD: NOAA Undersea Research Program; 1989.
14. Wells JM. Applications of atmospheric oxygen concentrators in the preparation of divers breathing media. In: MTS 90: Science and technology for a new ocean's decade. Vol 3. Washington: Marine Technology Society; 1990.

CHAPTER 4.4
Electrical Systems

Larry L. Wischhoefer, PE (Ret.)

The hyperbaric chamber environment imposes special demands on the safe use of electrical equipment. This chapter will explore factors that must be considered when electrical equipment is used in general situations and in the chamber environment. We will discuss how these factors influence creation of the codes and standards that govern the design and construction of hyperbaric electrical systems. The material covered is necessarily only a snapshot of the wide-ranging discipline of electrical systems. The reader is not expected to master hyperbaric electrical systems design and implementation; that is beyond the scope of this book and is best left to those who are experienced and licensed in electrical design and installation. The reader should gain an appreciation for the various elements that comprise an electrical system and of the importance of properly maintaining those elements.

Codes and Standards

ANSI/NFPA 70, National Electrical Code (NEC)[1] is a primary consensus standard governing many aspects of commercial and residential electrical design and construction practice in the United States. The *NEC* has been updated every few years since the first code document was published in 1897. The document covers the following: wiring design, protection, methods, and materials; equipment for general and special use; certain special conditions, occupancies, and equipment; and communications systems. To be sure, the National Fire Protection Association publishes many other documents that cover a wide range of situations requiring fire safety guidance. One of these is *NFPA 99, Standard for Health Care Facilities.*[2] *NFPA 99* Chapter 14: Hyperbaric Facilities treats the hyperbaric environment as a special occupancy from an electrical systems viewpoint, and specifies electrical requirements beyond those of the *NEC.* All references in the discussion that follows are based on the 2018 edition of *NFPA 99* unless otherwise noted.

The Hyperbaric Chamber as a Special Occupancy

What makes a hyperbaric chamber a special occupancy in electrical standards? Electricity is a source of ignition inside a chamber just as it is anywhere else. However, other things being equal, fires start more easily and spread more quickly in the elevated pressures and oxygen concentrations in hyperbaric chambers than in normal environments. The elevated oxygen atmosphere in a hyperbaric chamber is classified as an oxygen enriched atmosphere (OEA).[3] Next, hyperbaric chambers differ from most inhabited spaces in that the occupants cannot immediately exit in the event of an emergency. Fire inside a pressurized chamber could more likely result in serious injury or fatality. These and other factors make it necessary to impose extra layers of protection for electrical systems located within the chamber boundary. This chapter will examine hazards inherent in the use of electrical equipment in hyperbaric facilities and schemes and requirements developed to ensure that hyperbaric electrical systems are designed to an acceptable level of safety.

Electrical Safety Considerations

There are several hazards that must be considered in electrical systems design and safe use.

- Electric shock
- Physical burns from heated surfaces
- Fire from electrical ignition sources
- Explosion from electrical ignition sources
- Loss of critical hyperbaric functions

Electrical Safety Schemes

In general, methods of protecting against electrical hazards employ the following principles:

- Grounding
- Electric current limitation
- Physical isolation
- Physical containment

Electric Shock

Shock Principles

Electric shock occurs when a person is in simultaneous contact with two electrical conductors that are at different voltage potentials. The person acts as a conductive medium for the resulting electrical current. One of the conductors is generally, but not always, the ground or floor (often damp). The shock magnitude depends on numerous factors including the duration of contact with the conductors, the voltage difference between those conductors, the voltage frequency, and the amount of current available. Studies have shown that alternating current (AC) frequencies around 60 hertz usually produce the greatest shock effect, other factors being equal.

Shock Hazard Mechanisms

There are several ways that shock hazards arise in electrical equipment. One is from exposed live electrical circuits. Exposed circuits may be found inside electrical panels and boxes, or they may occur as a result of damage (frayed wires, electrical cords, bad plugs, etc.). A hazard can also occur when a live circuit contacts ungrounded equipment protective containment (casing, conduit, etc.). This is known as a short circuit or ground fault and can potentially turn the containment into an exposed live circuit. Another mechanism results from the buildup of electric charge from the atmosphere on isolated, ungrounded conductors. Static electricity can be a significant hazard in a hyperbaric environment and is discussed in Chapter 5.3: Static Electricity in this textbook.

Protection

Shock prevention is particularly important inside the cramped quarters of hyperbaric chambers, where it is easy to come into inadvertent contact with, and possibly damage, electrical equipment or cords. It is important to note that shock hazards inside the hyperbaric chamber also represent fire hazards, so it is essential to maintain the integrity of electrical equipment, devices, and grounding paths at all times. Because of this, the requirements for fixed wiring inside multiplace chambers is more robust than in normal areas. In addition, electrical conduit needs to be waterproof because of the required presence of a water deluge system for fire protection. Exposed conduit must be of the threaded metallic type, while conduit that is protected by physical barriers may be any waterproof type. Junction boxes, receptacles, and other enclosures must also be waterproof.

Burn Hazards

All electrical equipment emits heat to a varying extent. Some devices, light bulbs for example, operate normally at temperatures high enough to cause burns. Enclosures are used to protect against burn from hot-running electrical circuits in many devices. In some cases, equipment damage or malfunction can cause enough overheating to represent a burn hazard. It should also be noted that equipment hot enough to cause burns may also represent fire ignition sources, especially in the hyperbaric OEA. Hyperbaric codes limit the operational temperature rating of electrical equipment allowed inside the chamber. For multiplace chambers (*NFPA* 99-14.2.9.3.1.2), the limit is 85°C (185°F). For monoplace chambers (*NFPA* 99-14.2.9.6.3), where pure oxygen is likely the pressurizing medium and space is very confined, the limit is 50°C (122°F).

Fire From Electric Ignition Sources

Nature of Heat Source for Electrical Equipment

Sparking and hot surfaces are the two means by which electrical equipment can provide an ignition source for fire. Either of these conditions may occur in normally operating equipment or as the result of damage or wiring faults.

Sparking

Sparking, or arcing, occurs when electrical conductors of different voltage potential are in close proximity to one another. The voltage difference can cause electrons to jump the air gap between the conductors, resulting in the arc and a release of heat. The size and intensity of the arc depends on several factors, including the geometry of the conductors, conductor spacing, voltage difference, amount of electric current available, etc. The distance an arc can jump is generally proportional to the voltage difference. Lightning is probably the best known everyday example of an arc, involving millions of volts, thousands of feet of travel, and huge amounts of heat release. Examples of arcing in electrical equipment are as follows:

- Inserting or removing an electrical plug when the connected equipment is powered
- Opening or closing switch contacts in manual switches and in relays and motor starters
- Brushes in motor commutators
- Loose wiring connections
- Broken wires (especially hot wires) contacting other conductive surfaces

Hot Surfaces

Many electrical devices are, by their nature, hot enough during normal operation to pose an ignition hazard if they contact a fuel source. Such devices include light bulbs, hot plates, some motors, resistors, vacuum tubes, etc. Electrical fault conditions that can cause conductors and equipment to overheat to a dangerous level include the following:

- Overvoltage due to crossed or incorrectly connected wires.
- Overcurrent due to ground faults or stalled motor loads.
- Resistive heating in electrical switch contacts, joined wires, and wire terminations due to loose or corroded connections. Any mechanical joining of conductive surfaces will have a certain resistance. Since the heat dissipated by a resistance equals current squared times resistance (I^2R), the resistance of the connection needs to be as low as possible. Low resistance is a function of surface cleanliness, contact area, and the pressure holding the surfaces together. Poor wiring connections account for the majority of electrical problems. It is

important to ensure that terminal screws are properly tightened and that electrical circuits are properly protected from corrosive and dirty conditions.

Explosion from Electric Ignition Sources

General

Explosion can occur when an atmosphere containing a flammable gas or vapor comes into contact with a sufficiently energetic spark or sufficiently hot surface. The volume concentration of a gas or vapor in the air must exceed a value known as the lower explosive limit or LEL for the explosion hazard to exist. LEL is specific to each gas or vapor, as is the energy required to cause ignition. Places where explosive fuel mixtures might exist are classified as hazardous locations in *NFPA 497A*, which also defines classification criteria.[4] Hazardous locations are found in chemical plants, refineries and pipelines, paint shops, textile plants, coal mines, and many other places. Fuel in the vaporous form has the ability to migrate through the air via convection and diffusion and penetrate into electrical containment. Special construction methods are required for electrical equipment located in hazardous locations to prevent fire and explosion hazards. Methods include intrinsic safety, explosion proof enclosures, oil immersion, and purging. These methods are governed by standards for design and construction. Approval organizations such as UL (Underwriters Laboratories) and FM (Factory Mutual) use these standards to evaluate and list equipment for intended use. The standards are written to applications at one atmosphere pressure since that is where the equipment is used. The mining industry, where equipment may be exposed to elevated pressure atmospheres, has its own standards for electrical equipment. Since the hyperbaric chamber is no longer classified as a hazardous location as defined by code, these techniques will not be covered further here.

Applicability to Hyperbaric Facilities

The hyperbaric chamber *was* classified as a hazardous location for purposes of electrical design requirements for many years after the first hyperbaric standards were published. A review in the 1990s of electrical requirements led to the hazardous location classification being dropped in favor of recognition of the OEA, as the applicable criteria upon which to base hyperbaric electrical requirements. Under the OEA regime, solid fuels, not gaseous vapors, became the primary danger to guard against. This is much the same as in normal locations. However, the OEA and the restricted space and confinement of the hyperbaric environment still dictate a more robust approach for electrical requirements than is found for normal locations. Compared to the old regime, it is generally felt that the new requirements provide a more realistic framework by which hyperbaric patient treatment needs are balanced with the paramount requirement for safety.

Hazard Location Classification in the Hyperbaric Code

The hyperbaric code was written in the late 1960s in the aftermath of the *Apollo 1* fire that killed three astronauts. Medical procedures using flammable anesthetic gases had been performed in hyperbaric chambers up to that time. The first hyperbaric code and all subsequent ones banned the use of flammable anesthetics and other hazardous, flammable materials in chambers. However, it was felt that hazardous gases or vapors could not be kept out of the chamber with absolute certainty. For one thing, cleansing alcohol was used in the chamber. Oil-lubricated compressors were thought to be a potential source of volatile hydrocarbons, either oils or carbon monoxide. Additionally, it was felt that the potential existed for hazardous vapors to be present at the compressor air intake, despite the requirements that the air intake be placed away from potentially hazardous sources.

For reasons such as those above, multiplace chamber interiors were classified as a Class I, Division 1, Group C location for purposes of electrical installation.[4] Some of the requirements were copied word for word from the edition of *NFPA 56A, Inhalation Anesthetics,* that was in effect at that time. Hazardous area electrical equipment used in the chamber had to be rated for the effects of elevated pressures and oxygen levels found in hyperbaric atmospheres.

As mentioned previously, hazardous location equipment that was available on the market was intended for and utilized by industries that function in one atmosphere environments; it was not assured that such equipment would provide protection at the elevated pressures found in hyperbaric chambers. For example, explosive pressure varies roughly as the square of the pressure of the ambient atmosphere, meaning that explosion proof enclosures might not contain explosions in elevated pressure environments. Similar reasoning raised questions about the effectiveness of intrinsic safety in hyperbaric chambers. Furthermore, purging and oil immersion, while effective in theory, were expensive and in most cases, impractical to implement; the small clinical hyperbaric market could not support the cost to design, build, and test equipment for hyperbaric applications. Also, no research had been performed to establish the necessary criteria for testing and evaluating equipment for hazardous location hyperbaric conditions.

The UHMS supported a code overhaul effort in the 1980s that, among other things, attempted to address these issues. As a result, the 1993 edition of *NFPA 99, Hyperbaric Facilities,* contained revisions intended to ease some of these problems while maintaining an acceptable level of safety. The revisions can be summarized as follows:

- Equipment rated for Class I, Division 2 was allowed in the chamber if strict procedures were followed to prevent the entry of flammable agents into the chamber. This slightly expanded the selection of real world equipment available for use in the chamber.
- Intrinsically safe equipment had to meet Class I, Division 1, Group B requirements. Group B rating imposes stiffer requirements than does Group C, but the trade-off was dropping hyperbaric pressure and oxygen conditions.

- Explosion proof equipment was required to be listed for Class I, Division, 1, Group A or B locations. Again, ambient pressure and oxygen requirements were dropped by allowing equipment classified for more stringent (Group A or B) conditions.

The above changes made it easier for designers and installers to comply with the code in the case of fixed wiring and equipment inside the chamber. However, medical monitoring equipment would technically still have to be modified to be used in the multiplace chamber, potentially voiding FDA approval. Another problem was that intrinsically safe intercom equipment was not widely available. For these and other reasons, users were still forced to balance operational needs against the restrictions imposed by the code requirements.

Review of Hazard Location Classification

It was decided to reevaluate the basis for the hazardous location classification of multiplace hyperbaric chambers following adoption of the 1996 issue of *NFPA 99.* The criteria and examples of *NFPA-497A, Classification of Class I Hazardous Locations for Electrical Installations,* were used in the investigation.[4] The following were among the evaluation criteria:

- History of usage in the industry
- Availability of ventilation in enclosed spaces
- Types of potential liquids or vapors of concern
- Likelihood of explosive gas mixture in the chamber

Over 25 years of experience had been gained in hyperbaric operations since the original code adoption. There had been no reported incidents of fire or explosions in chambers due to flammable atmospheres. There had also been no reports of flammable air-gas mixtures in chambers equipped with hazardous gas monitors. Other considerations led to the conclusion that potential hazardous gases would be more of a toxicity hazard than an explosion hazard at hyperbaric treatment pressures.

- The LEL of hydrocarbons in air remains roughly constant over the range of hyperbaric treatment pressures.[5] This has been reiterated in theoretical and practical studies.
- NIOSH[6] publishes gas concentration limits called immediately dangerous to life or health (IDLH) for numerous gases. The IDLH for carbon monoxide is less than 1% of its LEL while the IDLH for isopropyl alcohol is 10% of its LEL. In addition, it can be stated with good confidence, when comparing LEL and IDLH of any flammable gas or vapor of interest, that these substances are toxic or irritating to humans well below their lower explosive limits (LEL).

Materials such as isopropyl alcohol, hairsprays, and flammable anesthetics were considered. It was found to be highly unlikely that these materials would be present in a chamber in quantities sufficient to form an explosive atmosphere. Aside from the toxicity hazard mentioned above, it would take least a pint of vaporized alcohol in most chambers at pressure to begin to pose a hazard (the lower explosive limit, LEL, for alcohol is about 2% by volume). Most facilities no longer use alcohol. Flammable anesthetics have been banned from use in chambers since the inception of the hyperbaric code and have been banned by The Joint Commission (TJC) from operating rooms in general for decades. It was also felt that mandated minimum chamber ventilation rates would also minimize concentration or stratification of gases within the chamber.

Air compressors were also considered, specifically the oil in oil-lubricated compressors. Oil is a flammable hydrocarbon. However, lubricating oils are not volatile below 200°F. Any oil vapor produced by heat of compression in the compressor cylinder would significantly condense in the cooler environment after discharge from the compressor. Oils do not represent a flammable gas hazard in any environment fit for human occupancy. Overheated compressors have been known to emit hydrocarbon byproducts, such as carbon monoxide. However, as stated above, carbon monoxide would become a deadly toxicity hazard long before it reached its LEL concentration in the chamber; toxicity is the reason that carbon monoxide monitors are required when oil-lubricated compressors supply air to the chamber.

A final concern was air drawn into the compressor intake. Air intakes must be located in open-air areas away from potential contaminants such as parking lots, gasoline engines, building exhausts, etc. Despite this, there have been incidents where gases from nearby asphalt laying operations, for example, have gotten into the air supply to the chamber. This, again, is more of a toxicity hazard than it is an explosion hazard. The compressor air intake would have to be located *in* a hazardous location in order to pick up a hazardous air-gas mixture. However, the experience of the API (American Petroleum Institute) and NFPA, as stated in their documents (e.g., *NFPA 497A*[4]), is that these agents would not be present in LEL concentrations in an open-air environment outside a *very* short distance (read 5 to 10 feet at most) from a culpable activity.

The conclusion drawn from the above review was that there is a negligible likelihood of a flammable or explosive gas mixture occurring in a multiplace chamber. In fact, the probability for hazardous gas mixtures being present is more on the order of that for normal areas. As a result, the hazardous area classification was dropped in favor of rules that recognize the well-studied hazards of elevated OEA in chambers. New rules, summarized later in this chapter, governing the installation and use of electrical equipment inside multiplace chambers were adopted for the 1999 issue *NFPA 99*. It is felt, based on the above analysis, that these rules better balance patient treatment needs with economics and equipment available in the market place without sacrificing safety.

Loss of Critical Hyperbaric Functions

Certain system functions are considered essential for the safe operation of a hyperbaric facility. These functions include chamber pressure control, intercommunications, and fire suppression. For example, loss of control of chamber pressure control could potentially result in personnel being locked in the chamber with no way to depressurize or result in uncontrolled rapid changes in pressure. Insofar as these functions rely on electrical power and equipment for their operation, remedial measures are required in the event that electric power is lost or equipment fails. The basic system design remediation principle is redundancy. Hyperbaric codes impose requirements for some form of functional redundancy. The redundant, or backup, function in general may only have to meet minimal requirements to safely finish a treatment schedule, depending on the types of treatments for which a facility is designed.

Grounding

Grounding is one of the most underappreciated and overlooked, yet most important, aspects of electrical systems. The NEC[1] deals with the subject at length for good reason. The ground system provides a path for electric current to dissipate safely into the earth in the event of an electrical fault or static charge buildup, thus preventing shock and spark hazards. A ground system also works in conjunction with electric current limiting devices to prevent overheating of wires and equipment. These are all *essential* fire prevention elements. A ground system consists of three elements: a ground, the grounded object(s), and a ground path.

A ground is essentially a large conductive object that can absorb a large amount of electric current with little change in its voltage potential. The voltage potential of the ground is usually at or near the voltage potential of the earth. This is because people are most often directly or indirectly in contact with the earth. For most applications the earth *is* the ground, hence the words "ground" and "earth ground." A ground also consists of electrically conductive medium in intimate contact with the earth that serves as a place to connect one end of the grounding path. The NEC carefully defines points that can serve as grounds. They include building steel structure, metal ground rods driven into the earth, metal grids buried in the earth, and steel water pipes. The use of water pipes has become restricted in recent years because of the practice of sometimes replacing pipe sections with nonconductive pipe, thus breaking the electrical path to earth.

Grounded objects include any electrically conductive surface in proximity to electrical circuits that a person could contact. These objects include metal enclosures mentioned above, hyperbaric chambers, etc. It is necessary that grounded objects remain at or near earth potential so that they cannot cause electrical shocks. This must be true even if a live electrical wire comes into contact with the object (short to ground).

A ground path is a low resistance connection between the ground and the grounded object. The ground path only conducts electrical current when there is a fault such as a short to ground. During such a fault, the voltage of the grounded object will rise in accordance with Ohm's law: $V_{object} = I_{fault} \times R_{path}$. The fault current, I_{fault}, can be many amperes and is limited only by the fusing in the upstream circuit. The grounding path resistance, R_{path}, must be an ohm or less to restrict the fault voltage to a low value that will minimize potential shock hazard. The resistance of the ground path is a function of the ground conductor and of the quality of the electrical connections in that conductor. Electrical connections must therefore use approved (e.g., UL) devices and methods. The mating surfaces must be clean. A good connection should have no more than a fraction of an ohm resistance. A poor or dirty connection may measure several ohms and result in a nonfunctional ground.

The ground path is usually a conductive wire or strap but can also be the metal conduit that protects the electrical wires. The most reliable path is generally the one with the fewest connections. Connections represent the most common source of faults in electrical circuits. Pipe joints in electrical conduit represent connections. Thus, special rules (NEC) apply for conduit installation if the conduit is the only ground path. It is important that the integrity of the conduit system be maintained in such cases. Wires used in grounding must be large enough to handle any potential fault current. The maximum fault current is usually governed by the amperage rating of the fuse in the associated electrical circuit. Ground wires may be bare (uninsulated) or insulated. Insulated ground wires must, by code, be identified by green insulation or have green banding at regular intervals.

Measuring Chamber Ground Resistance

General

The importance of grounding chamber hulls (monoplace and multiplace) needs to be stressed, given the need for hazard prevention in the OEA. This *especially* applies to monoplace chambers with their pure oxygen atmospheres and lack of fire suppression systems. It is suggested that ground integrity be checked at frequent intervals. A simple technique is presented here which should make this easy to do. The resistance of the chamber ground is mandated to be one ohm or less. Measurements in low resistance circuits of this nature require great care, since several unexpected factors can introduce small measurement errors that might indicate unacceptable results in an otherwise good ground path.

It is important to note that the one ohm resistance limit *only* encompasses the resistance between the chamber metal and its ground wire (the chamber connection), plus chamber ground wire resistance, plus resistance between the ground wire and the approved ground (the ground connection). The actual resistance in a structurally sound ground wire contributes a negligible amount of resistance in the ground path. For instance, 100 ft of #8 AWG (American wire gage) copper wire has a resistance of only about 0.064 ohms. Furthermore, the resistance in a clean, well-made electrical connection should be only .1 ohm to a few tenths of an ohm; the 1 ohm limitation is then, in effect, a requirement that all ground *connections* between the chamber hull and the ground point be in good condition. Note that ground integrity measurements should *not* be made between the chamber hull and a ground point *other than* where the chamber ground wire connects to the approved ground point; one might then be adding resistances from electrical connections that are *not* in the direct chamber ground path.

A Simple Measurement Method

The preceding discussion suggests that measuring the resistances of the connections in the direct chamber ground path should give a good indication of chamber ground integrity, assuming that the ground wire is in good condition. Use a digital multimeter in the following simple procedure to do this.

- Check the resistance reading with the multimeter probes firmly in contact with one another. This reading (normally 0.1-0.4 ohm) should be subtracted from each reading taken below to eliminate probe contact resistance from the connection measurement.
- At the mechanical connection points mentioned above, touch the meter probes firmly to the bare ground wire and to the adjacent structural metal (i.e. chamber metal at the chamber or ground metal at the grounded end of the wire). A good mechanical connection should have a resistance ranging from about 0.1 ohm to a few tenths ohm. Include measurements from any other connections in the ground wire path, if necessary (not usual).
- Resistance measurements obtained in this manner using the relatively short probes on most multimeters should preclude the possibility of measurement error due to any electromagnetic interference that might be present.
- Add the derived values for all connections to yield the nominal chamber ground resistance. If resistance values seem too high, check that the wire connections are clean and properly made. Consult an electrician, if necessary, to correct any problem that can't be easily resolved.

Electric Current Limitation

Current limiting is employed in conjunction with grounding in electrical systems to guard against overheating and electrical fault conditions. Overcurrent devices are designed to limit the current in downstream circuits and equipment to safe values by opening the electrical circuit when the current exceeds the device's rated value for a specified period of time. Overcurrent protection, grounding, wire sizing, and other protection techniques are covered in *NFPA 70* (NEC), Chapter 2: Wiring Design and Protection, and Article 430: Motors, Motor Circuits, and Controllers.[1] The selection and application of current limiting devices is best left to knowledgeable engineers and electricians.

Current limiting devices include fuses, circuit breakers, surge arrestors, ground fault protectors, motor overload devices, motor thermal protective devices, etc. Circuit breakers, for example, are designed to prevent fire hazard from overheated wiring by limiting the current that can flow in the protected wire. Another type of limiting device applicable to hyperbaric electrical design is the ground fault (circuit) interrupter or GFCI. This circuit, familiar in residential use as electrical receptacles required near water sources such as sinks and showers, is designed to shut off power to connected devices if a ground fault exceeding 3-6 milliamps is sensed, guarding against electric shock. It is felt that this also protects against fire in the OEA by limiting potential spark energy from faults in protected circuits to safe levels.

Intrinsic safety is another concept that has found use in hyperbaric systems design. Intrinsic safety seeks to limit the electrical energy in a given circuit to a value incapable of igniting specific hazardous gas-air mixtures when electrical faults occur in the protected circuit. The protective circuit is designed to guard against short circuits, open circuits, and application of overvoltage. ANSI/UL 913, *Standard for Intrinsically Safe Apparatus and Associated Apparatus for Use in Class I, II, and III, Division I, Hazardous (Classified) Locations,* presents criteria for equipment design and construction and gives limiting currents for various hazardous atmospheres and circuit configurations.[7] The intrinsic safety concepts were developed for the chemical industry where flammable, explosive gases are often present. Consequently, the current limits are generally fairly low, making intrinsically safe devices applicable in the OEA. Intrinsically safe equipment is limited to low energy devices such as passive switches, small solenoids and actuators, sensors, intercom components, etc. Intrinsically safe equipment may be installed in any type of enclosure otherwise suitable for the environmental conditions expected. Intrinsically safe wiring is required to be isolated from nonintrinsically safe wiring (ISA-RP12.6, *Installation of Intrinsically Safe Instrument Systems in Hazardous [Classified] Locations*).[8]

Physical Isolation

Containment

Electrical circuits are isolated from their physical surroundings by various types of enclosures. Virtually all electrical circuits are enclosed in some manner or other. Enclosures protect electric circuits and equipment from physical damage, guard against electric shock, prevent or hamper the spread of fires generated by circuit faults, and prevent electric arcs emitted from normal or faulty circuit operation from reaching fuel outside the enclosure. Enclosure types include wire and cord insulation, conduits and cableways, junction boxes, electrical panels, motor enclosures, equipment chassis, cabinets, control consoles, etc., as mentioned previously in the discussion on shock protection. *NFPA 70* (NEC), Chapter 3: Wiring Methods and Materials, specifies most enclosure and protective techniques.[1]

Enclosures may be constructed of either electrically conductive or nonconductive (insulating) materials. If the material is electrically conductive, it must be physically connected to the electrical ground system. This is why, for example, the electrical plug for a plastic-encased hand tool will not have a ground prong (two-pronged plug), while a metal encased tool will have a three-pronged, grounding plug.

Recessing

Some devices cannot be totally enclosed. Many motors and tools, for example, must have openings in their cases to allow for circulation of cooling air. In electrical receptacles, which *supply* power, the *female* electrical contacts are recessed behind a nonconductive, slotted face in the receptacle. The mating *male* plug/cord set is connected to the device that is to *receive* power. The exposed prongs of an unconnected plug cannot, therefore, have any voltage by which to cause a shock or spark hazard. This is an important principle of electrical construction: When using male and female electrical connectors, the female connector must be on the side of the power source and the male connector must be connected to the device that is to receive power. Modern terminal blocks are also designed whereby the screw terminals and wire receptacles are recessed in an insulating block. In all of these cases and others, the enclosure opening must be small enough to prevent intrusion of fingers to protect against shock, and live circuits must be recessed far enough that potential sparks (e.g., from connecting or disconnecting power plugs) cannot reach the outside environment and potentially initiate a fire.

Maintenance

The need to maintain the protective envelope of the electrical system must be appreciated. *Devices which are improperly installed, not maintained, or otherwise misused or damaged are unsafe.* Potential shock and fire hazard from poorly maintained equipment is increased and the functional reliability of the associated system is degraded. This applies especially inside the hyperbaric chamber where the consequences of fire are more serious than in normal locations.

Physical Containment

The term physical containment is used here in the sense of equipment enclosures designed to contain fire or explosion that might occur in the enclosed electrical equipment. This concept is found in hazardous area classifications where flammable or explosive vapors might be present. Since hyperbaric chambers are no longer classified as hazardous location by the criteria of *NFPA 497A*[4], this method is only mentioned in passing.

Hyperbaric Chamber Electrical Requirements

Multiplace Chambers

Current rules assume that potential fuel sources in the chamber are materials that cannot migrate into electrical circuits and equipment, similar to normal locations. There are certain characteristics that distinguish the oxygen enriched hyperbaric environment from normal areas.

- Lower ignition energy of materials in hyperbaric atmosphere
- Increased burning and flame spread rate in hyperbaric atmosphere
- Inability of chamber occupants to immediately exit chamber when necessary
- Limited chamber space exposes equipment to increased potential of physical abuse

These conditions increase the danger from fire and thus necessitate protective measures beyond those employed in normal locations for electrical equipment installed and used in the chamber. These measures are specified in *NFPA 99*-14.2.9.3. The basic principles followed in these rules is similar to, but more conservative than, rules for normal areas. The rules are summarized as follows:

- Equipment must operate safely at chamber operational pressures without failing.
- Only equipment needed for the procedure at hand is allowed in the chamber.
- Power control devices in the fixed electrical system, including overcurrent devices, motor controllers, relays, ballasts, panels, etc., must be located outside of the chamber. This is in keeping with the philosophy of limiting electrical equipment inside the chamber to the minimum necessary to perform required functions, to limit the number of potential problems.
- Signs must be posted prohibiting introduction of flammable liquids, gases, and other materials into the chamber.
- Permanently installed wiring must have flame-resistant insulation. Teflon generally meets this requirement.
- Threaded metal conduit and watertight methods are required for fixed wiring where exposed to physical contact. Liquid tight metal conduit may be used where guarded from physical harm. Intrinsically safe wiring techniques are allowed for intrinsically safe circuits. The presence of a water deluge system drives the watertight requirement.
- Cord connected devices rated at less than two amperes may use their normal cords if steps are taken to secure the cord out of traffic and the cord is otherwise protected from abuse. Otherwise, modifications need to be made to equipment to use cords and plugs rated for extra hard usage; these cords have special heavy-duty insulation.
- Receptacles must be waterproof with ground connection and must be supplied from isolated power circuits with ground fault monitoring. Provisions must be taken to ensure that the mating plug is not inserted or withdrawn under electrical load.

- Switches must be rated waterproof.
- Temperature of electrical devices is limited to less than 85°C (185°F) for fire and personnel burn protection.
- Requirements for lighting installed *inside* the chamber have been consolidated. Purging is not required for fixtures, but they must be rated for Class I, Division 2 areas with appropriate lens guards.
- The hazard location requirements no longer apply to low voltage, low power, installed equipment. Intrinsically safe devices are still allowed and are encouraged, where applicable. Such equipment must be isolated from mains power by design or by added means such as opto-isolation, etc. Exposed cables (e.g., headset cables and sensor leads) are limited to 28 volt, ½ amp circuits. Chamber speakers must have completely enclosed wiring and are limited to 28 volts and 25 watts.
- Electrical requirements have been added for the use of "Patient Care Related Electrical Appliances." These devices must meet design, construction, and maintenance requirements intended in *NFPA 99* (starting with the 2012 edition) Chapter 10: Electrical Equipment. Equipment utilizing oxygen must be designed to prevent the oxygen from contacting its electrical circuitry. Cord-connected devices must have an on-off switch, be rated 120 volts, 2 amps or less, or be inert-gas purged.
- Battery-operated devices are limited to 12 volts and 48 watts.
- Batteries must be sealed, nonoff-gassing types suitable for the chamber pressure, and must not undergo charging or replacement while in the chamber. The batteries must be fully enclosed and secured within the device. Lithium and Lithium ion batteries are generally prohibited from chambers (starting with the 2012 edition). The reported primary causes of battery overheating and resultant hazards (including explosions) are shorting of battery terminals and overcharging from faulty chargers or from chargers not designed for the battery type. This is why the rules do not allow changing or charging the batteries inside the chamber. While properly designed and operating battery chargers would be expected to pose no potential for overcharging a battery, it is faulty conditions that represent potential hazards.

Monoplace Chambers

The rules for monoplace chambers are far more restrictive than for multiplace chambers for the following reasons:

- Most monoplace chambers are pressurized with pure oxygen. This presents increased fire hazard when compared to a pressurized air environment.
- To date, *NFPA 99* has not required a fire suppression system in monoplace

chambers. This results from the limited space in the chamber and that fires spread so fast in the oxygen environment.

- The restricted volume of monoplace chambers does not allow for the presence of an attendant who could operate equipment or controls inside the chamber. This precludes the need for equipment and the accompanying rules located inside the chamber.

The rules in *NFPA 99*-14.2.9.6 Additional Wiring and Equipments Requirements Inside Class B Chambers are summarized below:

- Only intercom functions and patient monitoring leads connected to equipment *outside* the chamber are permitted inside the chamber.
- Electrical circuits are limited to 28 volts and 4 watts under normal *or* fault conditions. These are values that are within those that have been found safe by testing in pressurized pure oxygen environments.[9]
- Patient monitoring leads must be connected to approved electromedical apparatus. Such apparatus is designed to limit fault current and voltage for patient safety to levels also commensurate with fire safety in the pure oxygen atmosphere.
- Lighting inside the chamber must be from sources located outside the chamber. That monoplace chamber hulls are a least partly acrylic makes it easy to accommodate this rule.
- Temperature of materials and electrical circuits are restricted to 50°C (122°F) inside the chamber. This temperature is sufficient to accommodate, for example, a transcutaneous monitor.

Chamber and patient grounding is another extremely important point that must be considered in connection with monoplace chambers. This is discussed in Chapter 5.3: Static Electricity.

Facility Operational Safety

Facility operational safety is defined here to encompass the design of the hyperbaric facility support systems which ensure the safety and comfort of the patients and operating personnel during operation of the chamber. Many patients are in an infirm state and cannot tolerate physical or mental stress as well as healthy people can. Insofar as the electrical systems are involved in chamber support functions, it is necessary to achieve a necessary degree of reliability to protect patients and chamber operational personnel. The hyperbaric electrical code addresses such issues. A few of these are covered below (paragraph references are *NFPA 99*, 2018 edition):

- Chamber operators must be in constant visual and aural communication with the chamber interior to ensure the safety of the chamber occupants. *NFPA*

99-14.2.10.2.1 requires an intercom system. *NFPA* 99-14.2.10.2.2 requires a closed-circuit TV unless the outside operators can adequately view the chamber interior from their normal operational location.

- Chamber oxygen levels must be monitored whenever breathing mixtures containing elevated oxygen levels are used (*NFPA* 99-14.2.10.4) to guard against elevated oxygen levels in the chamber (increasing fire hazard) and whenever nitrogen or diluting gases are used to guard against low oxygen concentrations (an asphyxiation hazard).
- Chambers must be monitored for carbon dioxide levels whenever ventilation is *not* used, e.g., during saturation diving operations (*NFPA* 99-14.2.10.5).
- Electrical power outages must not pose a hazard to chamber occupants. The hyperbaric facility is required to have a backup power source in addition to the normal power from the electric utility (*NFPA* 99-14.2.9.2).

Electrical Service

Backup power is needed for hyperbaric facilities to ensure that critical life support functions are not interrupted during a power outage of the normal utility service. The requirements for backup power systems in health care facilities are given in *NFPA 99* (2018 edition), Chapter 6: Electrical Systems. The primary backup system components are a prime mover generator or generators, transfer switching equipment, and branch circuits. The size and complexity of the system depend on the facility and loads served. The electrical loads served by the backup power are generally limited to essential functions. Backup systems are thus called essential electrical systems.

Essential electrical systems are subdivided into separate subsystems that serve specific types of loads. The equipment system, or equipment branch, serves major electrical equipment including motors and other heavy loads. Such loads generally have high starting currents. The loads must be coordinated when they come online after a power outage so the generator is not overloaded. Thus, up to one minute is allowed for the restoration of power to equipment branch loads. The emergency system serves those functions of patient care depending on lighting and appliances. The emergency system is divided into two mandatory branches: the life safety branch and the critical branch. The life safety branch serves illumination for emergency building exit, exit signs, alarm systems including fire alarms, hospital emergency communication systems, etc. The critical branch serves numerous functions for task illumination, fixed equipment, selected receptacles, and specified functions related to patient care. Backup power should normally be restored to the emergency system within 10 seconds of a power outage.

Hyperbaric facility electric motor-driven compressors must be connected to the equipment system unless the air plant has sufficient stored air reserve capacity to maintain chamber pressure and ventilation (*NFPA* 99-14.2.9.2.4 through *NFPA* 99-14.2.9.2.6). Chamber atmosphere control equipment must also be connected to the equipment branch.

Other hyperbaric facility life support and safety functions are required to be connected to the critical branch (*NFPA 99*-14.2.9.2.3.2). These include chamber receptacles, chamber emergency lighting, intercom, alarm systems, fire suppression controls and equipment, some room lighting, and chamber pressure and ventilation controls. Control system design must prevent hazardous conditions such as loss of chamber pressure control, spurious alarms, deluge activation, etc., during power interruption or restoration (*NFPA 99*-14.2.9.2.1.1), i.e. between the time normal power goes out and backup power comes on and vice-versa. For example, pressure control valves, if dependant on electrical power, should fail closed on loss of power; failing open would cause uncontrolled pressure excursion. This comes under the category of good design practice and may be overlooked in systems design. The use of short-term battery-backed power (uninterruptible power supply [UPS] or standby power supply [SPS]) for selected functions is one method used to accomplish this objective. Even a small UPS can support intercom, control systems, and other small important electrical loads for the short amount of time that it takes for backup power to come online.

Maintenance of Hyperbaric Electrical Systems

The following list presents items that should be included in any electrical preventive maintenance program. The list is not meant to be exhaustive. It is based on years of observations in hyperbaric and other facilities of common electrical safety problem areas. *Particular care must be paid to electrical systems inside chambers* as mentioned previously. Many problems are easily correctable by the hyperbaric technician. Vigilance is required by all chamber operational personnel to recognize problems and undertake corrective actions before serious consequences arise. Electricians, engineers, or other knowledgeable individuals should be called upon when there is any doubt about the best course of action.

- Receptacles, switches, junction boxes, wireways, and electrical cabinets must have their covers secured or their doors closed at all times except when maintenance access is required. It is surprising how many fires are caused by electrical boxes being left open. It is equally distressing to find boxes without cover plates in too many facilities. Replacing a cover plate is an example of a large gain in safety at the expenditure of small cost and effort.
- Permanently installed wiring must be protected from physical hazard in accordance with the NEC. Cords for portable equipment should be kept out of harm's way. Special precautions must be taken to protect cords inside chambers. *Never* use equipment with a damaged cord.
- Wire connections are one of the primary sources of electrical problems. Connections must be properly made. Screw-down terminals can become loose, causing overheating when passing electrical current. Some connections may corrode and cause local overheating.

- Conduit and wireways protect wiring and must be properly installed. The integrity of conduit joints must be maintained. Some joining methods (e.g., threaded) are more robust and reliable than others (e.g., screw clamp), albeit more expensive.
- Use only the fuses intended for the purpose. Never substitute another fuse size or type unless approved by a knowledgeable (preferably licensed) individual.
- Maintain all equipment and instrument grounds in good working order. Pay particular attention to ground connection points. If in doubt about the condition of a ground, check that the path resistance is on the order of an ohm or less; otherwise, consult an electrician.
- Use only properly maintained and functioning equipment (which otherwise meets code requirements) inside the chamber. The hospital bioengineers are often the ones who maintain medical apparatus. Consult an experienced, knowledgeable person if in doubt about a particular application. Such people can often find a way to safely accomplish an objective that might not be otherwise apparent.
- Make certain that hot objects are kept out of the chamber interior. Anything too hot to touch should not be in the chamber.
- Follow preventive maintenance procedures on all equipment used inside chambers. The chamber is no place for equipment failure or malfunction. Incorporate manufacturers' recommended maintenance procedures and schedules for their equipment into the facility maintenance program.

Fire Prevention

The following general discussion is meant to present background knowledge for understanding and recognizing fire hazards from the use of electrical equipment in the hyperbaric environment.

Fire Principles

Fire is the result of an exothermic (heat-producing) chemical reaction. Such a reaction generally occurs when fuel, in the presence of an atmosphere containing oxygen, comes into contact with a source of heat. If the reaction produces sufficient heat and there is enough fuel and oxygen, the reaction can become self-sustaining, releasing heat, light, and pressure rise. With certain fuels such as gasoline vapors, hydrogen, acetylene, dynamite, etc., the reaction proceeds so rapidly that an explosive pressure wave is produced in addition to heat. This is known as detonation and can produce greater damage than fire. Numerous factors interact and affect the ease with which fire can start and the rapidity with which it can spread: type and quantity of fuel, fuel configuration, ambient oxygen concentration and partial pressure, and the nature of the heat source.

Fuels

Fuels can exist in the solid, liquid, or gaseous (vapor) phase. However, combustion most commonly occurs in the vapor phase. Thus, sufficient thermal energy must first be imparted to most solids and liquids to convert part of them to a vapor in order to initiate combustion. For such solids and liquids, the amount of heat needed to cause sustainable combustion is generally higher than it is for gaseous substances. Some liquids such as alcohol, gasoline, etc., are volatile. Volatile liquids can produce vapors (at room temperature) in the atmosphere in sufficient concentration to support combustion (usually explosive) with very little heat input.

Fuel Configuration

Some forms of solid fuels ignite more easily than others. For instance, loose strands of cotton fibers can ignite with very little heat input, whereas cotton textile fabrics containing no nap require a great deal more energy for ignition. Another classic example is when a paper cup filled with water will not ignite when held over the flame of a Bunsen burner because the water acts as a heat sink. The empty paper cup, of course, ignites easily. By the same token, paint properly adhered to the surface of a metal recompression chamber will generally not be a source of self-sustaining combustion due to the large heat absorption capacity of the metal.

Flammable gas vapors and dusts represent the most easily ignited fuels since they are so intimately mixed with the oxygen molecules in the atmosphere. Such fuels can spread to potential ignition areas by the natural processes of diffusion and atmospheric convection. Certain metals, coal, grain, starches, flours, and textiles can give rise to hazardous dusts.

Conclusion

After a hyperbaric facility is designed and built to standards that ensure a basic level of safety and reliability, it is up to those who run the facility to maintain and uphold those standards. All those who work in and around the chamber should have some knowledge of electrical hazards and their remedies. They should use that knowledge to remain vigilant for problems that arise in electrical equipment and wiring systems, to promptly report those problems, and to see that they are corrected.

References

1. ANSI/NFPA. NFPA 70-2017, National Electrical Code. Quincy, MA: National Fire Protection Association; 2017.
2. NFPA. NFPA 99-2018, Standard for Health Care Facilities. Quincy, MA: National Fire Protection Association; 2018.
3. NFPA. NFPA 53M-1990, Manual on Fire Hazards in Oxygen-Enriched

Atmospheres. Quincy, MA: National Fire Protection Association; 1990.
4. NFPA. NFPA 497A-1975, Class I Hazardous Locations for Electrical Installations in Chemical Plants. Quincy, MA: National Fire Protection Association; 1975.
5. Gexcon AS. Gas Explosion Handbook. Chapter 4.1: Flammability Limits. Available from: http://www.gexcon.com/handbook/GEXHBchap4.htm.
6. NIOSH Publication. Immediately Dangerous to Life or Health (IDLH) Values. 2014. Available from: http://www.cdc.gov/niosh/idlh/intridl4.html.
7. ANSI/UL. ANSI/UL 913, Standard for Intrinsically Safe Apparatus and Associated Apparatus for Use in Class I, II, and III, Division I, Hazardous (Classified) Locations. Northbrook, IL: Underwriters Lab.
8. ISA. ISA-RP12.6, Installation of Intrinsically Safe Instrument Systems in Hazardous (Classified) Locations. Research Triangle Park, NC: International Society for Automation.
9. Radiometer A/S. Safety Requirements for Electronic Sensors in Oxygen Enriched Atmosphere at Pressures up to 4 atm. [3 bar]. Brea, CA: Radiometer A/S.

Bibliography

1. NFPA. NFPA 56A-1971, Standard for the Use of Inhalation Anesthetics. Quincy, MA: National Fire Protection Association; 1971.
2. NFPA. NFPA 99-1993, Standard for Health Care Facilities. Quincy, MA: National Fire Protection Association; 1993.
3. Liptak BG, ed. Instrument Engineers Handbook, Process Measurement and Analysis, Chapter 7.3, Electrical and Intrinsic Safety. 3d ed. Radnor, PA: Chilton; 1995.
4. API. American Petroleum Institute 500A, Recommended Practice for Classification of Areas for Electrical Installations in Petroleum Refineries. 3d ed. Washington, DC: API; April 1966 (reaffirmed 1973).
5. Matheson Trigas, Inc. Lower and Upper Explosive Limits for Flammable Gases and Vapors (LEL/UEL). Matheson. Available from: https://www.mathesongas.com/pdfs/products/Lower-(LEL)-&-Upper-(UEL)-Explosive-Limits-.pdf.

CHAPTER 4.5
Fire Protection Systems

William C. Gearhart, BS, CHT, EMT, CRT, RCP, CFPS, FI 1, FI 2

The information contained in this second edition supplements the first edition and focuses on some of the advances in both hyperbaric medicine and fire protection as related to hyperbaric chambers. First, we should review some of the first edition information, which concentrated on an overview, design elements, maintenance, impairment programs and most importantly, fire prevention.

Fire protection systems are needed for use in multiplace hyperbaric chambers, with the necessity of these systems to be fixed in place, water supplied, properly designed, and maintained.

With the expanded delivery of hyperbaric medicine, the regulatory organizations of both health care and fire/life safety have become more aware and involved in oversight of hyperbaric facilities. These organizations share a common interest of protecting life and property and accomplish this mission through recognizing, adopting, and enforcing codes and standards relevant to life safety in the health care environment.

The development of fire protection codes and standards has long been a process of reaction to incidents, which have resulted in loss of life and property. Initial editions of codes and standards and their subsequent editions are based on knowledge and experience derived from situations many of which are rooted in tragic loss of life and extensive property damage.

While the requirements for the environment of care for the facility housing the hyperbaric medicine department are well documented with codes and standards, the actual multiplace chamber equipment also has requirements specifically detailing fire protection system standards. At this time, monoplace hyperbaric chambers are not universally included in the requirement for internal fire protection systems. However, this concept is changing.

Perhaps one of the most tragic hyperbaric chamber fire protection incidents comprising both fire-related fatalities and property damage occurred in Milan, Italy, in 1997. This incident resulted in the death of 11 individuals, 10 patients, and 1 staff member, all of whom were inside a multiplace chamber when ignition occurred, resulting in a rapidly spreading fire due to the increased concentration of oxygen, even though the chamber was designed as an air environment. Details of the incident lend important information regarding oxygen concentration, (percentage of oxygen), oxygen partial pressure, (PPO_2), ignition sources, etc.

What is especially relevant about this incident, with regard to life safety and fire protection, is the installed fire protection system was not operational at the time of the fire. Recognized procedures for safe operation of a multiplace hyperbaric chamber require that the fire protection system be in service or operational prior to and during compression of a multiplace hyperbaric chamber while it has human occupancy.

Multiplace Hyperbaric Chamber Fires – Two Incidents

With regard to fire protection systems, there are two hyperbaric chamber fires that represent both success and failure of the fire protection systems.

First is the aforementioned tragic incident in Milan, Italy, in 1997. The fire protection system was out of service (impaired), and yet the facility leadership allowed the chamber to be occupied and compressed. The details of allowing street clothing, ignition sources, contraband, etc., while contributory, are not part of this discussion.

What is important to this chapter is that the fire protection system was not being properly maintained and that it was out of service (impaired), while the chamber was being utilized for the delivery of patient care.

Maintenance of all systems is important, especially the fire protection system, which serves as a safeguard to life safety.

Second is a fire incident which occurred in a multiplace chamber in Pennsylvania when folded and microwave-heated blankets were introduced into the chamber through the medical lock. The blankets, which had been heated in a microwave device, were smoldering in their internal folds. When introduced into the increased oxygen partial pressure of the air-filled chamber, the smoldering combustible material began to burn more freely.

The inside attendant activated the internal fire protection system, which functioned and suppressed the fire. This would be considered a successful performance of the fire suppression system.

However, it should also be noted that several months later, in the same chamber, during a scheduled test of the fire protection system, the system failed to function. The lesson learned here is that mechanical systems are prone to failure or nonfunctionality despite maintenance, inspection, and testing.

Therefore, while we rely on the performance of these systems, we must always be aware that their operation is not guaranteed, and we should have backup systems in place. Redundant systems or systems not subject to single-point failure must be designed and installed, tested and maintained, and most importantly, work in conjunction with our fire prevention plans of minimizing potential hazards.

Inspection, Testing, and Maintenance Qualifications

The National Fire Protection Association (NFPA) standard for the inspection, testing, and maintenance of water-based fire protection systems is *NFPA 25*. This document has a section, which paraphrased, says that a service program should be provided by a qualified contractor or qualified property owner's representative in which all components unique to the property's system are inspected and tested at the required times and necessary maintenance is provided.[1]

One particular aspect of this requirement is qualified contractor, and that provision is often being stipulated by the authority having jurisdiction (AHJ), meaning licensed. In the United States, more AHJs, often at the state level, are requiring companies and individuals performing work on fire protection systems to be licensed within their working territory or domain.

Also, in conjunction with this requirement, is the increased professional qualification of personnel performing work on fire protection systems to earn and hold current certifications devoted to knowledge associated with fire protection systems. One of the most common certifications in the United States is the NICET (National Institute for Certification in Engineering Technologies). NICET offers several fire protection certifications under their Electrical and Mechanical Systems Engineering Technology Program.

When a hyperbaric facility is engaging a company to render contractor service for inspection, testing, and maintenance of their multiplace chamber fire protection system, it would be appropriate to engage a company that employs personnel holding appropriate NICET level certifications. Two of the most applicable certifications for hyperbaric facilities would be the certifications for inspection and testing of water-based systems and inspection and testing of fire alarm systems. Also, whenever possible, it would be advisable to develop a relationship with a company that has a fire protection engineer either on staff or available, if engineering questions come into question.

Utilizing a contractor holding these types of certifications makes it clear to reviewing and oversight AHJs, such as regulatory agencies including but not limited to local and state fire marshal offices, the Center for Medicare/Medicaid Services (CMS), insurance companies and others, that the hyperbaric facility is raising its own bar to a level of excellence.

Documentation

At the time of new construction or whenever a major renovation of the fire protection system is completed, all documentation pertaining to design parameters, inspection, and testing and the use and occupancy certificate should be retained on file. *NFPA 25* provides for electronic storage of these records.[2]

Another important factor to consider is obtaining a separate set of the fire protection system plans and specifications, hydraulic calculations, and cut sheets for components and placing them inside a PVC tube with the ends sealed by threaded fittings.

Often times, a 2-3" diameter piece of PVC will serve this mission. The PVC tube should be lettered and labeled, indicating the contents of the tube. The tube should be securely fastened to a major component of the fire protection system for safekeeping.

In the event of loss of the electronic file storage data, the original documentation will be available from this water-tight storage container. This simple but highly effective storage system will serve the hyperbaric facility safety director well, if he or she needs to view the original documentation. [3]

Testing Procedures

There are several basic concepts associated with the testing of the multiplace hyperbaric chamber fire protection system.The following is not meant to be a detailed procedural script but rather a conceptual approach of the essential elements. The facility safety director should develop his or her own policies and procedures, which may be unique to that facility.

First is preparation. One of the most important factors is to alert the necessary departments and personnel that a test is to be conducted. This should involve notifying the fire alarm supervisory service so that they are prepared to receive and document the incoming signals but not to alert responding units as they would for an emergency call. The usual procedure is to ask the supervisory service to monitor the incoming signals but to take the system off line and not to alert responding units. The essence of this step is to create a "planned impairment."[4]

There is a requirement that during an impairment of the fire protection system, an appropriate tag should be placed on the operator's console signifying that the system is out of service. (NFPA 25, 4.1.11.1)[5]

Second, have the necessary tools, equipment, and personnel on hand to complete the task. Equipment on hand should include gaskets, seals, special tools, etc., which are necessary to efficiently complete the task without unnecessary delay. Also, whenever possible, be prepared to maintain one section of the hyperbaric chamber in service so that patient care can be delivered, especially in the case of emergent procedures.

Third, the test should ensure at least the following elements:

1. Initiating devices (manual or automatic) function and actuate valves producing water flow. The initiating function test should include devices at both the operator's console and inside the chamber.

2. Alarm circuits function and send signals to the supervisory station. Also, any internal functions such as shutdown of nonessential electrical power inside the chamber should activate.

Fourth, following completion of the actuation phase of the test, all devices, circuits, equipment, etc. should be returned to the normal or baseline position and the fire protection system placed back "in service" and ready to function. If water has been flowed, storage tanks should be topped up to full and the water level indicators should demonstrate "full" storage capacity.

Once the system is returned to its fully functional status, the fire alarm supervisory service should be contacted and the fire alarm system placed back in its normal, "in service" condition. Also, the number of signals sent and received by the testing procedure should be confirmed with the fire alarm supervisory service.[6]

A sample of a system test document is provided at the end of this chapter. This sample should serve only as a guide and each facility should develop their own documentation which represents their own equipment, procedures, and policies (Figure 1).

Test Result Comparison

Records should be retained over the life of the system. The standard indicates that records shall be kept for a minimum of one year after the last inspection. However, if records can be kept for a longer period, they will demonstrate more data associated with the system, which may be helpful for maintenance activities and to demonstrate to various AHJs the completeness of the facility inspection, testing, and maintenance program.[7]

Frequency of Testing

The frequency of testing for hyperbaric chamber fire protection systems is stated in both *NFPA 99* and *NFPA 25.*[8-9] If the facility has a multiple lock chamber configuration, then this frequency schedule applies to each lock as a separate test. The NFPA documents state the frequency of tests and inspections for fire protection systems.

The concept of performing additional or more frequent tests, above the standard , may not ensure a higher degree of reliability or functionality; excessive testing of the fire protection systems may induce unnecessary wear on critical parts.

Staff Training

One of the opportunities afforded to the hyperbaric medicine team during a scheduled test of the fire protection system is to provide a training session where members of the unit can learn about the system and participate by activating the devices which initiate the fire protection system. Inside attendants should learn and demonstrate their ability to cycle the chamber interior actuating devices. Also, they should learn and demonstrate how to actuate the handheld hose systems, which supplements the deluge system.

Staff personnel responsible for operating the chamber console should be completely familiar with the all the emergency procedures related to operation of the fire protection system as well as duties associated with implementing the fire plan.

Fire Prevention

The daily practices, policies, and procedures associated with fire prevention in the hyperbaric chamber environment cannot be emphasized enough. Vigilance is imperative with regard to fire and life safety prior to each compression of the hyperbaric chamber. A fire that has not ignited does not need to be suppressed.

Also, due to the inherent design of compression chambers, the main component of life safety, that of egress, or evacuation to a safe site, is denied to the occupants inside a chamber under compression. Therefore, it is imperative that maximum efforts be applied to fire prevention, prior to each chamber compression. Practices associated with chamber safety must be learned, understood, and applied at all times, without exception!

Experience has shown that chamber operators must be constantly vigilant and attentive to their operator responsibilities during the entire therapy. Chamber operators who are easily distracted and do not pay attention to the chamber and patient during the therapy are a direct threat to early detection of any trouble with the patient, chamber equipment, or atmospheric monitoring.

Monoplace Hyperbaric Chambers

At the time of this writing, NFPA standards do not require the installation of a fire protection system in a monoplace hyperbaric chamber.

However, there currently is a requirement for fire protection systems to be installed in monoplace hyperbaric chambers in Australia. This requirement was brought about through the efforts of the HTNA (Hyperbaric Technician's and Nurse's Association) of Australia.

Although the effort was not subjected to laboratory or scientific testing, the HTNA group believes they are justified in their approach, and certainly there is merit to this consideration from a humanitarian viewpoint.

The efficacy of a fire protection system under live fire conditions and the collection of data points has yet to be studied in this smaller environment and in the face of a near 100% oxygen concentration. Perhaps under the most severe conditions and challenges, the system may be overwhelmed; future testing will demonstrate survivability in a monoplace chamber environment.

In 1999, a series of live fire tests were conducted in multiplace chambers at a facility in Germany, and data points were collected regarding oxygen concentration, ignition temperature, and conclusions were drawn regarding the need to control the percentage of oxygen concentration in the closed environment in order to allow the fire protection system to suppress the fire before the environment became untenable.

More work needs to be completed before we know the final answer to this question. However, there is the possibility that a fire protection system properly designed and installed in a monoplace chamber may prove effective, especially during the times when the oxygen concentration is in the lower limits.

Conclusion

A properly designed, installed, and maintained fire sprinkler system is the most effective and efficient method to mitigating property loss and ensure life safety. For many years, health care facilities have been required to be equipped with fire sprinkler systems for their environment of care areas. The requirement for hyperbaric chambers to be equipped with fire protection systems is a method of maintaining the same degree or level of protection found in other areas of the health care environment to be maintained in the chamber environment.

While it may be the direct responsibility of the safety director of the hyperbaric chamber facility to ensure the chamber fire protection system is functional and operational, it is the responsibility of all staff to ensure they support the efforts of the safety director and maintain their own level of knowledge and readiness to promote a high level of patient safety and a safe environment.

Fire protection is not singular in focus; it is a system of hardware components, scientific concepts, and management programs operating within the boundaries and challenges of a larger system, which seeks to mitigate the hazards developing from fires.

Figure 1. Example of Fire Suppression System Test.

Department of Hyperbaric Medicine
Hyperbaric Chamber
Fire Suppression System Test
Note: Test Conducted in Accordance with *NFPA 99,* Chapter 14 (14.2.5.5)

Test Date: **March 03, 2016**

Compartment Tested: **Therapy**

Number of Deluge Activation Devices Actuated:

Compartment:**1**

Console:**1**

Number of Deluge Activation Signals Received at UMMC Fire Alarm Panel: **2**

Time to Discharge: Seconds: **3**

Duration of Discharge: Seconds, Each Activation: **10 seconds**

Notes: FSS **NOT** Restored to In-Service Condition
Drain & Flush Flex Hoses and Check Valves, Respectively
Alarm System Cleared and In Service
False Activation, Flooded Chamber, Circuit, Valve Investigated
System Restored and In Service **03-14-2016**
Reviewed Operator Fire Incident Procedure
Deluge, Switch to Air, Rapid Decompression to 20 fsw

Test Conducted By:
BFPE Contractor
William C. Gearhart, CHT
Certified Fire Protection Specialist #902

Witness:
John Smith

*All three operators participated in review of **Code RED** for chamber.

References

1. NFPA. NFPA 25 Standard for Inspection, Testing & Maintenance of Water Based Extinguishing Systems. Quincy, MA: National Fire Protection Association; 2017. 3.3.24.
2. NFPA. NFPA 25 Standard for Inspection, Testing & Maintenance of Water Based Extinguishing Systems. Quincy, MA: National Fire Protection Association; 2017. 4.3.1.1.
3. NFPA. NFPA 25 Standard for Inspection, Testing & Maintenance of Water Based Extinguishing Systems. Quincy, MA: National Fire Protection Association; 2017. 4.3.3; 4.3.4.
4. NFPA. NFPA 25 Standard for Inspection, Testing & Maintenance of Water Based Extinguishing Systems. Quincy, MA: National Fire Protection Association; 2017. 3.3.21.2.
5. NFPA. NFPA 25 Standard for Inspection, Testing & Maintenance of Water Based Extinguishing Systems. Quincy, MA: National Fire Protection Association; 2017. 4.1.11.1.
6. NFPA. NFPA 25 Standard for Inspection, Testing & Maintenance of Water Based Extinguishing Systems. Quincy, MA: National Fire Protection Association; 2017. 4.1.11.2.
7. NFPA. NFPA 25 Standard for Inspection, Testing & Maintenance of Water Based Extinguishing Systems. Quincy, MA: National Fire Protection Association; 2017. 4.3; 4.3.5.
8. NFPA. NFPA 99: Standard for Health Care Facilities, 2018 Edition. Quincy, MA: National Fire Protection Assn; 2018. 14:3.4.3.3; 14.3.4.3.5.
9. NFPA. NFPA 25 Standard for Inspection, Testing & Maintenance of Water Based Extinguishing Systems. Quincy, MA: National Fire Protection Association; 2017. 4.5.

CHAPTER 4.6
Hyperbaric Chamber Control and Ancillary Support Systems

Jim Bell, CHT, EMT, CFPS, Stephen Fabus, CHT-A, and Greg Raleigh, CHT, RCP

Introduction

Typically clinical hyperbaric chambers are more complicated instruments than simpler pressure vessels used for diving and decompression. For our purposes we are defining clinical hyperbaric chambers as those built to meet the *American Society of Mechanical Engineers Pressure Vessels for Human Occupancy* (*ASME –PVHO-1*)[1] and operated in a pressure range of 1.4 atmospheres absolute (ATA) to 6 ATA.[2] The safe operation of a clinical hyperbaric chamber requires the coordinated operation of multiple control, monitoring, and medical and life support systems. The specific systems that will be addressed in this chapter are the following: chamber pressure control, environmental control, gas analysis, patient monitoring, communications, physiological monitoring, lighting, and patient entertainment. While there are significant differences between multiplace and monoplace chamber systems, the fundamental concepts of chamber operation remain quite similar. In this chapter all references to *NFPA 99* will be for the 2018 edition.

Chamber Pressure Control

Chamber pressure control systems are the tools that the chamber operator uses to pressurize, ventilate, and depressurize the chamber.

Terminology used by hyperbaric medicine practitioners to express these processes is inconsistent. It is not uncommon to hear or read in the literature the language of diving operations used in relation to clinical hyperbaric treatment. It is our opinion that terminology such as dives, ascending, descending, or up and down should not be used in clinical hyperbaric medicine practice as these can be confusing to patients and practitioners and are inaccurate. Clinical language such as treatments, chamber sessions, exposures, compression, and decompression (pressurize and depressurize) are more appropriate.

Chamber pressure is the term commonly used in clinical hyperbaric medicine when referring to the pressure of air or oxygen within the chamber. Chamber pressure is expressed in many different ways. (See Table 1.) The international system of units (SI) favors kilo pascal and bar as units of pressure measurement. This chapter will use the following units to express chamber pressure: atmospheres absolute (ATA), pounds per square inch gauge (PSIG), and pounds per square inch absolute (PSIA). Note that the clinical dosing of hyperbaric oxygen (HBO_2) is typically expressed in ATA or atm abs. Clinically, we are providing an oxygen dosage that is a combination of pressure, oxygen percent, and duration of exposure. It is important that we understand the various expressions of pressure in order to be as safe and accurate as possible.

Table 1. Absolute and Gauge Pressure Comparison (units rounded to the nearest integer)

Atmospheres Absolute (ATA)	Kilo Pascal (kPa)	Millimeters mercury (mmHg)	Pounds per square inch absolute (PSIA)	Pounds per square inch gauge (PSIG)	Feet of sea water (FSW)	Meters of sea water (MSW)
0.83 (5,000 ft altitude)	84.4	632.5	12.2	0	0	0
0.97 (1,000 ft altitude)	97.7	733	14.2	0	0	0
1.0	101.3	760	14.7	0	0	0
1.5	151.9	1140	22.0	7.3	16.5	5.1
1.8	182.3	1368	27.9	11.8	30	8.11
2.0	202.6	1520	29.4	14.7	33	10.1
2.5	253.2	1900	36.7	22.0	49.7	15.2
2.8	283.6	2128	41.2	26.4	60	18.2
3.0	303.9	2280	44.1	29.4	66	20.3

All hyperbaric chambers have the same basic operational functions: pressurization, ventilation, and depressurization. To pressurize the chamber, a valve controlling the compression gas supply (air or oxygen in oxygen-pressurized monoplace chambers) is opened, allowing the gas to enter the chamber. Opening or closing this supply valve regulates the rate at which the chamber will be pressurized. When the chamber reaches the desired chamber pressure, an exhaust valve is opened to provide ventilating flow through the chamber. The flow controlled by the pressurization valve is reduced to a point at which a constant flow of gas is provided to maintain both the chamber pressure and adequate ventilation. The exhaust valve can then be adjusted to maintain the chamber pressure at a constant flow.

The pressurization rate is based on the flow capability of the chamber gas supply, the chamber volume, and most importantly, on the chamber occupant's ability to equalize the pressure in ears and sinuses. Chambers can be pressurized at rates exceeding the ability of the occupants to adapt to the changes in pressure. Clinical pressurization rates vary from 1 PSIG per minute up to and exceeding 25 PSIG per minute, though it is rare to utilize rates in excess of 5 PSIG per minute. There is evidence that using a slow constant rate or a curvilinear compression rate facilitates middle ear pressure equilibration.[4-5] To use a curvilinear rate, the chamber is initially compressed at a slow to moderate rate which gradually increases as the chamber pressure increases. Essentially, a curvilinear compression tries to maintain a constant volume change rather than a constant pressure change. This maintains a more consistent pressure gradient change across the tympanic membrane. This method can be used within the same time frame as a slow linear pressurization using a constant rate.

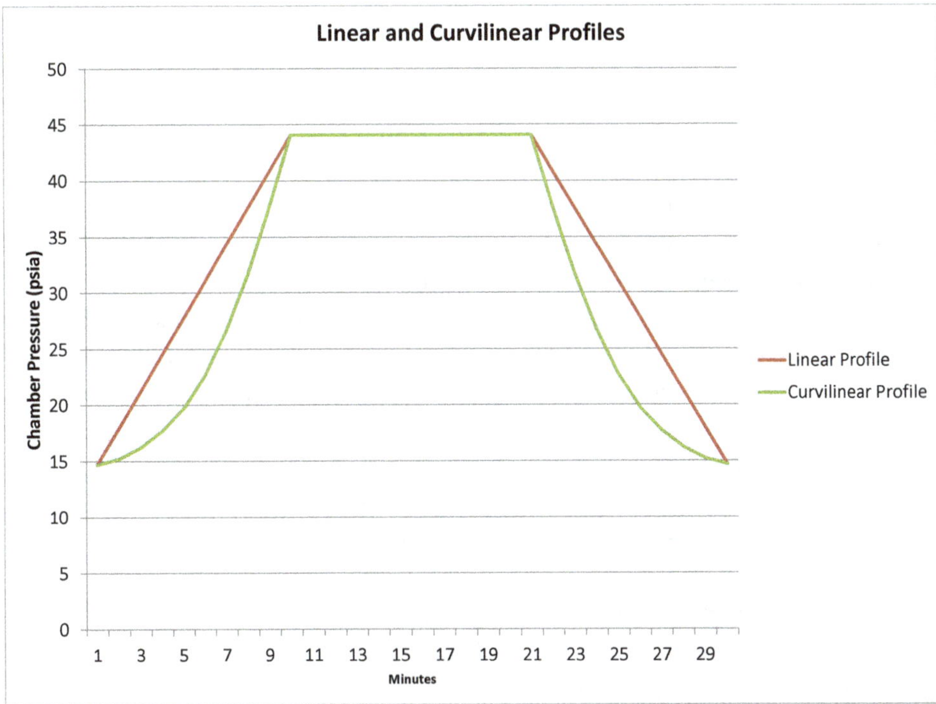

Figure 1. Curvilinear vs. linear compression.

To depressurize the chamber, the chamber exhaust valve is opened to provide an exhaust flow greater than the inlet flow provided by the pressurization valve. Depending upon the control system design, the inlet flow may be maintained or reduced while allowing continued ventilation of the chamber. Opening the exhaust valve slightly provides a slower depressurization rate, and fully opening it provides the maximum depressurization rate. To maintain a constant linear rate while depressurizing, the exhaust valve opening has to be increased as chamber pressure decreases to accommodate the reduction in the flow rate of the gas through the exhaust piping with this decreasing chamber pressure. With some chambers it may be impossible to maintain a constant decompression rate as the chamber approaches atmospheric pressure because of this reduced pressure differential.

The chamber is a sealed environment and ventilation is required to maintain attendant and patient safety and comfort. Chamber ventilation is the process of exchanging the air or oxygen inside the chamber with uncontaminated gas. Ventilating the chamber is necessary to control the oxygen and carbon dioxide levels and maintain adequate temperature and humidity control. The minimum threshold for ventilating a multiplace chamber is 3 actual cubic feet per minute (ACFM) for each person in the chamber who is not wearing a mask or hood equipped with overboard dump system (an exhaled oxygen scavenging system that collects residual oxygen and evacuates it out of the chamber). In monoplace chambers this threshold is 1 ACFM. Without proper ventilation, a person left in the sealed chamber would eventually deplete the oxygen and increase carbon dioxide level to a point of asphyxiation. Chambers designed for saturation diving are excluded from this ventilation standard as they commonly recirculate the chamber atmosphere and have filters and absorbents to maintain the atmosphere within safe levels.[3] In multiplace chambers where the occupants are breathing supplemental oxygen, proper chamber ventilation is necessary to keep the chamber oxygen percentage from increasing above the recommended fire safety level of 23.5%. The ventilation required to keep the oxygen levels below 23.5% may be higher than 3 ACFM.[3]

The size and design of the chamber, number, and type of patients all impact the chamber atmosphere. During a prolonged stay in a chamber, temperature, humidity and odor can become issues. Ventilating the chamber with fresh air helps to reduce these factors from becoming disagreeable. Ventilating a chamber while maintaining a constant chamber pressure is accomplished by opening either the exhaust or supply valve to a predetermined setting and then adjusting the opposing exhaust or supply valve to maintain the chamber at a constant pressure.

Multiplace Manual Pressure Control System

Basic pressure control systems use manually operated valves to control chamber pressure. This type of system can use either a quarter turn ball valve or some variation of a gate valve. In some chambers, pressurization can be controlled from inside and/or outside the chamber. In order for the chamber inside attendant to control the rate of pressurization, the external supply valve must be open allowing the inside attendant to control the rate while monitoring the other occupants. The chamber operator outside of the chamber observes chamber occupants and can assume control using the external valves if necessary. Normally, after the target pressure is reached, all chamber pressure control is relinquished to the chamber operator. This is done by ensuring that the exterior valves are closed, opening the interior valves, then re-opening the exterior valves as needed to ventilate the chamber and maintain a constant pressure. If a system does not have interior valves, the chamber pressure is completely controlled externally by the chamber operator. Once the chamber has reached treatment pressure the chamber operator must constantly monitor chamber pressure, particularly immediately following the initial pressurization of the chamber. As the chamber atmosphere cools, following the adiabatic heating caused by rapid pressurization, the chamber pressure will drop if the chamber operator does not compensate by adding more air with the supply valve.

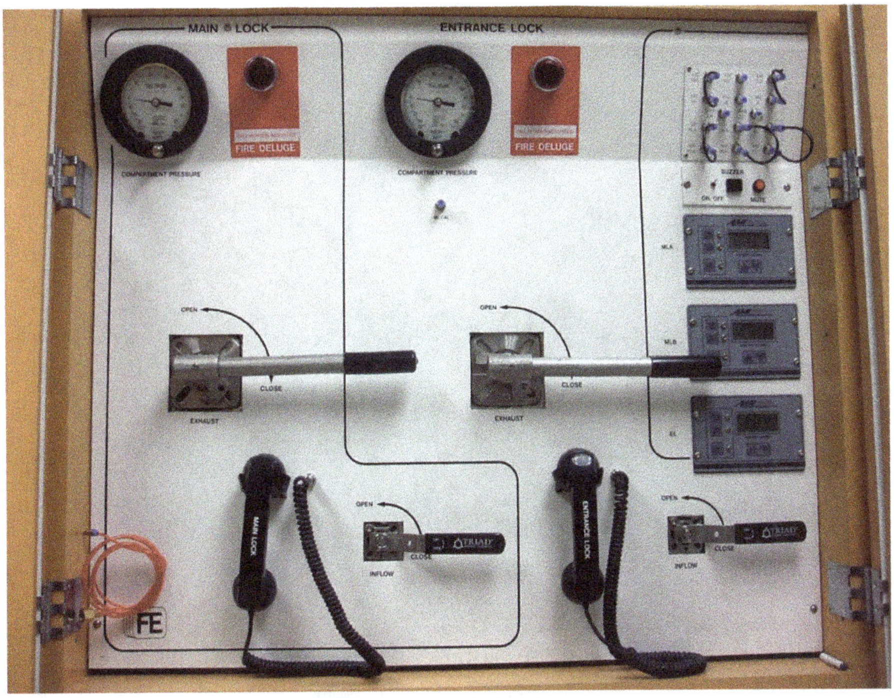

Figure 2. Manual control panel.

Manual control configurations commonly used on smaller chambers often have noisy air flow characteristics, making it uncomfortably loud when providing chamber ventilation. Mufflers can be added, but they may restrict gas flow, decrease the pressurization rate, and change gas flow characteristics. It can be difficult to maintain manual ventilation and stable chamber pressure for extended periods of time. Typically, when operating this type of system, a chamber ventilation schedule is prepared so that the ventilation of the chamber will be performed periodically instead of continuously. The ventilation timing and gas flow rates are based on formulas using the volume of the chamber, number of chamber occupants, and type of air supply and whether the occupants are breathing air or oxygen. These formulas can be found in the *U.S. Navy Dive Manual.*[6] In clinical hyperbaric chambers, where the chamber atmosphere is monitored for oxygen (O_2), carbon dioxide (CO_2), carbon monoxide (CO), temperature, and humidity levels, the ventilation will be performed as needed to keep the chamber atmosphere within prescribed limits. If the chamber uses quarter turn ball valves, there is often a scale on the supply and/or exhaust valves that shows the valve position that will provide the desired ventilation rate. The chamber may also be fitted with a flow meter in line with the supply valve that indicates the exact ventilation in standard cubic feet per minute (SCFM).

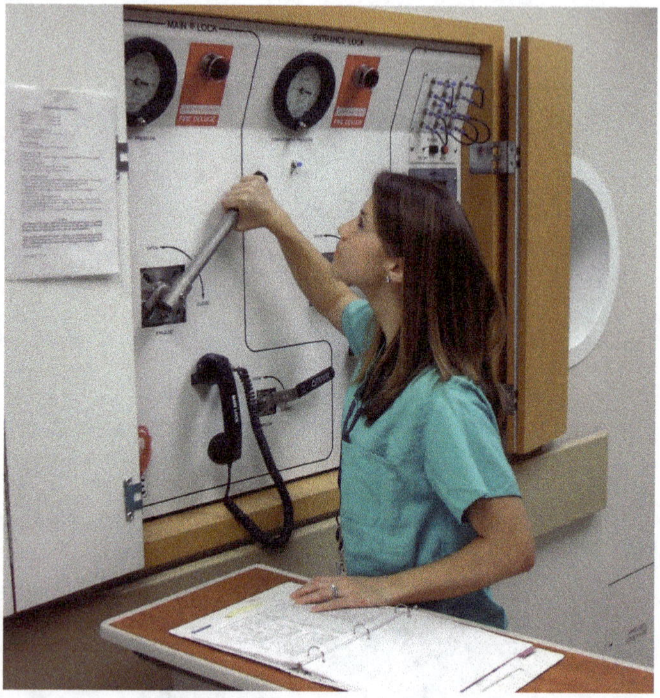

Figure 3. Manual chamber operations.

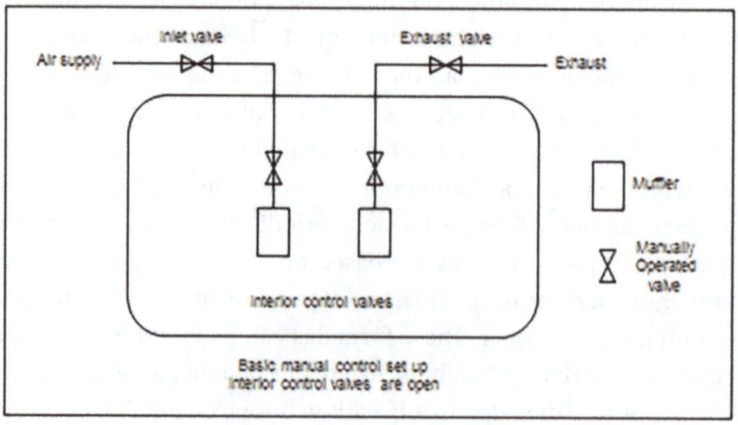

Figure 4. Diagram of manually controlled chamber.

Pressure Gauges

Clinical hyperbaric chambers may be equipped with both analog pressure gauges and digital pressure displays. Digital pressure displays are easy to read, and when properly calibrated, very accurate. One disadvantage of the digital pressure display is that it will normally indicate pressure to 0.1 PSIG or even 0.01 PSIG. A chamber operator can become frustrated while trying to manually maintain chamber pressure to the tenth of a PSIG during chamber ventilation. For this reason, many experienced chamber operators will use the analog gauge to monitor chamber pressure during manual chamber ventilation. Fluctuations in chamber pressure greater than approximately 0.5 PSIG can be uncomfortable for chamber occupants due to middle ear pressure changes.

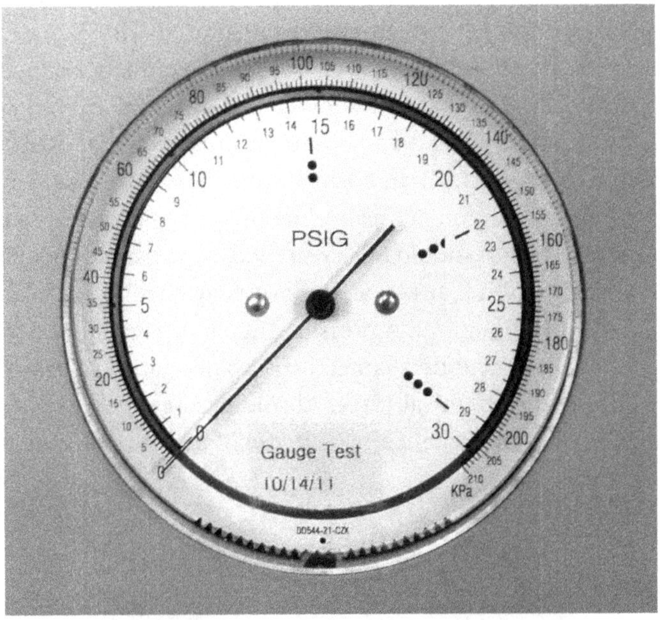

Figure 5. Analog pressure gauge.

An analog gauge is a pressure measuring device that uses an open tube or fitting connecting it directly to the chamber. The analog pressure gauge shown above has two scales to measure chamber pressure. The outside scale is in kilo pascals (kPa) and the inside scale PSIG. (The authors would like to point out that this is a common dual scale. PSI and kPa can be an absolute or gauge units of pressure depending on context. On the gauge demonstratsd they are gauge value.) Many test gauges and high-quality gauges will have a mirrored strip running around the face to ensure accuracy in reading the needle indicator by preventing parallax error. The chamber operator looks directly at the needle, using one eye. When properly done, one would see no visible reflection of the needle in the mirror strip.

A digital pressure display receives an electrical signal from a pressure transmitter that is located either inside the chamber or connected to the chamber by a thru-hull fitting. Pressure transmitters convert pressure into an electrical signal that is proportional to the pressure applied. A pressure transmitter is calibrated to output an electrical current in milliamps (mA) that will correspond to a given pressure range. For example, a pressure transmitter may read pressures between 0 and 100 PSIG, the corresponding output signal range will be 4 and 20 mA. The pressure transmitter for a chamber at sea level with 0 PSIG internal pressure should be outputting a 4 mA signal, and when the pressure in the chamber is at 100 PSIG, the pressure transmitter should be outputting a 20 mA signal. The pressure transmitter output is proportional to the pressure between sea level (zero) and 100 PSIG. The digital pressure display then interprets the electrical signal to display the chamber pressure in the desired gauge or absolute scale (i.e. fsw, msw, PSIG, kPa, PSIA, ATA, mmHg, etc). The pressure transmitter can also be used in conjunction with semiautomatic and automatic pressure controllers.

Most clinical hyperbaric chambers are manufactured with the gauges and pressure transmitters calibrated to sea level (1 ATA). Pressure reductions encountered when chambers are operated up to 1,000 feet above mean sea level are not considered significant enough to require further compensation, unless one is involved in research activities that require high precision in dosing of the HBO_2. To ensure accurate dosing of hyperbaric oxygen, the addition of an absolute pressure gauge or transmitter to your system, such as PSIA or kPa(a) should be considered. A pressure transmitter calibrated for absolute values such as PSIA or kPa at sea level may need to be recalibrated at altitude depending on the manufacturer. A pressure transmitter calibrated for gauge values such as PSIG or fsw will be accurate at any location since gauge values are not absolute measurements and start at 0 at any altitude. Absolute gauges can be purchased that do not need to be calibrated for a change in altitude. There are two concerns that must

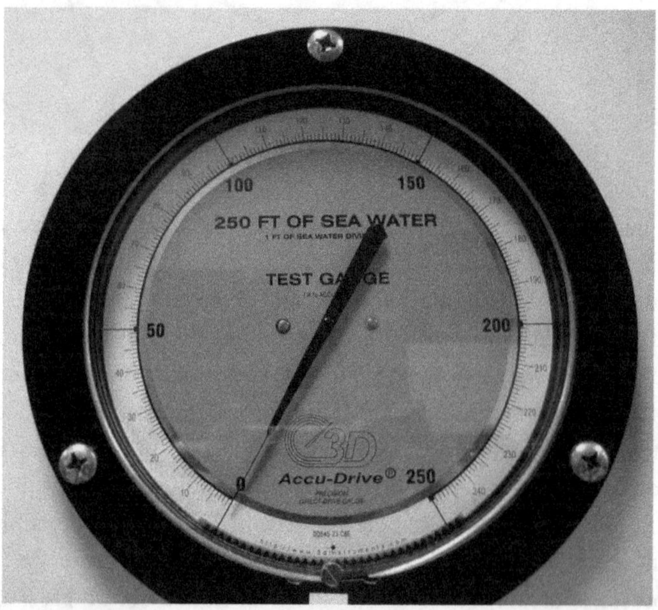

Figure 6. Analog pressure gauge in feet of sea water.

be addressed if you add absolute values. First, the operator needs to know the exact gauge pressure that air-breathing attending occupants inside the hyperbaric chambers are exposed to, regardless of altitude, in order to calculate safe exposure profiles and decompression procedures. Second, an absolute value is important to verify accurate treatment pressures for the correct dosing of HBO_2) as prescribed by the physician (example: 2.4 ATA for 90 minutes).

The analog pressure gauge shown in Figure 6 has one scale in feet of sea water (fsw) to measure chamber pressure. This is a common gauge face seen on multiplace chambers. Fsw is not an absolute unit of pressure and will start at 0 when at sea level or altitude. This gauge also has the mirrored strip running around the face to ensure accuracy in reading the needle indicator.

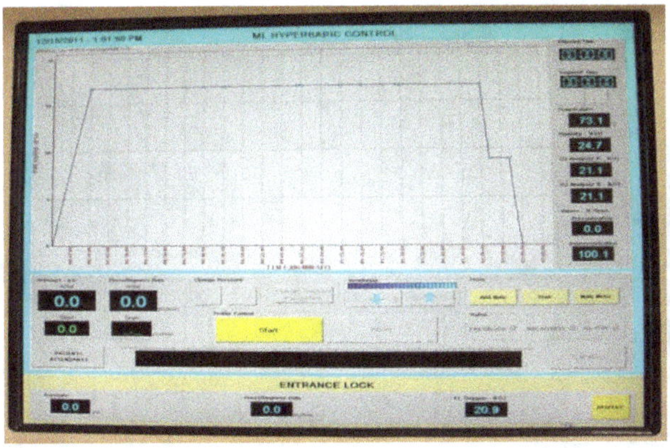

Figure 7. Digital pressure display.

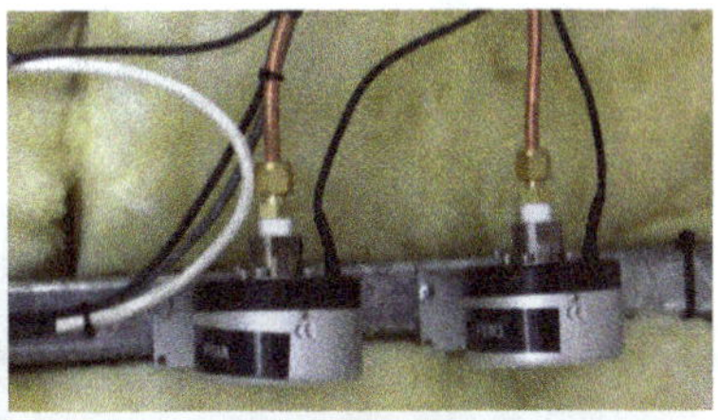

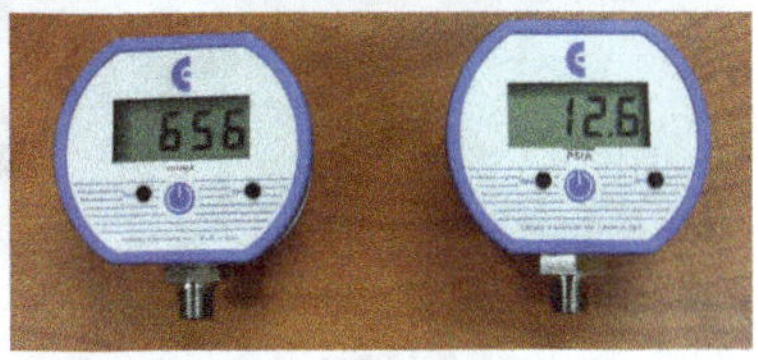

Figure 8. (top) Pressure transmitters. **Figure 9.** (bottom) Absolute pressure gauges.

It is good practice to test pressure gauges against a certified test gauge, dead weight tester, or have the manufacturer test them and certify their accuracy. It is important to verify the chamber gauge measurements to that of a calibrated test reference gauge periodically, at least annually. On multiplace chambers, a test port can be built into the system or a threaded fitting may be available on the hull that allows the test gauge to be fitted. A test gauge can be connected to a monoplace chamber through a door mounted gas port or an existing intravenous (IV) pass-through port. The gauge test should record data from stops at regular intervals throughout the rated pressure range of the chamber. The test data sheet will include details from the test gauge used, date, signature(s) of the tester, results, and pass/fail of the gauges. A dead weight tester is a mechanical device that uses calibrated weights to verify the accuracy of gauges.

At the time of this writing, we are not aware of a standard or code in the United States that requires this verification of gauge accuracy for clinical hyperbaric chambers. However, the U.S. Navy and Occupational Safety & Health Administration (OSHA) has regulations related to gauge accuracy verification for diving operations.[6-7] Although these rules do not specifically apply to the clinical hyperbaric chamber, the end user is responsible for maintaining the accuracy of their gauges. It is our recommendation that gauges be checked to a known source at least biannually or whenever there is a discrepancy between any two gauges on the same system and clearly if conducting research.

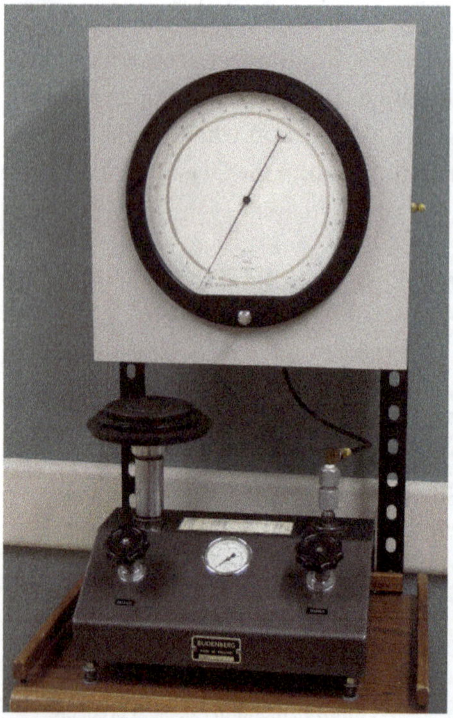

Figure 10. Dead weight tester.

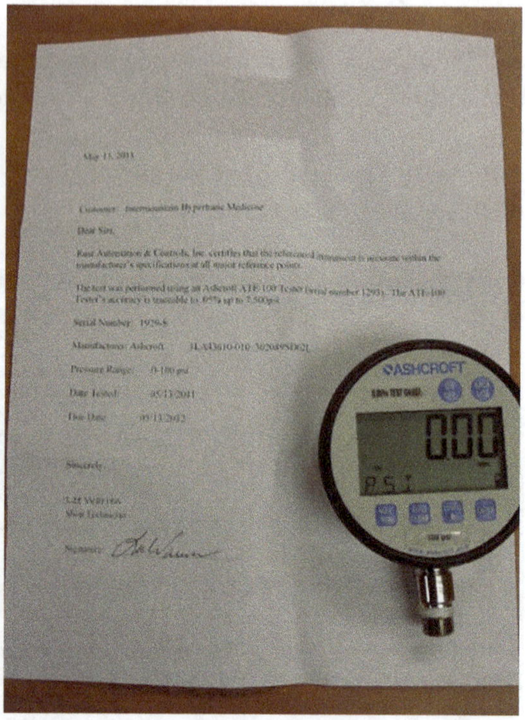

Figure 11. Test gauge and annual certificate of accuracy.

Pneumatic Control Valve

Pneumatic control valves use air pressure (also called control air) to open and close valves. A valve can be referred to as either normally open or normally closed. These terms describe the valve position when no control air pressure is supplied. Normally open means the valve is "at rest" in the open position and closed means the valve is "at rest" in the closed position. Most control valves are designed to be normally closed. Pneumatic control valves usually consist of an upper and lower dome with a diaphragm located between. The diaphragm has a metal plate in the middle. The metal plate will have a shaft or bolt attached to its center. This shaft runs through the lower dome to attach to the valve stem. The plate rests on a series of springs surrounding the bolt in the lower dome. When air pressure is applied to the upper dome, the diaphragm is pressed downward, compressing the springs in the lower dome, forcing the shaft or bolt in the center of the plate downward, pushing the valve stem downward, and opening the valve. The more air pressure that is applied to the upper dome, the more downward diaphragm movement, thus further opening the valve. Most valves operate in the control air pressure range of 3–15 PSIG. In a normally closed valve, if pressure on the upper dome is less than 3 PSIG, the valve remains closed. As pressure on the upper dome increases above 3 PSIG, the valve will open in proportion to the increased air pressure until the valve is fully opened at 15 PSIG. As the air pressure is reduced in the upper dome, the springs in the lower dome begin to return the diaphragm to its original position, pushing the shaft upward and closing the valve in proportion to the reduced pressure in the upper dome. When the pressure in the upper dome becomes less than 3 PSIG, the valve will be completely closed. One of the more common types of valve bodies used with the pneumatic controller is the gate valve. This valve allows for smooth proportional flow across the full range of pressures of the valve.

Some multiplace chambers have fast-acting valves placed in line with both the supply and the exhaust valves as a safety feature. These valves give the operator a method to instantly stop the flow of air in or out of the chamber. They can be either manually operated or controlled by a switch. Switch controlled activation can be plumbed in such a way to allow the inside attendant to stop pressurization or depressurization of the chamber. Quick-acting valves provide a greater level of safety, allowing the operator or inside attendant to stop pressure changes instantly in the event of a physiological or mechanical emergency. **Caution:** ***Ensure supply and exhaust valves are closed before reopening the safety valves. If either valve is open, a rapid unplanned pressure change will result!***

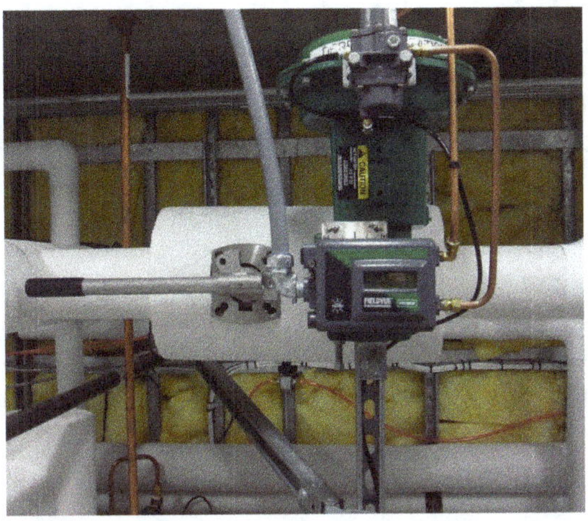

Figure 12. Pneumatic valve with manual safety valve.

Semi-Automated Pressure Control Systems

Multiplace chamber manufacturers and engineers are designing sophisticated automated and semi-automated pressure control systems. It would be challenging to review the differences between all of these systems. We will approach this issue by attempting to describe these systems in a generic fashion.

Semi-automated systems are designed to control two aspects of the chamber pressurization procedure: the rate of pressure change in the chamber (pressurization and depressurization) and the maintenance of consistent chamber pressure. There are a variety of designs that use semi-automated pressure control systems. The basic underlying operating concepts remain similar. The chamber is pressurized by opening the pressurization valve. Upon reaching the desired treatment pressure, this valve is adjusted to a predetermined setting designed to generate the proper ventilation flow rate. A pressure controller or loop processor then uses a reference point to monitor the chamber pressure. In the case of pressure controllers, the reference is provided by a tube that runs from the chamber to an automatic pressure controller. Because the tube is open to chamber air, as the air pressure increases in the chamber, it also increases in the tubing. The automatic pressure controller then tracks the actual chamber pressure changes and opens the exhaust valve to maintain consistent pressure. In the case of a loop processor, a pressure transmitter is located inside the chamber. A pneumatic-to-electrical signal is generated that is transmitted back to the loop processor. The loop processor tracks this electrical signal while referencing the internal chamber pressure. The loop processor can then send electric-to-pneumatic signal to the exhaust valve for fine adjustments to maintain the correct internal pressure.

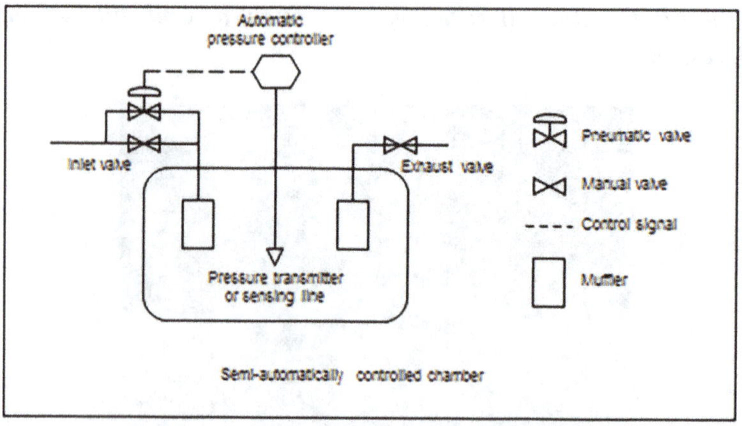

Figure 13. Diagram of semi-automatically controlled chamber.

Automated Pressure Control Systems

Automated pressure control systems are designed to control three or four aspects of the exposure: the rates of pressurization and depressurization; target pressure within the chamber; elapsed time of the exposure or segments of the exposure; and with some systems, the ventilation flow rate. The chamber operator is responsible for the exposure timing and ventilation of the chamber. An automated pressure control system relies on pneumatic valves for both the pressurization and depressurization of the chamber. Chambers are typically equipped with redundant manual supply and exhaust valves. Pneumatic valves can be controlled by the automated pressure controller or by the chamber operator using a valve actuator. In the manual mode, the operator controls the chamber as if using manual valves. To pressurize the chamber, the operator adjusts the actuator so that a signal, either pneumatic or electrical, causes the valve to open. The valve opening is proportional to the signal strength generated by the actuator—the stronger the signal, the greater the valve opens. As the operator reduces the signal strength, the valve will begin to close. In this manner the operator can control the pressure inlet and exhaust valves from an operations console remotely located from the actual valves. The chamber can also be ventilated in this manner, using the same method as described under manual pressure control. **Caution:** ***Unlike a hand-operated valve on a manually controlled chamber, which can be closed instantly, some pneumatic valves are slow to open and close. This valve characteristic must be considered by the operator.***

A programmable logic controller (PLC) is an electronic device that is capable of "driving" the hyperbaric chamber much like an auto pilot on an aircraft. Using a PLC, the chamber operator sets the desired pressure (set point) on the PLC. The PLC then opens or closes the pneumatic supply or exhaust valves to ensure that the chamber pressurizes to or remains at the set pressure. To change chamber pressure with the PLC, the set pressure is changed by the chamber operator at the rate of desired chamber travel. **Caution:** ***In some systems, if there is too great a distance between the set point and the actual chamber pressure, a radical change in pressure may occur as the controller rapidly opens the valve to reach the set point.***

Hyperbaric chamber systems use automatic and loop process controllers for many operations, such as controlling chamber pressure, temperature and humidity, and ventilation. To control these functions automatically, the systems need the following:

- A controller
- A process sensor or transmitter
- Pneumatic control valves

The operator sets the controller to the desired setting. For example, if this were a chamber pressure controller, the chamber operator would set it to the desired pressure that is to be maintained. This is the set point. The controller, through the chamber pressure transmitter, or a reference line, determines the actual chamber pressure. The PLC will open and close the inlet valve or exhaust valve as necessary to maintain the set point. Usually one of these valves is set at a fixed opening and actual control is maintained by the one that is not at the fixed opening setting. The PLC opens and closes this "non-fixed" valve by either directing control air to the pneumatic valve dome to open the valve or by sending an electronic signal to a device that will convert that signal to control air and pressurize the dome of the valve, opening the valve. The control valve is then opened and closed by automated regulation of the signal strength.

Multiplace Automated Pressure Control System with a Programmable Logic Controller (PLC)

There are programmable logic controller (PLC) devices that are capable of driving the hyperbaric chamber through a complete profile. The chamber operator selects a pre-programmed profile from a menu. The profile will dictate rate of compression, duration at treatment pressure, rate of decompression, and duration at stops, if necessary. Note: *Most systems have provisions for changing profiles or a method to take manual control during the treatment, if necessary.* Once the chamber door is closed, the PLC program is started. The PLC then drives the chamber through the profile. The PLC comes in several different configurations. Some units combine the PLC and the automatic pressure controller into one unit so that the PLC directly controls the chamber's pneumatic pressurization and exhaust valves. Others may have a personal computer (PC) that runs the profile. The PC sends a signal to the automatic pressure controller. This signal moves the set point on the automatic pressure controller up and down to correspond with the profile. The PLC moves the pressure controller set point at the rate specified. For example, if the profile calls for the chamber to pressurize from 0 PSIG to 20 PSIG in 10 minutes, the PLC will move the set point on the automatic pressure controller at a rate of 2 PSIG per minute. The automatic pressure controller will open the pneumatic inlet valve and compress the chamber to the set point, providing the chamber occupants with a smooth compression to the prescribed pressure. **Caution:** ***A PLC seems to simplify the job of the console operator, but the operator must be constantly vigilant of the PLC and chamber occupants and be ready to assume manual control of the chamber instantly in the case of emergency.*** The PLC can also be used as a central alarm center. Chamber temperature, humidity, oxygen percentage carbon dioxide, and carbon monoxide can all be monitored. Alarm parameters are set so that the operator is made aware of a situation prior to it becoming critical.

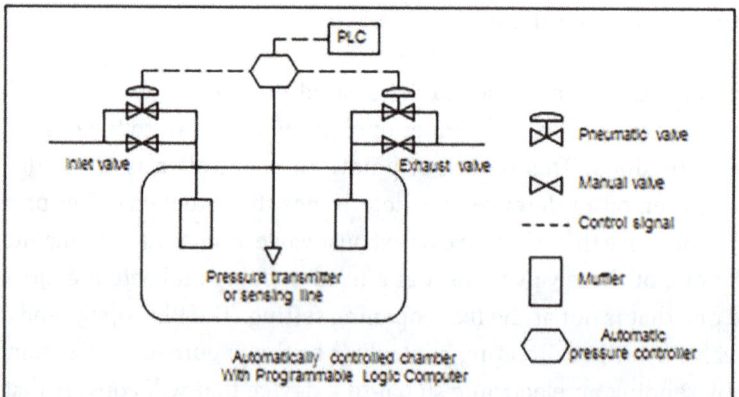

Figure 14. Diagram of automatically controlled chamber with programmable logic controller.

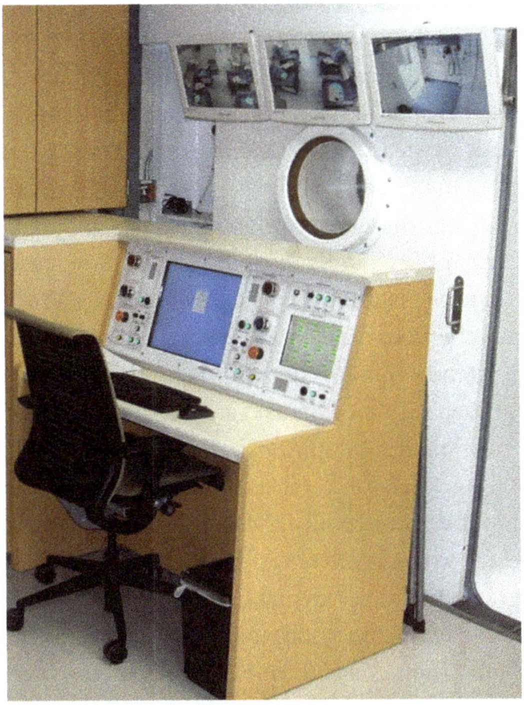

Figure 15. Automated control panel.

Another form of automated control is software-based as shown in Figure 15. Computer-based automatic systems are similar to the PLC. Pneumatic valves are still necessary as is some form of transmitter reference line. The software-based controllers allow a chamber operator to design profiles based on time and set point pressures and save them to be used repeatedly. These systems use the exhaust valve to control the chamber pressure and program the ventilation rate. The chamber operator can increase or decrease the ventilation rate as needed from the control panel. The controller will open or close the exhaust valve to maintain the set program, while adjusting ventilation rate as specified by the operator. The illustrated program has a touch screen or can be operated by a mouse or keyboard. Holding chamber pressure during compression and decompressing are all controlled by the operator. The automatic system can also be switched to semi-automatic where the set point is maintained by the controller and the chamber operator controls the interval of hold. This system can also be overridden completely and the chamber operator is able to control the chamber manually. *The caution to operators using a semi-automated system applies to the automated system as well. It would be easy to become complacent, as the automated system completes most, if not all, of the planned chamber profile.* ***Constant vigilance is imperative!***

Monoplace Chambers

Monoplace chambers are the most widely utilized type of clinical hyperbaric chamber in the world. The typical monoplace chamber is a well-engineered piece of equipment that is easy to operate. The majority of monoplace chambers in use today are pneumatically controlled devices, but some are computer controlled.

The patient or subject is placed inside the chamber, usually on a cart that mates with the chamber allowing the top mattress portion to be slid inside the chamber on rollers. The chamber door is closed and sealed. The chamber operator opens the oxygen supply valve and selects the treatment pressure and the rate of compression. The chamber is pressurized to the set pressure at the rate determined by the operator. Chamber ventilation is established with the supply coming in at the patient's head and the exhaust going out at the feet. There is a wide range of methods used to control the pressure and ventilation in monoplace chambers although most are automated.

Ventilation rates for monoplace chambers are typically between 90–400 LPM using approximately 10,800 to 48,000 liters of oxygen per session. Some chamber designs allow for the chamber to be pressurized with oxygen or air. If air is used it must be a minimum of Compressed Gas Association (CGA) Grade E and have no hydrocarbons.[3] A filter assembly is installed in line to protect the chamber from contamination by the air source. It is important to note that the size of the chamber and the exhaust flow rate set by the operator directly affect the rate that the chamber oxygen percent is at a therapeutic level. A 32-inch diameter monoplace chamber with an exhaust rate of 400 liters per minute (LPM) will reach 99% oxygen in 10 to 15 minutes depending on the pressure the chamber is being pressurized to. A chamber with an exhaust rate of 240 LPM may take quite a bit longer.[8-9] Some computer controlled monoplace chambers can be programmed to ventilate at a high rate during compression to accelerate the washout of nitrogen from ambient air initially in the chamber, then reduce the ventilation rate once the chamber is at treatment pressure to reduce oxygen consumption. NFPA 99 requires that each monoplace chamber have its own independent exhaust line.

An air supply is also necessary to provide an air breathing period using a mouthpiece, mask, demand regulator, or a ventilator. The air is commonly supplied from the

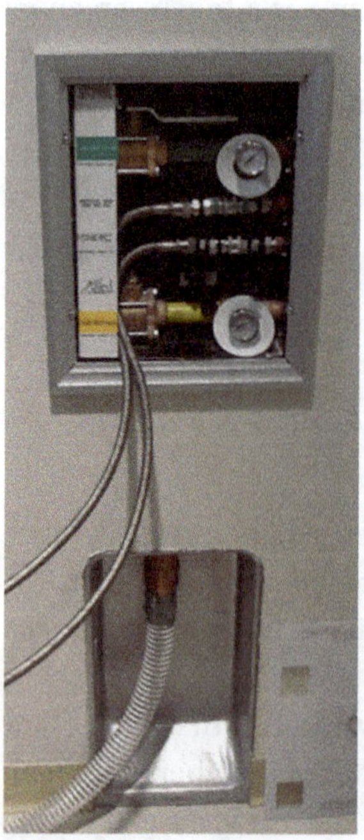

Figure 16. Oxygen supply and chamber exhaust connections for monoplace chamber.

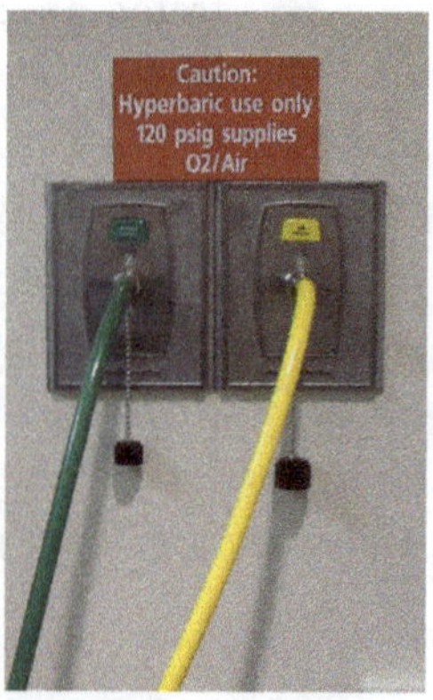

Figure 17. High-pressure connections for air breaks and ventilator use in a monoplace chamber.

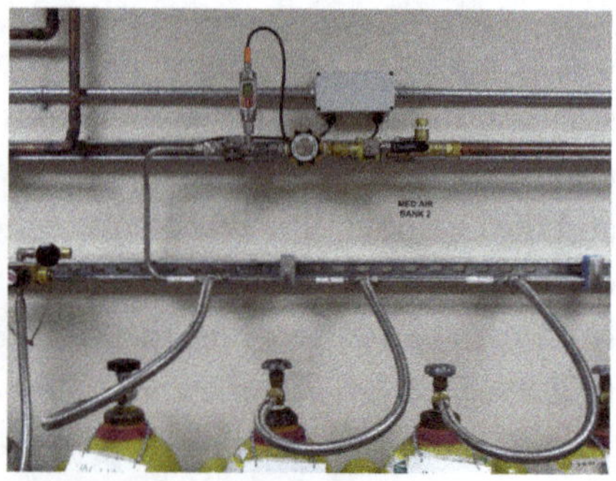

Figure 18. Micron filter location on commercially supplied cylinders.

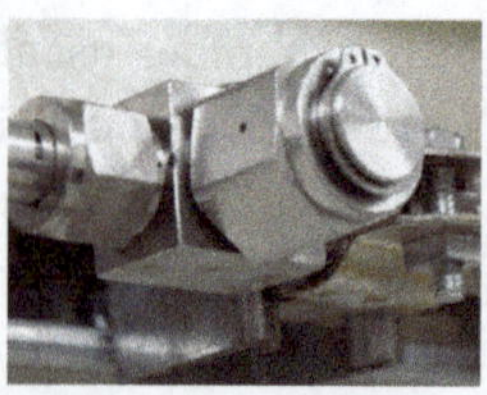

Figure 19. Micron filter.

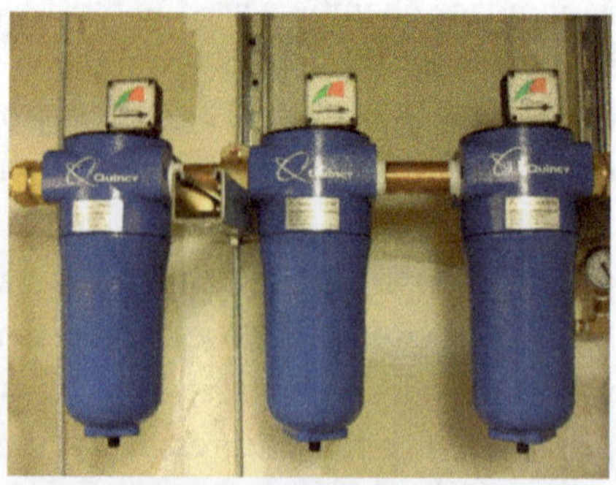

Figure 20. Filters on the medical air supply from the compressors.

hospital's medical air compressors or 200 cubic foot high-pressure cylinders called H or K cylinders. These cylinders are usually connected in series and the air is supplied through a manifold. High-pressure cylinders of air supplied from vendors must meet United States Pharmacopeia (USP) medical air and CGA Grade N requirements and should be delivered with the certificate of analysis from the vendor. Filtration of 66 microns is required on commercially procured cylinders. Filtration is also recommended on the air supply from compressors intended for the chamber.[3,10-13]

Monoplace Semi-Automated Pressure Control System

Monoplace chambers with semi-automated controls use both PLC technology and manual set valves. The pressure and rate are maintained by the controller as set by the chamber operator. A curvilinear pressurization is available as one of the settings on several of the electronic control options. The pneumatic controls are manual and the compression rate can be manipulated by the chamber operator to achieve a curvilinear or constant rate of compression or decompression.

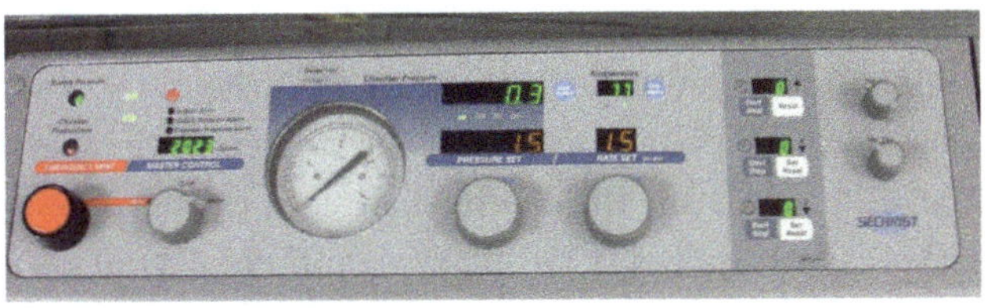

Figure 21. Semi-automated monoplace electronic control panel.

Monoplace Automated Pressure Control

The automated controls for the monoplace chamber operate in the same manner as the controls for multiplace chambers. The ability to enter duration, pressure, and save the profiles, patient, or subject information and other data from the treatment, electronically, is available from several manufacturers. Some automated systems also allow connection of the chamber to electronic medical record systems, eliminating the need for paper treatment records. There is also the ability to override the automated controls in a manner that is similar as the method described for multiplace chambers. The pressure, rate, and duration are all maintained by the controller unless manually overridden by the chamber operator.

Some monoplace chambers have analog and digital gauges. Most monoplace chambers are built and calibrated for sea level. Therefore, the gauges have the same issues that were previously described related to their use at higher altitudes. The analog and digital gauges set to display atmospheres absolute (ATA) at sea level will *not* be accurate at altitude. Using the terms ATA or atm abs without knowing the absolute pressure is a misnomer. Persons operating chambers at locations of altitudes greater than 1,000 feet should consider adding an absolute gauge such as PSIA or kPa, since the dosage of hyperbaric oxygen is a combined product of both the absolute pressure and concentration of oxygen.[14]

Environmental Controls

The chamber environmental control system provides the means to maintain temperature and humidity in the hyperbaric environment within a comfortable range. Normally, a temperature range of [22°C ± 2°C (75°F ± 5°F)] and 50 to 70% humidity are acceptable. During pressurization, the system should be able to maintain temperature below 29°C (85°F) and above 9°C (65°F) during depressurization.[3]

Some chambers may not have an environmental control system. In these chambers temperature and humidity can be partially modified by use of the ventilation rate and the ambient temperature of the room housing the chamber. One of the characteristics of energy transfer is that heat will transfer to cool until the temperatures are equal. Large metal chambers are large heat sinks, as the temperature of the chamber hull will cool to the temperature of the room. For both multiplace and monoplace chambers, consider the temperature of the room when trying to heat or cool the chamber(s). The ideal multiplace chamber would have an environmental control system designed to maintain the temperature at a comfortable level and humidity at a level sufficient to prevent the accumulation of static charges. The biggest challenge for a hyperbaric environmental control system is to maintain constant temperature during pressure changes. The increased heat of compression or the cooling during depressurization can overwhelm most systems. However, a comfortable level can usually be managed by using conservative rates of pressurization and depressurization and ventilating the chamber while at the set pressure.

A list of the typical components of an environmental control system (ECS) is as follows:

- Chilled water or water/glycol mixture (35°–45°F) and reheat water (165°–175°F) sources
- Chilled water and reheat water pumps
- Chilled water and reheat water flow control valves
- Heating and cooling coils, one for reheat water and one for chilled water (like radiators)
- Blower assemblies (blower motor normally outside chamber or venturi air "fan")
- Humidifier (air powered nebulizer)
- Temperature and humidity gauges (sensors/transmitters)
- ECS control methods, automated and manual

Warming inside the chamber is achieved by a blower assembly forcing chamber air over the heating coils while hot water flows through the coils. Cooling is achieved by the same method, only using cold (chilled) water. The reheat and chilled water pumps circulate the water through the corresponding heating and cooling coils. Some systems will have a bypass to protect the water pumps from overpressurizing when the flow control valves are only partially open or closed. Chilled and reheat water control valves can be manually controlled or operated by an automated system. To manually control the system, the chamber operator opens or closes the valves to adjust the flow rate of water through heat exchangers. If the chamber is slightly cool, the reheat water valve should be opened gradually, slowly warming the chamber; if the chamber is cold, more reheat water flow will be needed, especially during depressurization. (The faster the water flows through the coils of the heat exchanger, the quicker the chamber temperature changes.) To cool the chamber, the operator opens the chilled water valve in the same manner as when heating the chamber. Note: Usually, a higher water flow rate will be needed for the chilled water cooling coils to be as effective as compared to the reheat water side. Most systems will require maximum chilled water flow rate during the compression phase. **Caution:** ***As you change the temperature in the chamber, monitor chamber pressure closely, as temperature changes will affect the chamber pressure.***

The automated system requires a control loop to function properly. This automated system includes a thermostat, located at the operator station, and a temperature transmitter located inside the chamber. The chamber operator sets the desired temperature on the thermostat. The temperature transmitter sends a signal to the thermostat telling it what the actual temperature is in the chamber. The thermostat then opens or closes the chilled water and reheat water control valves and adjusts the blower as needed, to achieve the desired temperature in the chamber.

During pressure changes, an extreme workload is placed on the air conditioning system. Some chambers are equipped with multispeed blowers. Normally, during the pressurization phase, the blowers will be turned to high speed to try and keep up with the rapid heat build-up. Multispeed blowers will usually be set to automatically switch to slow speed before the chamber pressure reaches a point where the increased air density could cause the blower motor to overload. If the blower uses an electric motor, it may be mounted outside of the chamber and connected by a drive shaft through a hull penetrator or a magnetic coupler. Electric motors used inside the chamber should be especially designed for that purpose. As a rule, these in-chamber, NFPA-compliant motors should be brushless, spark proof, and equipped with circuitry that will shut the motor down in the event of an overload. If the motor is located outside the chamber, a sealed shaft can be used to drive the fan inside the chamber. Not all chambers use an electric blower; some incorporate a venturi "fan" or air mover. These systems commonly use the same air source as the compression air to move air across the coils.

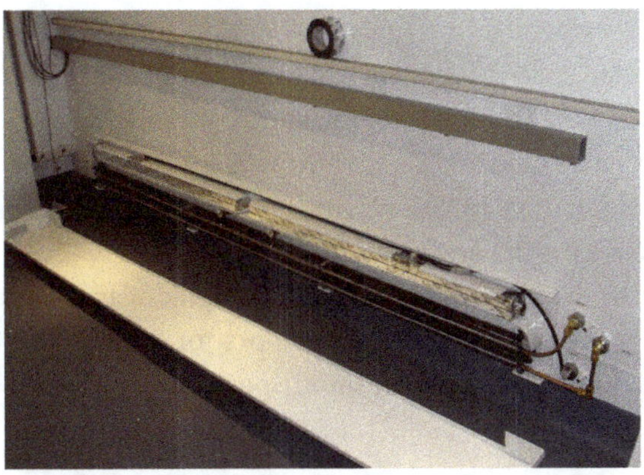

Figure 22. Cooling/heating coils in a multiplace chamber.

Humidity

Optimally, chamber humidity should be maintained in the 50 to 70% range for comfort and to reduce the risk of fire caused by a static electrical spark.[3,15] Depending on local climatic conditions, the efficiency of the air drier on the compressors and the number of chamber occupants, humidity may need to be raised or lowered. Some chambers use a pneumatic nebulizer that sprays a fine mist of warm water into the airflow from the blower to raise the humidity level. To lower the chamber humidity, the chilled water-cooling coils are used. As the air is forced over the cold coils, condensation forms on the coils, removing the moisture from the air. If the chamber becomes too cool during this procedure, the reheat water coils should be used to maintain proper temperature.

Humidity can be manually or automatically controlled. The reheated and chilled water flow is controlled in the same manner as when heating or cooling the chamber. To add humidity, the valve supplying water to the nebulizer is opened. Whether the system is automatic or manual, a method to measure humidity in the chamber is required to accurately monitor humidity levels. A hygrometer with or without a transmitter to send a signal to a remote display or controller can be utilized. An automated humidity control system may be linked to the ECS controls. The system will require a control loop, including a humidity sensor and transmitter in the chamber, a humidity controller, a control link through the ECS controller, or an independent control over the chilled and reheat water valves. A method to turn the humidity spray nozzle valve on and off is also necessary. The chamber operator sets the automatic humidity controller to the setting desired. The humidity sensor/transmitter sends a mA output signal to the controller that is proportional to the humidity level in the chamber. The controller then will automatically add or reduce humidity as needed to match the desired level. Monoplace chambers compressed with 100% oxygen rarely incorporate humidity control. Oxygen supplied to the chamber is anhydrous, so the only humidity in the chamber is that produced by patient's respirations and perspiration.

Gas Analysis

The gas analysis system gives the chamber operator the means to monitor the concentration of selected gases within the confined space of the hyperbaric chamber. There are single-use detector tubes that can be used for spot sampling for numerous gas contaminates, including carbon dioxide, carbon monoxide, oil mist, and water vapor. Sample gas is pumped into the tube by a handheld manual bellows pump, where the results are displayed on the tube in a scale appropriate for the gas being measured.

Air from compressors providing air to the chambers should be sampled biannually and certificates of analysis should be supplied by commercial vendors for the medical gas supplied to the chamber.[3,16] Table 2 describes some common specifications for air from the CGA.

Table 2. Common Specifications for Air and Uses; Data Obtained from CGA G-7.1

Grades, typical uses, and limiting characteristics (parts per million, ppm (V/V) unless otherwise noted)						
	A	L	D	E	J	N
Carbon dioxide			1,000	1,000	0.5	500
+ Carbon monoxide			10	10	1	10
Halogenated solvents					0.1	
Nitric oxide						2.5
Nitrogen dioxide					0.1	2.5
Nitrous oxide					0.1	
Odor		None	None	None	None	None
Oil (condensed)			5	5		None
Percent oxygen, balance predominantly nitrogen	19.5 -23.5	19.5 – 23.5	19.5 – 23.4	20 – 22	19.5 – 23.5	19.5 – 23.5
Sulfur dioxide					0.1	5
Total hydrocarbon content (as methane)				25	0.5	
Water Dew point F Dew point C		24 -65 -53.9			1 -105 -76.1	
Uses	**Industrial compressed** air	**Self-contained breathing** apparatus (SCBA)	**OSHA breathing** air	**Self-contained underwater** breathing apparatus (SCUBA)	**Specialty grade** air, analytical applications	**Medical air United States** Pharmacopeia (USP)

Oxygen Levels

Oxygen percentage is routinely monitored in the atmosphere of multiplace chambers. Chamber ventilation combined with an overboard dump system serves to maintain proper oxygen and carbon dioxide levels in the chamber. Carbon dioxide should be monitored in chambers where proper ventilation rates cannot be maintained.

To be in compliance with *NFPA 99*, multiplace hyperbaric chambers must maintain an environmental oxygen percentage of less than 23.5%.[3] When increased above this level, both the ignition temperature of flammable materials drops and the flame spread-rate increases to unacceptable levels. This standard also applies to monoplace chambers that pressurize with air and provide O_2 to the occupant by mask or hood. To ensure that this safety requirement is met, the chamber oxygen content must be constantly analyzed so that corrective action can be taken to decrease the excess O_2 level. An oxygen analyzer is connected to a chamber air sample-port by tubing. An inline flow meter is normally used to maintain a constant flow of sample gas across the analyzer cell. The analyzer should be located as close as practical to the chamber and the sample gas tubing should be ¼ inch in diameter, or smaller, to shorten the analyzer's response time to changing oxygen levels within the chamber, and/or the breathing device(s). Sample response times should be less than 30 seconds. We recommend that a fuel cell or paramagnetic oxygen analyzer be used if the intent is to use one analyzer to monitor both the oxygen levels in the breathing device(s) and air in the chamber. Once calibrated, the fuel cell and paramagnetic output are linear, and do not require recalibration between air and 100% oxygen. Not all analyzers use fuel cells or paramagnetic technology. The chamber operator should keep up with changing technology and use the best analyzer available for their specific application.

For example, there are analyzers that use a zirconium element which has proven very stable and has a 5–10 year life as opposed to the fuel cell, which usually lasts about a year, depending on the manufacturer. If the chamber is designed to utilize an inert gas diluent (such as nitrogen) as an alternative to air ventilation, oxygen levels must also be monitored to prevent chamber occupants from exposure to hypoxic oxygen levels. The minimum safe oxygen level is based on the partial pressure of the gas at the chamber pressure. (Dalton's Law). It should never go below the surface equivalent of 16%.[6] The oxygen analyzer should have visual and audio alarms that indicate when the chamber air is outside of the normal oxygen range. The chamber air sample-port should be located as close as possible to the chamber occupants. Chamber air should be circulated as much as possible during use to prevent local areas, or pockets, of high concentration of oxygen. Local oxygen pockets can form as a result of leaking oxygen equipment or equipment left on when not in use. By continuously circulating chamber air using the air conditioning blower and/or by ventilating the chamber, the production of these oxygen pockets is minimized. Keeping the chamber air thoroughly mixed ensures that the chamber air sample-port will quickly pick up any changes in the chamber's oxygen level. A local pocket of elevated oxygen may have contributed to a tragic chamber fire.[17]

Oxygen Analyzers

Oxygen analyzers are utilized to monitor the medical gas supplied to the chamber occupants. The chamber operator is able to observe the O_2 percent of the chamber atmosphere, the gas being delivered to the oxygen delivery devices, and the inside attendant's mask at the control panel. This practice is more common in multiplace chambers but some monoplace manufacturers provide this option as well. The addition of a portable O_2 analyzer to monitor the gas supplied to and/or to monitor the chamber atmosphere in the monoplace chamber should be considered.

The portable O_2 analyzer shown uses a galvanic sensor that generates an electrical current in proportion to the amount of oxygen to which it is exposed. To calibrate this analyzer, expose the cell to ambient air and adjust the display to 20.9% oxygen. On average, the sensor will last from 6 to 24 months depending on the sensor design and concentrations of oxygen measured. Each time they are turned on, they should be calibrated to 20.9% oxygen using room air.

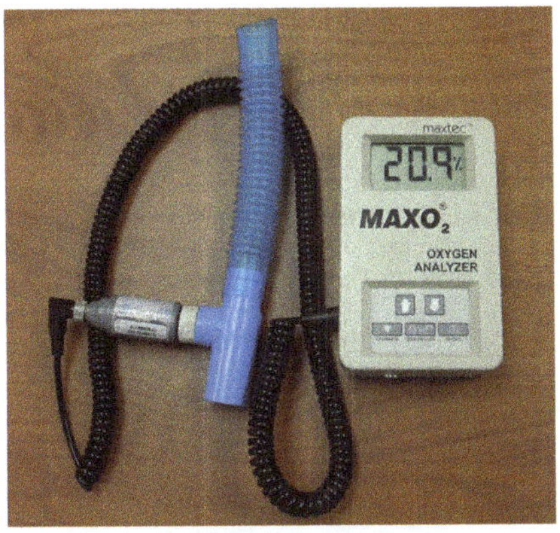

Figure 23. Portable oxygen analyzer.

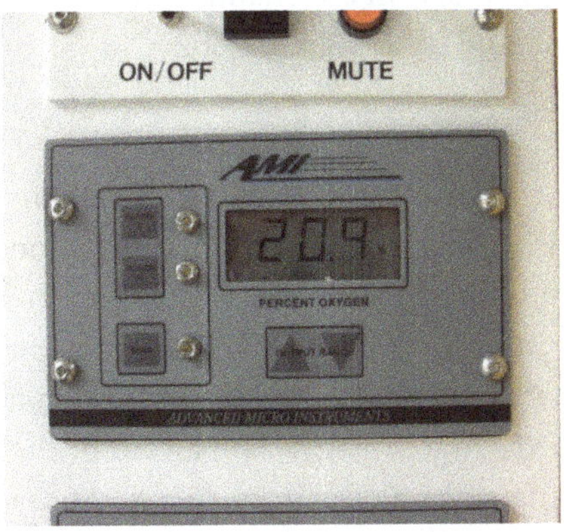

Figure 24. Panel-mounted oxygen analyzer.

The panel-mounted oxygen analyzer shown uses a zirconium oxide sensor that produces an output current in proportion to the amount of oxygen present. The zero output equals the absence of O_2 and there is no requirement to zero the analyzer. The calibration may be performed using a standard span gas or ambient air. Some analyzers will require a zero gas (nitrogen) and a full-scale gas (100% oxygen) to calibrate and a special calibration mix in the midrange of the analyzer scale, such as 50% oxygen with the balance nitrogen. There is a built-in critical orifice for automatic flow control over a wide range of pressures so a flow meter is not required. The sensor is stable, requiring calibration only a couple of times a year depending on use and has an expected life of 5 to 10 years. The analyzer is checked daily prior to chamber operation to ensure it is working correctly. If the facility uses carbon dioxide or carbon monoxide analyzers, it is possible to obtain all the calibration gases in one cylinder. For example, the calibration gas may contain 50% oxygen, 0.5% carbon dioxide, and 60 PPM carbon monoxide, with the balance nitrogen. In all of these analyzers, a consistent sample gas flow rate is required. Calibrate the oxygen analyzer with the calibration gas passing across the sensor at a given flow rate and ensure the sample gas coming from the chamber is flowing at the exact same flow rate. Without a constant sample flow rate, the analyzers reading of the chamber atmospheres oxygen percent will not be accurate. Inaccurate reading of the analyzer can cause the chamber operator to miss a high oxygen level in the chamber or to perceive that the oxygen level in the chamber was high, when it is not. These errors could prompt the chamber operator to unnecessarily decrease or increase the ventilation rate to try to bring the chamber atmosphere into prescribed limits.

If the oxygen level inside the chamber begins to increase, the following actions should be taken to keep the oxygen level below 23.5%:

- Increase chamber ventilation rate.
- Check the analyzer for proper gas sample rate and function.
- Have the inside attendant search for the source of possible oxygen leaks and stop the leak if possible. Typical sources are:
    - Loose hood connections or a torn hood or neck ring
    - Overboard dump system not on or set up incorrectly
    - Malfunctioning or failed oxygen regulator (or like equipment)
    - Leaking oxygen pipe fittings or unions
    - A sniffer line attached to the oxygen analyzer sample port of the chamber can be helpful in isolating oxygen leaks in the chamber.

If, after the above actions are taken, and the oxygen level in the chamber cannot be brought down below the 23.5% level, the chamber should be depressurized.

Carbon Dioxide Levels

Many clinical hyperbaric chambers are designed for constant ventilation. If the chamber cannot be ventilated or is not designed to use constant ventilation (saturation chamber), the carbon dioxide level must also be monitored.[3] Mechanical failure of the compressors, quality of the chamber's ambient air supply, or number of personnel in the chamber are all reasons to monitor the carbon dioxide (CO_2) level. CO_2 levels in a nonventilated chamber (typically multiplace) can exceed a safe level. Be aware of the concern while operating a monoplace chamber using air as a compression gas. At sea level, the maximum safe concentration of CO_2 is 40 mmHg or 5% by volume. As the partial pressure of CO_2 increases during chamber operation at increased pressure, the maximum safe CO_2 percentage decreases. At 2 ATA, the maximum safe partial pressure of CO_2 is still 40 mmHg but now only 2.5% by volume. This means, if the CO_2 analyzer reads in percentage by volume, that you must adjust the maximum allowable CO_2 percentage based on chamber pressure. The normal ambient concentration of CO_2 in the earth's atmosphere is approximately 400 ppm or 0.04 % by volume.[18] OSHA 29 CFR, 1910.1000 Table Z, limits CO_2 to 5,000 ppm (0.5% by volume over an 8-hour exposure).[19] Ideally CO_2 concentrations should be maintained as close to normal atmospheric levels as possible.[20] Oxygen breathing devices such as hoods, mask, etc. should be set to ensure sufficient flow to prevent a buildup of CO_2 greater than 0.05 ppm.[21] Higher levels of CO_2 will increase the likelihood of an oxygen toxicity seizure.[6]

We are aware of at least two occasions in 2013 during the Department of Defense clinical trials for head trauma and hyperbaric oxygen where the ambient carbon dioxide (CO_2) levels exceeded the USP medical air limit of 500 ppm (CGA Grade N).[16] This was due to local forest fires. The chambers in use were multiplace chambers and CO_2 scrubbers were added at the intakes for the compressors and in the chamber at the environmental control fan. The alternate source of medical air (H cylinders of USP medical air) was also utilized. *NFPA 99, 2018 edition,* Chapter 5, Table 5.1.12.4.12.3, limits the CO_2 in medical air to 500 ppm as does the specification for USP medical air (CGA Grade N).[3,16] *NFPA 99,* Chapter 14 does not require that air supplied to the chamber from compressors meet the USP medical air standard. Air supplied from high-pressure cylinders must be USP medical air. The hyperbaric facility is required to meet CGA Grade E which allows 1,000 ppm CO_2, unless the air from the compressors is shared with the hospital, in which case they must meet the requirements of *NFPA 99, 2018 edition* Chapters 5 and 14.[3]

Carbon Dioxide Analyzers

Carbon dioxide analyzers sample chamber air in the same manner as described for the oxygen analyzer. They are also calibrated in much the same manner.

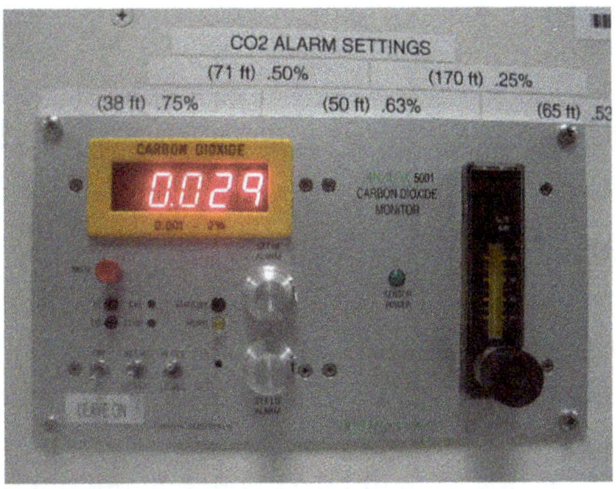

Figure 25. Panel-mounted carbon dioxide analyzer.

Carbon Dioxide Life Support Ranges

If the levels of CO_2 should become elevated, the following actions should be taken immediately:

- If possible, increase the chamber ventilation rate, or if using a staggered ventilation schedule, increase the frequency and duration of the ventilation.
- Have chamber occupants breathe from masks or hoods, preferably with an overboard dump system.
- If the chamber is equipped with a CO_2 scrubber[*], it should be used.

- If the CO_2 level cannot be controlled, and the built-in breathing systems (BIBS) system fails, chamber operation must be terminated.

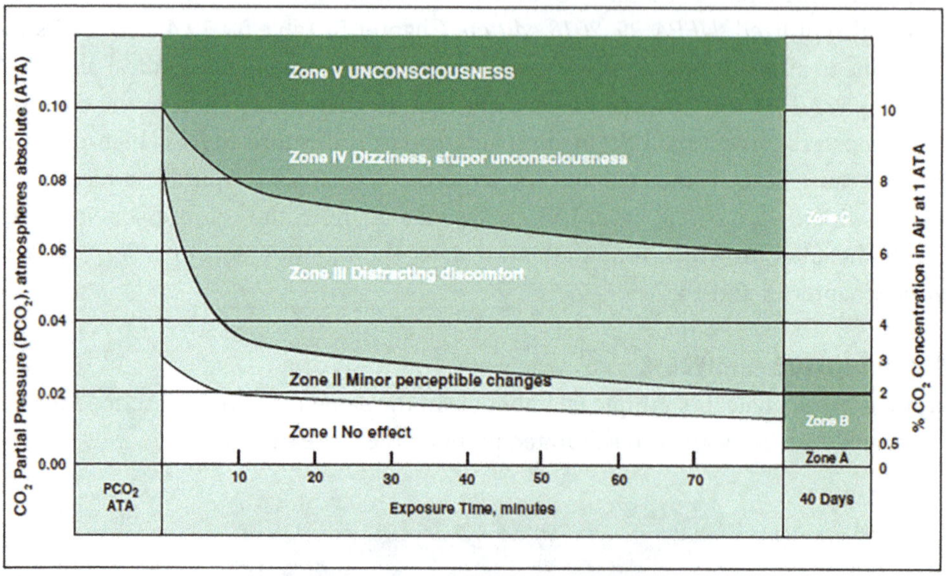

Figure 26. Carbon dioxide life support scale. Courtesy of Best Publishing Company, *NOAA 6th Edition*, 2017.

Carbon Monoxide Levels

The *NFPA 99* requires a minimum of CGA Grade E, USP medical air, or medical air as defined by the NFPA. The limit for carbon monoxide (CO) in all of these standards is the same. The CGA limit for CO in Grade E, Grade N, USP specification for medical air, and the *NFPA 99* definition of medical air in Chapter 5 (5.1.12.3.12.3) are all 10 parts per million.[3,16] As with CO_2, this is a multiplace concern unless a monoplace chamber is operated with air. The most likely source of CO is from the ambient source of air for the compressors. If the compressors are lubricated with a petroleum-based product, they must be equipped with a filtering and monitoring package designed to produce medical air. The effects of breathing CO while at increased pressure are greater than at ambient pressure. A CO level of 5 ppm would have the effect of 15 ppm at 3 ATA. The alarm limits can be set on some of the monitors, for example, 5 ppm, 10, ppm, or 15 ppm. It is good practice to monitor the chamber air supply for CO levels and abort chamber operations if the chamber atmosphere becomes contaminated and the monitors are working

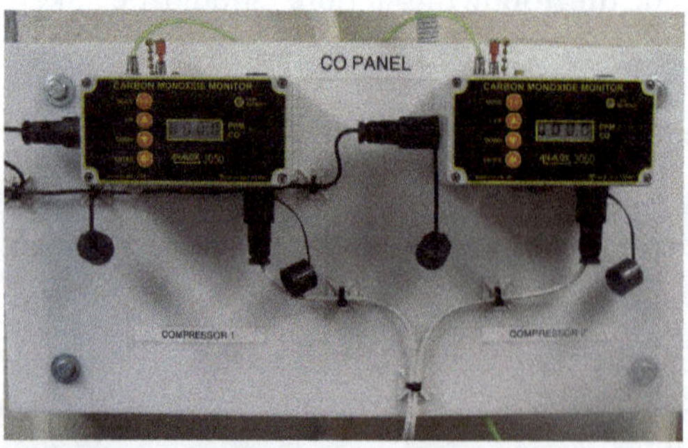

Figure 27. Carbon monoxide monitors set up to monitor the compressor air supply.

correctly. In our experience, the normal level is 0 ppm. There is a least one facility we are aware of that has installed the CO monitor at the intake for the compressors in order to monitor a high CO level before it contaminates the system. If the CO level in the chamber is above normal ambient or alarms at the set point, the inside attendant should have the patients or subjects leave their oxygen delivery devices on, don the alternative breathing air device, and prepare to decompress. The chamber operator should seek medical advice and prepare to decompress if the CO level remains elevated.

Carbon monoxide analyzers can be set up to sample chamber air in the same manner as described for the oxygen and CO_2 analyzers. They are also calibrated in much the same manner.

Patient Monitoring

Whether using multiplace or monoplace chambers, the chamber operator must be able to monitor the occupants of the chamber both visually and audibly.[3] Visual monitoring of a monoplace or small multiplace chamber is accomplished by the chamber operator observing the chamber occupants through the chamber viewport. On larger multiplace chambers, the chamber is operated from a console. To monitor the chamber occupants, video cameras are mounted either outside a viewport or inside the chamber. The chamber operator can then observe patients and inside attendants from monitors at the control console. If the chamber is sufficiently large, a pan and tilt video camera with a zoom lens may be installed. This camera allows the chamber operator to zoom in on a specific individual or piece of equipment. This feature can be useful when trying to evaluate a patient or coaching an inside attendant through an equipment problem. It may be necessary to mount multiple cameras for some chambers to be able to see all of the chamber occupants. Some monoplace facilities that operate several monoplace chambers simultaneously may utilize a video monitoring system to assist in patient monitoring.

If the visual monitoring system fails, the console operator should have another hyperbaric team member monitor the chamber occupants through the viewport and

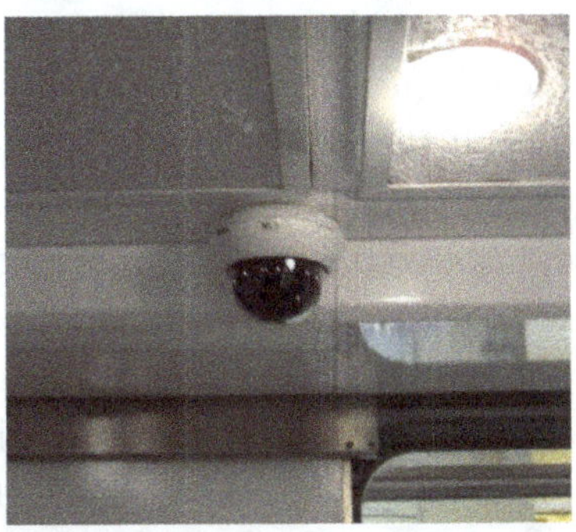

Figure 28. Interior mounted camera in multiplace chamber.

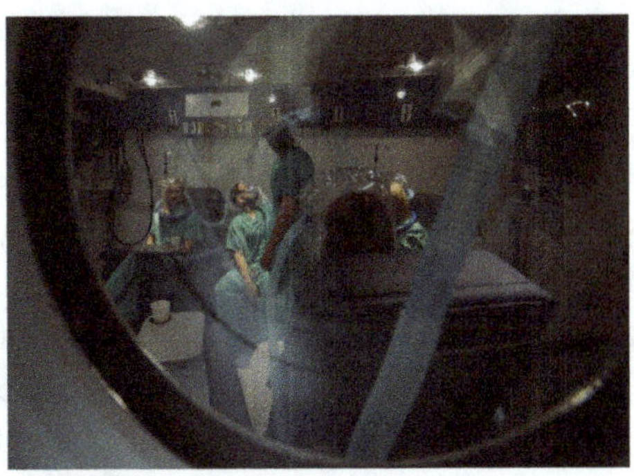

Figure 29. Viewport monitoring of a multiplace chamber.

relay their condition to the chamber operator. This aspect is especially important if communication is lost simultaneously or during chamber pressure changes.

Communications Systems

Monoplace

The acrylic hull and gentle sound of gas entering the chamber make for a quiet, peaceful treatment environment but restricts external sounds from reaching the occupant. Occupants inside a monoplace chamber would have a difficult time communicating with their chamber operator without an intercommunication system. The built-in, two-way communication system consists of an internally mounted hands-free microphone and electrically intrinsically safe speaker. The chamber operator uses a pushbutton microphone or telephone-style handset to talk to the patient. The operator depresses the button to talk and releases it to listen or a switch activates the handset microphone when it is removed from its storage cradle. A speaker and controls for volume in and volume out are located on the control panel. The chambers have an auxiliary input for entertainment audio to the internal speakers that are interrupted during patient and chamber operator communications.

Multiplace

The primary link between the chamber attendant and the chamber operator is the audio communication system. The communication system in most hyperbaric facilities is the intercom. It allows the chamber operator to hear all sounds coming from inside the chamber. The major drawback of this system is that patients can hear conversations between the chamber operator and the inside attendant. If an external speaker is mounted in the control panel, patient confidentiality can be compromised if visitors are near. Intercoms do not provide the clearest sound quality and if the chamber is noisy, voices may be unintelligible. Having the chamber attendant direct their voice toward the microphone and enunciate clearly helps facilitate clear communication. Power for the intercom system should be supplied from a hospital emergency power circuit and/or on an uninterruptible power supply (UPS).

Supplementing the intercom with a two-way radio provides a margin of safety through redundancy of systems. If the radio units include headsets, sound quality is usually improved and conversations are private. Ear muff style headsets can provide hearing protection in noisy chambers, but they may make it more difficult to hear what the patient is saying. The ear pads on this style may seal around the ears during pressurization, making ear equalizing difficult. This problem can be solved by drilling a small hole in the outer shell to allow air to pass freely in and out. Temple transducer headsets leave the ear canal free and transmit sound through the bones of the head. Sound clarity is excellent without muffling ambient sounds. If enough radios are available, the physician or other members of the hyperbaric team can help monitor and respond to the needs of the chamber attendant. Radios with access to multiple channels permit independent conversations when multiple chambers or locks are in use. Two-way radios may also be helpful when trouble shooting mechanical problems and performing maintenance tasks.

Wireless communications should meet the requirements for battery-operated devices as stated in *NFPA 99* and be pressure tolerant to the chambers maximum working pressure. They must be able to withstand rapid pressurization and depressurization as experienced in a medical lock. These devices are not considered intrinsically safe when the battery is being removed or installed so the entire unit will need to be locked out when battery changes are needed. Batteries must comply with *NFPA 99* requirements for battery-operated equipment. A concern has been noted for the rechargeable lithium ion type batteries.[3]

Hard-wired telephones can be used in the chamber if they are intrinsically safe or adequately nitrogen purged. The obvious advantage of telephones is the ability to converse with others outside of the hyperbaric facility. A nurse in the chamber can talk directly with the patient's nurse on the floor, to the pharmacy, or a consulting physician.

Sound-powered phones often are the default emergency communication system because they are reliable and do not require electrical power or batteries to function. These simple devices operate much like two tin cans on a string. The handsets contain a dynamic microphone that converts sound pressure from the user's voice into an electrical current that is converted back to sound by a transducer in the receiving handset. Many sound-powered phones do not have a ringer to alert the person on the other

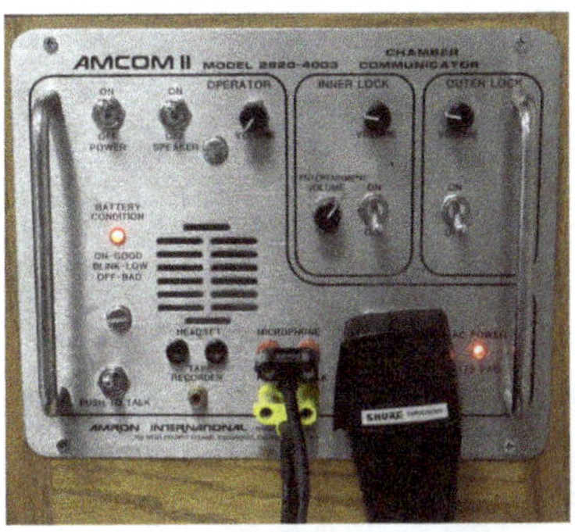

Figure 30. Intercom panel.

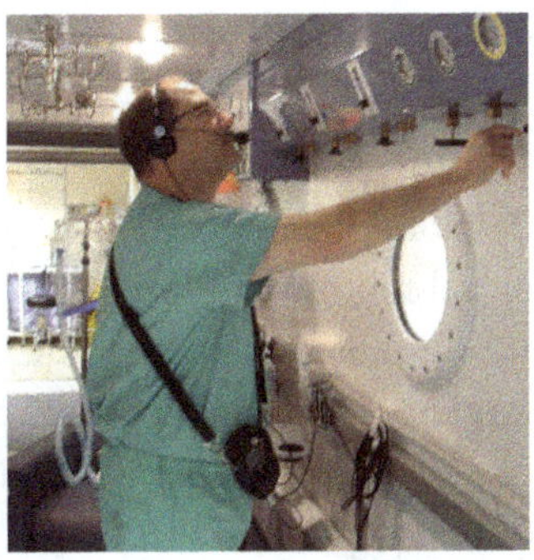

Figure 31. Wireless communications.

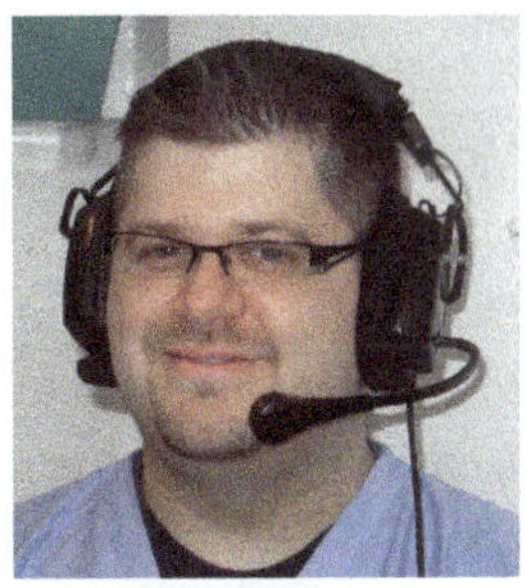

Figure 32. Earmuff-style headset.

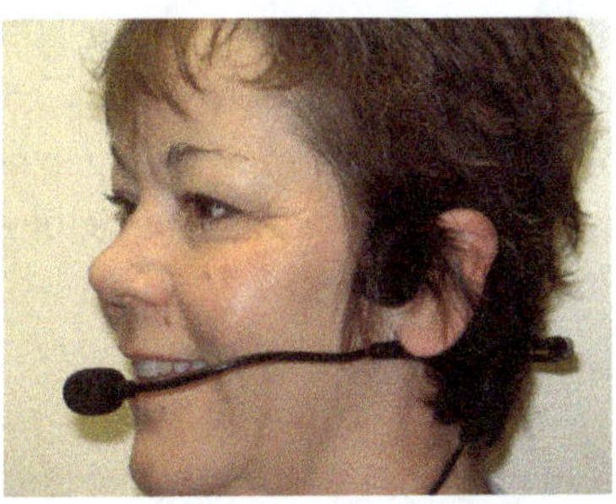

Figure 33. Temple transducer headset.

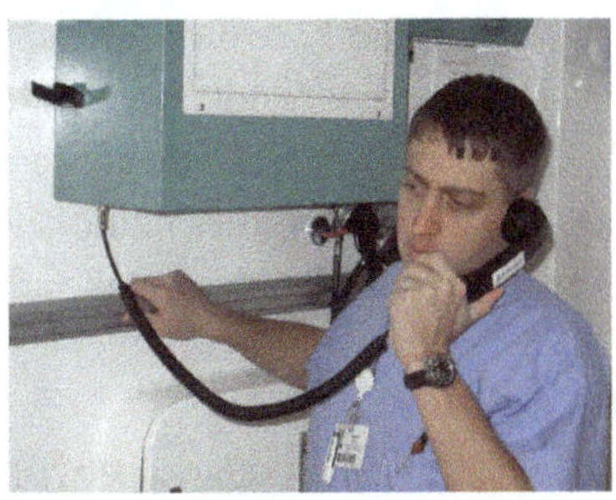

Figure 34. Sound-powered phone.

end of an incoming call, so some method of getting their attention, even knocking on the chamber hull must be used.

If redundant systems using independent power sources are available, it is unlikely that all should fail simultaneously. When all else fails, written notes can be held up to the chamber window.

Physiological Monitoring

Hyperbaric chambers usually do not come from the manufacturer outfitted with all the equipment necessary to monitor critically ill patients. Most monitoring equipment is not designed or rated for use within the hyperbaric environment. If acutely ill patients are to be treated, monitoring equipment will need to be adapted by the chamber owner. The NFPA has recognized this dilemma and provides a method for the end user to accomplish the task. *NFPA 99*, 14.2.9.3.2, 2018 edition, states that all equipment is rated, tested, and the process documented for the intended hyperbaric conditions prior to use. *NFPA 99* also provides valuable information for developing a systematic program to evaluate and test equipment for compatibility within the hyperbaric environment. Not all hyperbaric facilities have chosen to equip their chambers with monitoring capabilities. A high level of commitment is needed to safely adapt equipment, train, and maintain staff competency with the equipment. Some of the physiological parameters that have had equipment adapted for monitoring include electrocardiogram (ECG), electroencephalogram (EEG), transcutaneous oximetry monitoring (TCOM), intracranial pressure (ICP), invasive and noninvasive blood pressure, central venous pressure (CVP), end tidal CO_2, and respiratory variables.[22-24]

Monoplace

Electrical equipment inside monoplace chambers is restricted to communications functions and patient physiological monitoring leads. All other equipment that is necessary to facilitate patient monitoring must be located outside the chamber. Chamber manufacturers provide pressure tolerant electrical pass-through ports that allow clinicians to adapt and connect existing monitoring equipment to the patient leads inside the chamber. Whenever possible, the same equipment that is used in the rest of your facility should be adapted for chamber use. Familiarity with equipment will instill confidence in its use, decrease learning time, reduce errors, and streamline patient preparation for HBO_2. At the time of this writing, Radiometer is the only manufacturer of transcutaneous oximetry leads that are approved by Underwriters Laboratory (UL) for use in 100% oxygen at pressures of up to 4 ATA.[25] Other manufacturers of transcutaneous oximetry machines may utilize Radiometer electrodes to take advantage of the UL rating.

Multiplace

Multiplace chambers have a variety of solutions for meeting monitoring needs. Some multiplace chambers have the physiological monitors located outside of a chamber window, making it visible to the chamber attendant. Cables for the patient leads are passed through the hull via pressure tolerant electrical pass-through ports similar as done with the monoplace chambers. Portable transport monitors have been utilized as have monitors installed inside the chamber using inert gas purging of the internal electronics. Others have split with both internal and external uses, locating some of the equipment inside and some outside of the chamber. Telemetry devices have been found to work from inside the multiplace chamber; however the location of the antenna is critical. Telemetry boxes are battery-powered devices and must conform to *NFPA 99* requirements for battery-operated devices. The batteries must not be changed in the chamber while the chamber is pressurized. *Telemetry devices are not allowed inside the monoplace chamber.*

For a comprehensive discussion of physiological monitoring in clinical hyperbaric medicine, refer to *The Physiology and Medicine of Hyperbaric Oxygen Therapy*, Thom and Neuman, editors, and *Hyperbaric Medicine Practice, 4th edition*, Whelan and Kindwall, editors.

Vacuum System (Suction)

Vacuum is used clinically for nasogastric tubes, thoracostomy tubes, surgical wound drains, negative pressure wound therapy, oropharyngeal suctioning, and deep suctioning of endotracheal tubes and tracheostomy tubes included during HBO_2 exposures. Vacuum pumps that power standard wall vacuum usually generate about 450 mmHg to 600 mmHg vacuum, but most clinical tasks can be accomplished with less than 200 mmHg vacuum. Vacuum inside the hyperbaric chamber is generated by the pressure gradient across the chamber hull with chamber pressure relative to atmospheric pressure. The amount of vacuum is controlled by a vacuum regulator located inside the chamber. Once the chamber has been pressurized past 4 PSI, the vacuum generated is sufficient for clinical purposes. Caution should be exercised when utilizing in-chamber suction as the pressure gradient at normal treatment pressures is several times that of standard wall suction. At a chamber pressure of 6 ATA, approximately 3800 mmHg vacuum is potentially available.

Weaver described a method for providing suction for nasogastric tubes, thoracostomy tubes, and surgical wound drains inside a monoplace chamber.[26] In this system, a Boehringer Model 3704 suction regulator, cleaned and lubricated for oxygen service, and a collection canister is mounted inside the chamber door. An externally mounted three-way stopcock connected to the vacuum regulator via an IV pass through port or custom bulkhead fitting is used with an external flow meter to turn on or off and adjust the amount of vacuum. Ensurance against excessive vacuum is provided by presetting the vacuum regulator and securing the regulator's adjustment knob. Standard hospital wall suction is temporarily connected to the externally mounted stopcock while the chamber is at atmospheric pressure so that the internal vacuum regulator can be adjusted.

Raleigh et al. devised a vacuum device for monoplace and multiplace chambers to provide continuous negative pressure wound therapy (0-150 mmHg) during hyperbaric oxygen therapy.[27] The essential features of this unit include the Boehringer vacuum regulator that can be preset and locked in place and an inline adjustable vacuum relief valve that ensures vacuum cannot exceed prescribed limits in the event of a regulator failure. When constructed for monoplace use, the vacuum regulator should be disassembled and cleaned for oxygen service prior to its installation and use.

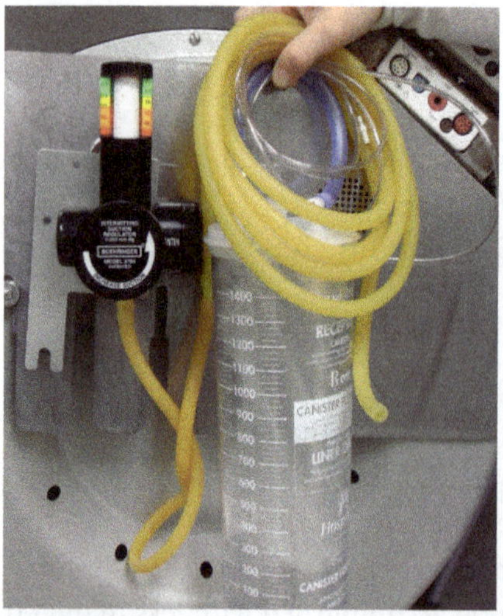

Figure 35. Weaver suction assembly for the monoplace.

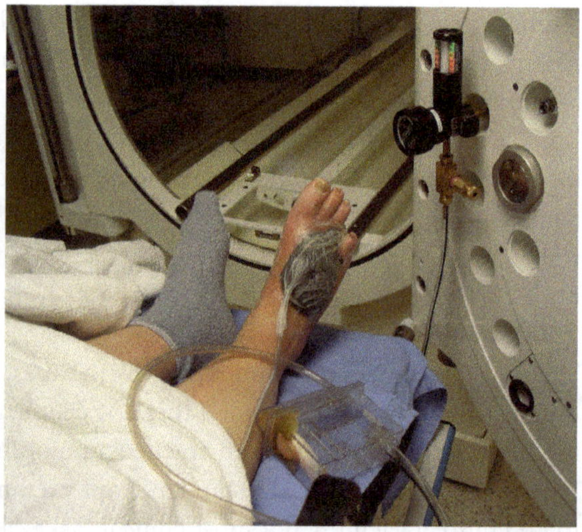

Figure 36. Monoplace negative pressure wound therapy.

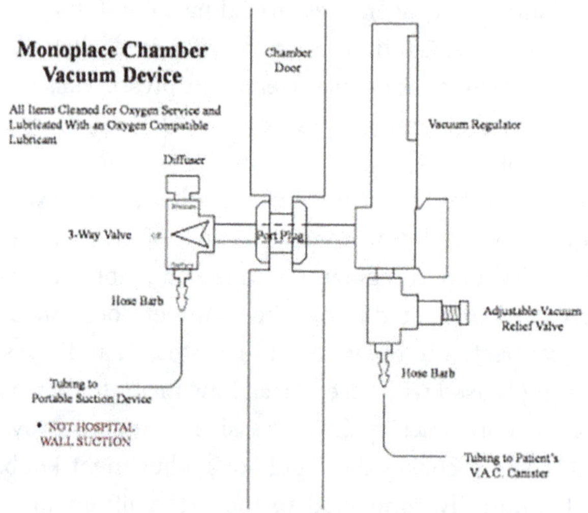

Figure 37. Diagram of monoplace chamber vacuum device.

Chamber Lighting

Monoplace Chambers

Most monoplace chambers have incorporated an extensive cylindrical viewport/hull in their design. The large surface area of the cylindrical viewport allows an adequate amount of light into the chamber from the surrounding room. Additional lighting is seldom required and often a reduction is appreciated by chamber occupant(s) who want to rest or sleep during the time the chamber is pressurized. The acrylic viewport/hull should be protected from ultraviolet sunlight that will, with time, deteriorate the acrylic.[28] Emergency backup lighting should be provided and can be as simple as a flashlight that is stored nearby; however, local, state, and national codes may require the installation of automated emergency lighting in the hyperbaric room.

Multiplace Chambers

There are several methods to provide illumination of the interior of multiplace chambers. Natural light can be allowed to shine through viewports if the number and arrangement of viewports is adequate. However, provisions must be made if the chamber is operated when sunlight is not present. Exposure to ultraviolet light will deteriorate acrylic viewports. Most clinical chambers will need some form of artificial light. External lighting systems may be as simple as a light fixture shining directly into the chamber through the chamber viewports. While effective, the viewports are not then usable for observation in or out of the chamber. Heat generated from external lights can damage temperature sensitive acrylic viewports. The light source should be kept a safe distance from the viewport, and it should be protected by infrared filters, fans, dichroic mirrors, or some other means of dissipating heat. There have been windows damaged by heat from external light sources such as chamber lighting. The danger of incandescent lighting too close to the acrylic viewports is well known in the clinical and diving industries. Even fluorescent lighting can produce temperatures in excess of 140°F. The Association of Diving Contractors, International (ADCI) issued a safety alert on this issue in February 2008.[29] An incandescent drop light was placed too close to the viewport of a deck decompression chamber. The resulting radiant heat exceeded the design temperature of the viewport (125°F/51.6°C). The acrylic became soft due to the heat and the window failed. Chamber pressure was vented through the viewport to atmospheric pressure.

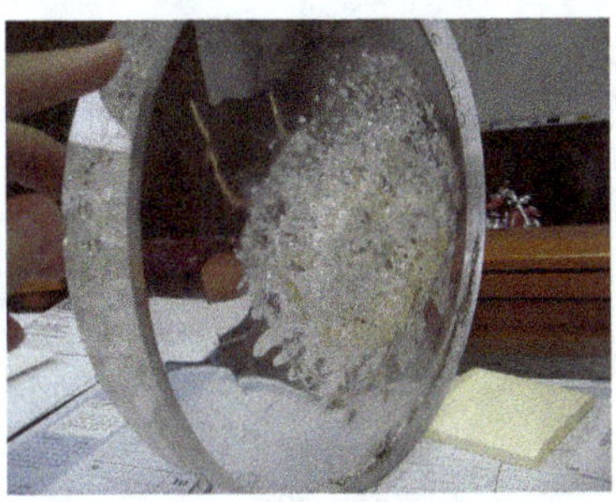

Figure 38. Failed acrylic viewport.

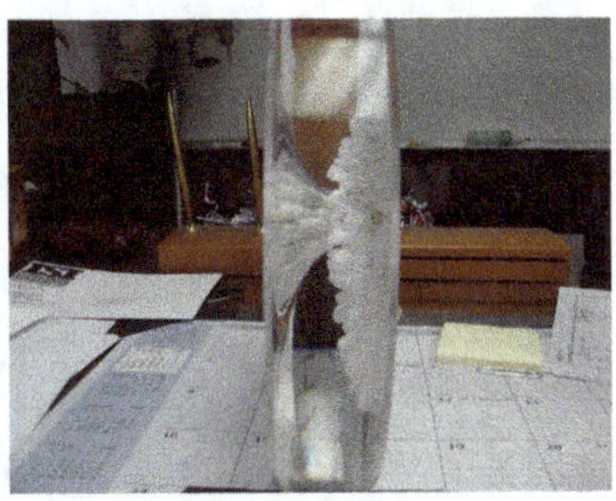

Figure 39. Failed acrylic viewport.

Permanently mounted electric or battery powered lighting fixtures can be located inside the chamber. Incandescent and fluorescent fixtures are giving way to light emitting diode (LED) fixtures as this technology continues to develop. Permanent internal lighting systems should meet the requirements in *NFPA 99* and built to withstand 1.5 times the maximum allowable working pressure (MAWP) of the chamber. All ballasts and other energy storage components must be located outside the chamber. The light fixture should have lens guards and be situated so they are protected from physical damage during normal chamber operations.[28]

Acrylic light pipe systems that use an external light source focused onto an acrylic tube in a through-hull penetrator are used to provide lighting in the chamber. Canty [30] patented the first such light in 1974, and this style has since become the standard for pressure vessel illumination. The advantages of acrylic light pipe systems include no heat radiation inside the chamber, ease of changing bulbs even when the chamber is pressurized, unobtrusive with minimal protrusion into the chamber, no risk of fire or electrical shock to chamber occupants, and structurally sound to 1,000 PSIG. These fixtures are not totally without risk. We are aware of an incident where the light support came loose and the high intensity bulb came in close proximity to the acrylic tube causing the acrylic to bubble and deform.

Acrylic light pipe systems usually have at least three components. A high intensity light source mounted on the outside of the chamber, and an acrylic tube in a through-hull penetrator. A diffuser may or may not be present inside the chamber to disperse the light. The housing for the light is usually fan cooled to dissipate heat and some method of thermal switching is provided to turn off the light if the fan malfunctions or the fixture becomes too hot. Acrylic light pipe systems are an integral part of pressure boundary and as such, they should be inspected and maintained in the same manner as the acrylic viewports.

Chamber lighting should be powered by the hospital emergency power circuit and/or on an uninterruptable power supply (UPS). Even with these preemptive strategies to avoid loss of the chamber's primary lighting source, a readily available emergency backup should be in place. Flashlights that are rated for hazardous environments and are

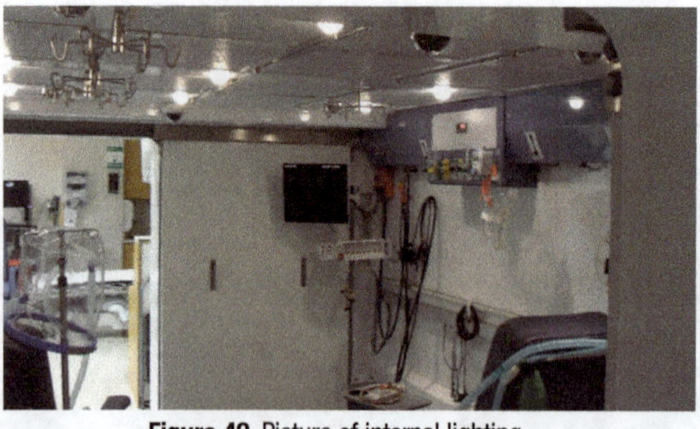

Figure 40. Picture of internal lighting.

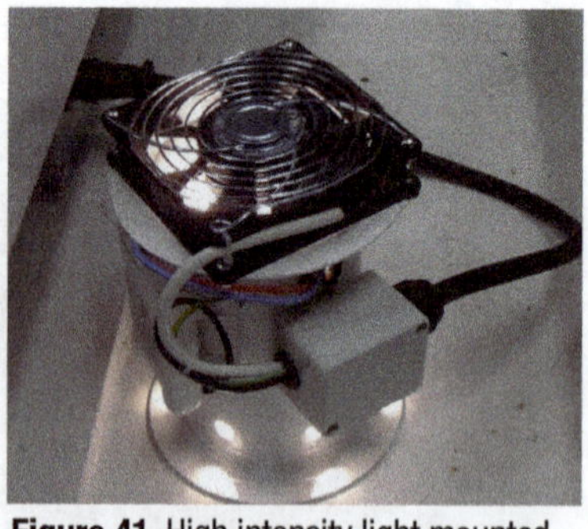

Figure 41. High intensity light mounted over acrylic light pipe.

pressure tolerant or diving flashlights are excellent for backup lighting. Flashlight batteries should not be lithium ion type and must be less than 12 V, fully enclosed, tolerant of maximum chamber pressure, and sealed to not off-gas during normal use. A simpler alternative is to have chemical light sticks available to hang in the chamber or outside viewports. Chemical light sticks are plastic tubes that usually contain two chemicals that when combined produce light. They are waterproof, pressure tolerant, inexpensive, and disposable, generate negligible heat, and do not spark or require batteries.

Whatever lighting system is utilized to illuminate the chamber interior, the lamps used should have spectrum characteristics similar to the lighting used throughout the rest of the clinical facility. This will provide visual consistency for color judgments of cyanosis.[31]

Patient Entertainment System

Monoplace

Most monoplace chambers have an internally mounted, electrically intrinsically safe speaker that is used for both communication and entertainment. Entertainment devices, such as radio, television, DVD players, etc. must be externally located since they are not allowed inside the monoplace chamber. Sound inside the chamber is achieved via auxiliary audio jacks. The clear acrylic hull allows patients to view movies or television if a monitor screen is properly situated above the chamber. Sound input through the auxiliary jack will be silenced when the intercom is in use. UL-labeled, hospital-grade devices should be chosen for safety and durability as they will see considerably more use than standard home units.

Multiplace

NFPA 99 limits equipment in the multiplace chamber to what is necessary for safe operation of the chamber or required for patient care. Many practitioners are deciding that, as for monoplace chambers, there should be some sort of entertainment provided for the chamber occupants. A patient entertainment system helps improve patient satisfaction, comfort, and compliance, especially with pediatric patients, when treatments can be hours in length. The decision whether to provide an entertainment system is made by the owner of the chamber.

Existing entertainment systems for multiplace chambers range from radio broadcast through the intercom speakers to 48-inch-wide screen liquid crystal displays (LCD) to chambers where each chamber occupant can chose to watch and/or listen to their own choice of TV shows, movies, or music on individual screens. As technology changes, we will have more entertainment options available to us. Entertainment monitors can be installed as remote displays with the DVD players located outside of the chamber. The monitors can have dual use as a display of the patient's physiological parameters or to display the movie of the day. There is value in considering both 12-volt electrical supply and inert gas (nitrogen) purging of the monitors. Monitors have a transformer that boosts electrical energy high enough for the screen to work. The larger the screen, the more energy is required. In many cases if the back cover is removed from the monitor, you will see a caution sign indicating high voltage on the circuit board. Do not underestimate the value of limiting electrical energy in the chamber.

Another type of entertainment system utilizes a projector located outside of the chamber that projects through a chamber window onto a screen inside the chamber. In this case no electrical energy from the device is located inside the chamber. There are several methods for providing the sound for the movie to the occupants in multiplace chambers. Some systems utilize speakers installed in the chamber and others use air-powered ear phones similar to the ones provided in the past by the airlines. Whichever system is used, it must not interfere with the communications between the chamber operator and the inside attendant and must meet *NFPA 99* requirements for equipment in chambers.

Books and magazines can be provided in limited quantities for the patients in a multiplace chamber; however, because of its low flashpoint and high combustibility, newsprint should never be permitted inside the chamber! **Caution:** ***Limit the amount of material allowed inside the chamber. Don't permit combustible material to accumulate. Reading material as well as combustible medical supplies should be removed from the chamber or stored in metal containers when not in use.***[3]

Conclusion

The designs of both multiplace and monoplace chambers and their supporting systems have seen exceptional development and creativity over the past few decades. From manually operated pressure vessels typically designed to support diving and research operations, chambers have developed into sophisticated patient care and research devices. The Food and Drug Administration (FDA) considers the clinical chambers Class II medical devices.[32] Modern clinical chambers utilized to provide hyperbaric oxygen therapy need to be capable of providing state of the art care to a variety of patients from the routine to the most critical. This rapid growth in technology is sure to continue. The sophisticated level of patient physiological monitoring, controlled medication administration, and other equipment needs necessary to assure continuity of patient care and research will challenge development of chamber systems and support devices that will be able to keep pace with rapidly changing medical technology.

Acknowledgments

We would like to thank the following persons:

- Lindell K. Weaver, MD, Medical Director and Division Chief, Hyperbaric Medicine, LDS Hospital, Salt Lake City, UT and Intermountain Medical Center, Murray, UT; Professor of Medicine, University of Utah School of Medicine for his critical review.
- Kayla Deru, medical writer for her help with preparing the figures.
- Tom Schmidt for his help with *ASME-PVHO-1* language.
- We are grateful to Tom Workman and Steve Wood for the opportunity and their constructive comments and all of our co-workers who put up with us using them as models for this chapter. The authors have received no financial support for this project.

References

1. ASME. Safety Standard for Pressure Vessels for Human Occupancy (ANSI/ASME PVHO-1: 2016). New York: American Society of Mechanical Engineers, 2016. Available from http://www.asme.org [cited 2018 August 3].
2. Weaver L. (ed). Hyperbaric Oxygen Therapy Indications, Undersea and Hyperbaric Medical Society, 13th Edition. NPB, Florida: Best Publishing Company; 2016.
3. NFPA. NFPA 99, Health Care Facilities Code. Quincy, MA: National Fire Protection Association; Available from https://www.nfpa.org/ [cited 2018 August 14].
4. Zwart BP. The "smooth ride" profile: development, implementation, and evaluation of a hyperbaric chamber descent and ascent based on a constant rate of volume change with time. Davis Hyperbaric Laboratory Report. Brooks AFB, Texas. 1998. [Available from http://www.tanktigers.net [cited 2018 August 14].
5. Chhoeu AH, Conard JL, Chen M., Freiberger JJ; Carraway, MS; Dear, et al. [Abstract] Reducing compression rate during clinical hyperbaric therapy will reduce the rate of otic barotrauma. Undersea and Hyperbaric Medical Society, Inc. Available from http://rubicon-foundation.org [cited 2018 August 14].
6. US Navy. US Navy Diving Manual, Revision 7**,** Direction of Commander, Naval Sea Systems Command, 01 December 2016. Available from http://www.supsalv.org/00c3_publications.asp [cited 2018 August 8].
7. OSHA. Occupational Safety and Health Administration (OSHA), Code of Federal Regulations, (Standards-29 CFR), part number 1910, part title Occupational Safety and Health Standard, subpart T, commercial diving operations, standard number 1910.430, title, equipment. Available from http://www.osha.gov [cited 2018 August 3].

8. Weaver LK, Churchill S, Deru K, Haberstock, D. Hyperbaric oxygen in chronic stable brain injury (HYBOBI): Interval to achieve 100% oxygen of monoplace chamber pressurization to 1.5 ATA. *Undersea Hyperb Med.* 2011;38(5):462. Available from http://rubicon-foundation.org [cited 2018 August 24].
9. Worth ER, Cochran SK, Dale HM. [Abstract] Oxygen concentration rise in a monoplace chamber. Available from http://rubicon-foundation.org [cited 2018 August 24].
10. Raleigh GW. Air breaks in the Sechrist Model 2500-B monoplace hyperbaric chamber. *J Hyperbaric Med.* 1988;3(1):11-14. Available from http://rubicon-foundation.org [cited 2018 August 14].
11. NBDHMTI. National Board of Diving & Hyperbaric Medical Technology, Intermittent air breathing: (2009-04) August 2009. Available from http://www.nbdhmt.org [cited 2018 August 14].
12. Weaver, LK. Air breaks with Sechrist 500A monoplace hyperbaric ventilator. *J Hyperbaric Med.* 1988;3(3):179-186. Available from http://rubicon-foundation.org. [cited 2018 August 14].
13. Weaver LK. Monoplace hyperbaric chamber use of US Navy Table 6 – a 20-year experience. *Undersea Hyperb Med.* 2006;33(2):85-88. Available from http://rubicon-foundation.org [cited 2018 August 14].
14. Undersea and Hyperbaric Medical Society. Definition of hyperbaric oxygen therapy: Indications for hyperbaric oxygen therapy. Available from https://www.uhms.org/resources/hbo-indications.html [cited 2018 August 14].
15. NFPA. NFPA 77, Recommended Practice on Static Electricity. Quincy, MA: National Fire Protection Association; 2019. Available from https://www.nfpa.org [cited 2018 August 14].
16. CGA. CGA G-7.1-2018: Commodity Specification for Air, Seventh Edition. Compressed Gas Association, Inc. 14501 George Carter Way, Suite 103 Chantilly, VA: CGA, Inc. Available from [cited 2018 August 24] available from https://blog.ansi.org [cited 2018 August 24].
17. Sheffield PJ, Hewitt M, Sheffield RB. Fire risk in hyperbaric facilities: could oxygen pooling be a factor? In: Proceedings of the Fourteenth International Congress on Hyperbaric Medicine. 2002;305-311. Available from http://rubicon-foundation.org [cited 2018 August 24].
18. NOAA. U.S. Department of Commerce, National Oceanic & Atmospheric Administration, NOAA Research, Earth System Research Laboratory. Available from: http://www.esrl.noaa.gov/gmd/ [cited 2018 August 24].
19. OSHA. U.S. Department of Labor, Occupational Safety & Health Administration. Available from https://www.osha.gov/index.html [cited 2018 August 24.
20. National Oceanic and Atmospheric Administration. NOAA Diving Manual, Sixth Edition. Best Publishing Company, 631 U.S. Highway 1, Suite 307, North Palm Beach, FL: Best Publishing Company; 2017.

21. Reimers SD. Flow dynamics of patient hoods. In: Proceedings of the Fourteenth International Congress on Hyperbaric Medicine, 2002. 80-87. Available from http://rubicon-foundation.org [cited 2018 August 24].
22. Weaver LK. Monoplace hyperbaric chambers. In: Thom SR and Neuman T, (ed). The Physiology and Medicine of Hyperbaric Oxygen Therapy. Philadelphia: Saunders/Elsevier. 2008:27-35.
23. Weave, LK. Critical care of patients needing hyperbaric oxygen. In: Thom SR and Neuman T, (ed). The Physiology and Medicine of Hyperbaric Oxygen Therapy. Philadelphia: Saunders/Elsevier. 2008:117-129.
24. Weaver LK. Hyperbaric oxygen in the critically ill. *Critical Care Medicine.* 2011;39(7):1784-1791.
25. Undersea and Hyperbaric Medical Society. Definition of hyperbaric oxygen therapy: Indications for hyperbaric oxygen therapy. Available from https://www.uhms.org/resources/hbo-indications.html [cited 2018 August 24].
26. Weaver LK. A functional suction apparatus within the monoplace hyperbaric chamber. *J Hyperbaric Med.* 1988;3(3):165-171. Available from http://rubicon-foundation.org [cited 2018 August 24].
27. Raleigh GW, Niezgoda JA, Fabus SV. A vacuum regulation system for continuing vacuum assisted closure therapy (V.A.C.) in multiplace and monoplace hyperbaric oxygen chambers. *Undersea Hyperb Med.* 2002; 29. Available from http://rubicon-foundation.org [cited 2018 August 24].
28. Stachiw JW. Illumination of vessel interiors. In: Handbook of Acrylics for Submersibles Hyperbaric Chambers and Aquaria. Flagstaff, AZ: Best Publishing; 2003. 775-832. [Out of print 8-8-2018].
29. Association of Diving Contractors, International (ADCI). ADC Safety Alert, Lamps on Viewports. February 2008. Available from http://membership.uhms.org/?page=Safety_Articles .[cited 2018 August 24].
30. Canty JM. Light piping unit for supplying radiant energy to the interior of a pressure vessel. U.S. Patent No. 3,813,514. 1974.
31. AS/NZS 1680.2.6:1997. Interior lighting. CodeHub. Available from: https://codehub.building.govt.nz/home/resources/asnzs-1680-2-51997 [cited 2018 September 4].
32. U.S. Department of Health and Human Services, U.S Food and Drug Administration, Produce Classification, Medical Devices. Available from: http://www.fda.gov [cited 2018 August 24].

CHAPTER 4.7
Introduction to Acrylic Windows in Hyperbaric Chambers

Kevan Corson, CHT, CHWS, DMT-I and Guy Richards, MA, CChem, FRSC

This chapter is dedicated to Mr. Jerry Stachiw, PhD. He was a great man and mentor who spent numerous hours with us both in person and on the phone. His dedication to this field is legendary and his ability to teach and share this information is the foundation of this chapter.

What Is Acrylic?

Acrylic is the thermoplastic polymer made from methyl methacrylate (MMA) with some additives to enhance strength, chemical, and UV resistance. Acrylic is made by heat-initiated radical polymerization, which produces cross-linked interpenetrating molecular network—equivalent molecular weight of 4 million—of 46,000 MMA molecules, chemically bonded and "woven" together in a three-dimensional net.

Acrylic was invented independently by ICI, Rohm & Haas, & I G Farben in the 1930s. It is widely used as an engineering plastic in signs, aircraft, submarines, aquariums, and medical devices—chromatography columns, dental moulds, and hip replacements. MMA is manufactured in huge quantities in plants worldwide and is the key raw material for windows. Acrylic is produced in different grades, dependent on its intended use. Do NOT think that the grade of acrylic supplied to the hyperbaric industry has the same properties as extruded or some store-bought acrylic. Current manufacturers use the same building blocks but put them together in such a way that makes the acrylic much, much stronger and longer lasting.

This chapter will focus on the unique properties of acrylic used in hyperbaric chamber window construction and how to evaluate, maintain, and repair these vital chamber components.

Figure 1.

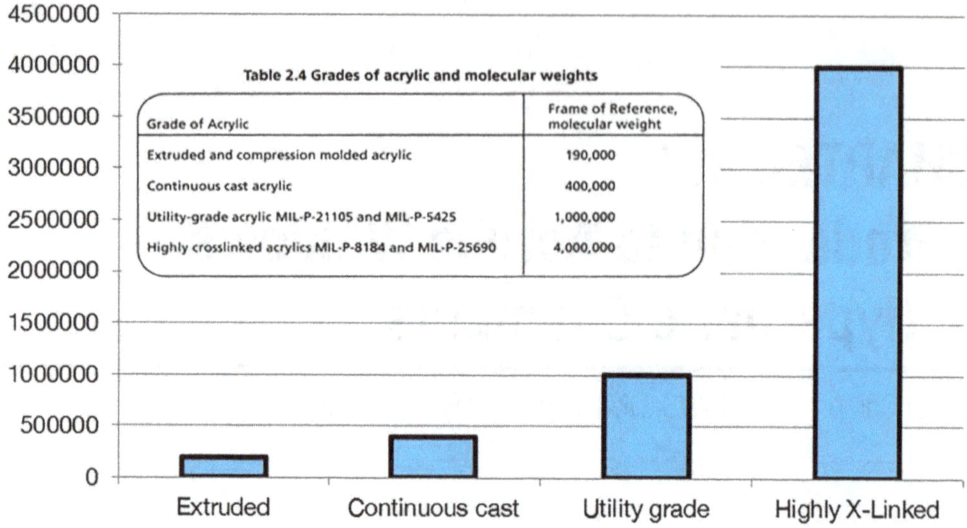

Table 2.4 Grades of acrylic and molecular weights

Grade of Acrylic	Frame of Reference, molecular weight
Extruded and compression molded acrylic	190,000
Continuous cast acrylic	400,000
Utility-grade acrylic MIL-P-21105 and MIL-P-5425	1,000,000
Highly crosslinked acrylics MIL-P-8184 and MIL-P-25690	4,000,000

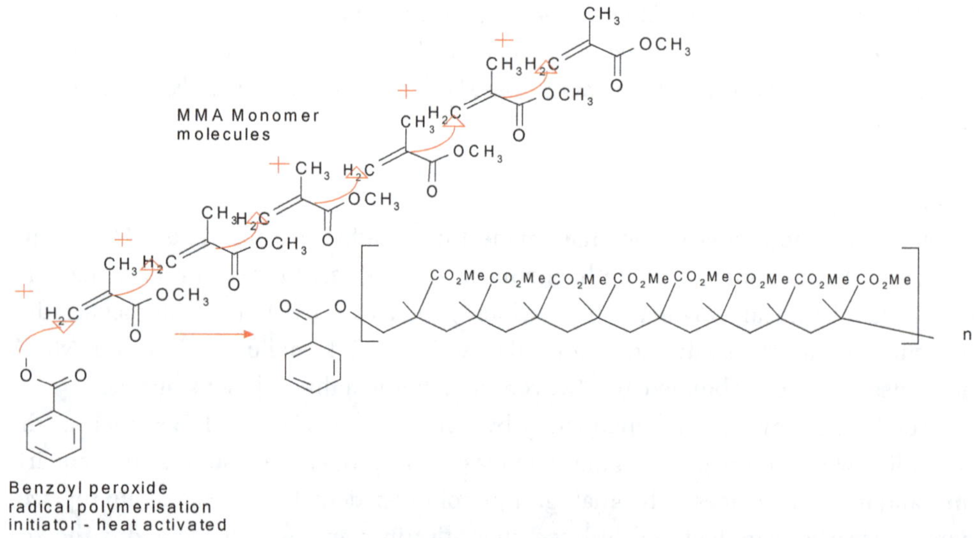

Figure 2.

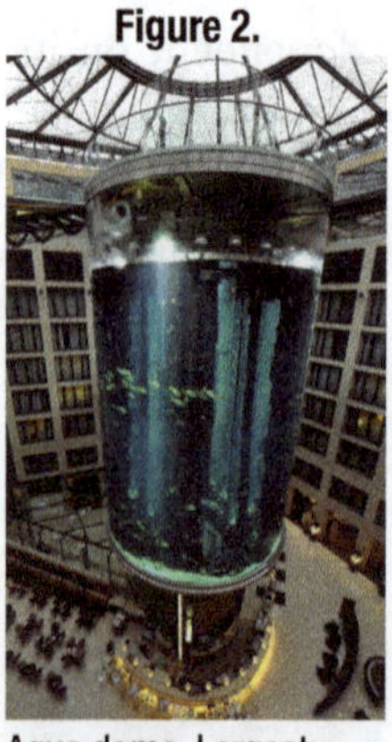

Aqua dome. Largest aquarium in the world. 2003, Reynolds Polymer.[4]

Figure 3.

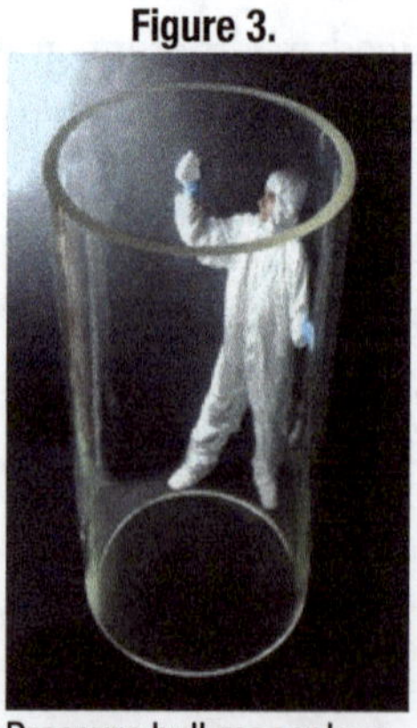

Pressure hull monoplace chamber. Photo courtesy of Blanson archive.

Figure 4.

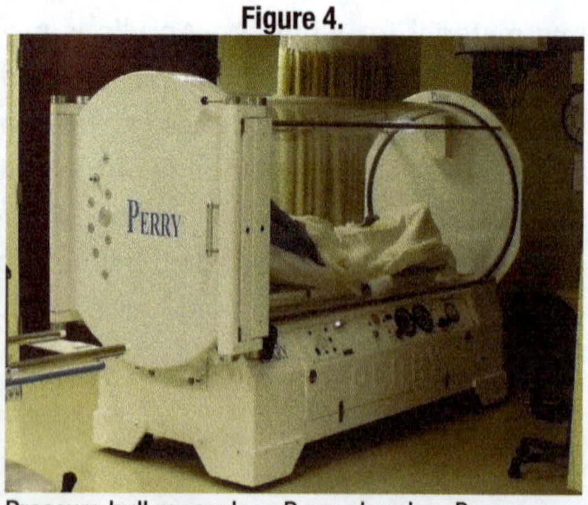

Pressure hull monoplace Perry chamber. Perry Baromedical. Photo courtesy of Blanson archive.

Type of Acrylic Windows used in Hyperbaric Multiplace and Monoplace Chambers

In today's clinical and diving hyperbaric chambers, acrylic windows with *PVHO-1* defined standard geometries and design criteria are used.[1] Acrylic window shapes vary with chamber type and the window requirement of the specific chamber type.

Multiplace chambers operate with a wide range of maximum allowable working pressures (MAWP) ratings, ranging from approximately 35 PSIG to 150 PSIG for clinical-based chambers. Chambers used for the support of commercial and military diving operations may operate at MAWP ranging from approximately 35 PSIG to over 1,000 PSIG.

Multiplace chambers generally use the following types of acrylic window geometries:

- Flat disk windows
- Conical frustum windows
- Double-beveled disk windows
- Acrylic light pipes (ALPS)

Most monoplace and some smaller multiplace chambers use a large cylindrical window built for internal pressure with a MAWP of approximately 35 PSIG. Though the tubular acrylic structure utilized in these chamber designs may be the largest component of the chamber, under construction codes, the acrylic section is classified as a window. Some monoplace chambers that are constructed with a predominately metal hull utilize window geometries similar to those used in multiplace chambers.

Design Life for Acrylic Windows Used in Clinical Hyperbaric Chambers

Acrylic windows utilized in hyperbaric chambers have a limited lifespan. The lifespan of a given window is established by the designer and is influenced by multiple factors ranging from the window environment to pressure exposure. *ASME PVHO* standards establish specific lifespans and provide guidance for chamber operators who may wish to extend the service life of chamber windows. Operators of hyperbaric chambers must understand the life limitations of these windows.

We first must understand the difference between design life and service life as it pertains to acrylic windows.

Design Life

Cylindrical Windows for Internal Pressure and Flat Disc Windows

The **design life** of cylindrical windows for internal pressure applications and flat disc windows meeting the requirements of *ASME PVHO-1 Standard* is 10 years from the date of fabrication.[1]

Service Life

The **service life** of windows in a PVHO operated in a *protected service environment* may be extended beyond the chronological or cyclical design life on the basis of visual inspections alone, carried out by a qualified maintenance inspector. However, no window may remain in service for more than 10 years beyond its design life (i.e. for a total of 20 years in operation) or for cylindrical window chambers, these may be operated for an additional 10,000 cycles maximum, prior to replacement.[1] (Storage of the window in the fabricator's crate for a maximum of 10 years does not contribute to its design or service life, as noted in *PVHO-2.*)[2]

Under no circumstance shall a window found to be in need of repair be permitted further use without making the needed repair. Similarly, under no circumstance shall a window found to be nonrepairable be permitted to be used again. These limitations shall be strictly adhered to, regardless of how short the actual service duration and/or number of accumulated cycles may have been at the time of the subject inspection.

Inspection of PVHO Windows and Viewports

When the end user receives a hyperbaric chamber with PVHO windows, the inspection process starts at the time of installation and commissioning. There are three types of inspections that are required for the end user under *ASME PVHO-2* in order to certify the safe operating condition of the pressure vessel and window.

1. Operational window inspection: This inspection must be completed as part of any pre-operational procedure. Operational inspections should be performed prior to pressurization by the operators who have been trained in what to check for and whom to contact should a window fault or flaw be observed. Chambers that are pressurized several times daily need to be inspected only before the first pressurization on that day. This inspection, which does not require removal of the window from its mounting, is limited to the viewing faces. This inspection allows the end user to establish the safety and serviceability of the PVHO system.

2. Maintenance window inspection: This type of inspection is to be performed at periodic intervals by a qualified maintenance inspector. It is more comprehensive than operational inspections and may possibly require removal of the window to satisfy the user or the agent that no hidden damage is present. Maintenance inspections should also be performed on windows in PVHOs that have been out of service for 18 months or longer, prior to putting the PVHO back into service.

3. Viewport seat and seal inspection: This type of inspection applies when (a) a window has been removed for maintenance inspection or repair, or (b) a new replacement window is being installed. At this time all related viewport components, seating surfaces, seals, etc. should be checked for conformance.

Table 1.

Maximum Intervals for Seat/Seal Inspection and Refurbishment	
TYPE	**Maximum Interval**
Cylindrical window chambers	After 10 years, carry out a detailed visual seat and seal inspection in accordance with PVHO-2 Case 1- Alternative 10-year maintenance viewport inspection for PVHO cylindrical windows which allows the window to remain in place (under defined conditions).[2]
Medical (all other types)	Completely refurbish at expiration of the extended service life, which is typically after a total of 20 years of operation.
Minimum intervals between maintenance window inspections	
During design life	Past design life
(Protected environment) indoor location 3 yrs.	(Protected environment) indoor location 2 yrs.

The visible surfaces shall be inspected in enough detail to detect all flaws of critical severity that require immediate removal of the window or PVHO from service. Inspection for the presence of crazing, cracks, discoloration, blisters, scratches, and pits shall be made during the operational inspections.

Remember: Your window inspection form **must** reflect the inspection of all the following: crazing; cracks; discoloration; blisters; scratches; and pits.

Training and Competency of Inspectors

Training of inspectors is the responsibility of the user or the third-party inspection organization acting on behalf of the user. A formal training program should be used in the training of inspection personnel.

Training programs: Inspection personnel shall have competent knowledge of Section 2 of *PVHO-1* and a complete knowledge and understanding of *ASME PVHO-2*. The inspection personnel should have practical training and competency in the use of measuring instruments. The training program should provide adequate exposure to the principles of quality control and quality assurance documentation to allow the inspection personnel to perform the inspections required and document those inspections in accordance with this standard.

The training program shall prepare inspection personnel to properly identify various window conditions and the acceptance criteria and required actions as detailed in this standard.[2]

Testing requirements: Upon completion of training, inspection personnel should be formally tested for competency and understanding of Section 2 of *PVHO-1* and a complete knowledge and understanding of *ASME PVHO-2* and results shall be maintained for the duration of the inspector's employment. Where the maintenance inspections are performed by the user, such data should also be retained for the duration of the service life plus an additional year of the being windows inspected. Regardless of who performs the inspection, it is the responsibility of the inspector's employer to determine when periodic retesting of inspection personnel is required.

Certification of inspectors: Certification of inspectors and use of third-party inspectors are the responsibility of the end user or the third-party agent of the user. When a third party is engaged as the window inspection agency, the end user is responsible for selection of a knowledgeable organization. Bottom line: You as the end user are responsible for all inspection being done on the pressure vessel or window in your facilities.

Documentation and record retention: All window maintenance inspection results and findings shall be documented using the correct forms. These forms must accompany the pressure vessel or window, and the forms shall be retained by the user for the duration of the window's service life plus one year.

Each facility will document all performed inspections, maintenance, and repairs utilizing the appropriate PVHO forms.

- Window Maintenance Inspection Form
- Acrylic Window Repair Certification Form for windows repaired by the user (or authorized agent)
- Acrylic Window Repair Certification Form for severely damaged windows
- Material Testing Certification for repair by spot casting
- Annealing Process Certification Form
- Pressure Testing Certification Form
- Material Testing Certification for Continued Service Form
- Material Testing Evaluation for Continued Service Form
- Facility Generated Forms
- Operational Window Inspection Tracking Form
- Window Flaw Tracking Sheet

The facility will maintain a file on each window.

- Original *PVHO-1* documentation package
- All applicable *ASME PVHO-2* forms
- Facility's window flaw tracking sheet

The facility will document all performed inspections, maintenance, and repairs utilizing the appropriate forms.

- PVHO-2 Forms
    - Window Maintenance Inspection Form
    - Acrylic Window Repair Certification Form for windows repaired by the user (or his authorized agent)
    - Acrylic Window Repair Certification Form for severely damaged windows
    - Material Testing Certification for repair by spot casting
    - Annealing Process Certification Form
    - Pressure Testing Certification Form
    - Material Testing Certification for Continued Service Form
    - Material Testing Evaluation for Continued Service Form
- Facility-Generated Forms
    - Operational Window Inspection Tracking Form
    - Window Flaw Tracking Sheet

Records retention:

- Each window file will be kept for the service life of the window plus one year.
- All documentation not retained in the window file will be retained for the service life of the oldest window plus one year.
- All staff training and certification will be retained for the length of their employment.

PVHO Window Markings

The window fabricator must apply markings to each window that provides information about the window's production, pressure rating, and identifying number. Marking shall be located on the window's seating surface or where specified by *ASME PVHO-1*. Identification shall consist of ½ in. (12.5 mm) letters and numbers made by the window fabricator with an indelible black felt marker (Sharpie) or ⅛ in. (3.2 mm) letters and numbers applied with epoxy ink.

The identification shall contain information per the following example:[1]

Figure 5. New Window

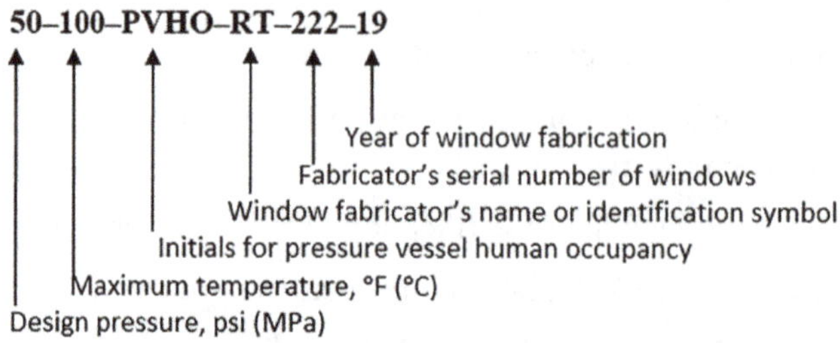

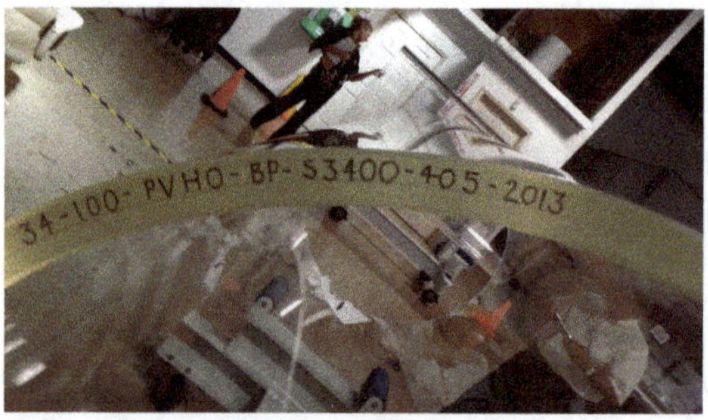

Photo courtesy of Blanson archive.

At the time of marking, the window fabricator shall certify the overall fabrication of the window by completing window certification PVHO-1 Form VP-1. Only after completion of PVHO-1 Form VP-1 shall the window be considered to have met the requirements of this standard, and the window can be marked in accordance with *ASME-PVHO*. This window certification shall be forwarded to the purchaser or used as part of the window certification package.[1]

Repaired Window

Repaired windows shall be marked with the identification of the window fabricator performing the repair. The repair identification shall consist of ½ in. (12.5 mm) letters and numbers made with indelible black marker or ⅛ in. (3.2 mm) letters and numbers made with epoxy ink located on the window's seating surface.

The repair identification shall contain the following information as noted in this example: [1]

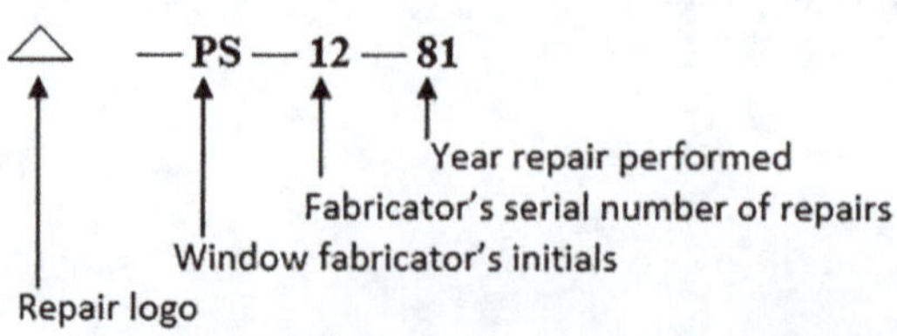

If the window has been repaired, a subsequent set of numbers or markings must be present on the window along with all accompanying documentation. The repair identification shall not obscure in any manner the original window identification. All the above documentation must be present for any facility or chamber inspection by the fire marshal, The Joint Commission (TJC), Undersea and Hyperbaric Medical Society (UHMS) hyperbaric facility accreditation survey, or other authority having jurisdiction (AHJ) over the facility/chamber.

Categories of Damage

Damage to the pressure vessel or window can occur at any point, from mishaps during manufacturing through shipment to the end user or during chamber installation. Most, if not all, damages or discrepancies that have occurred at or by the manufacturing process should be addressed and corrected before the chamber reaches the end user. Errors occur, and damage can be missed, therefore, before putting a chamber into service, the operator must perform a window inspection even on a new chamber or window to ensure that no damage has occurred during transportation or in the manufacturing process that was not caught by the company's internal quality assurance program. It is rare to find a damaged window, but it can and has occurred. Most of the possible damages that can occur to the acrylics happen from, and at the hand of, the end user. For this reason, we all must be cognitive that all personal, equipment and cleaning protocols may affect our acrylics. Each facility must have a policy and procedure in place that addresses the care of your acrylic windows and everyone needs to be familiar with it.

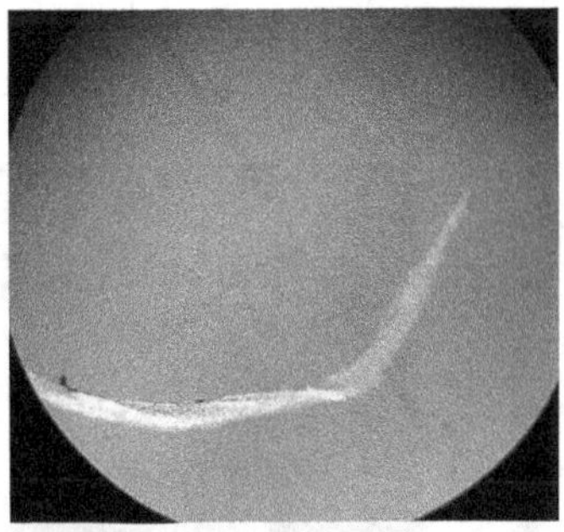

Figure 6. 3.8mm acrylic sliver inclusion under magnification. Photo courtesy of Blanson archive.

Flaw: Any imperfection in the acrylic present from manufacture or service that affects the cosmetic or structural capability of the window. Note that during manufacturing, foreign bodies (inclusions) may be introduced into the acrylic that may be present in the finished product.

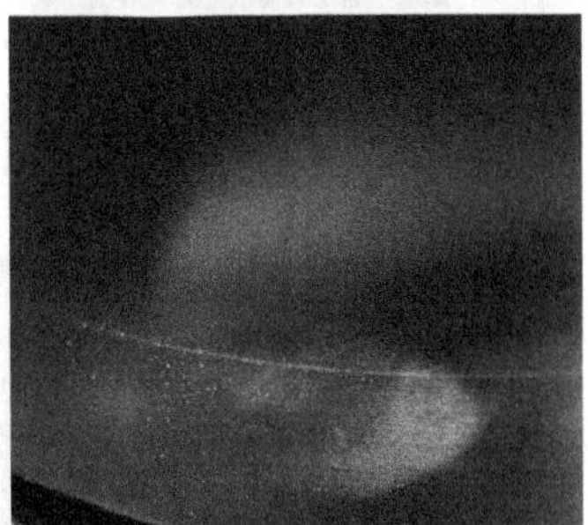

Figure 7. Machining marks on bearing surface – conical frustum. Photo courtesy of Blanson archive.

Scratches and inclusions: When supplied by the window fabricator, scratches (or machining marks) on the surfaces of and inclusions in the body of the window shall not be acceptable if they exceed the specified critical dimension, critical spacing, critical size of population, or critical density of population, or are found in a critical location. Smaller inclusions in an operational window are allowable if the conditions specified within Section 2 of *ASME PVHO-1* are met. Monitoring of any such inclusions should be a part of the daily operational inspection.

Things to remember about acrylics are as follows:

1. It is a pressure barrier, but it is not as robust as the metallic portions of the pressure vessel and easier to damage. Take care of it.
2. It is susceptible to external mechanical damage (i.e., something being dropped on it, scratching it, or gouging it), heat, solvents, solvent vapors, age, ultraviolet light (i.e., direct sunlight, sun lamp, mercury vapor lamp, ultraviolet [UV] disinfection robots), X-rays, and pressure.
3. Its responsiveness to a load (pressure) is a function of environmental temperature, rate at which the load is applied, duration of the load, previous loads, previous load cycles, exposure to solvents, solvent vapors, UV light with a wavelength of <400 nm, and the age of the acrylic.

Before we can prevent any damage from occurring to our chambers' windows, we must first understand what can happen, why it happened, and what effect it will have on the acrylics. Any flaw larger than those specified in *ASME PVHO-2* will act as a stress concentrator and lead to irreversible damage to the acrylic window.

Crazing: A microfeature (consisting of voided and orientated material formed at crack tips or inclusion particles) that are associated with the fracture and failure of polymers. With localized crazing, no action required other than ongoing monitoring.

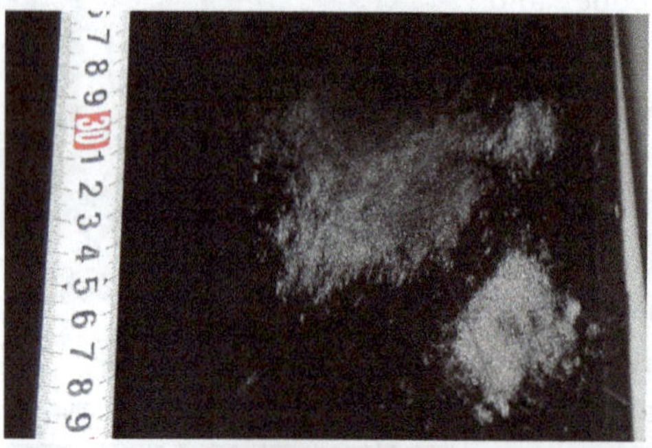

Figure 8. Crazing. Photo courtesy of Blanson archive.

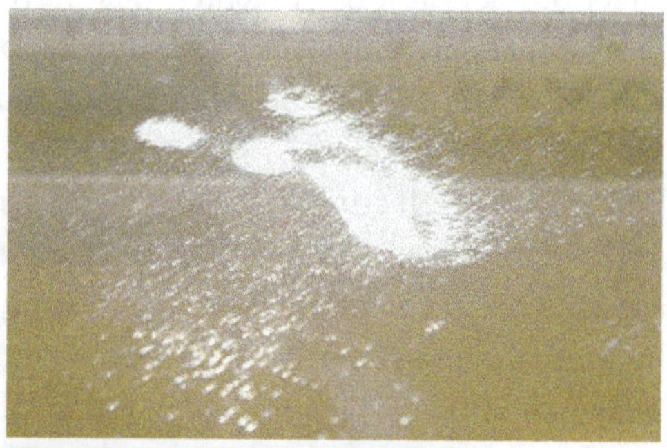

Figure 9. Crazing. Photo courtesy of Blanson archive.

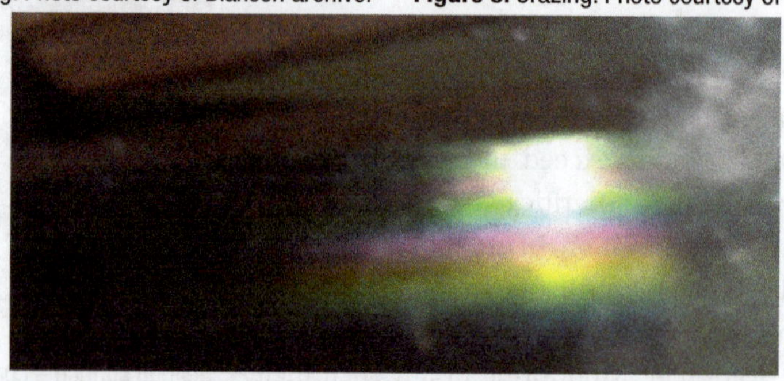

Figure 10. A submersible window showing rainbow colors due to excessive induced stresses. Photo courtesy of Blanson archive.

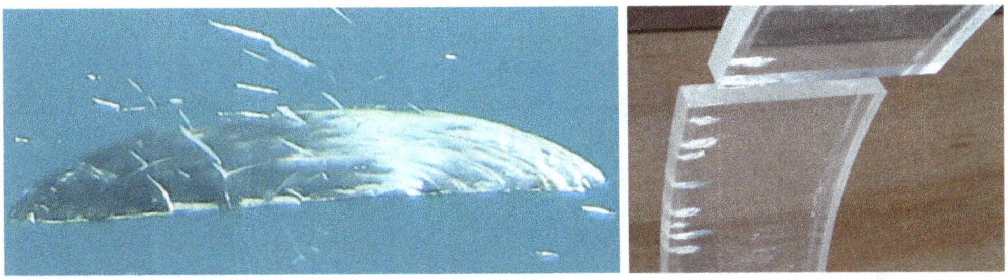

Figure 11. Cracks, especially those in the mid-plane of the window can lead to catastrophic failure even at pressures well below their design MAWP. Photos courtesy of Blanson archive.

Discoloration: A change in the window's natural color or an altered color.

Crack: A narrow opening or a fracture originating at the surface.

Chip: A small fracture flaw in the window surface, most typically the result of impact with a hard object.

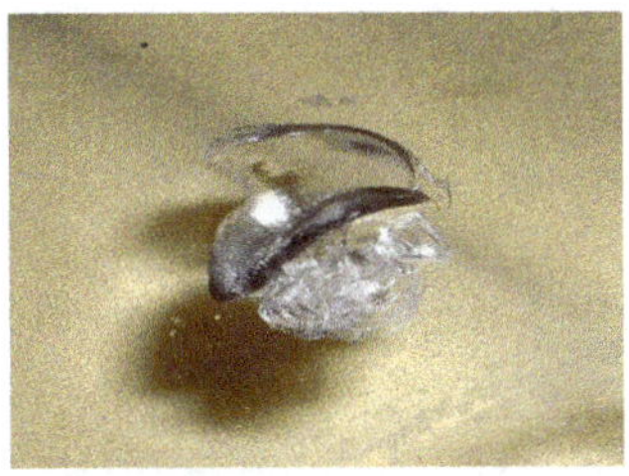

Figure 12. Chip. Photo courtesy of Blanson archive.

Scratch: A mark on the surface of a window. The origin may be a deep cut by machining tool or contact with a sharp object during transporting, movement, installation, or as a result of patient care.

Gouge: A narrow trench without cracks on the surface of a window, deeper and/or wider than a scratch.

Thermal shock: Damage to the window due to excessive heat. The affected area looks caramelized, highly crazed, and/or blackened. Most common cause is an incandescent light, steam hose, or other heat-producing equipment too close to the window.

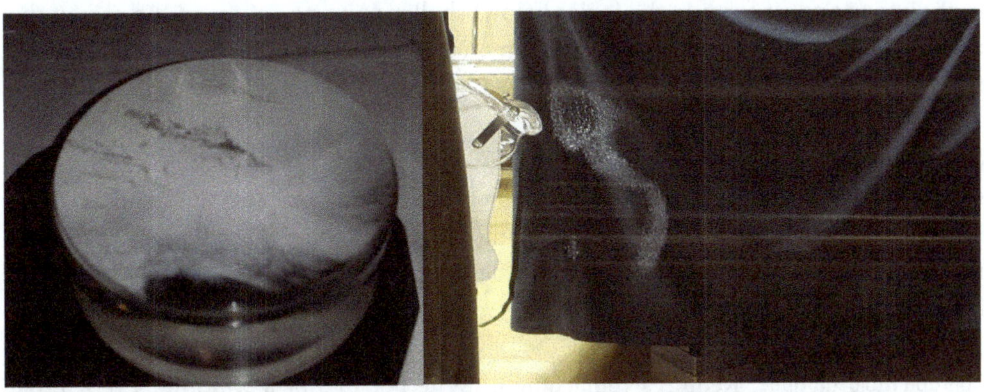

Figure 13. Wood's Hole remotely operated vehicle (ROV) window that got too close to a 400°C "smoker." Steam hose impact on a chamber. Photo courtesy of Blanson archive.

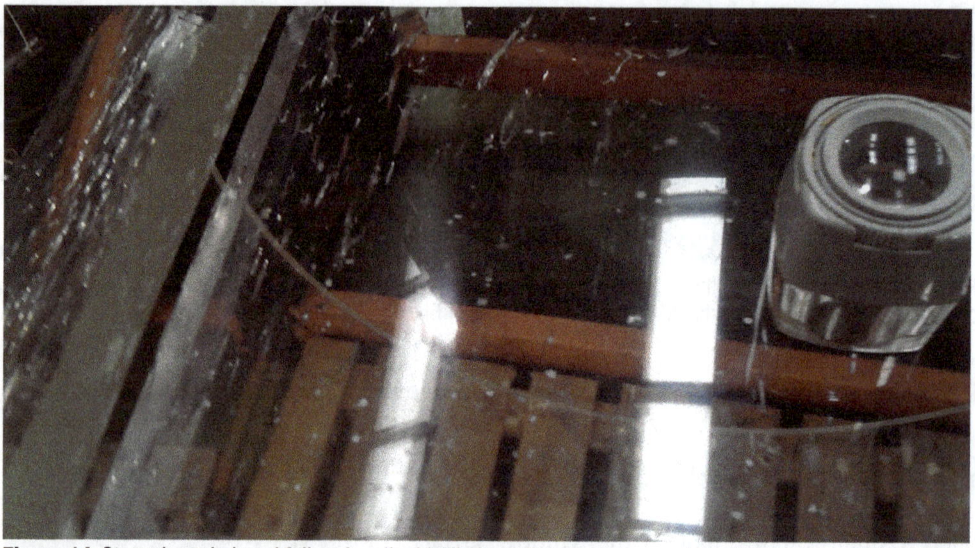

Figure 14. Steam hose induced failure in a liquid-filled acrylic pressure vessel. Photo courtesy of Blanson archive.

Pit: A circular crater without cracks.

Blemish: A small flaw on the surface of the window.

Defect: A flaw in the window usually present from the time of manufacture.

Blister: A swelling of the acrylic at the surface of the window due to excessive heat, usually accompanied by a burn. Typically caused by incandescent light or other heat-producing equipment too close to the window.

Superficial damage: Does not require action. Damage or a scratch that is superficial in nature (i.e. affecting only the optical clarity of the window and/or is below the significant dimensions set forth in the tables below) shall require no action on the part of the user other than the logging of the condition on the inspection documents at the time of the discovery of the condition and continued monitoring thereafter.

Significant damage: Requires action. Damage that is not superficial (i.e. exceeds the significant dimensions set forth in the tables below) shall require the window to be red-tagged (being placed out of service), and action on the part of the user to either repair or replace the window shall be undertaken. Logging of the condition on the inspection documents at the time of the discovery of the condition shall be made.

Nonrepairable damage: Requires replacement. Whether or not a window is repairable depends, in part, on the thickness, as indicated in Appendix I, Enclosure 1 of *PVHO-1*.

Can the repair be accomplished with the final thickness equal to or greater than the thickness required for the design pressure rating of the window? The other consideration is cost. It might appear that a window whose service life has already exceeded its design life should simply be discarded. Replacement windows shall meet the requirements for PVHO windows as described in Section 2 of *ASME PVHO-1* (i.e., materials, manufacturing processes, quality assurance, material testing, pressure testing, inspection, and certification).[1] Replacement windows shall have all necessary PVHO certifications (design, manufacture, and pressure test).

Table 2.

Limits for blemishes of flaws on window surfaces

Type of window	Location	Type	Size	Corrective Action
Plane (flat disc); conical with t/Di <0.5; double bevel disc with t/Di<0.5; spherical sectors with square edges; and hemisphere with flanges (GROUP A)	HPS	Pit	k>.02t*	Red Tag
	HPS	Scratch/gouge	k>.02t*	Red Tag
	HPS	Crazing	Visible	None**
	HPS	Crazing/cracking	k>.02t*	Red Tag
Type of window	**Location**	**Type**	**Size**	**Corrective Action**
Plane (flat disc); conical with t/Di <0.5; double bevel disc with t/Di<0.5; spherical sectors with square edges; and hemisphere with flanges (GROUP A)	LPS	Pit	k > .01	Red Tag
	LPS	Scratch/gouge	k > .01	Red Tag
	LPS	Crazing/cracking	k > .01	Red Tag
Plane (flat disc); conical with t/Di <0.5; double bevel disc with t/Di<0.5; spherical sectors with square edges; and hemisphere with flanges (GROUP A)	BS	Pit	k > .06	Red Tag
	BS	Scratch/gouge	k > .06	Red Tag
	BS	Crazing	Visible	None**
	BS	Crazing/cracking	k > .06	Red Tag

Definitions

HPS High-pressure side
LPS Low-pressure side
BS Bearing surface
k = Depth of flaw or blemish, inches
t = Thickness of window, inches
Di = Inside diameter of window, inches
** When t =2.25
depth of flaw > .045
When t = 1.5
depth of flaw > 0.3

General Notes:

a) Although visible surface crazing per se is not cause for immediate action, if the crazing pattern forms a "closed circle" concentric with the bearing surface, then the window shall be red-tagged.

b) Other criteria that may require the acrylic to be red-tagged include significant reduction in clarity, burns, blisters, and significant internal flaws.

Important note: Acrylic has a benign failure mode. If abused or stressed beyond its design limits, the acrylic will show early symptoms of imminent failure. If large areas or circumferential crazing, mid-plane or surface cracking, or large discolorations are observed or impact/thermal damage occurs, then cease operation (red-tag the chamber) and seek advice from the safety director or a qualified maintenance inspector. Tests show that acrylic windows, without flaws, even beyond their service life still have a large safety margin. An 8" diameter double beveled, PVHO-1 time-expired window rated at 100 PSI was tested to destruction and achieved 7,100 PSI before failure, within 100 PSI of what was predicted (7,200 PSI).

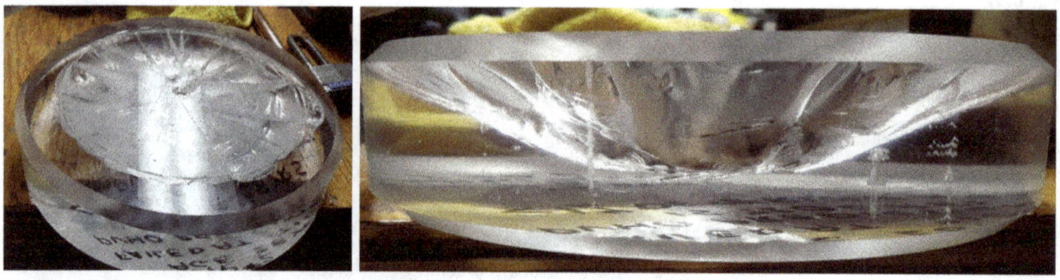

Figure 15. Stachiw Associates, Duke University. Photo courtesy of Blanson archive.

Any of the above flaws can be caused by the following:

- External damage (dropping something on the pressure hull)
- Internal damage (from external orthopedic medical device)
- Heat (photo lamp)
- Solvents (improper cleaning, i.e. alcohol or ammonia)
- Ultraviolet light (wavelength <400 nanometers) (i.e. disinfection robots)
- X-ray
- Excessive pressure (combination of heat, solvent, age, and UV)

Window Repair

When and how to determine if a PVHO window can be repaired on site or needs to be sent back to the original equipment manufacturer (OEM) for replacement or repair requires assessment and documentation. The extent of any damage and its impact on chamber operations and safety of all personnel and patients must be assessed.

Whether a surface defect is determined by the inspection to be a safety hazard depends on three factors:

1. The type of defect
2. The size of the defect
3. Location of the defect

The types of **surface defects** can be grouped into six categories: scratches, dings, gouges, crazing, depressions, and cracks.

When ranked in terms of **severity**, the most severe are cracks, while the most benign are depressions.

In terms of **size**, the critical factor is the sharpness of the penetration edge and its depth below the surface. Cracks have the sharpest edge and thus are more likely to initiate fracture, even when they are shallower than gouges or dings.

The **length** of a crack, scratch, or gouge has only a minor influence on the possible progression of the fracture. Similarly, the number of defects can be ignored in most cases in the evaluation of the structural condition of the window since its condition is determined by the single most severe defect and its location that will cause the progression of the fracture during pressure loading.

The **location** of the defect on the window has a direct bearing on the structural performance of the window under pressure. The scale of the consequence on the structural integrity of the window depends primarily on the type of stresses found on the damaged window surface during pressurization of the window. Generally speaking, damage to the low-pressure side of the window are more likely to progress to structural failure than those on the high-pressure side. If the stresses on the damaged surface are positive (< pressure), the defect will have a significant effect on the structural performance of the window and therefore will reduce its short- and long-term critical pressures. If the damaged window stays in service without being repaired, the continuing use of the window will cause the crack in a window to progress under repeated pressure cycles until catastrophic fracture takes place with instantaneous pressure release resulting in loss of equipment and life.

The courses of action available to the chamber technician for removing the surface defects whose depth exceeds the critical magnitude defined in the *ASME PVHO-2 Standard* are as follows:[2]

- Disassemble the viewport, remove the window from the viewport assembly, and replace it with a spare on a permanent basis.
- Disassemble the viewport, remove the window from the viewport assembly, and replace it temporarily with a spare.

The damaged window is either repaired by the chamber technician if the damage is slight or is sent to a window fabricator for repair. Upon return from the fabricator, the spare window is removed from the viewport assembly and the repaired window is reinstalled.

If the damage to the window surface is slight (i.e. < 0.02 in or 0.5 mm), the chamber technician may repair the window on site. Upon completion of repair, the window may be immediately put back into service.

Detailed discussion of the defects and their location on window surfaces is found in *ASME PVHO-2*.[2] Surface defects in the form of faint crazing, scratches, and dings that are between 0.01 in and 0.02 in depth are considered **slight damage** and may be removed by hand sanding and polishing without removal of the window from the viewport. Such a repair of the window surface can be performed by chamber technician if properly trained to do so. Manual sanding and polishing does not require re-annealing of the window. Surface defects with >0.02 in depth, however, are **severe damage** and the window should be removed, sent to a window fabricator who refinishes the damaged surface using power tools, followed by annealing, dimensional inspection, and pressure testing prior to reinstallation. Some windows with severe damage may require excision of the damaged area and spot casting, which mandates re-annealing of the window. Windows with severe damage may be refinished in the field, provided that the work is performed by a technically qualified representative of the window fabricator utilizing only manual sanding and polishing techniques. Upon completion of repair, the window must be pressure tested to original design pressure prior to resuming regular service.

Extent of Damage Evaluation and Possible Repair Process

When assessing the extent of damage to a PVHO window, the following can be helpful in determining the extent of the damage:

- *Crazing:* A series of very fine shiny lines, stars, or haze when viewed at an angle in bright light. Crazing is located below the surface and usually cannot be felt with the fingernail. Requires aggressive hand sanding to remove. Begin with 120 grit open coat sandpaper.
- *Deep scratches:* Readily detected with fingernail. Begin with 220 open coat sandpaper.
- *Minor scratches:* Readily detected with fingernail. Begin with 400 wet/dry sandpaper.
- *Hairline scratches with light scruffs, light scratches, and hazing:* Begin with a fine wet/dry sandpaper or plastic polish.
- *Acrylic repair:* Two common products used to repair acrylics are Micro-Mesh® and Novus plastic polish. Micro-Mesh is a sanding product that differs from sandpaper. Its backing is made of flexible cloth and latex and comes in a number of different grades that are finer than traditional sandpaper. Novus plastic polish is a three-step system that can remove hazing, discoloration, and light-to-moderate scratches from acrylic surfaces that will help with fogging, repels dust, and eliminates static.

Pre-Operational Daily Inspection Procedure: Pre-operational inspections are the most common window inspections performed by hyperbaric technologists, who inspect for the presence of crazing, cracks, discoloration, blisters, scratches, and pits. See definitions section for description of each type of flaw. These inspections can be conducted without the need for highly specialized tools. For daily inspections, use a high intensity light (nonheat-producing flashlight) with a magnifying glass to help identify possible damage. If damage is discovered, it must be measured and documented. There are two classes of instruments for measuring acrylic damage: mechanical and optical. Each of these has its advantages. The primary advantage of the mechanical instruments, such as feeler gauges and rulers, is their cost. Optical devices, such as the optical micrometer, can provide an accurate measure of defect depth.

1. Start from the outside of the chamber, with the room and chamber lights off, and shine the light at various angles across the entire surface of the window. Practice is the best way to understand what angle works best. The proper angle will eliminate the glare and bring out any flaws. You will need to refocus your eyes between inspecting the low-pressure surface and the high-pressure surface.

    a. If you find flaws not previously recorded or the results of your inspection are questionable, remove the protective cover if in place, clean both sides of the window, and repeat the inspection without the protective cover.

    b. If a flaw is confirmed (one not already on the data tracking sheet for that specific window), record your findings on that window's tracking sheet. The sheets are in individual files (one for each window) and can be found in various locations, but should be kept with the maintenance files in some form of accessible storage.

    c. Use the facility supplied measuring devices to get accurate data. Examples of possible measuring devices are business card, your fingernail, small needle, magnifying glass, ruler, and the above commercial devices (depth micrometer or optical micrometer). If the measurements fall outside of the safe dimensions for that given window, red-tag the window.

    d. If a window is red-tagged, put that lock or chamber out of service and notify the appropriate administrative and medical staff.

2. Document with your initials that you have completed the daily operational window inspection.

Documentation and Records Retention

Figure 16 is a few examples of windows forms used in both inspection and maintenance for multiplace monoplace chambers.

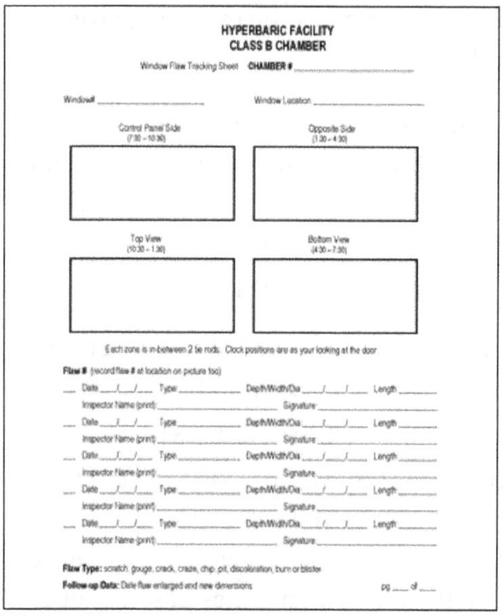

HYPERBARIC FACILITY
CLASS B CHAMBER

Window Flaw Tracking Sheet CHAMBER # ______

Window# ______ Window Location ______

Control Panel Side (7:30 - 10:30)

Opposite Side (1:30 - 4:30)

Top View (10:30 - 1:30)

Bottom View (4:30 - 7:30)

Each zone is in-between 2 tie rods. Clock positions are as your looking at the door.

Flaw # (record flaw # at location on picture too)

__ Date __/__/__ Type ______ Depth/Width/Dia __/__/__ Length ______
Inspector Name (print) ______ Signature ______

__ Date __/__/__ Type ______ Depth/Width/Dia __/__/__ Length ______
Inspector Name (print) ______ Signature ______

__ Date __/__/__ Type ______ Depth/Width/Dia __/__/__ Length ______
Inspector Name (print) ______ Signature ______

__ Date __/__/__ Type ______ Depth/Width/Dia __/__/__ Length ______
Inspector Name (print) ______ Signature ______

__ Date __/__/__ Type ______ Depth/Width/Dia __/__/__ Length ______
Inspector Name (print) ______ Signature ______

Flaw Type: scratch, gouge, crack, craze, chip, pit, discoloration, burn or blister

Follow-up Data: Date flaw enlarged and new dimensions pg __ of __

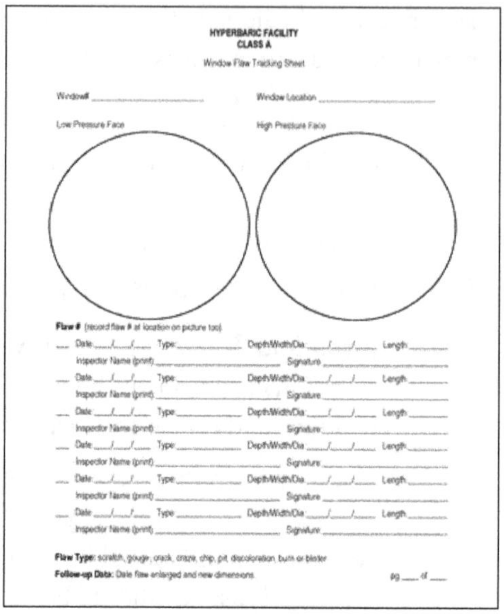

HYPERBARIC FACILITY
CLASS A

Window Flaw Tracking Sheet

Window# ______ Window Location ______

Low Pressure Face

High Pressure Face

Flaw # (record flaw # at location on picture too)

__ Date __/__/__ Type ______ Depth/Width/Dia __/__/__ Length ______
Inspector Name (print) ______ Signature ______

__ Date __/__/__ Type ______ Depth/Width/Dia __/__/__ Length ______
Inspector Name (print) ______ Signature ______

__ Date __/__/__ Type ______ Depth/Width/Dia __/__/__ Length ______
Inspector Name (print) ______ Signature ______

__ Date __/__/__ Type ______ Depth/Width/Dia __/__/__ Length ______
Inspector Name (print) ______ Signature ______

__ Date __/__/__ Type ______ Depth/Width/Dia __/__/__ Length ______
Inspector Name (print) ______ Signature ______

__ Date __/__/__ Type ______ Depth/Width/Dia __/__/__ Length ______
Inspector Name (print) ______ Signature ______

Flaw Type: scratch, gouge, crack, craze, chip, pit, discoloration, burn or blister

Follow-up Data: Date flaw enlarged and new dimensions pg __ of __

Figure 16.

Hyperbaric Light Pipes

Light pipes, which are acrylic tubes used to conduct light from external sources through the hull of a chamber, also fall under the same requirements as any window pertaining to the frequency and type of inspection. These inspections are continuous during the life of the light pipe and shall be part of any pre-operational procedures the user institutes to establish the safety and serviceability of the PVHO system. Inspect all surfaces readily visible daily and surfaces not readily visible should be inspected annually by removal of the acrylic pipe. The retaining clamp or ring and pressure-sealing surfaces may not be readily visible. Removal of the light pipe allows for both the high- and low-pressure surfaces to be fully examined. All visible surfaces shall be inspected in enough detail to detect all flaws of critical severity that require immediate removal of the light pipe or PVHO from service. Inspection for the presence of crazing, cracks, discoloration, blisters, scratches, and pits shall be made during the operational inspections. This process is critical, due to the possibility of the user overlooking the acrylic light pipes during the dally inspection. In addition, we must be aware of the possibility of improper operation of lighting equipment. When replacing the light source for the light pipes, we must ensure that the new bulb has the same rating (wattage and temperature) as the old one. Light pipes shall not be operated with light bulbs of a wattage greater than the rated capacity of the lighting system, faulty temperature sensors, or with the cooling fan inoperative or disabled. Under no circumstances shall the surface of the acrylic light pipe, due to the use of a lighting system, be permitted to exceed the window's maximum temperature rating.

Hyperbaric Acrylic Pressure Vessel and Ultraviolet Light

All hyperbaric chamber windows, regardless of chamber class, can be affected by ultraviolet light. Direct sunlight can cause crazing and hazing on the chamber pressure boundary. Fortunately, laminated glass absorbs all harmful UVA radiation and most UVB. Therefore there is no need other than patient comfort and ability to watch TV for monoplace chambers to be shaded by blinds or curtains.

Hospital acquired infections (HAIs) are a major safety concern for both health care providers and the patients. Considering morbidity, mortality, increased length of stay and the cost, efforts should be made to make the hospitals as safe as possible by preventing such infections. In the ongoing battle of infection control, many hospitals are using whole-room robotic disinfection systems that bathe a room in high-intensity ultraviolet light produced by xenon lamps. These systems have been shown to be effective in killing microorganisms, but they may prove damaging to hyperbaric chamber acrylics. In his acrylics handbook, Dr. Stachiw warns that the danger zone for UV damage begins at wavelengths below 400 nm. UV disinfection systems operate in the UVC spectrum, which peaks at 254 nm, so chamber acrylics can be at risk.[3]

Though some acrylic manufacturers include UV protectant agents or stabilizers in their formulations, the high levels of UV radiation produced by disinfection systems have the potential to overwhelm these protective agents and accelerate degradation of acrylic windows. Until there is evidence to the contrary, prudent practice would be either to prohibit the use of UV disinfection systems in chamber areas or to provide some form of protective covering for chamber acrylic components.

Acrylic Cleaning and Maintenance

Acrylic is sensitive to many chemicals that, upon contact with the material, deteriorate its surface. The deterioration may take the form of crazing, softening, and dissolution. The prevalent form of chemical attack is surface solvent crazing. Softening and dissolution may occur without prior crazing if the surface of the acrylic is stress-free.

Crazing can take place even upon a very short contact with the chemical substance if the surface of the window is under tensile or flexure stress. Crazing generally occurs in service during cleaning or disinfections of the windows with organic solvent or alcohol-based germicides.

Even if the contact between the chemical and acrylic lasts only a few seconds, this may be of enough duration to initiate crazing if there are stresses on the acrylic surface. This is further reason for keeping the level of residual stresses low and avoiding contact with unapproved cleaners and germicides. The compatibility of cleaners, germicides, oils, adhesives, and sealants with acrylic plastic have been established and is presented here for the benefit of the personnel servicing the PVHOs.

In many hospitals that treat hyperbaric patients, the task at hand is getting the infection control policy makers to understand that many of the hospital-based disinfectants cannot safely be used on the acrylics of both multiplace and monoplace chambers. The most-asked question is, "What can now be used to disinfect acrylic chambers?" With the increasing concern over nosocomial infections and the possible effect they have on patient outcomes, keeping the hyperbaric chamber infection free is a major concern for all. Below is the most current list of disinfectants that can used on the acrylic portion on both multiplace and monoplace chambers.

Remember, it is the responsibility of the safety director to ensure that disinfectants used are compatible with the acrylics. The products that have been identified acceptable for use on acrylic hyperbaric chambers for infection control are listed below.

Table 3. Approved Acrylic-Compatible Disinfectants

PRODUCT NAME
Amphyl Professional®
Benckiser Asepti-HB
Dispatch
Neutral Disinfectant Cleaner
Pro Spray®
LLC
Pro Spray C-60®
Quaternary Disinfectant Cleaner
Sani-Cloth HB
Sani-Master 4
Hi-TOR Plus Disinfectant (1:256)**
Matar Disinfectant
Stat III TB Disinfectant (1:128)**
Beaucoup Disinfectant
Amphyl Disinfectant (1:128)**
Benckiser
LpH se Disinfectant

**Dilute or use as per manufacturer's direction. To prevent surface damage, concentrates must be diluted with water at the given recommended ratios.

The role of infection control of acrylic monoplace chambers has proven to be prickly due to many commercial biohazard-cleaning agents containing alcohol or ammonia that have a direct effect on the serviceability of the acrylics. While alcohol is adequate to kill many pathogens, it is destructive to acrylic. Therefore, the procedure recommended here uses sodium hypochlorite (bleach) for high-level disinfection. The Center for Disease Control (CDC) also recommends the use of sodium hypochlorite for durable surfaces contaminated with Clostridium difficile (C-diff) because no commercial or Environmental Protection Agency (EPA)-registered products exist at this time. Sodium hypochlorite in a concentration of 10% free chlorine was also chosen because it has been found to show no damage to acrylic.

When using any disinfectant, one must remember that all cleaners will at some point off-gas, and when placing a patient into a closed environment regardless of the ventilation rate one must take this into consideration and be mindful of the potential problems that could occur.

Table 4. TOR-HB (Made by Ecolab) Contact Times

Product Name:	Contact Time to Recommended Effect
HIV	30 seconds
HCV (Hepatitis C Virus)	10 Minutes
HBV (Hepatitis B Virus)	10 Minutes
Cytomegalovirus	10 Minutes
Enterococcus faecalis—Vacomycin-resistant (VRE)	10 Minutes
Staphylococcus aureus—Methicillin-resistant (MRSA)	10 Minutes
Pseudomonas aeruginosa	10 Minutes
Herpes simplex type 2 virus	10 Minutes
Serratia marcescens	10 Minutes
Acinetobacter calcoaceticus	10 Minutes
Streptococcus pyogenes	10 Minutes
Salmonella choleraesuis	10 Minutes
Polio Virus Type 1	30 Minutes

References

1. The American Society of Mechanical Engineers. PVHO-1 safety standard for pressure vessels for human occupancy. New York, NY: The American Society of Mechanical Engineers; 2019.
2. The American Society of Mechanical Engineers. PVHO-2 safety standard for pressure vessels for human occupancy in-service guidelines for PVHO acrylic windows. New York, NY: The American Society of Mechanical Engineers; 2019.
3. Stachiw JD. Handbook of Acrylics for Submersibles, Hyperbaric Chambers and Aquaria. Flagstaff, AZ: Best Publishing Company; 2003.

CHAPTER 5
Fire in the Hyperbaric Environment

CHAPTER 5.1
Clinical Hyperbaric Chamber Fires: To What Extent Is the Problem?

Paul J. Sheffield, BS, MS, PhD, CAsP, CHT-A

Introduction

Fire in a hyperbaric chamber is rare but usually catastrophic. Once a fire occurs in the oxygen enriched environment, patient injury or death is the likely outcome. As compared to air at one atmosphere absolute (ATA), hyperbaric chamber fires ignite at a lower temperature, generate more heat, and burn more rapidly. Since fire is such a devastating occurrence in a hyperbaric facility, the emphasis must be on fire prevention. Medical and technical staff at the clinical hyperbaric facility must know the potential for hyperbaric chamber fires and must be especially vigilant to prevent its occurrence.

On January 27, 1967, the death of three NASA astronauts in the *Apollo I* Command Module fire at Cape Canaveral, Florida, drew world attention to fire risks in oxygen enriched hyperbaric environments. The oxygen-filled capsule was only pressurized to 16.7 pounds per square inch absolute (PSIA) [863.6 mmHg, or 115 kPa, or 4.5 fsw]. In 1997, Sheffield and Desautels reviewed and analyzed reports of 39 hypobaric (spacecraft simulators, altitude chambers) and hyperbaric (decompression chambers, research chambers, clinical chambers) fires that occurred during 1923–1996 in Asia, Europe, and North America.[1] In 1999, data from 59 hypobaric and hyperbaric chamber fires with 117 fatalities, including 10 USSR fires,[2] were reported in *Workman's Hyperbaric Facility Safety, 1st Ed.*, 1999.[3] At the 2012 Undersea and Hyperbaric Medical Society (UHMS) Annual Scientific Meeting, the clinical chamber fire data were updated with additional fires from China.[4]

This chapter summarizes 42 reported clinical hyperbaric chamber fires that occurred inside the chamber during the 50-year period (1967–2016) in Africa, Asia, Europe, North America, and South America. Also selected for discussion are four fires that occurred outside the chamber requiring evacuation of chamber occupants, the earliest of which occurred in 1923.[5-7] During 2006–2015, there were also reports of four fires in hyperbaric chambers that killed the animals being treated in the chamber. In one equine chamber fire, the temperature was so intense that the elevated pressure caused chamber structure failure and the explosion also killed the chamber operator and injured another person in a nearby hallway.

Reports were obtained from news reports, personal contacts, scientific publications, and from the UHMS Chamber Experience & Mishap Database.[8] Ignition sources are as provided in the reports, most of which did not discuss the thoroughness of investigation. Thus, it is possible that some reported causes could have been what seemed to make sense to the evaluator at the time rather than the actual cause of ignition.

Fires Occurring Inside Clinical Chambers

The first report of a fatal clinical hyperbaric chamber fire occurred in 1967 shortly after the *Apollo I* Command Module fire. This fire occurred in Japan, when a patient took a concealed benzene hand warmer into an oxygen-filled monoplace chamber. During the ensuing 50-year period (1967–2016), reports were obtained for 42 fires that have occurred inside clinical hyperbaric chambers, causing 101 fatalities and nine injuries, as summarized chronologically in Table 1. Chamber fire characteristics by ignition source and oxygen percentage are in Table 2.

Clinical Hyperbaric Chamber Fires in the First 25 Years (1967–1991)

Clinical chamber fire reports obtained over the 50-year period are analyzed in two 25-year increments. During the first 25-year period (1967–1991), there were 16 clinical hyperbaric chamber fires (28 deaths) reported in six nations for an international average of 0.6 fires and one fatality annually. Because of the quick actions of the hyperbaric chamber operator, there were surviving chamber occupants in one pressurized clinical hyperbaric chamber fire, which is discussed in a following section titled "Survivors of Fires Occurring Inside Clinical Hyperbaric Chambers."

Clinical Hyperbaric Chamber Fires in the Second 25 Years (1992–2016)

During the more recent 25-year period (1992–2016), there were 26 clinical hyperbaric chamber fires (74 deaths) reported in 13 nations, for an international average of one fire and three fatalities annually. There have been no surviving chamber occupants of pressurized clinical chamber fires that occurred in the more recent 25-year period.

Fires were analyzed based on the three components needed to produce a fire: burnable material, oxygen concentration, and ignition source. Analysis of clinical chamber fires confirms the need to exclude ignition sources from the chamber. Since there will always be burnable material and oxygen in the chamber, controlling ignition sources becomes the crucial factor and the largest challenge for hyperbaric facilities.

Burnable Materials

Three fires in monoplace chambers (Japan 1996; South Africa 2004; China 2004) contained enough burnable material that the fire's temperature increased the chamber pressure to the point that the chamber structure failed. In Japan (1996) fatal burns killed the patient and projectiles from the chamber killed the spouse and injured two others outside the chamber. In South Africa (2004), the homemade chamber explosion killed the outside attendant and propelled the fatally burned patient through the opening to land about 33 feet (10 meters) away from the chamber. In China (2004), a patient was fatally burned and the chamber explosion killed one person and seriously injured another outside the chamber. Note that the chamber in Japan was designed and built to *ASME-PVHO* standards, but the design standards of the South African and Chinese chambers were not reported.

Oxygen Concentration

Over the 50-year period (1967–2016), oxygen-filled chambers experienced 25 fires (43 fatalities) and air-pressurized chambers with variable oxygen concentrations experienced nine fires (45 fatalities). Oxygen concentration was not reported in eight fires (13 fatalities). In the recent 25 years (1992–2016), clinical chamber fires occurred in both monoplace chambers (16 of 26 fires, 20 fatalities) and multiplace chambers (10 of 26 fires, 53 fatalities). Table 2 summarizes the chamber fire characteristics by ignition source and oxygen percentage.

Ignition Source

Over the 50-year period (1967–2016), there were 42 clinical hyperbaric chamber fires of which 23 (55%) were ignited by items taken into the chamber, nine (21%) were by electrical ignition, seven (17%) were ignited by miscellaneous causes (electrostatic, oxygen piping), and three (7%) were unreported.

Of the 26 more recent (1992–2016) clinical hyperbaric chamber fires, 15 (57%) were ignited by items taken into the chamber; seven (27%) were by electrical ignition; two (8%) were ignited by miscellaneous causes (oxygen piping system, static), and two (8%) of ignition sources were unreported.

Comparing the more recent 25-year period with the previous 25-year period, chamber components caused about eight fires in each period, but fires caused by items taken into the chamber approximately doubled from eight to 15 in the more recent period.

Electrical ignition: Electrical ignition was cited for seven more recent fires resulting in 33 fatalities. Electrical short in air conditioner was cited for four multiplace chamber fires with eight fatalities (China 1993), seven fatalities (China 1994), 11 fatalities (China 1994) and one fatality (China 2001), respectively. Electrical short in loudspeaker/intercom was suspected for two monoplace chamber fires with one fatality each in Russia (1993) and in Peru (2006). The site of the electrical short was not reported in one multiplace chamber fire with four fatalities in Indonesia (2016).

Electrostatic charge: Static charge was reported as the cause of one more recent monoplace chamber fire that caused two deaths, but it was not confirmed and the source of the static charge was not reported (China 2004). There were also reports of static charge as the probable cause of five fires in the previous 25-year period, but none of them were confirmed. A static electricity ignition study by Steve Wood showed it was difficult to ignite materials with static charge in the absence of a hydrocarbon vapor, such as alcohol. (See Chapter 5.3: Static Electricity for more information.)

Oxygen piping system: The oxygen piping system was thought to cause a more recent fire with three fatalities (Turkey 1998). The reporter originally thought ignition was caused by a cigarette lighter found inside the chamber, but later investigation identified fire in the oxygen piping system as the likely cause.

Igniters taken into the chamber: Ignition sources were taken into the chamber in 15 more recent fires, resulting in 32 fatalities.

Cigarette lighters or smoking by inside occupants caused five fires resulting in 10 fatalities. In Belgium (1993) the patient ignited his clothing with a cigarette lighter, which was ruled a suicide. In China (1993) smoking in the multiplace chamber resulted in five fatalities. In the United Kingdom (1996), a patient died while smoking inside his home-based chamber. In China (2003), a lighter taken into a multiplace chamber caused two fatalities. In China (2015), a patient was fatally burned while attempting to smoke in a chamber pressurized with 100% oxygen.

Hand warmers caused three of the fires resulting in 14 fatalities. A benzene hand warmer (Japan 1993) caused a monoplace chamber fire that killed the occupant. An exothermic (chemical) hand warmer (Japan 1996) caused a monoplace chamber fire that killed the occupant, and the resultant chamber structural failure killed his spouse and injured an outside attendant and another person. A butane hand warmer (Italy 1997) caused a multiplace chamber fire during pressurization on air that resulted in 11 fatalities.

Children's toys caused two of the fires resulting in two fatalities. A child's toy (Cuba 1997) caused a fire with one fatality in the last few minutes of the treatment. A child's toy (China 2011) inside an infant monoplace chamber caused a fire that fatally burned the infant.

A child received a call on the cell phone that was taken into the chamber (China 2002). The battery overheated and ignited the patient's clothing and bedding resulting in fatal burns.

Electrostatic charge (USA 2009) was cited in a monoplace chamber fire that killed a child and an adult. An intercom speaker was originally suspected, but later investigation listed electrostatic charge from static-producing fabrics and baby wipes containing alcohol that was reportedly taken into the chamber.

Igniters taken into the chamber were not specifically identified in three fires. A multiplace chamber fire (China 2002) resulted in one fatality and two monoplace chamber fires (China 2003, China 2006) resulted in one fatality each.

Unreported cause: Ignition sources were unreported in two fires (Russia 1995; South Africa 2004) that resulted in three fatalities.

Fires Occurring Outside the Chamber

In 1997, Sheffield and Desautels[1] reported 19 fires during the period 1968–1996 that occurred outside the chamber with no fatalities. The fires were from a variety of causes, such as failure of ball valves and other components in high-pressure oxygen lines (12 events), compressor failure (two events), welding or soldering (two events), electrical component failure (one event), short in battery charger (one event), and failure of a high-pressure airline that fanned the flame of an existing building fire (one event).

Three fires that occurred outside the chamber are selected for discussion (Table 3). Two clinical monoplace chamber fires (USA 1976; UK 1978) occurred in the chamber stretcher unit following the 100% oxygen treatment after the stretcher unit had been withdrawn from the chamber. Both stretchers had damaged or missing earth grounding clips. Investigators (USA 1976) concluded electrical discharge at the site of the ground circuit discontinuity ignited the wire insulation in the reinforced plastic (fiberglass) stretcher. The patient had already been removed when smoke and flame was seen emanating from within the chamber stretcher unit. After the second similar fire (UK 1978), investigators attempted to reproduce the ignition source of the two incidents and suggested that inadequate grounding caused the stretcher to be electrically isolated from the chamber and the gurney, and the resulting electrostatic charge had caused the fire in an ignitable atmosphere within the fiberglass stretcher unit. Subsequently, grounding clips became more robust and fiberglass stretcher units were replaced by metal.[6] The third fire (USA 2001) was not related to the chamber but required evacuation of the chamber and premises. The Hyperbaric Department in New York was evacuated when a fire occurred in the adjacent intensive care unit. A patient on nasal cannula oxygen lit a cigarette, causing the hospital fire that also required evacuation of patients from all four intensive care units (ICUs)— medical, surgical, cardiac, and pediatric.[7]

Fires Occurring in Hyperbaric Chambers Used to Treat Animals

During the period 2006–2015 there were reports of four fires in hyperbaric chambers pressurized with 100% oxygen in which the animals being treated perished. Three fires occurred in oxygen-enriched hyperbaric chambers treating horses. It was speculated that in each case, a horse shod with metal shoes had kicked the chamber wall creating a spark or frictional heat that ignited vapors/materials in chamber. One dog perished in a chamber fire caused by a battery operated fan. There were no humans inside the chambers at the time the fires occurred.

- Canada (2006) - Four horses died in a chamber fire.
- United Kingdom (2008) - One horse died in a chamber fire.

- USA (2012) - One horse died in a chamber fire. The temperature was so intense, the elevated pressure caused the chamber structure to fail and the resultant explosion killed the chamber operator and injured another person in a nearby hallway.
- USA (2015) - One dog died in a hyperbaric chamber fire started by a battery--operated fan that the veterinarian had placed in the chamber.

Fire Extinguishment and Escape

Many test fires have shown time is available for fire extinguishment and escape, particularly in air-filled chambers. As previously reported,[1] within the collected reports, a variety of fire extinguishing methods were mentioned as being available, including slapping with hands, stamping with feet, asbestos fire blankets, buckets of sand or water, carbon dioxide extinguishers, water-filled fire extinguishers, handheld water hoses, and water deluge fire extinguishing systems (FES).

Even though a water deluge FES existed in two multiplace chamber fires, it was either not operable (Italy 1997) or not used (Turkey 1998). In the 1997 fire in Italy, the chamber operator attempted to activate the FES to extinguish the chamber fire, but there was no water in the system and 11 chamber occupants perished. In the 1998 fire in Turkey, three people perished and it is not clear why the outside chamber operator did not attempt to activate the FES.

Regardless of the fire extinguishing method available, there have been no reports of successful fire extinguishment in a pressurized chamber by an inside chamber occupant. However, there were survivors in one chamber fire (USA 1989) when the outside chamber operator activated the water deluge FES.

Survivors of Fires Occurring Inside Clinical Hyperbaric Chambers

In the 50-year period (1967–2016), 42 fires were reported to have occurred inside clinical hyperbaric chambers. However, there are known survivors in only one occupied chamber that was pressurized when the fire occurred (USA 1989). Following the hospital's standard procedure at the time, a cotton blanket was warmed by microwave and sent into the chamber via the entry lock intended to keep a four-week-old infant warm during decompression to surface. The chamber operator had just completed venting the chamber so the chamber environment was known to be 22% oxygen at 2.0 ATA. On exposure to the oxygen-enriched chamber environment, the blanket burst into flame. The inside attendant immediately sounded the alarm. The outside chamber operator's quick response to activate the water deluge FES and control chamber pressure spared the lives of four patients and two inside medical attendants. The fire was extinguished and the patients were removed without injury.[9] In 2012, the Gulf Coast Chapter of the UHMS presented the prestigious Wilbur T. Workman Safety Award to the chamber operator, Betty Knox Brown, acknowledging her heroic actions that saved the lives of the chamber occupants.

Chamber Fire Reporting

Despite the limited number of reported chamber fires, the risk of fire is ever-present. In 1992, Christy Pirone and associates at the Royal Adelaide Hyperbaric Medicine Unit in Adelaide, Australia, implemented the Hyperbaric Incident Monitoring Study (HIMS) as an international study of incidents occurring in hyperbaric medicine units.[10] By 2001, the HIMS Fire Risk Database contained 112 reports over an eight-year period where reporters thought there was a fire risk even though there was no fire and no one was injured or killed. Events reported were the following: elevated oxygen levels in the chamber environment; prohibited items inside the chamber; faulty electrical wiring; items installed in chamber systems by nonhyperbaric trained staff; and fire hazards in the area surrounding the chamber. On 16 occasions, patients took forbidden items in the chamber including cigarette lighters, matches, unauthorized equipment, alcohol, oil-based products, unapproved clothing, shoes, and watches. On one occasion, a nursing attendant halted the chamber pressurization to pass a cigarette lighter through the medical lock. She had done a thorough check of the patients but forgot to check her own pockets.[11]

Conclusion: To What Extent Is the Problem?

In 1974, U.S. Congress passed the Federal Fire Prevention and Control Act which created the U.S. Fire Administration (USFA) as an entity of the U.S. Department of Homeland Security's Federal Emergency Management Agency (FEMA). Because of emphasis on fire prevention, the clinical hyperbaric medicine community has a remarkable fire safety record. There were 13 nations contributing to this dataset. Of the fires reported, the annual average was one clinical chamber fire causing three fatalities worldwide. The incidence of hyperbaric fires was so small that the USFA does not include hyperbaric fires in their statistics.

In contrast, the National Fire Protection Association (NFPA) reported that, for the period 2002–2005, home medical oxygen fires in the United States occurred at an annual average of 182 fires, causing 46 deaths and 1,190 thermal burns seen in emergency rooms, primarily caused by smoking while using oxygen.[12] NFPA also reported that, for the period 2011–2015, U.S. fire departments responded to an estimated annual average of 5,750 (or 16 per day) health care facility structural fires (48% in nursing homes; 20% in hospitals and hospices, and 32% in other medical facilities). The fires resulted in an annual average of two deaths and 157 injuries caused primarily by cooking, electrical or heating sources, and smoking. Six percent of the health care facility fires were intentionally set.[13]

Although the number of hyperbaric chamber fires is small, when a fire has occurred, it has been devastating. It is such a serious concern that the NFPA requires appointment of a hyperbaric safety director at each clinical hyperbaric facility.[14] Each hyperbaric medicine team member must be trained, know the potential for fire mishaps, and use that information to safely operate the chamber and its support equipment.

References

1. Sheffield PJ, Desautels DA. Hyperbaric and hypobaric chamber fires: A 73-year analysis. *Undersea Hyperbaric Medicine.* 1997;24(3):153164.
2. Tyurin VI. Fires and fire prevention in diving and therapeutic pressure chambers. St Petersburg: Russian Federation Defense Ministry Main Military-Medical Administration. 1998;1-30.
3. Sheffield PJ. Hyperbaric chamber fires: To what extent is the problem? In: Workman WT (ed). Hyperbaric Facility Safety: A Practical Guide. Flagstaff AZ: Best Publishing. 1999;487-493.
4. Sheffield PJ, Sheffield RB, Sheffield JC. Review of Recent Clinical Hyperbaric Chamber Fires (1992-2011). UHMS ASM, (Abstract E86). UHM 2012:1014-15.
5. Trimble VH. The Uncertain Miracle: Hyperbaric Oxygenation. Garden City, NY: Doubleday. 1974;62-63.
6. Hughs JF, Bright AW. Electrostatic charge control on hyperbaric chambers – a case history. IEEE Transactions on Industry Applications, Vol IA-16(6); 1980:762-766.
7. Kelly PT. Fire in the ICU: A description and analysis. *Pressure.* 2001;30(6):11.
8. Undersea & Hyperbaric Medical Society. UHMS Chamber Experience & Mishap Database. North Palm Beach, FL: UHMS.
9. Youn BA, Gordon D, Moran C, Brown B. Fire in the multiplace hyperbaric chamber. *J Hyperb Med.* 4(2);1989:63-67.
10. Pirone CJ. HIMS Fire Risk Database. Adelaide, Australia: Royal Adelaide Hyperbaric Medicine Unit; 2000.
11. Sheffield PJ. Equipment and chamber related incidents: HIMS fire risk database, In: Barach P & Mueller PHJ, Patient Safety: Prevention & Treatment of Complications in Hyperbaric Medicine. UHMS 52nd Workshop Report. UHMS; 2002.
12. Flynn JD. Structure fires in medical, mental health, and substance abuse facilities. NFPA: Feb 2009.
13. Campbell R. Structure fires in health care facilities. Quincy, MA: National Fire Protection Association; Nov 2017.
14. National Fire Protection Association. NFPA 99, Health Care Facilities, Chapter 14, Hyperbaric Facilities. 2018;108-118.

Table 1. Fires Inside Clinical Hyperbaric Chambers 1967 - 2016

TOTAL CLINICAL CHAMBER FIRES OCCURING DURING 50-YEAR Period 1967 – 2016

42 Fires (27 Mono, 15 Multi); 101 fatalities;9 injuries

A. FIRES OCCURING DURING FIRST 25-YEAR Period 1967 – 1991

16 Fires (11 Mono, 5 Multi); 28 fatalities;6 injuries

Date/ Nation	Chamber Type	% of O_2	Casualties Fatal	Injury	Probable Cause
1967JA	Mono-Tr	50%	1	0	Butane hand warmer ignited clothing
1967CH	Multi-Tr	100%	2	0	Patient smoking inside chamber
1969JA	Multi-Res	73%	4	0	Sparks from camera cord ignited newspapers
1973FR	Mono-Tr	100%	1	0	Cause unreported
1974RU	Multi-Tr	20+%-Air	3	0	Electric speaker ignited chamber at 3.8 ATA
1979JA	Mono-Tr	100%	1	6	Patient tried to light a cigarette. 6 injured outside chamber
1983CH	Mono-Tr	100%	1	0	Static electricity (unconfirmed)
1984CH	Mono-Tr	100%	1	0	Static electricity (unconfirmed)
1986CH	Mono-Tr	100%	1	0	Static electricity (unconfirmed)
1986CH	Mono-Tr	100%	1	0	Electrical short in phone
1987CH	Mono-Tr	100%	1	0	Static electricity (unconfirmed)
1987CH	Multi-Tr	100%	8	0	Sparks for a child's electrical toy
1987IT	Mono-Tr	100%	1	0	Spark-generating friction toy ignited bedding
1989JA	Mono-Tr	60-90%	1	0	Butane hand warmer ignited clothing
1989US	Multi-Tr	22%-Air	0	0	Microwave-heated blanket ignited when sent via medical lock into chamber. Outside operator extinguished fire with water deluge FES saving 4 patients and 2 inside medical attendants.
1989CH	Mono-Tr	100%	1	0	Static electricity (unconfirmed)

Legend: BE = Belgium; CH = China; CU = Cuba; FR= France; IN = Indonesia; IT = Italy; JA = Japan; PE = Peru; RU = USSR; SA = South Africa; TR = Turkey; US = United States; UK = United Kingdom; Tr = Treatment Chamber; Res= Research; Unk= Unknown % O_2; Unrpd = Unreported % O_2

B. FIRES OCCURING DURING SECOND 25-YEAR PERIOD 1992 – 2016

26 Fires (16 Mono, 10 Multi); 73 fatalities; 3 injuries

Date/ Nation	Chamber Type	% of O_2	Fatal	Injury	Probable Cause
1993BE	Mono-Tr	100%	1	0	Patient ignited his clothing with cigarette lighter. Ruled suicide.
1993JA	Mono-Tr	100%	1	0	Butane hand warmer ignited clothing
1993CH	Multi-Tr	100%	5	0	Smoking
1993CH	Multi-Tr	Unk-Air	8	0	Electrical short in air conditioner
1993RU	Mono-Tr	100%	1	0	Electrical short in loudspeaker
1994CH	Multi-Tr	Unk-Air	7	0	Electrical short in air conditioner
1994CH	Multi-Tr	Unk-Air	11	0	Electrical short in air conditioner
1995RU	Mono-Tr	Unrpd	1	0	Cause unreported 12 YO shirt caught fire
1996JA	Mono-Tr	100%	2	2	Chemical hand warmer ignited blanket killing patient. Chamber structure failed killing spouse and injuring 2 outside chamber.
1996UK	Mono-Tr	Unk-Air	1	0	Smoking inside home-based hyperbaric chamber
1997CU	Mono-Tr	100%	1	0	Child's toy in last few minutes before ending treatment
1997IT	Multi-Tr	21%-Air	11	0	Butane hand warmer; 8 burned, 3 others asphyxiated. FES activated but there was no water in it.
1998TK	Multi-Tr	Unk-Air	3	0	Initial report suspected cigarette lighter found inside chamber. Later investigation found fire in O_2 piping system was likely cause. FES was installed but not used.
2001CH	Multi-Tr	Unk-Air	1	0	Electrical short in air conditioning
2002CH	Mono-Tr	100%	1	0	Child received call on cell phone taken inside chamber
2002CH	Multi-Tr	Unrpd	1	0	Unidentified source of fire taken into chamber
2003CH	Mono-Tr	Unrpd	1	0	Unidentified source of fire taken into chamber
2003CH	Multi-Tr	Unrpd	2	0	Cigarette lighter taken into chamber

Table 1. Fires Inside Clinical Hyperbaric Chambers 1967 - 2016 (continued)

B. FIRES OCCURING DURING SECOND 25-YEAR PERIOD 1992 – 2016					
26 Fires (16 Mono, 10 Multi); 73 fatalities; 3 injuries					
2004CH	Mono-Tr	Unrpd	2	1	Static caused fire that killed patient. Chamber explosion killed one person and seriously injured another outside chamber.
2004SA	Mono-Tr	Unrpd	2	0	Cause unreported. Fire in homemade chamber killed patient; chamber explosion killed the outside attendant
2006PE	Mono-Tr	>50%	1	0	Intercom suspected to cause fire that burned door seal releasing pressure that blew out windows of building
2006CH	Mono-Tr	Unrpd	1	0	Unidentified source of fire taken into chamber
2009US	Mono-Tr	>50%	2	0	Adult & child in monoplace chamber received fatal burns. An intercom speaker was originally suspected, but later investigation listed electrostatic charge from static producing fabrics and baby wipes containing alcohol reported to have been taken into chamber.
2011CH	Infant Mono-Tr	Unrpd	1	0	Child's toy taken into chamber
2014CH	Mono-Tr	100%	1	0	Patient attempted to smoke while pressurized in the 100% oxygen chamber
2016IN	Multi-Tr	Unrpd	4	0	Initial report was that the fire was suspected to be caused by electrical short circuit. Final investigative report not received.

Legend: BE = Belgium; CH = China; CU = Cuba; FR= France; IN = Indonesia; IT = Italy; JA = Japan; PE = Peru; RU = USSR; SA = South Africa; TR = Turkey; US = United States; UK = United Kingdom; Tr = Treatment Chamber; Unk= Unknown % O_2; Unrpd = Unreported % O_2

Table 2. Chamber Fire Characteristics by Ignition Source & Percent Oxygen

	1967 - 2016		1967 - 1991		1992 - 2016	
IGNITION SOURCE	Total Clinical Chamber Fires	Total Fatalities	Clinical Chamber Fires	Fatalities	Clinical Chamber Fires	Fatalities
CHAMBER COMPONENT	16	47	7	9	9	38
Electric Arc/Spark	9	37	2	4	7	33
Electrostatic	6	7	5	5	1	2
O2 Piping System	1	3	0	0	1	3
TAKEN INTO CHAMBER	23	50	8	18	15	32
Smoking/ Lighter	7	13	2	3	5	10
Hand Warmer	5	16	2	2	3	14
Child's Toy	4	11	2	9	2	2
Cell Phone	1	1	0	0	1	1
Camera	1	4	1	4	0	0
Blanket (heated)	1	0	1	0	0	0
Static producers	1	2	0	0	1	2
Unidentified	3	3	0	0	3	3
UNREPORTED	3	4	1	1	2	3
TOTAL	42	101	16	28	26	73
OXYGEN PERCENTAGE						
Known 21-24%	3	14	2	3	1	11
Unknown- Air	6	31	0	0	6	31
Known ≥ 24%	25	43	14	25	11	18
Unreported	8	13	0	0	8	13
TOTAL	42	101	16	28	26	73

Table 3. Fires Outside Chamber Requiring Evacuation of Chamber or Removal from Premises

Date/ Nation	Chamber Type	% O_2	Casualties		Probable Cause
			Fatality	Injury	
1976US	Mono-Tr	21% Air	0	0	Electrostatic spark in unoccupied chamber fiberglass stretcher unit following treatment of a child. Fire occurred in chamber stretcher unit following HBO_2 at 2 ATA after stretcher unit was withdrawn from chamber. Earth grounding clips were damaged or missing. Patient had already been removed when smoke and flame was seen emanating from inside the stretcher unit.[6]
1978UK	Mono-Tr	21% Air	0	0	Electrostatic spark in unoccupied chamber fiberglass stretcher unit following treatment of an adult. Fire occurred in chamber stretcher unit following HBO_2 at 2 ATA after stretcher unit was withdrawn from chamber.[6]
2001US	Multi -Tr	21% Air	0	0	Patient on O_2 (nasal cannula) in the adjacent ICU lit a cigarette causing the hospital fire. Hyperbaric Department and 4 ICUs were evacuated.[7]

Legend: US = United States; UK = United Kingdom; Tr = treatment.

CHAPTER 5.2
The Role of Oxygen in Hyperbaric Chamber Fire Safety

Harold D. Beeson, PhD, Gwenael Chiffoleau, PhD, and R.W. "Bill" Hamilton, PhD (DECEASED)

Editor's note: Dr. Hamilton was a co-author of the original chapter on the role of oxygen in hyperbaric chamber safety. Unfortunately, he has passed away. While the entire second edition is dedicated to him, his name is being retained as a primary contributor to this chapter in his honor.

Introduction

Fire is the heat, light, and reaction products resulting from an exothermic chemical reaction between a fuel and an oxidizer. The reaction initiation and rate are subject to the laws and principles of chemical kinetics and thermodynamics. The configuration of the fuel source and the fluid dynamic aspects of the combustion event heavily influence the initiation and progression of a fire.

This chapter discusses the fire hazards associated with the oxygen-enriched atmosphere that exists in hyperbaric chambers. In particular, methods that can reduce or protect against the fire hazards are discussed, including materials and ignition control and fire suppression.

The Fire Triangle and the Special Role of Oxygen

In general, fire prevention is described in terms of the Fire Triangle model (Figure 1). For a fire to occur, a fuel, an oxidizer, and an ignition source must be present. Fire prevention in a hyperbaric chamber must account for an increase in the oxygen component of the atmosphere in terms of both oxygen fraction and partial pressure. The resultant increase in oxygen renders what might be inactive fuels and ignition sources in a "normal" air environment active, which increases the risk of a fire.

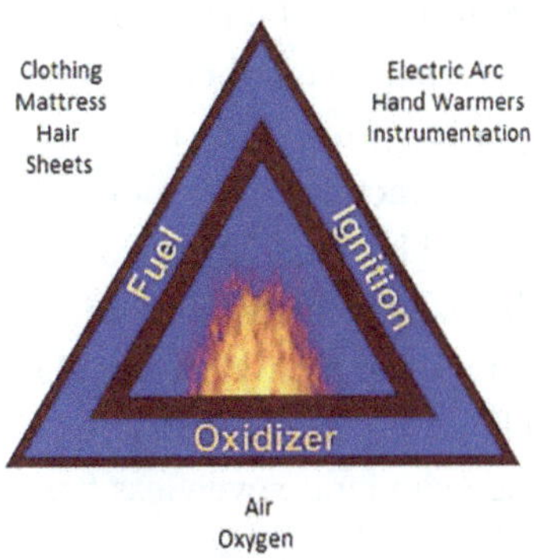

Figure 1. Fire Triangle.

The oxidizer in a hyperbaric environment is generally "air" which has a remarkably constant oxygen concentration of 21% but can, by standard, vary from between 19.5% and 23.5%. In certain applications and treatments, the oxygen concentration can increase and can be as high as 100%. In addition to the increased oxygen concentration, the oxygen partial pressure will increase as a direct function of the total pressure such that at two atmospheres the partial oxygen pressure or PO_2 is twice that at one atmosphere. At a given pressure, when the oxygen fraction or percentage of an atmosphere is changed, the partial pressure is changed as well.

Two terms are commonly used to refer to the environment within a hyperbaric chamber as it relates to the definition of the amount of oxygen. First, in an **oxygen-enriched atmosphere**, the concentration of oxygen exceeds 21% by volume or its partial pressure of oxygen exceeds 21.3 kPa (160 torr).[1] Second, an **atmosphere of increased burning rate** is any atmosphere containing a percentage of oxygen, or oxygen and nitrous oxide, greater that the quotient of 23.45 divided by the square root of the total pressure in atmospheres.[2] While both of these definitions have wide subscription, are the basis of standards, and are conservative when applied to the normal range of hyperbaric environments, both definitions may not fully define the hazards associated with the hyperbaric environment. Certain oxygen-enriched atmospheres can exhibit combustion-supporting properties similar to ambient air, while others are incapable of supporting the combustion of normally flammable materials. For example, a 4% oxygen mixture in nitrogen or helium with a total pressure of 12 atm (1.2 MPa) will not support combustion of paper, even though the partial pressure of oxygen is 0.48 atm (48.6 kPa).[3] The second definition is based on results for filter paper burning at 1 atm (101.3 kPa) and does not fully address the variety of materials whose ignition and burn rate may have a greater or lesser dependence on oxygen concentration and pressure effects.[2]

The fuel in a hyperbaric environment can be any unoxidized material within the environment, including metals, plastics, fabrics, salves, dressings, anesthetic agents, wire insulation, and composite materials. Whether a material will sustain combustion is a function of the specified environmental conditions and the material's configuration.

Ignition sources include any energy source capable of providing sufficient energy to overcome the reaction activation energy and initiate the combustion reaction. In a hyperbaric chamber, common ignition sources include electrical arc, friction, thermal ignition from hot surfaces, and possible static discharge. In piping systems, particle impact and adiabatic compression are also considerations. In the past, fires were caused by open flame from cigarette smoking, and in the future, fires may be caused by "high-tech" instrumentation. Oxygen fires in general are caused by ignition of a small amount of highly flammable material (often a contaminant), which then progresses in a kindling chain fashion to ignite less flammable bulk material such as polymers, which then can ignite even less flammable metallic system components.

Effects of Increased Pressure and Oxygen Concentration: The Cook Diagram

As noted, the term "oxygen-enriched atmosphere" is often used to describe an atmosphere in which a fire is easier to start and will rapidly spread. It is occasionally assumed, however, that if the fraction (or percentage) of oxygen is no greater than that of air, the atmosphere is not "enriched." This could be a costly mistake because rapid flame spread and easy ignition can take place in an atmosphere of compressed air. Thus, this should also be regarded as an oxygen-enriched atmosphere. Caisson and tunnel workers are well aware of this fact.

Historically, much of the work on the role of oxygen in fire safety has been based on the performance of materials in pure or nearly pure oxygen. The hyperbaric chamber, however, involves mixtures of varying fractions of oxygen over a range of pressures; this describes a complex distribution of flammabilities.

For most biological responses to oxygen, the response increases almost linearly with the oxygen partial pressure. For fires, the situation is different. Fires tend to be affected by both partial pressure and fraction and are more strongly influenced by the fraction or percentage of oxygen. The reason for this is derived somewhat intuitively. As the oxygen fraction changes, the inert fraction which acts to "blanket" the fire changes as well, but of course in the opposite direction. While the effects may be arrived at intuitively, the quantitative aspects are not.

When a fire killed two divers in a chamber at the U.S. Navy Experimental Diving Unit in 1965, the pressure and oxygen concentration in the chamber at the time called attention to this phenomenon and the fact that little was known about it.[4] The U.S. Navy sponsored a research program at the Tonawanda, NY, laboratory of Union Carbide Corporation to attempt to describe this quantitatively. The investigators, under the leadership of Gerhard Cook and later Victor Dorr, learned that filter paper strips held at a 45° angle from the horizontal and ignited by a hot wire would burn at a reproducible rate under the same conditions. With this setup they were able to compare burning rates in different gas mixtures at different pressures.[5]

Cook and Dorr used mixtures of oxygen and nitrogen with oxygen ranging from 15 to 50%, and pressures from 1 to 10 atm (101 to 1013 kPa) and measured the burn rates of filter paper strips.[5] The authors included a graph that summarized the results, which acquired the name Cook Diagram.

The curves rise steeply at first as pressure increases from 1 to 3 atm, then begin to flatten out. The authors believed that these curves would eventually turn back down as pressure continues to increase, especially for the lower oxygen fractions. It can be seen that the burning rate in air at the pressure of a treatment for decompression sickness, 2.8 atm, is about 1.6 times as fast as that in air, and at the treatment depth of 6 atm is well over twice that at sea level. On the same scale, an atmosphere of 100% oxygen has a burning rate of a little over 4 times that of air at 1 atm (101.3 kPa).

Cook and Dorr also noted that ignition temperatures are reduced as the oxygen fraction increases in a pattern similar to that of the increase of burning rates.

A similar diagram shows equivalent burning-rate curves derived in a helium atmosphere.[5] In general, burning rates are slightly greater in helium, but ignition temperatures are higher.[6] Much of the information on helium is moot because when a chamber is filled with helium, the oxygen is too low for fire to be a possibility.

Cook, Dorr, and co-workers produced most of the data on which conventional chamber fire safety is based.[6-7] The Cook Diagram has been reproduced in many places, including the *Underwater Handbook.*[2,8-9] Several of these also contain references to other work on materials and ignition sources.

Another important concept from Cook and Dorr was the zone of no combustion. This is a diagram that shows the zones of complete combustion, partial combustion, and no combustion for different oxygen fractions (in nitrogen) as a function of depth.[10] It also shows overlap with the zone where the PO_2 is compatible with normal respiration. These diagrams, including a companion one for helium, are useful for operations such as welding where there is a guaranteed source of ignition, and the only way to maintain fire safety is to work in the zone of no combustion.

Fire in the Hyperbaric Chamber Environment

Classical fire prevention relies on the separation of elements of the Fire Triangle to prevent fires from occurring. In a hyperbaric chamber, separation of the elements of the Fire Triangle is of critical importance and is quite difficult because the hazard is inherent in the environment. High-pressure air or an oxygen-enriched atmosphere exists by necessity in an area where fuels are present and ignition sources are prevalent. For many materials, the energy for ignition is so small that ignition is more likely. In addition to the increased ignition probability in a hyperbaric environment, the resultant fire will be more intense, consuming more material while producing more heat and higher temperatures than fires in normal air environments. Fires in hyperbaric chambers have been described as explosive in nature due to the severity of the burning and the speed at which the fire propagates.[4]

Methods of Controlling Fires in Human Occupied Chambers

The fact that the elements of the Fire Triangle are necessary for a fire to occur does not guarantee that a fire will occur. It is possible that either the probability of a fire occurring may be low or the consequences may be insignificant. Examples of low probability include regions and environments where materials are "situationally nonflammable," such as 2% hydrogen in oxygen (which is below the flammability limit for hydrogen) or environments in which sufficient separation exists between the ignition source and the fuel so that ignition will not occur (e.g., not smoking within 50 feet of a gas pump and shutting off your engine while putting gasoline in your automobile). Examples of insignificant consequences include areas where the fuel loading and propagation pathways for a fire are sufficiently controlled that if a fire were to occur, it would be small and would not propagate to surrounding materials. Therefore it does not present a hazard to either personnel or equipment. The National Aeronautics and Space Administration (NASA) has been applying these concepts in control of manned space environments successfully since the 1960s, after the tragic *Apollo I* fire.

Industry courses on the subject of controlling fire hazards in oxygen systems teach the following approaches to avoid fires in these systems:[11]

- Minimize the severity of the environment
- Withstand the environment
- Do it all

The concept of **minimizing the severity of the environment** focuses on system design and includes such things as decreasing the oxygen concentration and pressure and controlling ignition sources. **Withstanding the environment** pertains to control of materials that are nonflammable in the environment, are not susceptible to ignition by the ignition mechanisms present or, when ignited, do not propagate the fire to surrounding materials because of slow flame spread rate and low heat of combustion. **Do it all** incorporates the other two concepts in the day-to-day operation of the hyperbaric chamber such that the hazards are continuously recognized and dealt with. This includes training of personnel and patients, housekeeping, written procedures around critical equipment, and attention to detail in operation and maintenance of the chamber and its associated facility.

Another similar training approach uses the following three principles:[32]

- Maximize compatible materials
- Minimize ignition mechanisms
- Utilize best practices

This educates the designer or user to select the most ignition-resistant, burn-resistant, and low fire-damage potential materials available (e.g., most oxygen compatible), while still fulfilling material suitability requirements. Minimizing ignition mechanisms focuses on controlling the potential for heat generating sources to become active by targeting specific characteristic elements of each potential ignition mechanism. Utilize best practices includes cleaning for oxygen service (from initial cleaning to assembly to maintenance) and best design and operating principles.

In the event that design and materials selection fail in the prevention of fires in hyperbaric chambers, then fire extinguishment systems must be present to control and extinguish the resulting fire. A greater demand is placed on extinguishing systems in hyperbaric chambers than for a nonoxygen-enriched environment. Fire suppression systems will be discussed in more detail later in the chapter.

Effects of Oxygen on Material Flammability

It is generally accepted that increasing the oxygen concentration in an environment will increase material flammability. To fully describe the flammability of a given material in an environment, one must consider the following:

- Whether the material of interest is flammable given a positive ignition source
- Whether the material will ignite, given the strength of active ignition sources
- If the material is flammable and is ignited, how fast will it burn and how much heat will be given off in the burning

The information presented in the next two sections examines the effect of an increased oxygen environment on these variables.

As noted, material flammability as a function of both oxygen concentration and pressure is complex and dependent on kinetic and thermodynamic control of the ensuing chemical reactions. The Cook Diagram represents this complex behavior by describing the flame spread rate for a given material, i.e. filter paper.[5] There exists in theory an equivalent diagram for every material, each of which will exhibit its own relative behavior with respect to increases in pressure and oxygen concentration; however, the research has not yet been accomplished to determine the set of curves for all materials. In many cases, only single data points are available, and care should be taken when extrapolating these results to the environment of interest. Hirsch, Bunker, and Janoff present an excellent review of previous work.[12]

Flammability of materials is determined using several test methods developed for specific materials and configurations. When considering design and material selection for a particular application, it should be determined whether the data are conservative in the intended application. Complex configuration effects influence flammability. An example of this is the lighting of a fire in a fireplace, in which first paper is ignited, followed by twigs, then the kindling that ignites the logs. All are cellulose materials but their configuration affects their flammability, and all of this is affected by whether or not the damper is open. In the same manner, configuration effects will also influence material flammability in a system. For example, cotton sheets with "pills" are more flammable than "unpilled" sheets, and stainless steel in a wire mesh configuration is flammable in atmospheric pressure oxygen, whereas a thicker stainless steel sheet configuration is not.

Configuration effects influence all stages of combustion, from ignition to flame spread rate to extinguishment. Therefore, when applying data to a particular environment, it is critical to understand the conditions under which the data were taken so that they may be conservatively applied. For example, many people mistakenly assume that a flash point represents a flammability limit and that a material below its given flash point will not ignite. However, if the material is sprayed across an ignition source because of a hose rupture (for example, atomized), or if a stronger ignition source is present, then the material can ignite, and once ignited, continue to burn.

The Nonflammable Becomes Flammable

In general, it is assumed that a material will be made more flammable by increasing the fraction of oxygen in a gas mixture than by increasing the total pressure at a constant fraction of oxygen. Therefore a 42% oxygen environment (balance nitrogen) at 1 atm (101.3 kPa) is more hazardous than a 21% air environment at 2 atm (202.6 kPa). Despite the fact that both atmospheres contain the same number of moles of oxygen, materials that will not burn in the 2 atm environment will burn at 1 atm. This is shown clearly in the Cook Diagram.[5]

The oxygen index of a material (as determined by a standard test method such as ASTM D2863,[13] ASTM G125,[33] or equivalent) can be used to determine if a material will burn in a given environment. The oxygen index of a material may be given as a fractional amount or as a percentage; for example, the oxygen index of cotton fabric is 0.184[14] and polytetrafluoroethylene (PTFE or Teflon) is 1.0[15] or 18.4 and 100 respectively when referred to as a percentage. These values imply that in a standard test the materials will not support sustained combustion until the oxygen concentration reaches 18.4% and 100%, respectively, at 1 atm (101.3 kPa).

Several references give extensive tables of oxygen indices for a variety of materials.[1,14-16] Table 1 provides the results of testing by the Naval Research Laboratory on the flammability of fabrics and demonstrates the general trend for a variety of materials that as the oxygen concentration increases, the material will become flammable.[17] Ikeda showed an inverse relationship exists between oxygen index and heat of combustion; the lower a material's heat of combustion, the higher its oxygen index.[15] Ikeda also demonstrated that no such inverse relationship exists for ignition properties such as autogenous ignition temperature (AIT). This finding by Ikeda supports the contention that because a material may readily burn in oxygen does not necessarily mean it will readily ignite.

Table 1. Flame Resistance of Materials Held Vertically at One Atmosphere Pressure in O_2/N_2 Mixtures[7]
Table courtesy of U.S. Naval Research Laboratory.

NRL Sample Number	Material	Combustion in O_2/N_2 Mixtures		
		21 % O_2	31 % O_2	41% O_2
FM-1	Rosin-impregnated paper	Burned		
FM-3	Cotton terry cloth	Burned		
FM-28	Cotton cloth, white duck	Burned		
FM-4	Cotton terry cloth, Roxel-treated	No	No	Burned
FM-5	Fleece-backed cotton cloth, Roxel-treated	Surface[1]	Burned	Burned
FM-14	Cotton, O.D. Santeen, Roxel-treated	No	Burned	
FM-15	Cotton, green ripcord, Roxel-treated	No	Burned	

Table 1. (continued)

NRL Sample Number	Material	Combustion in O_2/N_2 Mixtures		
FM-16	Cotton, white duck, Roxel-treated	No	Burned	
FM-17	Cotton, King Kord, Roxel-treated	No	Burned	
FM-29	Cotton, white duck, treated with 30% boric acid-70% borax	No	Burned	Burned
FM-30	Cotton terry cloth, treated with 30% boric acid-70% borax	No	Burned	Burned
FM-6	Fire resistant Cotton Ticking	No	Burned	
FM-7	Fire resistant foam rubber	No	No	Burned
FM-9	Nomex temperature resistant nylon	No	Burned	
FM-10	Teflon fabric	No	No	No
FM-11	Teflon fabric	No	No	No
FM-12	Teflon fabric	No	No	No
FM-13	Teflon fabric	No	No	No
FM-19	Verel fabric	No	Burned	Burned
FM-22	Vinyl-backed fabric	No	Burned	Burned
FM-23	Omnicoated Dupont high-temperature fabric	No	Burned	Burned
FM-24	Omnicoated glass fabric	No	No	Burned[2]
FM-20	Glass fabric, fine weave	No	No	No
FM-21	Glass fabric, knit weave	No	No	No
FM-25	Glass fabric, coarse weave	No	No	No
FM-26	Glass fabric, coarse weave	No	No	No
FM-27	Aluminized asbestos fabric	No	No	Burned
FM-32	Rubber from aviator oxygen mask	Burned	Burned	Burned

[1] Only the surface of the sample burned

[2] Burned only over the igniter

Benning studied the effect of pressure on oxygen index and determined that generally the oxygen index of a given material decreases as a function of increased pressure.[18] However, materials appear to preserve the same ordering with respect to oxygen index as obtained from the standard atmospheric pressure test. The data in Table 2 show the relative change in oxygen index for PTFE and neoprene as a function of increased pressure.[18] Note that the change appears to be more dramatic for PTFE than for neoprene. This is probably because neoprene has a fairly low oxygen index to begin with, so that the reaction is proceeding under thermodynamic control more than kinetic control. Therefore, increased pressure represents a heat sink as much as an increased availability of oxygen for the reaction. Hirsch and Bunker[19] extended this data for some materials to pressures as high as 3,000 PSI (20.1 MPa) where they observed PTFE to be flammable at 21% oxygen in nitrogen.

Table 2. Oxygen Index and Burning Rate at the Oxygen Index Given as a Function of Pressure for Polytetrafluoroethylene (PTFE) and Neoprene[18]

Material	Pressure, atm absolute	Oxygen Index, Mole percent oxygen
PTFE	1.7	81.2
PTFE	1.8	80.0
PTFE	4.1	62.0
PTFE	7.1	53.5
PTFE	14.9	46.0
Neoprene	1.0	35.3
Neoprene	4.1	33.0
Neoprene	7.1	32.0
Neoprene	14.9	27.0
Neoprene	20.4	25.5

Benning[18] also measured material burn rate at the measured oxygen index. For a given constant pressure, he observed an increased burn rate with increasing oxygen concentration, similar to that observed by Cook et al.[5]

Oxygen indices exist for metals as well as polymers. Typically, reactive metals which are flammable in air such as magnesium, lithium, sodium, and potassium are not used in hyperbaric environments. Common structural metals such as carbon steel, aluminum, and stainless steel that are used in and around hyperbaric chambers may be flammable at the environment that exists within a chamber. This is particularly true for certain configurations such as wire screens, tubing, thin diameter wire (e.g., instrumentation wire), or thin sheet. Zabrenski, Werley, and Slusser determined the effect of pressure on oxygen index for several common metals including stainless steel, carbon steel, and aluminum.[20] The data was collected with argon as the diluent (argon is a common fixed-gas in many oxygen enrichment processes); however, the trends are applicable to nitrogen diluent atmospheres. The data, as expected, shows that as the pressure increases, the oxygen index decreases. For example, carbon steel rod which is flammable in 100% oxygen at 25 PSIG (172 kPa) is also flammable in 90% oxygen at 100 PSIG (689 kPa).

The data in Zabrenski et al.[20] also shows the effect of configuration on the oxygen index, where 304 stainless steel rod, which was recorded as not flammable in pure oxygen at pressures up to 500 PSIG (3.4 MPa), was recorded flammable in 90% oxygen at 150 PSIG (1.03 MPa) when configured as a tube. The effect of configuration can be dramatic. For example, Monel (a copper-nickel alloy), which is not flammable at 10,000 PSI (69 MPa) in 100% oxygen, is flammable in 100% oxygen at ambient pressure (14.7 PSIA [101.3 kPa]) when configured as a fine wire-mesh filter screen.[34]

For vapors and gases, the material flammability is generally expressed in terms of flammability limits. The lower flammability limit (LFL) is the minimum concentration of fuel that will ignite and propagate a flame in a particular atmosphere; below this point, a mixture is considered "fuel lean." The upper flammability limit (UFL) represents the maximum concentration that will ignite and propagate a flame in a particular atmosphere; above this point the mixture is considered "fuel rich." For example, the LFL and UFL for methane are 5.0 and 15% by volume in air at atmospheric pressure, respectively. As the atmosphere changes, flammability limits also change. Typically, the LFL does not change significantly as a function of a change in atmospheric conditions; however, the UFL will change drastically, extending the region of flammability for a given atmosphere. *NFPA 53* includes data that shows the change in lower and upper flammability limits as a function of increased oxygen concentration for several common gases and vapors.[1] The data indicates, among other things, that a change from air to oxygen has little effect on ignition temperature or lower flammability limits but can reduce the necessary ignition energy a hundredfold and raise the upper flammability limits by approximately a factor of 3.

Flame Speed and Burn Rate

Other key aspects that describe the change in material flammability are related to the rate at which the fire develops (flame spread rate), the material is consumed (burn rate or mass loss rate), and the heat is released to surroundings (heat release rate). These parameters are essential for determining the potential for fire spread and time characteristics for fire control.

Flame spread rates over surfaces have been measured and reported in the literature for a variety of materials. *NFPA 53* also includes data that compares flame spread rates in air versus pure oxygen at 258 mm Hg (34 kPa) (a pressure of interest in early manned space environments).[1] It shows many materials that will not ignite in air will ignite readily in oxygen, and flame-spread rates across the surface increase by up to 20 times in oxygen compared to air. The flame-spread rate over the surface may or may not correspond to the burn rate of the material. For thin materials there is typically a better correlation between the rates than for thick materials. For example, nylon Velcro (0.125-inch (3.2 mm) thick) has been observed to burn at nearly the same rate as the flame propagates over the surface, while Pyrell foam (1-inch [25.4 mm] thick) exhibits a rapid surface flame spread and then the sample is consumed at a much slower rate.[21] In terms of fire risk, the more rapid the flame spread the greater the area of fire development.

Burn rate is also affected by increase in pressure and/or oxygen concentration, which was consistent with the Cook Diagram.[5] The magnitude of the effect will vary depending on the material and the configuration of burning. Figure 2 shows the effect of pressure and oxygen concentration on the upward burning of three materials: nylon Velcro, polyester/cotton cloth, and Pyrell foam (0.25-inch thick).[21] Figure 2 also shows that the magnitude of the effect can vary from material to material and, in general, the effect of a change in oxygen concentration is greater than that for a change in pressure.

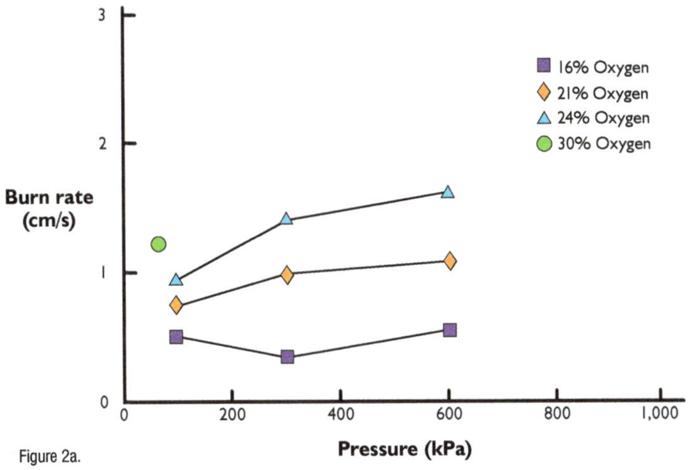

Figure 2a.

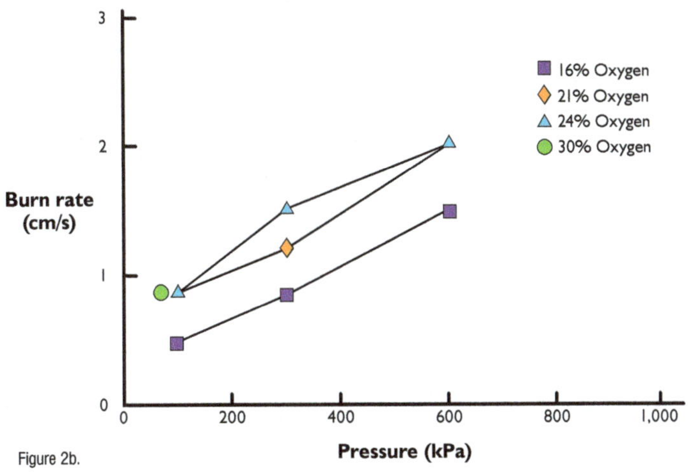

Figure 2b.

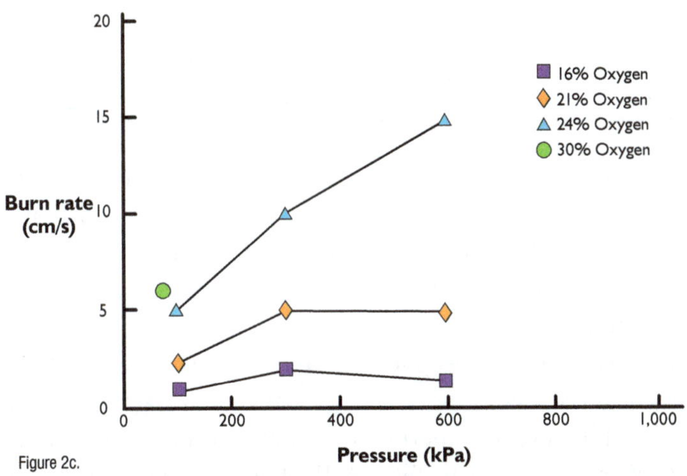

Figure 2c.

Figure 2. Burn rate as a function of pressure at four oxygen concentrations for the following: 1) Nylon Velcro; 2) polyester/cotton; and 3) Pyrell foam. The purpose of this is to show that both pressure and oxygen concentration may act differently on different materials. Note that the scales are different.

Investigations into the effects of oxygen concentration on material flammability have been carried out using a controlled atmosphere cone calorimeter. This device, which has been described in detail in the literature,[22-24] allows material flammability determination as a function of incident heat flux on the materials, simulating the radiant heating responsible for fire progression. Measurements include peak and average heat release rate, total heat released, average effective heat of combustion, average specific extinction (smoke obscuration), peak and average mass loss rate, CO and CO_2 production, and time to ignition. Table 3 shows the effect of increased oxygen concentration at constant pressure on these measured parameters for untreated cotton fabric.[23] The data indicate a direct relationship between several of these parameters and increased oxygen concentration.

Table 3. Effect of Oxygen Concentration on Combustion of Untreated Cotton Fabrics at 25 kW/m^2 Heat Flux

Combustion	O_2 Concentration (vol. %)				
Parameters	15	18	21	25.9	30
Peak heat-release rate (kW/m^2)	285	313	334	338	384
Average heat-release rate (kW/m^2)	142	171	191	190	240
Total heat released (MJ/m^2)	6	6	6	7	8
Average effective heat of combustion (MJ/kg)	14.1	12.9	12.2	12.8	11.7
Effective heat of combustion at peak heat-release rate (MJ/kg)	11.2	12.0	12.2	11.9	13.0
Average specific extinction area (m^2/kg)	22	30	38	34	21
Peak mass-loss rate (g/s· m^2)	25.35	26.11	27.4	528.43	29.65
Average mass-loss rate (g/s· m^2)	13.43	16.86	17.93	19.48	22.09
Average CO production (kg/kg)	0.0410	0.0236	0.0095	0.0099	0.0046
Average CO_2 production (kg/kg)	1.1698	1.2348	1.2077	1.2286	1.2838
Time to ignition (sec)	26.5	26.3	24.0	25.9	22.7

Note that the data presented in Table 3 indicate little change in the total heat released. This is expected because total heat released should be constant for a given mass of material, given complete combustion. The completeness of combustion can be related to two factors measured in the cone experiment: the relationship between CO and CO_2 production and the amount of soot produced, which is related to the average specific extinction area and in this case shows a steady decrease from 21 to 30% oxygen. Given that the total heat released is essentially unchanged, the fact that the heat release rates increase through the range of experiments is a function of the material's increased burning rate, given by mass loss rate in Table 3. The higher a material's heat release rate, the more effective heat transfer to surrounding materials becomes, and the greater the risk of fire propagation.

The total heat released by a material is derived from the material's heat of combustion. Given a choice of materials, properties for use in hyperbaric environment and all other things being equal, a material with a low heat of combustion is preferred. A common test standard to determine the heat of combustion of materials is ASTM D4809.[35] Gross heats of combustion for several common materials are listed in *ASTM G63*,[16] *ASTM Manual 36*,[36] and in Hsheih, Beeson and Stoltzfus.[25]

Ignition

Elimination of ignition is a primary means of controlling the fire hazard in hyperbaric environments. If there is "no ignition," there is "no fire," even if the material is flammable. In order to effectively control ignition, one must understand that many ignition mechanisms can exist in a hyperbaric environment and that the environment affects the ignition mechanism.

An ignition source can be any energy release capable of raising the local temperature above the activation energy required to initiate the combustion reaction. This required initiation energy can be lowered by any mechanism that effectively lowers the activation energy, such as an increase in reactant concentration, increase in free radical concentrations, and catalytic surface effects. The details of these effects are not well understood except for a very few reactions, such as those involving hydrogen and oxygen.

In general, at a given pressure the minimum ignition energy decreases with an increase in oxygen concentration. For many ignition sources at a fixed oxygen concentration, the minimum ignition energy decreases with an increase in pressure at least for the range of pressures associated with hyperbaric chambers. The exception is for ignition mechanisms that rely on effective heat transfer, such as friction.

Ignition Sources

Table 4 lists several potential ignition sources for hyperbaric fires. The two most common types of ignition sources for fires occurring within the hyperbaric chamber, or those not associated with the external facility oxygen systems, are from hot surfaces and electrical sparks and arcs. Electrical sources require particular attention because large energy densities are delivered to the flammable material over a relatively short period of time.

Table 4. Some Possible Ignition Sources for Hyperbaric Environments

Electrostatic sparks	Friction
Frictional or impact sparks	Failed motor
Sparks or arcs from electrically powered devices	Hot gases
Hot Surfaces	Gas Flames
Warming devices for towels and hands	Shock waves
Electrical wiring overload	Compression heating of gases

Ignition Temperature

The potential for a material to ignite in a hyperbaric environment is related to its ignition temperature or to its AIT. The difference between the two measurements relates to the way that the experiment is conducted. In a typical ignition temperature test, such as a flash point determination, the sample is heated until the vapors generated above the sample are ignited by an external ignition source. To determine the AIT, the sample is heated until the vapors ignite without an external ignition source. Therefore, the AIT will always be greater than the flash point ignition temperature. The AIT is also called the auto-ignition temperature. This is not to be confused with "spontaneous combustion" or "spontaneous ignition," where the fuel itself is the source of the heat.

Generally, the AIT and ignition temperature of a given material will decrease with either increasing oxygen concentration or pressure, and the magnitude of the effect will vary from material to material. For example, test results indicate that the AIT of nylon Zytel 42 in 21% oxygen decreased by approximately 60°C when the pressure increased from 500 PSI to 1,000 PSI (3.4 to 6.9 MPa).[26] Similarly, the AIT decreased by 75°C when tested at 500 PSI (3.4 MPa), and the oxygen concentration increased from 21 to 100%. This can be compared to results for PTFE which demonstrated only an approximately 20°C decrease in AIT resulting from changes in oxygen pressure and demonstrated no appreciable change in AIT based on changes in oxygen concentration. AITs and ignition temperatures for many polymers are tabulated in the literature.[1,16,37,27] The AITs and flash points of several combustible liquids and gases are given in *NFPA 53*.[1]

AIT for Hyperbaric Oxygen

In recent years, the hyperbaric industry has become more intentional about understanding the oxygen compatibility of chamber designs, as well as wound care products and other materials for used in hyperbaric service and research. Collaboration between the Undersea & Hyperbaric Medical Society (UHMS), ASTM International Committee G04 (Committee G04 on Compatibility and Sensitivity of Materials in Oxygen Enriched Atmospheres) and WHA International, Inc., led to the development of a test approach to measure the AIT of nonmetallic materials specifically in hyperbaric oxygen (HBO_2) conditions.[38-39] This led to the modification of an existing AIT ASTM test standard: ASTM G72.[37] Bernatchez, Tucker, and Chiffoleau presented the AIT of a wide range of wound care products and other materials according to this test standard.[40]

The 2018 version of *NFPA 99* indicated that ASTM G72 can be used to determine the AIT of materials intended for a hyperbaric chamber (*NFPA 99*, Annex A, section A.14.3.1.6.4.3). Although there is currently no pass/fail criteria listed in either *ASTM G72* or *NFPA 99*, the test results of their materials can be compared with test results of materials currently being used in HBO_2. This comparative approach can also be performed with the oxygen index and heat of combustion tests described previously.

Ignition Energy

A material's ignition energy is another important consideration when assessing the hazard of a hyperbaric environment. However, ignition energies are reliably determined only for gases and vapors. The lack of data for other materials points out the lack of a test method to determine the ignition energy for other materials because of the difficulty of measuring ignition energy such as spark energies. *NFPA 53* lists minimum ignition energies for several gases and vapors.[1] The data suggests that there is a significant decrease in ignition energy when the atmosphere is changed from air to oxygen. The reduction of energy by three orders of magnitude, results in an ignition energy so low, such as 3 μj for methane, that one has to assume an ignition source is available that will ignite the material.

Time to Ignition

Time to ignition also decreases with increasing oxygen concentration and pressure, although the influence of pressure is more complex because of the heat sinking ability of the gas. Table 3 provides the time to ignition for cotton fabric as measured from the cone calorimeter at the prescribed test conditions and at atmospheric pressure. While the data in Table 3 indicate only a modest reduction in time to ignition, other materials tested between 18 and 30% oxygen demonstrated a 50% reduction in time to ignition.[24]

Additional Guidance and Testing

NFPA 99 (Figure A.14.3.1.6.4.3 Risk Assessment Process) offers guidance to perform a risk assessment to help determine whether candidate materials can qualify for hyperbaric service. The process includes answering questions such as, "Does the material produce heat?" and, "Does the material have a low flash point?" The flash point is a material property that is inconsistently found on safety data sheets (SDS) and, if available, is typically associated with testing in atmospheric pressure air. Although these test conditions are not as severe as HBO_2, the test still provides valuable information regarding the material's ignitability. If the flash point of a material is not available, the AIT of the material can be used to help evaluate the "Low flash point?" question because the materials with low flash points typically exhibit low AITs, relatively. The oxygen exposure test, developed by WHA International, Inc. and described below, is a simple test concept (currently nonstandard) available to help evaluate the "Produce heat?" question.

Oxygen exposure test: This test can be applied to both materials and components. Test articles are exposed to severe HBO_2 conditions (severe in duration and temperature) by first positioning them in a test chamber (approximately 6" diameter by 1.5' long) and positioning thermocouples directly against or proximate to the test articles. The chamber is pressurized to 3 atm with static oxygen and heated to 60°C. These conditions are held constant for six hours and thermocouples are monitored for any temperature increases that may indicate exothermic activity with the test article. The pretest and posttest mass are measured to calculate mass loss. Since low flash points are also associated with materials that can lose mass overtime (e.g., volatility), the supplemental mass loss measurement is also valuable information. There are no pass/fail criteria for this test but it can be an important test option to consider before placing a new item into HBO_2 with a patient.

Fire Causes and Responses

This section does not directly examine fire prevention or its rules, but instead draws on the cause of actual chamber fires to derive some ideas for prevention.

Oxygen is always present in a chamber; thus we cannot entirely remove the oxygen leg of the Fire Triangle. (See Figure 1.) Fuel is normally kept to a minimum in chambers, except for the monoplace hyperbaric chamber in which the oxygen concentration is high and the effort is entirely on prevention of ignition.

The EDU Fire

An overheated motor started the fatal 1965 fire at the U.S. Navy Experimental Diving Unit. The fire got out of hand because the filter to the chamber was soaked with jet fuel and the oxygen fraction in the chamber was higher than it should have been, creating what proved to be a very hazardous situation. This highlights a particular hazard, that of a volatile or finely divided flammable material. The use of this type of material in a hyperbaric chamber should be strictly prohibited.

Fire suppression was not available at that time; back then, deck chambers often had only a bucket of sand for that purpose. To some extent there was an overreaction to the motor, and many facilities will not use internal motors at all, or use fans or blowers with magnetic couplings or hydraulic drive. Well-enclosed brushless motors can be used safely if they are properly designed.

Several Monoplace Fires with Ignition Introduced

There have been several fires in monoplace chambers caused by sparking toys, hand warmers, or smoking materials taken in by the occupants. Although the hazard should be obvious, this type of accident has happened all too often. Safety in the monoplace chamber depends **entirely** on prevention of ignition. Current practice is to use cotton clothing and bedding in the chamber with the concept that this material is less likely to cause a static spark. The consequence of this is that there is usually a great deal of easily ignited fuel, making a fire guaranteed to be catastrophic, often for people outside the chamber as well.

Countermeasures to prevent this situation include intensified training efforts to ensure that patients and staff understand the risks, careful searches for banned materials, or having patients wear only hospital garments. This can be considerably more trouble in places where normal hospital garments contain some synthetics because it may not be possible to put the HBO_2 garments into the normal hospital laundry. The importance of static sparks that might be generated by cotton-polyester materials is not yet well understood.

Another countermeasure is to fill the chamber with air and avoid the 100% oxygen. For compliant patients and treatment situations that permit it, filling the chamber with air and using a hood or mask to administer the oxygen is preferred.

The Milan Fire

A hand-warming device was suspected of causing this tragic fire that killed 11 people.[28] Normally a fire from such a device would start small and be controlled before it spread. In this case, a deluge system was installed but it did not work. It turned out that the chamber personnel thought the maintenance department was checking the system, and the maintenance department thought the chamber crew was doing it; the tragic result is that no one checked it. Incidentally, events like this have prompted the NFPA to specify a hand-held hose and a deluge system; in the Milan fire such a hose was probably not available. Further, the way this fire spread so quickly suggests that the oxygen level was much higher than that of air; analyses have not shown clearly how this may have happened, but the increased oxygen most likely came from the breathing system.

Many chambers in the U.S. require patients and inside attendants to wear fire resistant clothing. The fairly expensive Durette Gold from Monsanto is often specified, and this has been shown to be quite flame resistant even in high oxygen mixes.[6] Although this is probably the best material, other less expensive materials like Nomex® might be an effective compromise; the idea of flame resistant fabric should not be abandoned just because Durette seems too expensive.

Fire Suppression Systems in Hyperbaric Chambers

Fire suppression system requirements for hyperbaric chambers are given in *NFPA 99* and will not be repeated in detail here.[2] The preferred extinguishing agent for hyperbaric chambers is water. Water acts primarily by reducing the heat in the fuel, thereby inhibiting ignition and combustion. In some cases, a foaming agent is added to the water to increase the wetting ability of the water, which may increase the effectiveness of water as an extinguishing agent. Gaseous extinguishants such as CO_2 and nitrogen, which primarily extinguish fires by reducing the oxygen concentration, are ineffective for extinguishing hyperbaric fires. Chemical fire extinguishants such as halogenated hydrocarbons may require as much as five times the amount of agent to extinguish a fire in a 40% oxygen environment.[29] Also, the combustion products produced by halogenated hydrocarbons when it is ineffectively applied to a fire represent a severe toxic hazard in an enclosed environment.

The average spray density required for the fixed deluge system in a hyperbaric chamber is 2 gal/min/ft^2 (82 L/min/m^2). Recent testing to determine critical application rates in hypobaric chambers indicates that a 2 gal/min/ft^2 (82 L/min/m^2) spray density is sufficient for oxygen concentrations below 30%.[30] However, at concentrations of 40% and at pressures above 14.7 PSIA (101.3 kPa), the required demand rate for water to extinguish a fire exceeded 2 gal/min/ft^2 (82 L/min/m^2). It was also noted during this testing that at concentrations greater than 40%, direct impingement of water on all burning surfaces was required to reliably extinguish the fire. For these reasons it is recommended that a hand-held hose be used in hyperbaric environments to supplement the fixed deluge extinguishing system. The hand-held hose allows the operator to direct the water at the burning surfaces, thereby increasing the local water density.

In addition to increased water density, the extinguishing system should be automatic with a minimal delay before discharge. This is because of the increased flame spread, burning rates, and heat release rates of materials involved in hyperbaric chamber environments. Any delay in effecting extinguishment can mean that the extinguishing system will be quickly overwhelmed with potentially disastrous consequences.

Future Trends

The use of hyperbaric chambers is increasing as the effectiveness of hyperbaric treatment of disease is further explored. The trend, however, is to move the use of these chambers out of highly controlled environments and into clinics, private-treatment centers, health clubs, and private residences. Training and certification programs are not consistent throughout the industry, and the approach to materials and ignition control may be haphazard at best. With these challenges comes the responsibility of operators and manufacturers of chambers to understand the hazards as well as the benefits involved with the use of hyperbaric chambers.

There are three areas for recommended improvement in hyperbaric fire safety as related to the role of oxygen.

1. One needs to understand the hazards involved in hyperbaric environments; once understood, control measures should be put in place for materials and ignition sources to preclude compromising the safety of personnel and equipment. This can be accomplished through the use of an oxygen system hazard analysis described in *NASA TM 104823*,[31] *ASTM Manual 36*,[36] and other publications.[41]
2. There is a particular need for intensive instruction on how oxygen increases the flammability of the materials in a hyperbaric environment and how to design and select materials to minimize the operational risks. ASTM International offers two such courses: one for oxygen system designers and the other for system maintenance personnel. It appears to be more important than ever that experts in oxygen safety be involved in hyperbaric system design. WHA International, Inc. also offers a range of oxygen safety courses from basic oxygen safety awareness to advanced application of oxygen system and component analysis. These courses include specific guidance for operators of oxygen equipment and for maintenance or oxygen cleaning personnel.

3. A major area that requires further study is fire extinguishment. The effect of pressure at increased oxygen concentration on water demand rates is relatively unstudied.

References

1. NFPA. NFPA 53, Recommended Practice on Materials, Equipment and Systems Used in Oxygen Enriched Atmospheres. Quincy, MA: National Fire Protection Association; 2016.
2. NFPA. NFPA 99, Health Care Facilities Code. Quincy, MA: National Fire Protection Association; 2018.
3. Dorr VA. Fire studies in oxygen-enriched atmospheres. *Journal of Fire and Flammability, Vol. 1.* 1970;91-106.
4. Harter JV. Fire at high pressure. In: Proceedings of the Third Symposium on Underwater Physiology. Baltimore: Edited by, Williams and Wilkins; 1967.
5. Cook GA, Meierer RE, Shields BM. Screening of flame-resistant materials and comparison of helium with nitrogen for use in diving atmospheres. First Summary Report Under ONR Contract N00014-66-C-014. Tonawanda, NY: Union Carbide; 1967.
6. Dorr VA. Compendium of hyperbaric fire safety research, final report on combustion safety in diving atmospheres. Contract N0014-70-C-0169. Tarrytown, NY: Ocean Systems, Inc.; 1971.
7. Dorr, VA, Schreiner H.R. Region of non-combustion, flammability limits of hydrogen-oxygen mixtures, full scale combustion and extinguishing tests and screening of flame-resistant materials. Second Summary Report.ONR Contract N00014-66-0149. Tonawanda, NY: Ocean Systems, Inc.; 1969.
8. Shilling CW, Werts MF, Schandelmeier NR. The Underwater Handbook: A Guide to Physiology and Performance for the Engineer. New York: Plenum Press; 1976;646664.
9. Schmidt TC, Dorr VA, Hamilton RW. Chamber fire safety. Technical Memorandum UCRI-721. Tonawanda, NY: Ocean Systems, Inc; 1973.
10. Cook GA, Dorr VA, Shields BM. Region of noncombustion in nitrogen-oxygen and helium-oxygen diving atmospheres. I&EC Process Design and Development. 1968;7(2):308-311.
11. Werley BL, editor. Fire hazards in oxygen systems. Technical Professional Training Course. West Conshohocken, PA: ASTM; 1991.
12. Hirsch DB, Bunker RL, Janoff D. Effects of oxygen concentration, diluents, and pressure on ignition and flame-spread rates of nonmetals: a review paper. Flammability and Sensitivity of Materials in Oxygen-Enriched Atmospheres: Fifth Volume, ASTM STP 1111, Joel M. Stoltzfus and Kenneth McIlroy, Eds. West Conshohocken, PA: ASTM; 1991;179-190.

13. ASTM. ASTM D2863 Standard Test Method for Measuring the Minimum Oxygen Concentration to Support Candle-like Combustion of Plastics (Oxygen Index). West Conshohocken, PA: ASTM International; 2017
14. Hilado CJ. Flammability Handbook for Plastics, Third Edition. Westport, CT: Technomic Publishing Co.; 1982.
15. Ikeda GK. Oxygen index tests to evaluate the suitability of a given material for oxygen service. Flammability and Sensitivity of Materials in Oxygen-Enriched Atmospheres, ASTM STP 812, Werley BL, Ed. West Conshohocken, PA: ASTM; 1983;56-67.
16. ASTM. ASTM G63 Standard Guide for Evaluating Nonmetallic Materials for Oxygen Service. West Conshohocken, PA: ASTM; 2015.
17. Johnson JE, Woods FJ. Flammability in unusual atmospheres, part 1 - preliminary studies of materials in hyperbaric atmospheres containing oxygen, Nitrogen, and/or Helium. NRL Report 6470. Washington, DC: Naval Research Laboratory; 1966.
18. Benning MA. Measurement of oxygen index at elevated pressures. Flammability and Sensitivity of Materials in Oxygen-Enriched Atmospheres, ASTM STP 812, Werley BL, Ed.West Conshohocken, PA: ASTM; 1983; 68-83.
19. Hirsch DB, Bunker RL. Effects of diluents on flammability of nonmetals in high-pressure oxygen mixtures. Flammability and Sensitivity of Materials in Oxygen-Enriched Atmospheres: Sixth Volume, ASTM STP 1197, Janoff D, Stoltzfus JM, Eds. West Conshohocken, PA: ASTM; 1993;74-80.
20. Zabrenski JS, Werley BL, Slusser, JW. Pressurized flammability limits of metals. Flammability and Sensitivity of Materials in Oxygen-Enriched Atmospheres: Fourth Volume, ASTM STP 1040, Stoltzfus JM, Benz FJ, Stradling JS, Eds. West Conshohocken, PA: ASTM; 1989;178-194.
21. Sircar S, Dees J, Gunaji MV, Beeson, HD. Evaluation of fire extinguishants for space station freedom. TR-650-001. Las Cruces, NM: NASA Johnson Space Center White Sands Test Facility; 1992.
22. ASTM. ASTM E1354 Standard Test Method for Heat and Visible Smoke Release Rates for Materials and Products Using an Oxygen Consumption Calorimeter. West Conshohocken, PA: ASTM; 1990.
23. Hshieh F, Beeson HD. Evaluation of the controlled-atmosphere cone calorimeter for determining fire properties of materials according to NASA handbook 8060.1C Test 2. NASA Technical Memorandum 104809. Washington, DC: NASA; 1995.
24. Hsheih F, Beeson HD. Flammability testing of flame-retarded epoxy composites and phenolic composites. Fire and Materials. 21:1997;41-49.
25. Hsheih F, Beeson HD, Stoltzfus JM. Note: autoignition temperatures of selected polymers at elevated oxygen pressure and their heat of combustion. Fire and Materials. 20:1996;301-303.

26. Hirsch DB, Hsheih F, Beeson HD, Bryan CJ. Ignitibility in air, gaseous oxygen, and oxygen-enriched environments of polymers used in breathing-air devices. Flammability and Sensitivity of Materials in Oxygen-Enriched Atmospheres: Eighth Volume, ASTM STP 1319, Royals WT, Chou TC, Steinberg TA, Eds. West Conshohocken, PA: ASTM; 1997;359-369.
27. Chou TC, Fiedorowicz A. Oxygen compatibility of polymers including TFE-Teflon, Kel-F 81, Vespel SP-21, Viton A, Viton A-500, Fluorel, Neoprene, EPDM, Buna-N, and Nylon 6,6. Flammability and Sensitivity of Materials in Oxygen-Enriched Atmospheres: Eighth Volume, ASTM STP 1319, Royals WT, Chou TC, Steinberg TA, Eds.West Conshohocken, PA: ASTM; 1997;319-349.
28. Cali-Corleo R.Chamber fire in milan. European Underwater and Baromedical Society Newsletter (Aberdeen). 1998:4(3);1.
29. Zallen DM, Morehouse ET. Fire extinguishing agents for oxygen-enriched atmospheres. Flammability and Sensitivity of Materials in Oxygen-Enriched Atmospheres: Third Volume, ASTM STP 986. Schroll DW, Ed.West Conshohocken, PA: ASTM; 1988;391-412.
30. Beeson HD, Forsyth E, Hirsch DB. Total water demand for suppression of fires in hypobaric oxygen-enriched atmospheres. Flammability and Sensitivity of Materials in Oxygen-Enriched Atmospheres: Eighth Volume, ASTM STP 1319, Royals WT, Chou TC, Steinberg TA, Eds.West Conshohocken, PA: ASTM; 1997;17-24.
31. Stoltzfus JM, Dees J, Poe RF. Guide for oxygen hazards analyses on components and systems. NASA Technical Memorandum 104823. Washington, DC: NASA; 1996.
32. Forsyth E, Newton B. O2 analyze: oxygen hazards and fire risk applications. Technical Engineering Course. WHA International, Inc.; 2018.
33. ASTM. ASTM G125 Measuring Liquid and Solid Material Fire Limits. West Conshohocken, PA: ASTM; 2015.
34. Stoltzfus J M, Lowrie R, Gunaji MV. Burn propagation behavior of wire mesh made from several alloys. Flammability and Sensitivity of Materials in Oxygen-Enriched Atmospheres: Fifth Volume, ASTM STP 1111, Stoltzfus JM, McIlroy K, eds.Philadelphia, PA: ASTM; 1991.
35. ASTM. ASTM D4809, Standard Test Method for Heat of Combustion of Liquid Hydrocarbon Fuels by Bomb Calorimeter (Precision Method). West Conshohocken, PA: ASTM; 2018.
36. ASTM. ASTM Manual 36, Safe Use of Oxygen and Oxygen Systems: Handbook for Design, Operation, and Maintenance. Eds. Beeson HD, Smith SR, Stewart WF, eds. West Conshohocken, PA: ASTM; 2007.
37. ASTM. ASTM G72/G72M - 15, Standard Test Method for Autogenous Ignition Temperature of Liquids and Solids in a High-Pressure Oxygen-Enriched Environment. West Conshohocken, PA: ASTM; 2015.

38. Chiffoleau G, Barry R, Newton B, Linley N. Autogenous ignition test approach for hyperbaric oxygen (HBO_2) and other low-pressure oxygen applications. ASTM STP 1569. Flammability and Sensitivity of Materials in Oxygen-Enriched Atmospheres: Fourteenth Volume. ASTM International; 2016.
39. Barry R. Material Safety Testing. PowerPoint Presentation presented at the Undersea and Hyperbaric Medical Society's Northeast Chapter Meeting; Atlantic City, NJ: 2018.
40. Bernatchez SF, Tucker J, Chiffoleau G. Hyperbaric Oxygen Therapy and Oxygen Compatibility of Skin and Wound Care Products. Advances in Wound Care, Wound Healing Society; 2017.
41. Forsyth E, Newton B, Rantala J, Hirschfeld T. Using ASTM standard guide G88 to identify and rank system-level hazards in large-scale oxygen systems. Flammability and Sensitivity of Materials in Oxygen-Enriched Atmospheres: Tenth Volume, ASTM STP 1454. Steinberg TA, Beeson HD, Newton BE, eds. West Conshohocken, PA: ASTM; 2003.

CHAPTER 5.3
Static Electricity

J. Steven Wood

"Fire in the chamber" are the most feared words in hyperbaric operations. Though the incidence of fire in hyperbaric facilities is low, fire is never far from the minds of chamber operators. When oxygen concentrations increase in an atmosphere, the risk of fire increases. Flammable materials ignite at lower temperatures and burn more energetically as oxygen concentrations rise. Sparks caused by discharges of static electricity have been implicated as ignition sources in fires and explosions and consequently, many industries have undertaken stringent static control measures to reduce risks. Yet static still remains a concern. The hyperbaric chamber, with its abundant fuel and elevated oxygen content coupled with slow egress, poses a particularly hazardous environment.

To prevent fires in any environment, the three legs of the classic Fire Triangle must be considered: fuel, ignition source, and oxygen. In the hyperbaric environment (particularly the oxygen-pressurized monoplace chamber), maintenance of a near-ambient pO_2 (159 mmHg) is not possible. Fire prevention in hyperbaric environments focuses on reducing the amount of available fuel and eliminating sources of ignition.

Though the majority of fires in clinical hyperbaric chambers have been caused by the introduction of an ignition source (hand warmers, cigarette lighters, etc.), static sparks have been implicated in some fires,[13] though the original data source for a number of these fire reports is suspect.[12] To date, there have been no chamber fires in which static discharges have conclusively been shown to be the ignition event.

This chapter will review the nature of static charges and discharges and the risk they pose as ignition sources in normoxic and enriched oxygen atmospheres. The primary consideration will be the generation of static charges by humans engaged in hyperbaric oxygen therapy, though this chapter will discuss some general health care and industrial applications.

Static Electricity – Nature and Causes

Static electricity is a routine part of our lives. Hardly a day goes by without experiencing the familiar snap and pop of static when you reach for a doorknob, particularly after walking across a carpeted floor. These sparks are so common, we often forget that in certain situations, a static discharge can lead to disaster. This chapter will review the nature of static charges and discharges and the risk they pose as ignition sources in normoxic and enriched oxygen atmospheres. A primary consideration will be the generation of static charges by humans engaged in health care activity, with a secondary discussion of some industrial applications.

Electrons accumulate on the surfaces of objects (including the human body) and can result in significant voltage potentials (up to 20,000 volts for a human) under certain conditions. These surface electron accumulations (voltages) are usually unnoticed as they "flow" from object to object through conductive pathways. Sparks are generated only when the voltage accumulations exceed the "bleed-off" rate and the electrons find a path to ground via an air gap. In order to understand this phenomenon, we must review the factors that contribute to the accumulation of static charges and their discharge as sparks.

Materials may fall into one of three electrical classes: 1) *Conductors* allow electrons to move from atom to atom easily (i.e. metals); 2) *Nonconductors* (or insulators) have molecular structures that offer great resistance to the flow of electricity (i.e. glass, stone rubber, plastics, and textiles); 3) *Semiconductors* are neither good conductors nor good insulators (i.e. certain silicon devices utilized in computers).

Whenever objects move and contact other objects (even air), electrical energy is transferred through an electron shift. If dissimilar materials (a conductor and a nonconductor) are pressed together, electrons may shift from one material to the other. If the materials are then separated, there may be an imbalance in the charge distribution, particularly if one of the materials is a nonconductor. The amount of the electron shift is dependent on the nature of the materials. There may be a continuous transfer of electrons which, due to low resistance, multiple contact points, and low energy, is unnoticed. In most cases, accumulated charge levels are very low as long as objects frequently come into contact with grounding paths. Rubbing or friction accelerates transfer of electrons.

Static charges accumulate on the surface of objects. As negative electrons accumulate on an object, it is said to have a negative charge. Objects that lose electrons develop positive charges. Both insulators and conductors are capable of becoming electrically charged but insulators, due to their high resistance, can accumulate larger charges. The accumulated charge on an object is termed a static charge; it is virtually at rest. A potential is the difference in charge accumulated. The amount of the potential is expressed in voltage and is proportional to the amount of work or energy necessary to separate the positive and negative voltages.

Dissimilar charges attract. When objects with dissimilar charges are brought near to each other, they are acted upon by a force that tends to reunite them. This phenomenon can be observed when combing your hair on a low-humidity day. Hair strands are attracted to the comb by the charge imbalance (around 1,000 volts). If a low-resistance circuit is provided, the charges will be reunited and charge equilibrium will be reestablished with minimal physical evidence of the current flow, due to the low voltages developed. When large potential voltages are developed, the attraction between dissimilar charges can be strong enough to overcome the insulating (dielectric) properties of air or other nonconductors. When the electric field strength (volts/distance) between charged conductors becomes sufficiently intense, some of the ions normally present in the air are able to initiate a process known as collision ionization. Electrons will flow through the air when the materials are brought close enough together for the attraction between the dissimilar charges to overcome the insulating properties of the air. The movement of electrons is evidenced by a rapid (10^{-8}sec)[1] discharge which exhibits light, heat, and sound (the spark and snap seen when you touch a doorknob after walking across a carpeted floor).

Static charges typically develop when dissimilar materials rub together; however, charges can also develop when charges slowly transfer from insulated conductors that are in intimate contact. In nature, the movement of rain droplets in clouds can generate tremendous (>1 million volts) potential voltages which, when discharged, evidence themselves as lightning. Conveyor belts, spinning drums, and materials applications devices utilized in industry can also develop significant static charges, which, if allowed to discharge, can cause havoc. In the hospital setting, static discharges have been observed emanating from operating tables, anesthesia machines, stools, beds, anesthesia circuits, and personnel.[1]

The potential energy of a given static charge is typically expressed in the voltage accumulated. The human body is a conductor and can become charged by movement such as rubbing or scuffing feet or by removal of clothing or other materials. The voltage accumulated may range from 5,000 – 8,000 volts[2] to as high as 18,000 volts,[3] though some investigators have projected a maximum potential of as much as 90,000 volts.[4] Hospital beds have been shown to accumulate voltages as high as 20,000 volts.[5] If the charged body then comes into close contact with a metal object or other suitable ground, the charge will dissipate, often in the form of a spark.

To reduce the potential for sparks, static charges must have pathways to flow through to a suitable ground before the charge can reach a sufficient voltage to allow a spark discharge. This can be accomplished by providing suitable conductive pathways (grounds). Conductive footwear, devices such as cables, chains, or elevated relative humidity levels (>50%) can provide an appropriate path to ground to dissipate the accumulated charge.

Static Sparks as Ignition Sources

Static sparks have been implicated as ignition sources in a wide range of environments.[1,5,7,12-13] In order for a fire to start, three factors must be present:

1. A flammable material
2. Oxygen
3. The flammable material must be heated above its flash temperature. In addition, the temperature of the flammable material must be kept above its flash

temperature either from some external source of heat or by its own heat of combustion or the fire will immediately go out.

For a static spark to start a fire, the spark must have enough heat energy to heat some of the material above its flash temperature. If the heat energy of the spark is below a critical level, the amount of material burned is too small to heat any further material above its flash point and the fire goes out immediately.[5]

One factor in determining the risk of ignition from a static spark is the flammability of the material into or through which the spark discharges. If fuel and oxygen molecules are to react, sufficient energy must be imparted to these molecules to result in a chemical transformation. The minimum energy that the molecules must possess to permit chemical interaction is the energy of activation. For many fuel-oxygen combinations at room temperature, the activation energy is much greater than the average energy of the constituent molecules. As the temperature of the materials increases, the amount of spark energy necessary to ignite the material decreases. The reaction rate increases with temperature until enough thermal energy is released to enable a combustion reaction (fire) to become self-sustaining or the reactants are consumed.[8]

Oxygen content and atmospheric pressure primarily influence the likelihood of ignition. For a given percentage of oxygen, the ignition temperature of a material decreases with increases in pressure. Conversely, for a given pressure, the ignition temperature decreases as oxygen content increases.[9] Once the combustion reaction becomes self-sustaining, the rate of combustion is largely influenced by the amount of oxygen available. Comparison of 100% oxygen and air at one atmosphere shows that there is a thousandfold increase in the ignitability of most substances and a fivefold increase in burning rate.[10]

Knowing the influence of oxygen concentration on ignition energy, the question still remains: Do static sparks impart enough energy to ignite fires in hyperbaric environments? In response, one must consider the electrical energy liberated during a static spark discharge and the flammable nature of the material studied.

The discharge energy of a static spark is a function of the voltage accumulated and the capacitance of the object holding the charge. Discharge energy can be calculated using the formula W=1/2 CV2 where W=charge energy in joules, C=capacitance of the charged body in farads and V=charge potential in volts.[1] For example, a hospital bed with a capacitance of 100 picofarads accumulates a charge of 20,000 volts which is discharged as a 0.7 inch spark. The maximum energy expected of the spark would be 0.02 joules (20 millijoules).[5]

Experimental Data – Normobaric Hyperoxic Environments

There is limited data available concerning the spark ignition energies of materials other than gases or vapors, particularly when one considers variations in oxygen concentrations. (Note: From an industrial standpoint, such data is vital not only for safety, but also for calculation spark energies necessary for ignition in devices such as internal combustion engines) For example, the minimum spark ignition energy (millijoules) for propane in air is 0.25 mj vs 0.001 mj in oxygen, whereas the minimum spark ignition energy for cotton is 800 mj under both conditions and dust is 10 mj in air.[9]

Plano and Guest[5,11]studied a variety of textile and plastic materials to determine ignitability under oxygen concentrations ranging from 21–100%. Their work was stimulated by concerns over static-caused fires in oxygen tents. Materials were subjected to single (20 and 800 mj) and repetitive (90 mj—roughly equivalent to an automotive ignition spark energy at 60 sparks/sec and 20 mj at 30 sparks/min) sparks. Materials studied were those typically found in or around oxygen tents and include cotton and dacron-cotton fabrics, wool, cotton balls, and vinyl plastic.

Plano's study showed that no single spark was able to ignite the clean tested materials. In the series utilizing a 90 mj spark at 60 sparks per second (30 second test = 1,800 sparks) in 21 and 100% oxygen, the investigators were able to cause ignition of clean materials only in the 100% oxygen environment. No ignitions were noted in the air environment studies, though Plano observed that although large holes were slowly burned in some of the samples, no open flames resulted. All materials studied in the 100% oxygen environment could be ignited after multiple sparks, but a single spark was insufficient to ignite any of the samples. The number of sparks required for ignition in the 100% oxygen environment ranged from 5 (wool and vinyl plastic) to 100 (cotton and dacron-cotton).[5] Note that discharge energies in this study were up to 4 ½ times greater than human body generated discharges.

A separate series by Guest studied the effect of petrolatum contamination of cotton and acetate fibers on flammability using lower spark energies (2.5 - 20 mj) at 30 sparks/minute. In this series, through clean cotton, there were 8 ignitions out of 2,800 sparks in a 100% oxygen atmosphere and no ignitions out of 4,000 sparks in a 64% oxygen environment. When the cotton was impregnated with 5.1% petrolatum by weight and placed in a 52% oxygen atmosphere, there were 15 ignitions out of 1,300 sparks. Guest also noted ignitions of contaminated (5.1% and 34% petrolatum) cotton fibers with spark energies of 2.5 mj at 5,000 volts in 64% oxygen environments and acetate fibers impregnated with 5.6% petrolatum exposed to 5 mj sparks in oxygen, though he did not specify the ratio of sparks to ignitions in the low voltage series nor the percentage of oxygen.[11] One should consider that the spark rate used in these studies was considerably more frequent than might be encountered in a clinical setting.

Experimental Data – Hyperbaric Environments

After reviewing the available literature, the author began to suspect that static sparks encountered in the course of human activity did not generate sufficient discharge energy to initiate ignition of the typical fuel sources found in hyperbaric chambers. To test this hypothesis, an experimental series was designed and a test cell constructed. A review of the experimental protocol and report results from the initial test series follow.

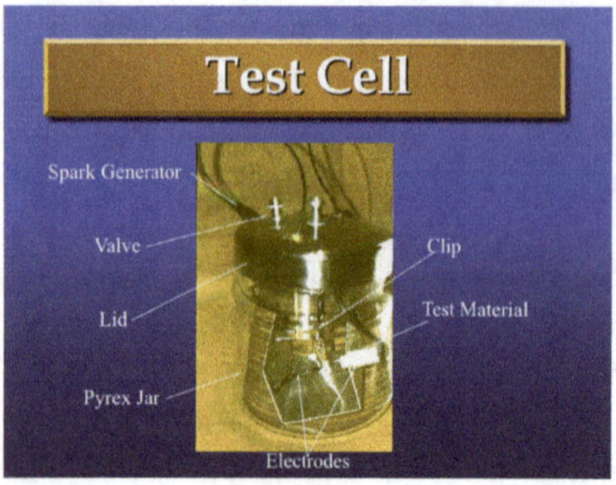

Figure 1.

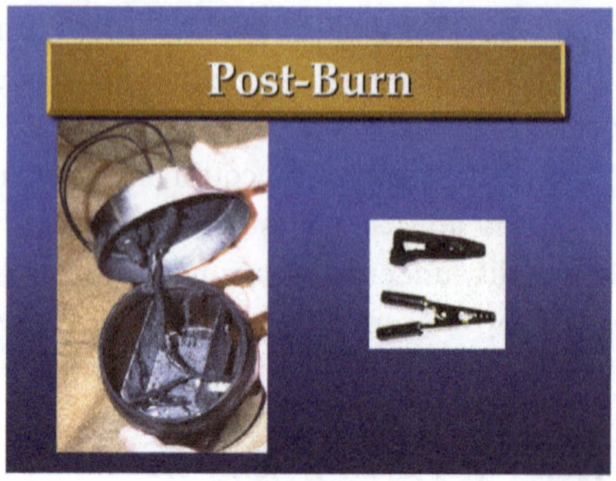

Figure 2.

In a multiplace hyperbaric chamber pressurized with air at 2.4 atmospheres absolute (ATA) (45 feet of sea water [fsw]), one-centimeter square samples of test materials were placed between electrodes in a test cell charged with 100% oxygen (pO_2: 1824 mmHg). Electrodes were connected to a piezoelectric spark generator that produces a 15,000-volt spark with discharge energy of 15–20 millijoules (upper limit of discharges from a human). Sparks were generated by manually activating the generator at a rate of 1 spark/second until either 30 sparks is reached or ignition occurs.

The test cell (Figure 1) consists of a 250 ml Pyrex container with a loose-fitting metal lid. Lead wires from the spark generator and a one-way valve for oxygen introduction are mounted in the lid. A U-shaped aluminum frame inside the cell contains electrodes with an adjustable spark gap and an arm/clip assembly to suspend test materials in the spark gap. The cell is charged with oxygen by attaching tubing from a flowmeter to the one-way valve and flowing oxygen at 5 liters/min for one minute.

Materials tested in the initial series were the following: 100% cotton (from pillowcase); 100% polyester (underwear); facial tissue; cotton gauze; Vaseline gauze; human hair; and alcohol prep pad. Initial difficulties with the spark generator forced us to reduce the spark gap from 6 mm to 3 mm in order to get reliable sparking at 2.4 ATA. (the initial test plan was to test at 3 ATA, but due to spark limitations resulting from increased atmospheric density, the pressure was reduced to 2.4 ATA). All materials with the exception of the alcohol prep pad were tested in a 100% oxygen environment and no ignitions were noted after 30 sparks.

The alcohol prep pad test was added after noting no ignitions of the other materials. During setup, the pad was placed in the cell per procedure, but prior to charging the cell with oxygen, the spark generator was actuated once to ensure proper function. Upon generation of the test spark, the alcohol ignited, igniting the pad material and a plastic grip retained on the alligator clip (Figure 2). Duration of the fire was approximately 20 seconds. The pad material and plastic grip were completely consumed. Insulation on the lead wires was charred, but there was no extension of the fire outside the test cell.

Risk, Energy, and Materials – Contributing Factors

Now we return to our original question. What is the risk of a static electrical spark igniting a fire in an enriched oxygen atmosphere? It depends upon two factors—the flammability of the material the spark contacts and the energy contained in the spark.

If one considers flammability as the amount of energy (in millijoules) required to ignite a given material, then the risk of a single static spark igniting a flammable gas or vapor is very high, even in an atmosphere with little or no oxygen enrichment (i.e., propane and dust in room air at 0.25 and 10 millijoules respectively or the alcohol prep pad noted above). Conversely, clean cotton fabric will not ignite even when exposed to multiple 800 mj sparks in a normobaric 100% oxygen environment.

Limitations on in-chamber fuel loads, i.e. linens, dressing materials, and other patient care items, are important, particularly in helping reduce charge accumulation as well as the intensity and duration of a chamber fire. However, they are unlikely to be the initial point of ignition. Though NFPA code allows the introduction of flammable materials that can produce vapors (alcohols) into multiplace chambers, such practices should only be conducted under the strictest of conditions. No flammable vapor producing materials should ever be introduced into a monoplace chamber pressurized with 100% oxygen.

The two fire cases described by Hughes and Bright[13] and the subsequent investigation provide the best case to support ignition by a static spark. Both cases involved fires in the bed assembly of an early monoplace chamber design that utilized a box section of the bed constructed of fiberglass. Fires occurred in the distal end of the bed following removal from the chamber at the conclusion of a treatment. Investigation revealed the presence of styrene and benzaldehyde in the box section and missing grounding clips on the bed assembly. Though initial studies of charge accumulation did not appear to produce static charges with enough energy to ignite these materials, the act of pulling the bed out of the chamber onto the trolley resulted in a substantial voltage increase, sufficient to produce a spark that could cause ignition. Subsequent to these incidents, the bed and grounding system was modified by the manufacturer, and modern monoplace chamber beds were constructed of conductive metal.

Spark energy levels accumulated by humans can exhibit a wide range of variance, but charges large enough to ignite gases can easily be generated through routine activities. A charge of sufficient energy to ignite a flammable gas may accumulate and discharge via physical contact without the person sensing the discharge, yet another individual may feel, see, and hear the spark discharge into a textile or other material without any ill effect.

Static Control

Measures to control static are primarily focused on prevention of charge accumulation. If adequate low-resistance paths to ground are provided, charges are dissipated to ground as fast as they are created.[2]

Attention has been given to installation of conductive flooring in static-critical areas. Efficacy of such flooring may be influenced by factors such as relative humidity, residual moisture remaining from cleaning, and the conductivity of footwear.[1]

Increasing the relative humidity (RH) in the environment can reduce charge development on personnel. Introducing water vapor into the work environment allows textile fibers to pick up a film of water, giving the material a slight degree of conductivity that provides conductive paths for dissipation of charges. Antistatic materials may be applied to fabrics. Organic antistatics (materials that attract moisture from the air and increase conductivity) may be applied to fabrics.

For environmental humidity to be effective, the relative humidity must be maintained at a minimum of 50% (below 30% RH, there is a rapid increase in static generation in all textiles), though to be really effective, RH must be >60%. A textile industry standard of 65% RH at 70°F practically eliminates static.

The conductivity of textiles can also be improved by blending fine (8 micron) metal or carbon fibers into yarn prior to weaving. The small size of the fibers renders them unnoticeable, yet impart conductivity to the cloth. Impregnated textiles may prove useful as static-control measures in environments in which high humidity is not practical or desirable.[2] These textiles are not readily available for clinical hyperbaric use.

In some instances, grounding straps, wires, mats, or related devices may be desirable to prevent charge accumulation and discharge. Personnel who assemble or repair sensitive electrical devices, such as computers (straps and mats) or work encountered when refueling aircraft (wires), commonly employ these devices in hazardous or potentially hazardous atmospheres.

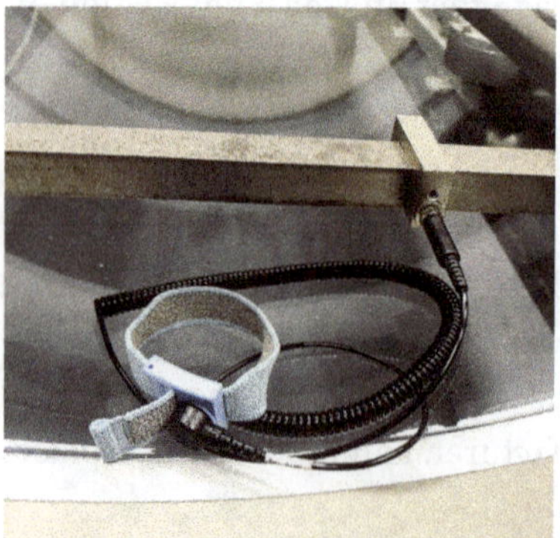

Figure 3.

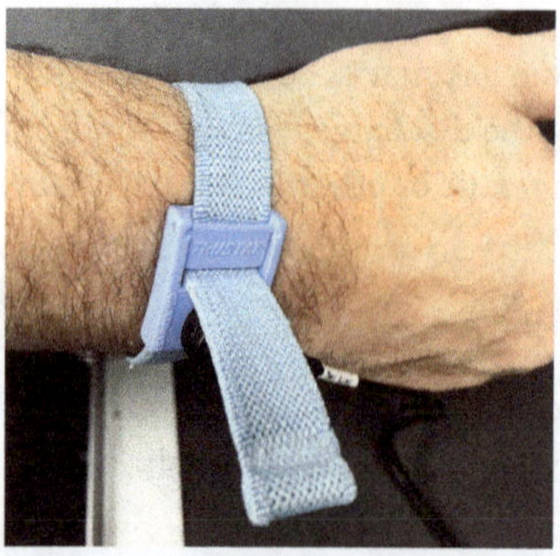

Figure 4.

There are specific grounding requirements for hyperbaric chambers and occupants defined in *NFPA 99*, Chapter 14. In addition to the chamber grounding requirements of section 2.7.4, section 3.1.5.3 (c) requires grounding of all hyperbaric chamber occupants when oxygen concentrations exceed 23.5%. The ground system must provide a high impedance conductive pathway in contact with the patient's skin.[6] Grounding straps used in hyperbaric chambers are usually attached to the patient's wrist or to an adhesive ECG-monitoring pad. Wrist straps may be made of metal (similar to a watchband) or carbon-impregnated plastic. The ground wire should contain a 1 megohm resistor to convert the wire from low to high impedence. A typical monoplace chamber patient grounding system is shown in Figures 3 and 4.

Certain industrial environments combining static generating devices with flammable materials (printing, tire making, etc.) may combine environmental controls and grounding devices with active static control. Active static control consists of insulated positive and negative needle electrodes charged to potentials of several kilovolts. Positive charges generated by the device are attracted to the target negative charge (which has the potential for discharge), neutralizing it, while the accumulated target charge tends to repel the generated negative charge which dissipates to ground.

Conclusions and Summary

Static charges and sparks are common. Spark energies produced by, or in the course of normal human activities, can reach levels high enough to ignite fires in some materials. If one considers sparks generated by the human body, the risk of ignition by static sparks in normal and enriched oxygen environments is predominately influenced by the nature of the material into which the spark discharges. Gases and vapors typically require extremely low energy levels compared to solid materials. Increases in oxygen concentrations lower ignition energy requirements in all materials.

The hyperbaric environment poses an increased fire hazard primarily due to elevated oxygen concentrations. Under typical hyperbaric conditions, it would be extremely rare to see the discharge of more than a single spark, particularly if the patient was properly grounded. The potential for a single static spark to ignite a fire in a hyperbaric chamber is very low, unless volatile vapors or gases are introduced into the chamber environment. All personnel working with hyperbaric chambers should be aware of the hazards posed by volatile materials and should be vigilant to prevent the introduction of those materials into the chamber.

Safely treating patients in enriched oxygen environments requires close attention to flammable materials control, maintaining oxygen levels as low as possible in the multiplace chamber, and controlling the development of hazardous static charge levels through grounding and humidity control. Increasing relative humidity and providing adequate conductive paths can significantly reduce the likelihood of charge and spark development.

References

1. Guest PG, Sikora VW, Lewis B. Static electricity in hospital operating suites: direct and related hazards and pertinent remedies. Bureau of Mines Bulletin 520; 1953.
2. Thompson R. Static electricity - causes and controls. *AORN Journal.* Oct 1970:81-83.
3. Marble A, MacDonald A, et.al. A measurement of the electrostatic voltage, capacitance and energy storage characteristics of the human body. *Phys Med Biol.* 1977;22(2);365-367.

4. Heron M. Capacitance and static electricity in the human body (letter). *Bhys Med Biol.* 1977;22(4);1208.
5. Plano R. Tests evaluate fire hazard of static sparks. *Modern Hospital.* Sept 1960;95:154.
6. National Fire Protection Association. (2018). NFPA 99: Health Care Facilities Code. Quincy, MA: NFPA; 2018.
7. Beach R. Preventing static electricity fires. *Chemical Engineer.* Dec 21, 1964;73-79.
8. Aerospace Medical. Proceedings of fire hazards and extinguishment conference. Aerospace Medical Division. Brooks AFB. Directorate of R&D, Aerospace Medical Division, Air Force Systems Command; May 23, 1967.
9. Workman W. Report to space station freedom. Hyperbaric Medicine and Safety Ad Hoc Committee; Jan 1989.
10. Denison D, et.al. Fire and hyperbaric oxygen. *Lancet.* Dec 24, 1966:1404.
11. Guest P. Oily fibers may increase oxygen tent fire hazard. *Modern Hospital.* 1965;104:180.
12. Sheffield PJ, et.al. Hypobaric and hyperbaric chamber fires. UHMS Gulf Coast Chapter Annual Scientific Meeting; March 1998.
13. Hughes JF, Bright AW. Electrostatic charge control on hyperbaric chambers - a case history. IEEE Transactions on Industry Application: Vol IA-16, No 6; Nov/Dec 1980.

CHAPTER 5.4
Hyperbaric System Fire Risk Assessments and Failure Analysis

Barry E. Newton, PhD, PE

Gaseous oxygen will vigorously support the combustion of most common engineering materials, especially at high pressure, and very few practical engineering materials available today are inert to ignition in oxygen systems. There is presently no known method to "turn off" the reactivity of oxygen under the common operational conditions within hyperbaric chambers and supply systems. Consequently, oxygen practitioners generally consider the hazard of ignition and sustained combustion as an inherent hazard, and the challenge to designers/operators is to cope with the hazard by reducing the risks to acceptable levels.

Risk reduction is usually aided by concepts associated with the familiar Fire Triangle (Figures 1 and 2). The Fire Triangle is a memory aid indicating that at least three necessary elements must come together simultaneously for a fire to occur: an oxidant, a fuel, and a source of ignition. If any of these elements are eliminated, the Fire Triangle is broken, as shown, and a fire cannot occur. Clearly, however, for most oxygen systems, neither the oxidant nor the fuel can be removed. Oxygen is inherent to the system and virtually all system materials can support combustion under certain conditions, even the metals, if the pressure is sufficiently high. Hence, in order to minimize the fire hazard, reducing the influence of active ignition mechanisms by design optimization and materials choices is the only practical approach. Unfortunately, the positive identification of potential ignition mechanisms and precise assessment of when they are, or will be, active is not possible with the current state-of-the-art. Hence, no valid "cookbook"

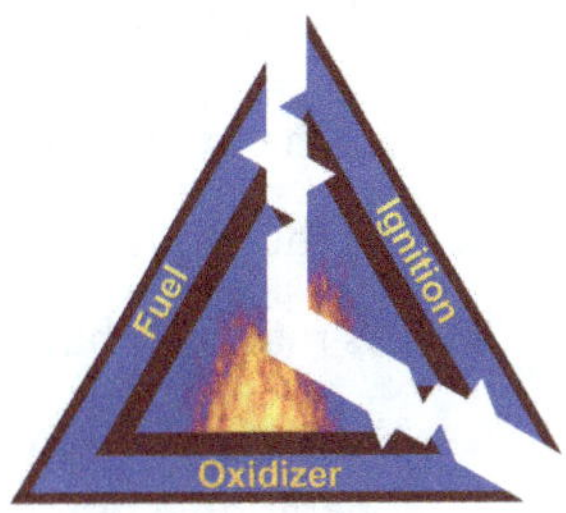

Figure 1. Broken Fire Triangle.

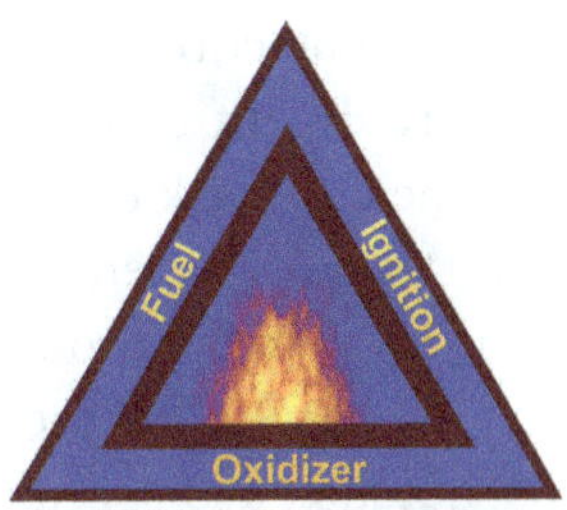

Figure 2. Completed Fire Triangle.

approach exists for either designing an oxygen system or eliminating all potential ignition sources. Most oxygen designs must tolerate an operational condition wherein all elements of the Fire Triangle are present.

Although ignition and combustion hazards are present in most oxygen systems, testing and experience have shown that designs having a low probability of ignition and a low consequence of ignition can be achieved. The combination of these two conditions provide a practical means to reduce the risks to acceptable levels. Low probability of ignition hinges on the reduction of active ignition mechanisms by design optimization and careful operational practices. Low consequence of ignition hinges on the utilization of materials having inherently superior oxygen compatibility based on standardized compatibility testing and good history of use.

With these concepts in view, oxygen practitioners have defined the oxygen compatibility of a material as the ability of a substance to coexist with both oxygen and a potential source of ignition within a predetermined level of risk.[1] An approach to evaluating the oxygen compatibility of a material and the risks of ignition of a component or system design is referred to as a hazard analysis or oxygen fire risk analysis and has been developed by the American Society for Testing and Materials (ASTM) Committee G04.[2] This chapter describes the hazards analysis approach as it has been implemented by personnel from WHA International, Inc.[3]

Understanding the Hazards

Part of the challenge of designing an oxygen system is in correctly assessing the fire hazards associated with the materials used in the design. Minimizing the fire risk requires careful assessment of the overall hazard level due to the design constraints. In general, the hazard level in oxygen systems increases with the following factors:

1. As the oxygen concentration is raised
2. As the oxygen partial pressure is raised
3. As materials having high heats of combustion are used
4. As the active ignition mechanisms become stronger due to system demands or operational practices, including the hazards of contamination.

Active ignition mechanisms exist in most oxygen systems. It has long been realized by oxygen practitioners that many ignition mechanisms can be reduced (i.e. influence minimized), but they cannot be eliminated. For instance, any time a cylinder valve is opened, the risk of ignition by adiabatic compression heating (defined later on) of downstream polymers is present. Testing has indicated that common coarse-threaded cylinder valves can produce pressurization times to full pressure of less than 200 msec (i.e. ~10,000 PSI/sec pressurization rate) in downstream components (depending on configuration and speed of opening). Testing also indicates that virtually all common polymers will ignite with these pressurization rates, at cylinder pressures, if the heat of compression cannot be rejected by the component design. Likewise, friction occurs at valve/regulator seats, mechanical impact occurs in moving parts, and particles entrain in gas flows and are accelerated at choke points. Less well-defined ignition mechanisms can also occur, including electrostatic discharge when flowing through electrically ungrounded components with particulates, during triboelectric charging of materials, electrical arcing in powered components, and plastic deformation of polymers (i.e. with flow-induced heating) due to throttling flow past a polymer (common hazard for some valve designs). These are some of the ignition mechanisms that are known to be active in oxygen systems. Their ability to initiate a sustained reaction depends on the level of hazard existing in the oxygen system design (i.e. oxygen concentration and partial pressure) and how much energy they release as compared to the minimum ignition energy required for the environmental conditions that exist.

In order to manage the hazard of an oxygen system design, bear in mind the interrelationship between the variables that work to increase risks. As was previously indicated, the oxygen concentration greatly influences the risk of ignition of all common engineering materials. The oxygen index (OI),[4] heat of combustion (ΔHc), and autogenous ignition temperature (AIT) for various common materials utilized in oxygen system design is described in this chapter. Additional data for selected materials is provided in Appendix A at the end of this chapter. These data apply to nonmetallic materials and provide a measure of their compatibility in gaseous oxygen. For instance, Figure 3[5] and Figure 4[6] show the variation in the OI and AIT for several common nonmetallic materials used in oxygen systems and Figure 5 depicts the increase in burning rate as concentration increases.

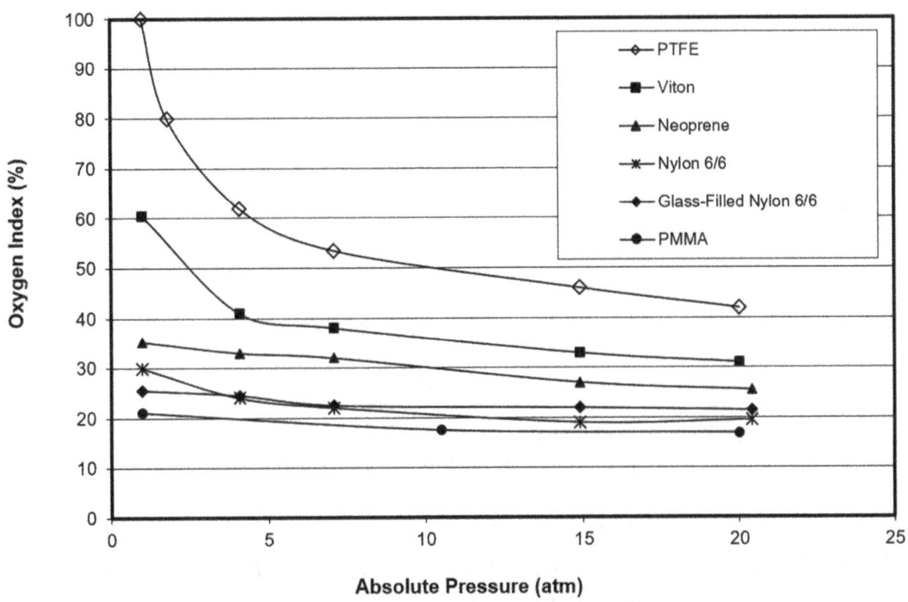

Figure 3. Variation of oxygen index with absolute pressure.

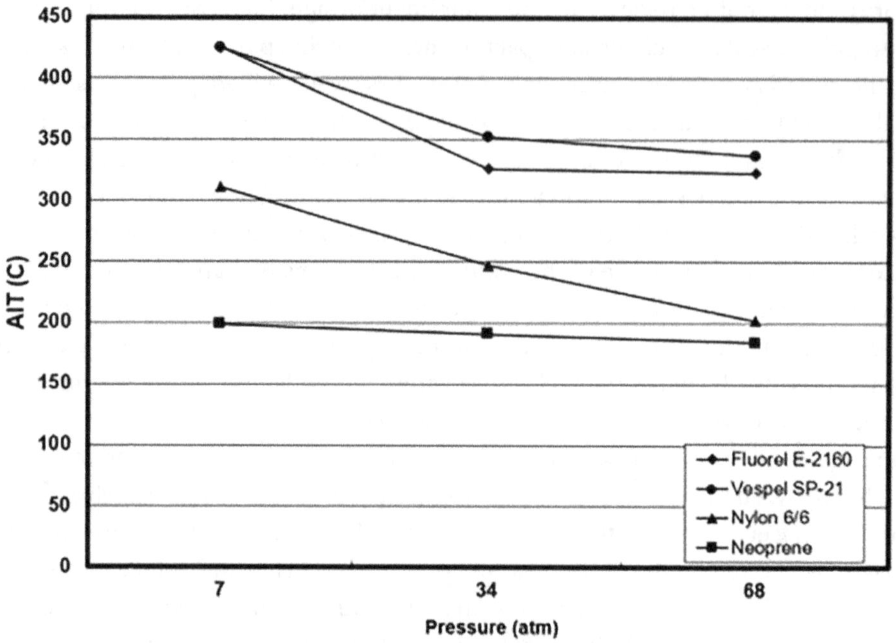

Figure 4. Variation of AIT with pressure.

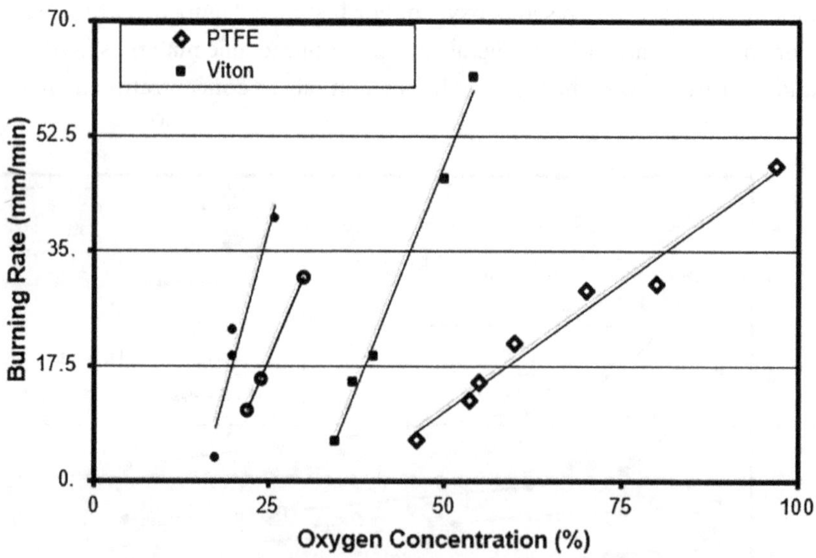

Figure 5. Variation of burning rate with oxygen concentration at 10.5 atm. (Nylon data taken between 1 and 7 atm.)

The OI provides an indication of whether a material is flammable (will support combustion) under the oxygen concentration that exists. For example, polyacetal plastics like Delrin® will support combustion at oxygen concentrations below standard 20.9% oxygen in air. However, PTFE plastics like Teflon® require near 100% oxygen before self-sustained combustion at one atmosphere pressure will take place. Therefore, materials having lower oxygen indices are generally considered more flammable. The OI and AIT of a material decreases by various amounts, depending on material, with increasing pressure as shown in Figure 3 and Figure 4. For a given pressure, the burn rate of a material generally increases as the oxygen concentration increases as shown in Figure 5. Experience has shown that materials with an OI above 55% are generally preferred. Materials with OIs below 20% are considered unsuitable for all but the mildest applications.[7]

The AIT of a material is the temperature at which liquids and solids will spontaneously ignite in a high-pressure oxygen-enriched environment without the application of an external ignition source (i.e. a spark or flame). The AIT of a material is generally measured by standard test methods such as ASTM G72 or BS 3N-100.[8] The AIT of a material generally decreases with pressure as shown in Figure 4.[9] For the vast majority of materials, pressure has its greatest effect at lower levels, below 7 MPa. For instance, the AIT of nylon decreases from 311° C to 226° C between 0.68 MPa and 3.4 MPa, but only decreases to 202° C between 3.4 MPa and 6.8 MPa. The autogenous ignition temperature test measures a highly behavioral property of a material, especially among polymers. Variations in the measured AIT of a material may be observed with variations in geometry, heating rate, flow rate, and temperature history of the material. As a result, *a safety margin of 100° C is generally recommended between the measured AIT (based on standard testing at a pressure above the use pressure) and the maximum foreseeable use temperature of the material.*[10]

The ΔHc of a material is the amount of energy released per unit mass when it is burned in oxygen and the combustion products are returned to essentially the original temperature. [11] This property is generally measured according to standard test methods such as ASTM D4809. This parameter provides a means for estimating the damage potential of a material once ignited and is an intrinsic property of the material. The total heat release, on a mass basis, is directly proportional to the heat of combustion. As the pressure increases, the total heat release stays the same if the reacted mass remains constant. While the heat release may stay the same as the pressure rises, the rate of combustion generally increases and therefore the damage potential increases due to the higher total energy density (i.e. heat released per unit time). General guidelines based on heat of combustion have been developed by oxygen practitioners as follows: 1) ΔHc < 2500 cal/grm are generally considered acceptable in most oxygen systems; 2) 2500 < ΔHc > 7500 cal/grm require scrutiny of ignition mechanisms; 3) ΔHc > 10,000 cal/grm are unsuitable except for the mildest applications.[12]

Fire Risk Assessments and Hazards Analyses

An approach to evaluating risks and developing an understanding of the inherent oxygen hazards requires balancing a design's inherent ignition risks against the compatibility of the materials used in the design as indicated by the OI, AIT, and ΔHc. A useful approach has been developed by ASTM committee G04 on the Compatibility and Sensitivity of Materials in Oxygen-Enriched Atmospheres. The G04 approach is specified by ASTM standards G88, *Designing Systems for Oxygen Service*, G63, *Evaluating Nonmetallic Materials for Oxygen Service*, and G94, *Evaluating Metals for Oxygen Service*. Figure 6 summarizes the WHA application of this approach to evaluating the risk of fire in an oxygen system design.

The hazard analysis is a formal process of evaluating an oxygen system design that focuses on known ignition mechanisms, materials choices, and good operating practices. As depicted in Figure 6, the process starts with defining the reasonably foreseeable operating conditions (i.e. temperature, pressure, etc.) to determine the severity of the design environment. Experience indicates that the strength of the active ignition mechanisms is directly proportional to the severity of the environment. For instance, as the design pressure is raised, the AIT of nonmetallic materials generally decreases while the temperature achieved by compression heating increases, leading to higher ignition risk. These trends lead to higher probabilities of ignition as pressure is increased.

Once the severity of the environment is defined, the components and materials of construction are evaluated for flammability based on the results of standardized tests. The pressure thresholds for sustained combustion of metals is generally evaluated based on ASTM G 94.[13] The concentration required for sustained combustion of nonmetals is generally evaluated based on the OI (ASTM D 2863). The materials that are flammable are identified at this stage of the analysis. The ignition probabilities for these materials are then ranked based on the perceived severity of the known ignition mechanisms (i.e. particle impact, adiabatic compression, friction, etc. See definitions in the section Fire Risk Assessments and Hazards Analyses – Ignition Probability Ratings.) Flammability data for these materials are then collected to evaluate the relative compatibility as compared to materials having a good history of use. The fire damage potential (reaction effect), should the material ignite, is evaluated based on the mass of each material and its ΔHc.

Risk management by the hazard analysis process described seeks to produce a design that is tolerant of the common ignition mechanisms. As shown in Figure 6, after reviewing the operating conditions and flammability of the materials, the design is evaluated based on the influence of various known ignition mechanisms.

In a hazard analysis, the potential for ignition is subjectively ranked, based on experience and applicable test data. Each ignition mechanism that is potentially active is evaluated individually for each component/material in the system design. The process just described, along with the detailed information that can be derived, is illustrated in the example provided in Table 1. While the ignition and reaction effect rankings are subjective, if the process is carefully followed, experience indicates that the highest components or areas of risk are usually identified and steps to mitigate these risks can be applied to the design. The process shown in Figure 6 and Table 1 is described as follows:

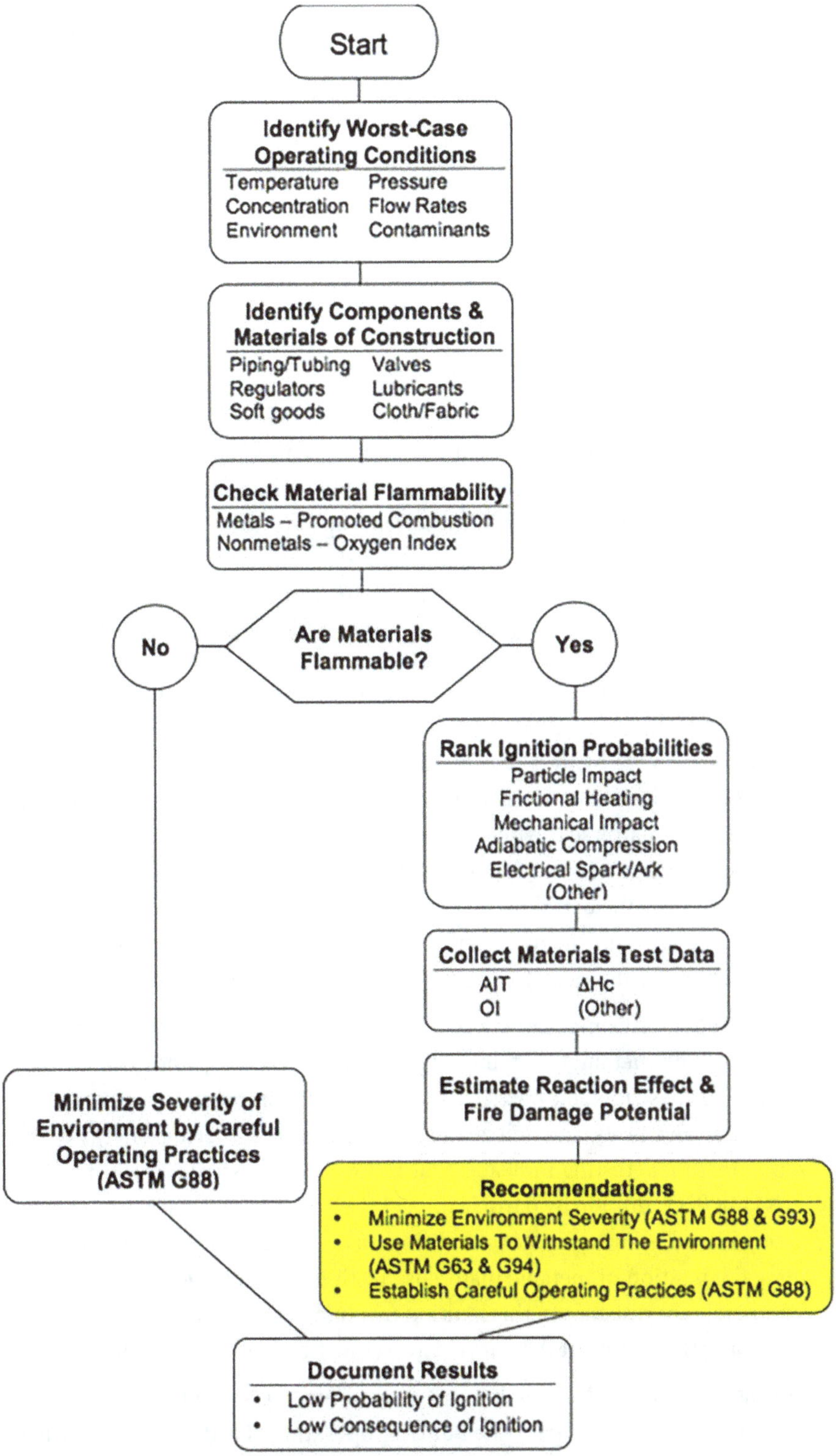

Figure 6. Flowchart illustrating ASTM hazards analysis process.

Fire Risk Assessments and Hazards Analyses – Ignition Probability Ratings

After defining the worst-case operating conditions, the flammability of each material is evaluated from the available compatibility data previously. Each component having situationally flammable[14] materials is ranked as to its exposure to ignition energy on a scale ranging from 0 to 4. These probability-ranking categories are defined as follows:

0 = Almost Impossible

1 = Remotely Possible

2 = Possible

3 = Probable

4 = Highly Probable

Both the identification and risk of an ignition mechanism is best evaluated by experience and application of characteristic elements that have been developed for each ignition mechanism.[15] However, while these rankings are subjective, they are useful in identifying the most active ignition mechanisms and combinations of bad circumstances.

The following ignition mechanisms have demonstrated their presence in many oxygen systems and should be understood and considered during any hazard analysis:

- Adiabatic compression: This mechanism represents the potential for ignition from rapid compression of gases within the system. Rapid compression of gases is usually associated with a rise in gas temperature, potentially beyond a material's AIT, and exhibits itself most commonly at a flow stagnation point (such as a valve/regulator seat while subjected to pressurization transients or a closed valve downstream of another valve that can be rapidly opened). This ignition mechanism is considered by many oxygen practitioners to be the most efficient at kindling ignition of nonmetallic materials. Testing indicates, however, that metals are not vulnerable to direct ignition by this mechanism.
- Particle impact: This mechanism represents the potential for ignition of small particles (usually metallic) entrained in the gas flow causing the ignition of system materials. These metallic particles may ignite upon impacting another solid target, such as a valve body, and will efficiently transfer their thermal energy to the rigid target material. Testing indicates that if flow velocities are greater than about 45 m/s (148 ft/s), ignition by particle impact is plausible.[16-17] This ignition mechanism is considered by many oxygen practitioners to be the most efficient at directly kindling the ignition of metallic materials. Testing indicates, however, that most soft nonmetals are resistant to this ignition mechanism since they are more capable of absorbing the energy of the particle impact without producing particle ignition.
- Mechanical impact: This mechanism represents the potential for ignition from materials that strike each other during operation. Heat is generated from the transfer of kinetic energy to strain energy when the momentum of one mass is

Table 1. Example of Hyperbaric System Hazard Analysis Worksheet (Analysis Footnotes at Bottom)

Component	Material	Max Use Conditions (Temp, oC)	(Press, MPa)	F/NF	PI	AC	FH	MI	ARC (ESD)	O	PC	RE	AIT (oC)	OI/PC (%, MPa)	ΔHc (cal/grm)
Supply System															
Valve Body	Brass	50	13.8	NF[1]									N/A	>68.9 MPa	825
Valve Seat	Nylon	50	13.8	F	0	0	2	0	0[2]	2[3]	1	C	178	30%	7900
Manifold	Brass	50	13.8	NF[1]									N/A	>68.9 MPa	825
Manifold Valve 1															
Body	Brass	50	13.8	NF[1]									N/A	>68.9 MPa	825
Seat	Nylon	50	13.8	F	0	3[4]	1	0	0	2	2[5]	C	178	30%	7900
Seals	Silicone	50	13.8	F	0	1	0	0	0	1[6]	1	B	270	33%	3700
Regulator 1															
Body	Brass	50	13.8	NF[1]									N/A	>68.9 MPa	825
Seat	Viton	50	13.8	F	0	3	1	2	0	2[7]	4[8]	B	297	56%	3350
Spring	Steel	50	13.8	F	3	0[9]	1	0	0	0	3[10]	C	N/A	0.17 MPa	1800
Diaphragm	Neoprene	50	1	F	0	0	1	1	1	0	4[11]	C	200	32%	6523
Manifold Piping	Brass	50	1	NF[1]	0	0	0	0	0	0	0	A	N/A	>68.9 MPa	825
Chamber															
Bedding	Cotton and Urethane Foam	20	0.2	F F	0	0	0	0	3[12]	3[13]	3	D	325 250	<21% 25%	4000 6500
Pt. Clothing	Polyester	20	0.2	F	0	0	0	0	3	3	3	D	210	41%	4300

F/NF	Flammable or Nonflammable (under service conditions)	ARC/ESD	Arc/Spark or Electrostatic Discharge (ESD)
PI	Particle Impact	O	Other (Dynamic Chatter, Flow-Induced Heating, or Other)
AC	Adiabatic Compression (Compression Heating)	PC	Promoted Combustion (or Promoted Burning)
FH	Frictional Heating (Mechanical Rubbing/Gouging)	RE	Reaction Effect
MI	Mechanical Impact	AIT	Autogenous Ignition Temperature
OI/PC	Oxygen Index (Nonmetals); Promoted Combustion (Metals)	ΔHc	Heat of Combustion

1 Standard testing indicates that metallic materials like brass will not sustain combustion in bulk configurations below 68.9 MPa.

2 Electrical discharge is minimized for system components that are electrically grounded or bonded.

3 Flow-induced heating potential is increased for weeping/seeping flow and for valves with nonmetallic seats used in throttling conditions.

4 Calculations indicate that theoretical temperatures of 1042°C (ideal gas assumption) and 879°C (real gas assumption) can be achieved by compression heating downstream of fast-opening valves.

5 Ignition of supply system contaminants or upstream components are sufficient to kindle downstream nonmetallic materials.

6 Ignition of the seals from shaving/cutting by mechanical interference during assembly (sharp edges, etc.) is a remote possibility. Shaving/cutting of mold surfaces on seals may lead to higher ignition probability at the seal and contamination in downstream components.

7 Vulnerable to ignition from simultaneous application of several ignition mechanisms (e.g., adiabatic compression, friction, and impact from seat/poppet stroke), which increases ignition energy.

8 Promoted combustion of the regulator seat is probable for ignition of an upstream manifold valve seat or an upstream contaminant.

9 Adiabatic compression is efficient for igniting nonmetallic materials, but testing has not led to direct ignition of metals by this mechanism.

10 Promoted combustion of this component is probable for ignition of an upstream contaminant or component. Testing indicates that spring steel will support combustion above 2 atmospheres oxygen pressure and stainless steels (300 series) may support combustion above 14 atmospheres, depending on thickness.

11 Regulator burnout from kindling of contaminant/seat-to-spring-to-diaphragm may occur for regulator seat/contaminant ignition by any heating mechanism.

12 Human body electrostatic charging develops readily under low-humidity conditions and movement over certain materials. Testing indicates that ignition can develop by ESD discharge if oxygen pressures/concentrations are elevated and flammable fabrics are in the discharge path if a patient is not bonded/grounded properly.

13 Heating devices normally not authorized in chambers under elevated oxygen pressures/concentrations may self-ignite or cause ignition of flammable fabrics, skin creams, or flammable wipes.

transferred to another. This mechanism is unlike particle impact in that the two striking masses are large and intended to contact each other during service (i.e., valve seat, poppet, etc.). Experience indicates that this mechanism may be active if the target is gouged/deformed/fractured, exposing fresh metal to oxidation.

- Elevated temperature: Elevated temperature represents the potential for ignition due to extreme exposure temperatures usually generated from heating components or locked rotors on motorized components. The thermal capacity of the various components and their heat transfer characteristics were also evaluated with this mechanism to estimate the ability of a material to reach its ignition temperature. High environmental temperatures increase the risk of all ignition mechanisms since the margin to the AIT of a material is reduced.
- Frictional heating: This mechanism represents the potential for ignition due to the rubbing of two solid surfaces together. Heat is generated by this mechanism due to frictional rubbing (mechanical interaction) and the exothermic re-oxidation of a material after removal of any protective surface oxides.
- Galling: This mechanism represents the potential for extreme surface disruption and sudden unoxidized metal exposure due to abrasive interaction (or chemical adherence of surfaces) between two metallic components (usually threaded fasteners). Heat is generated through strain energy and re-oxidation mechanisms at the affected surface. Two ignition mechanisms closely related to galling are the following:
  - *Mechanical fracture:* This mechanism represents the potential for ignition due to the sudden release of strain energy when a mechanical failure/fracture occurs.
  - *Fresh metal exposure:* This mechanism represents the potential for ignition due to the exothermic re-oxidation of unoxidized metal surfaces that were produced by any abrasive interaction or mechanical failure of metal parts.
- Electrical arc/spark: This mechanism includes electrical arcing ignition from a powered electrical source. This mechanism also includes the likelihood of electrostatic discharge principally due to triboelectric charging.
  - *Electrostatic discharge (esd):* Electrostatic discharge is usually a low energy arc/spark caused by the flow of electricity between two objects that are at different charge potentials. Charging may occur due to frictional contact, rubbing, between objects (triboelectric charging), or electrostatic induction (redistribution of charges due to nearby energy). When differently charged objects are brought together and the difference in charge is sufficiently high, a dielectric breakdown of the air separating the objects may occur, often creating a visible spark (ESD). If the ESD spark has sufficient energy, ignition of flammable materials exposed to the spark may occur.

› *Triboelectric charging:* Triboelectric charging may develop when materials interact (i.e., rub across one another). A common illustration of a materials vulnerability to triboelectric charging is shown in Figure 7. The farther two materials are apart on the "triboelectric series", the more readily they will develop charge from interaction/rubbing.

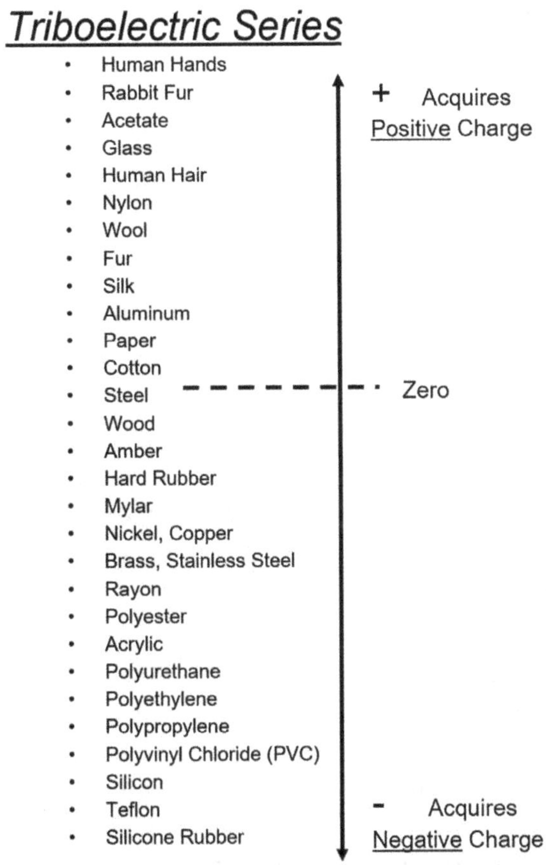

Figure 7. Triboelectric series for various materials (Desco Industries, Inc.).

- Promoted combustion: This mechanism represents the potential for ignition due to exposure to a material already ignited. This mechanism assumes that an ignition has already occurred and considers the vulnerability of the material in question to ignite and sustain combustion due to exposure to another kindling source. "Kindling chain" ignition[18] is a key concept and usually begins as a small event that grows into a fire through a kindling chain sequence. A small amount of energy ignites a material having a low ignition temperature or a particle with a large surface area and small mass. Once ignited, the material gives off enough heat to ignite the bulky surrounding materials that have higher ignition temperatures and generate more heat until the process is self-sustaining. This mechanism can be exacerbated by flow of oxygen across the ignition/burning site, much like the "bellows" effect on a forge.

- **Chemical reaction:** This mechanism represents the potential for chemical reactions that would lead to mechanical failure or heat generation such that an ignition could occur. For instance, some of the chemical reactions known to produce potential ignitions or mechanical failures are hydrocarbon/oxygen exothermicity, halocarbon/aluminum reactions leading to mechanical fracture due to chlorine-aluminum reactivity, and formation of shock sensitive gels when liquid oxygen is exposed to hydrocarbons.
- **Other:** This is a catch-all category to represent the potential for ignition due to other ignition mechanisms that experience indicates could be present. For instance, dynamic flow in gaseous systems often results in instability of moving components causing rapid cyclical striking of one solid object against another. This mechanism is analogous to mechanical impact but is different in that it is a rapid cyclical event not intended to occur. Valve and regulator designers commonly refer to this mechanism as dynamic chatter. This event can readily cause ignition and can be active in spring-balanced components such as regulators and high capacity relief valves. Another example is flow-induced heating, which causes heating as gas flow impinges directly on a polymeric material, especially under throttling flow, such that the flow work causes slight deformation (microchannels and/or finely divided surfaces) in the material.

Ignition Ranking Summary

Table 1 shows that for the example system being considered, adiabatic compression in manifold valve(s) downstream of the main supply developed a concerning ignition risk (probable) for conditions where the upstream supply isolation valve was opened rapidly. Frequently, an ignition risk of probable (3) or greater requires a mitigation action. Therefore, a mitigation step would be suggested to ensure that personnel are trained to open valves slowly or that slow-opening valves are installed to avoid this ignition risk and written procedures be implemented. The ignition level that requires mitigation is usually established by company management.

For the components considered, the system regulator was highlighted as having a high number of flammable materials, both metals and nonmetals, and as being vulnerable to several ignition mechanisms including particle impact, adiabatic compression, and promoted burning from contaminants or upstream components. Therefore, ignition within the regulator could lead to higher reaction effects. Regulators are known to operate with a highly dynamic internal flow, causing several ignition mechanisms to be active. Regulator burnout (i.e. discharge of fire from the regulator bonnet) is a common reaction effect for regulators that include flammable metals in close proximity to flammable nonmetals, such as a large diaphragm. Several mitigation steps would be suggested, such as installation of a nonflammable particle filter upstream of the regulator to reduce particle migration and hinder contaminant promoted ignition as well as positioning the regulator so personnel are protected from a possible burnout event.

Finally, the ignition analysis revealed that ignition energy within a hyperbaric chamber was generally low, except for ESD from triboelectric charging and the potential presence of heating devices that are normally prohibited from a chamber environment. The analysis also recognized that a high number of flammable materials would be expected to also burn if ignition were to occur, leading to the catastrophic "D" reaction effect. This assessment relates to chamber installations that are not complicated by extenuating circumstances, such as self-heating materials or reactive chemicals. The analysis also recognizes that highly flammable materials such as alcohol wipes and some flammable skin creams be minimized or avoided.

ESD conditions worsen under hyperbaric conditions, complicated by the human body being a good charge accumulator. ESD ignition potential has been shown to increase as oxygen pressure increases, while simultaneously, the ignition energy for flammable nonmetallic materials, such as cotton, decrease. Figure 8 illustrates this potential in some recent testing by WHA and is compared to historical testing by NASA. While the data is not intended to represent absolute or minimum energies, the pressure trends indicated above are evident. Therefore, ESD ignition potential and risk both increase in a hyperbaric chamber environment. ESD is effectively mitigated by proper grounding/bonding of chamber components and occupants as required by international standards and control of materials allowed inside the chamber. This guidance effectively mitigates against ESD and should be followed.

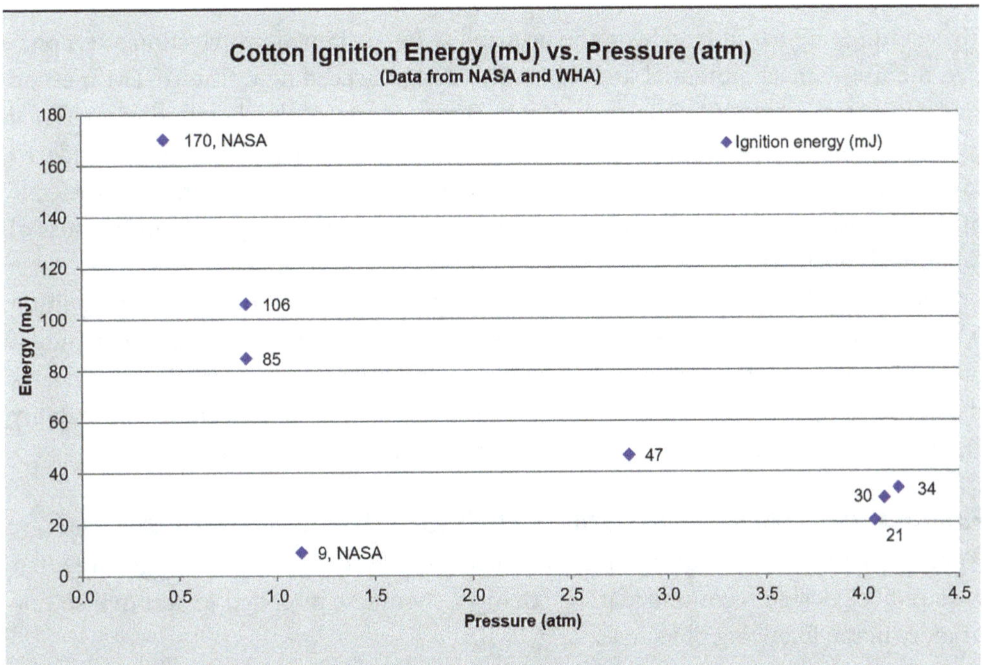

Figure 8. Ignition energy testing by electrostatic discharge on cotton by NASA and WHA.

Fire Risk Assessments and Hazards Analyses – Reaction Effect Ratings

The reaction effect rating shown in Table 1 represents an assessment of the probable result of ignition for the materials that were considered flammable in the ignition assessment. In order to estimate the probable reaction effect, the energy that a material and/or component can release (heat of combustion and material mass) under the exposure conditions, and the potential of that energy release to involve other adjacent materials or components, is ranked. The A to D rankings that are used to develop reaction effect ratings are defined as follows:

A. **This rating represents a NEGLIGIBLE effect.** For the effect of an ignition to be considered negligible, ignition probabilities and propagation potential must be minimal.

B. **This rating represents a MARGINAL effect.** For the effect of an ignition to be considered marginal, ignition probabilities must be possible or less and the configuration must not favor propagation. A configuration not favoring propagation would be one in which the polymers are of low mass, pressure conditions are low, oxygen concentration is low, and/or thermal mass of metallics is high.

C. **This rating represents a CRITICAL effect.** For the effect of an ignition to be considered critical, sustained propagation must be considered probable. Propagation is considered probable if polymers are felt to be of sufficient mass to kindle the adjacent metallics or if the expected combustion are felt to produce a sustained flame.

D. **This rating represents a CATASTROPHIC effect.** For the effect of ignition to be considered catastrophic, sustained propagation that involves the risk of death or multiple injury and/or heavy loss of infrastructure occurs.

These ratings are based largely on the probability for sustained propagation to emphasize the fire-damage potential and adjust the design accordingly. The ASTM method (see *ASTM G 63* and/or *G 94*) uses a slightly different approach wherein the functional capability, system mission objectives, and potential injury potential are also considered in evaluating the reaction effect. This procedure may be preferred if intimate knowledge of the operation is obtained since it emphasizes the potential for injury and/or loss of functional capability.

Reaction effect ratings less than critical are preferred, if the probability of ignition is low, possible, or less. While the action taken as a result of these ratings is dependent on the degree of risk that can be tolerated by the design objectives, experience indicates that an acceptable level of risk is usually developed for a combined ignition probability and reaction effect rating of possible and marginal or less, respectively.

Fire Risk Assessments and Hazards Analyses – Mitigating Hazards

After evaluating the ignition and reaction effect potential of a design, changes are often required. All design recommendations/changes should be intended to accomplish one or more of the following objectives:

- **Minimize** the severity of the environment by reducing the influence of active ignition mechanisms.
- **Maximize** the best materials that can withstand the environment based on applicable test data and good history of use.
- **Utilize** proven design practices to avoid known ignition mechanisms and combinations of bad circumstances.

Minimizing the Severity of the Environment

This principle entails actions that reduce the magnitude of the known ignition mechanisms or other variables that are known to add to the consequence of fires. This step focuses on ignition mechanisms from the standpoint of the environment, the operating conditions, and the maintenance practices. The design parameters generally affected in this step are usually environmental in nature (i.e. lowering pressure/temperature to the lowest practical levels, limiting the pressurization rates and flow rates by design, etc.) but also include maintenance issues such as cleaning. In fact, scrupulous cleaning prior to the initial installation, and then maintaining the cleanliness of a system are often the most important factors in reducing the risk of fire in the system.[19-20]

Within any system the design environmental factors are key parameters that can increase the overall hazard and make ignition more likely. The influence of several important environmental parameters is discussed in *ASTM Standard G 128.*[21]

These parameters and their influence on system severity are summarized as follows:

- **Role of oxygen concentration:** As oxygen concentration increases, the hazards of ignition and fire intensity increase as more materials become flammable (i.e. the OI) and more oxygen is available for combustion. Testing has indicated that the type of diluent gas can have a significant effect on the overall hazard. Inert diluents of large molecular weight are most effective at reducing the hazard. In a few cases, even small amounts of diluents (tenths of a percent) can reduce the flammability of some materials.[22]
- **Role of pressure:** As pressure increases, so do the hazards of ignition and fire intensity. Pressure increases the density of the gas and has the same effect as increasing the oxygen concentration. More oxygen is available to the fuel, so materials are relatively more flammable and burn at a faster rate. Pressure also increases the gas flow velocity at restrictions such as valves, regulators, and tubing intersections, which increase particle impact[23] and compression heating hazards.

  In general, <u>as pressure increases</u>:

  - The AIT of a material decreases.
  - The OI of a material decreases.

- The ΔHc of a material stays the same but the burning rate increases rendering a combustion event more capable of promoting surrounding materials.
- The hazards of ignition by adiabatic compression heating increase.
- Particle impact ignition probability increases as flow velocity increases and metals become flammable.
- Fire damage potential increases due to higher combustion intensity and greater energy release upon compromise of the pressure containment.

As pressure increases, progressively stringent oxygen service practices should be considered, in the following order:

- *Cleaning:* When oxygen concentration and pressures are low, the ignition hazard is also low, and cleaning may be the primary control necessary. (Accepted definitions of low or high concentration and pressure have not been agreed upon within the industry; however, testing indicates that concentrations above air [20.9% O_2] and pressures above ambient increase oxygen ignition hazards of most materials including contaminants.)
- *Compatible lubricants:* As oxygen concentration and pressure increase, careful cleaning is required, and more compatible lubricants should be selected.
- *Compatible polymers/nonmetals:* At higher pressures, careful cleaning, selection of lubricants, and selection of more compatible nonmetals is important.
- *Compatible metals:* At levels of greatest severity (generally at the highest pressures), metals must also be selected based on their flammability, in addition to all the preceding measures.

- **Role of temperature:** Common use temperatures have little effect on the intensity of combustion and the resulting fire damage. However, as the environmental temperature increases, the likelihood of ignition increases because less energy must be added to reach the ignition temperature of a material. High temperatures can accelerate the aging of polymers and reduce their compatibility with oxygen.
- **Role of time and aging:** Fires sometimes occur the first time oxygen is introduced into a system. However, more often, fires occur in equipment that has been used for many years. Experience indicates that the longer a system is in use, the more likely a fire event may be if conditions change or if proper maintenance is not performed. In these systems, a fire may occur only if a special or additional factor increases the hazard (for example, a rub in a machinery item or a hydrocarbon contaminant introduced). The event can occur early in the life cycle but, more likely, will occur late in the life cycle after the attention to the system hazards are relaxed, especially if complacency about the inherent oxygen fire hazard develops.

  Experience indicates that material compatibility is the key to the consistent limitation of fire hazards.[24] Aging increases the fire risk due to the degradation of polymers and the accumulation of contaminant debris. As systems get older, polymers age and may become brittle or porous and begin to slough off debris from their surfaces. This both creates contaminant debris migration in the system and provides a surface morphology more favorable to ignition. The quantity of contaminants generally increases over time, increasing the risk of kindling chain ignition. Mechanical failures become more likely, thereby providing additional ignition opportunities.

- **Role of phase:** Liquid oxygen at standard pressure exists at –183° C, and low temperatures generally result in a decreased likelihood of ignition. However, liquid oxygen is virtually 100% pure oxygen (only trace amounts of atmospheric contaminants). The high purity liquid phase introduces two new hazards that greatly increase the risk. First, the density of liquid oxygen is hundreds of times (~860 times ambient) greater than that of the gas, which results in more oxygen available to support combustion than does 100% oxygen in the gas phase at high pressure. Combustion generates enormous pressures as the liquid changes to a gas. Experience has also shown that combustion intensity can be far more intense. Liquid oxygen with carbon or hydrocarbon particles or metal fines, which are high-surface area flammable materials, has been considered for use as a high explosive due to the increased combustion intensity. For this reason, liquid oxygen with finely divided porous particles represents an exceptionally severe explosion hazard. Second, if liquid oxygen is mixed with hydrocarbons, such as for an inadvertent spill onto asphalt, the resulting mixture can form a shock-sensitive explosive gel, which can be present for some time after the initial spill.
- **Role of velocity:** Oxygen velocity increases in flowing systems lead to higher particle velocities and an increased risk of ignition by particle impact. For hazard assessments, the particle velocity is usually considered to be at or near the gas velocity. Velocity is a hazard that is controlled primarily by system design, including metals that tolerate particle impact (i.e., copper/nickel alloys) and the use of appropriate filtration to limit particulate migration in a system. Line sizes should be selected to minimize system gas velocities. Abrupt size changes should be avoided, and the location of particle impingement points can be controlled by system design to minimize the risks associated with particle impact. The Compressed Gas Association[25] recommends that velocities should be limited wherever possible and means should be provided to increase the resistance to ignition (by materials choices) at locations where high velocity may exist.

Maximizing the Use of Compatible Materials

This principle involves selecting materials that will both accommodate the design objectives and are fire resistant. Fire prevention in oxygen-enriched systems requires a material focus since the three essential elements for a fire cannot be eliminated, as discussed previously. In addition to minimizing the severity of the environment, fire prevention in oxygen systems also requires a material focus to reduce the risk to a tolerable level. Combustible materials (such as clothing, insulation, bedding, skin creams, flammable wipes, etc.) inside chambers cannot be eliminated, but their selection can be controlled.

Similarly, ignition sources in the system must be identified and controlled. A material's fire resistance is typically measured by its ability to resist ignition, resist propagation when ignited, and contribute to limiting the damage potential of an event, as follows:

- Materials that resist ignition are typically those that have high ignition temperatures, high impact ignition thresholds, and require high oxygen concentrations and/or pressures to support sustained combustion.
- Materials that resist propagation are those that tend to self-extinguish when ignited under the expected service conditions.
- Materials that reduce the damage potential are those that have limited heat release potential during combustion (i.e., low ΔHc).

The design objectives, which dictate pressure, temperature, flow, and oxygen concentration, must often be weighed against the known fire resistance of the available materials. Hence, the choice of a suitable material is based on weighing the available materials against their measured behavior in specific oxygen compatibility tests. Standard tests to measure the behavior of materials in oxygen, such as those indicated in Table 1, have been developed and are utilized to evaluate the performance of one material against another.

Utilizing Proven Design Practices

This principle uses known good practices to reduce/avoid known ignition mechanisms and combinations of bad circumstances and is often the basis of the mitigation recommendations developed in a hazard assessment. *ASTM Standard G88* provides several design considerations that have been proven by experience and are worth consideration. The hazards analysis process provides a tool for identification of ignition mechanisms that may be active and assessing whether they are operative for the applicable service conditions. The good practices provided in *ASTM Standard G88* help to reduce a system's severity and its active ignition mechanisms. These principles are not considered absolutes in the sense that they must always be followed, but experience has shown that system safety is improved as more good practices are implemented. Generally, a successful oxygen design will incorporate as many of the following steps and practices described below as possible:

- **Avoid unnecessarily elevated pressures:** Where possible, reduce the pressure near the supply point. Since pressure aggravates the ignition probabilities of virtually all mechanisms, the use of high pressures, where low pressures can serve equally well, increases the risk of fire.

- **Avoid sumps, dead ends, and cavities:** This helps ensure cleanliness is maintained as the oxygen system is operated. Sumps, dead ends, and cavities produce collection points for contamination and are particularly difficult to clean and maintain clean. Contamination that is not removed from an oxygen system or that is introduced and collected during its service life can be easily ignited and will serve to promote fires in other materials.
- **Use filters to limit gas-entrained particulate:** Filters are typically recommended ahead of components in which the gas velocity cannot be controlled (i.e. valve seats or orifices) and after components that have moving parts that can produce particulate during operation. Filter media are generally of sintered bronze or nickel-copper mesh because of their superior ignition properties of these metals.
- **Avoid particle impact and limit gas velocities:** Where filters are intended to limit particles, this principle is intended to reduce locations of unduly high velocities and potential particle-impact-impingement points. Absolute removal of particulate is seldom realistic; hence the severity of particle collisions can be reduced by limiting gas velocities and sharp transitions where high velocity gas flow changes direction. Ninety-degree bends, elbows, drill points and other gas flow stagnation points are vulnerable to impingement of gas-entrained and collected particulate.
- **Limit pressurization rates:** This reduces the effect of compression heating. Design limiting of pressurization rates is best addressed by using slow opening valves and/or incorporating restrictive orifices or capillary tube flow devices.
- **Avoid impingement of gas flow on polymers:** When gas flow impinges directly on polymers, flow-induced heating is rendered more severe. While this mechanism is weak, as compared to compression heating, it has been implicated in ignition events. Impingement of flow on polymers may also lead to erosion and production of contaminants. Since polymers are usually the most readily ignited elements in the kindling chain, their minimal use and protection are keys to designs that can tolerate dynamic conditions.
- **Design to manage fires:** Avoidance of fires in oxygen systems is not an exact science and fires can result from mechanisms that cannot be predicted with certainty. However, this principle highlights the need to take steps to cope with fires at the design stage in order to deal with these uncertainties. These steps can include the following:
    - Installation of remote shutoff valves to interrupt oxygen flow to a fire
    - Minimizing the use of polymers that help to initiate, sustain or promote fires
    - Minimizing the volumes of oxygen passages so as to reduce the available oxidizer
    - Utilization of shields, barriers, and fire stops near vulnerable components

The design principle of managing fires assumes that an ignition may occur. It then considers the design for areas of greatest hazard and identifies design elements that inherently limit fire progression. Most commonly, the key element in terminating an oxygen fire is quickly shutting off unhindered oxygen flow. This consideration should be especially evaluated where components have developed a critical reaction-effect rating. Where possible, unrestricted flow should be terminated automatically and incorporated as an integral part of the design. It is also considered important that personnel be properly trained to immediately terminate oxygen flow during an incident, without exposing personnel to greater risk, and that emergency procedures be developed.

Fire Risk Assessments and Hazards Analyses – Summary

The hazard analysis tool described previously provides a proven process of evaluating an oxygen system design that focuses on known ignition mechanisms, materials choices, and good operating practices. Figure 6 and Table 1 illustrated the process for a contrived system. The process systematically evaluates a design and assigns rankings to the likelihood of ignition and the reaction effect that could develop, so that hazards can be mitigated for the highest ignition probabilities. The systematic approach, if performed carefully, has been shown to effectively recognize the design-specific hazards and allow for mitigation of these hazards through implementation of the "minimize, maximize, utilize approach."

However, the risk of fire is an inherent hazard for oxygen systems, and occasionally unintended fires develop. In these circumstances, the hazard analysis is also an indispensable tool to quickly reevaluate what may have gone wrong and/or what unexpected propagation path developed.

Oxygen Fire Failure Analysis

Analyzing an oxygen system fire may seem daunting due to the considerable destruction of the structural components comprising the oxygen system. Where high-pressure oxygen is involved, the fire can burn through valve bodies consuming large quantities of the metallic and nonmetallic components within fractions of a second. For a hyperbaric chamber, operating at just a couple of atmospheres pressure, rapid fire spread may lead to catastrophic results. See Figures 9, 10, and 11 that show the aftermath of an unintended oxygen fire.

Physical Evidence "Tells the Story"

At first glance, the physical evidence appears to be a dirty mess of soot, char, and melted metal. These photos depict the fire damage that occurred during actual operation of an oxygen system. However, for a trained investigator, the fire patterns indicated by the physical evidence "*tell the story*" about where the fire originated and how it propagated.

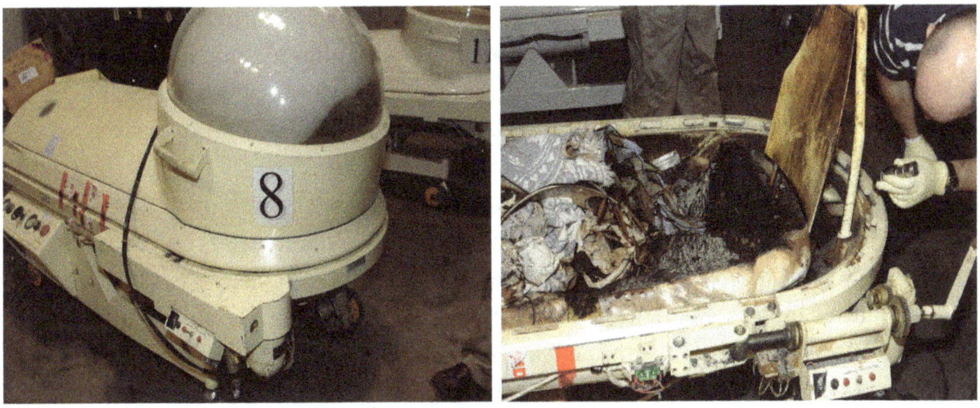

Figure 9. Photographic views of monoplace hyperbaric chamber fire.

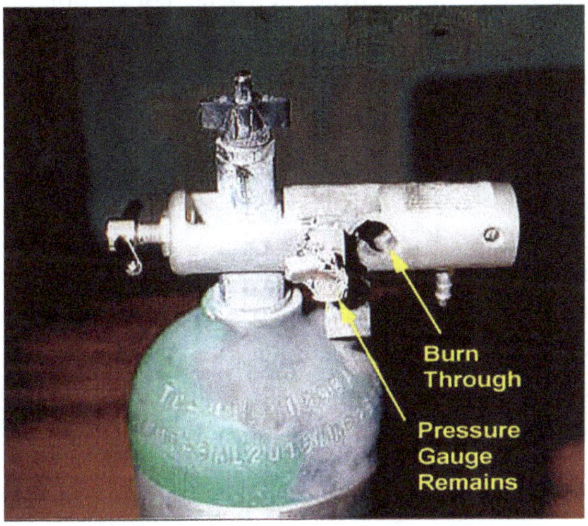

Figure 10. Aluminum medical regulator burnout.

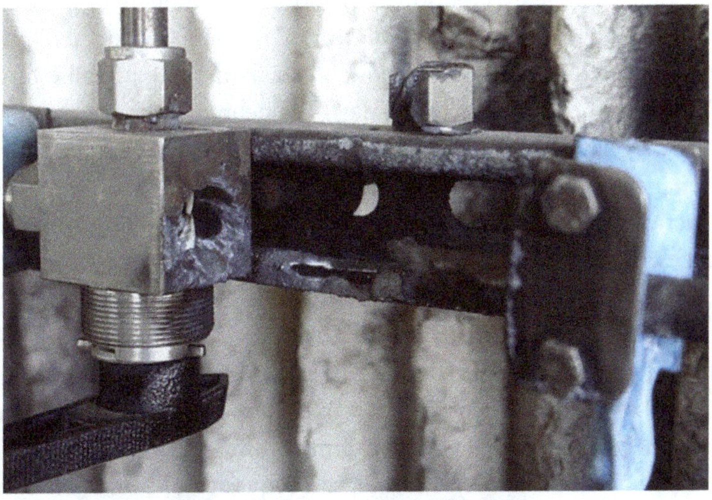

Figure 11. Oxygen supply manifold fire.
Photos courtesy of the author via the Broward County Sheriff's office.

In any fire investigation, it is extremely important that the evidence be documented thoroughly as early as possible. Collection of the evidence would include both burned and unburned components and documentation of the fire patterns by macro-photographs and video before changing the appearance of any component. The fire patterns and propagation clues are very important to the fire investigator.[26]

Oxygen fires develop and propagate within oxygen systems, at low pressures, and in ways analogous to ambient pressure fires already detailed in numerous texts on this subject.[27-28] However, the oxygen-enriched fire investigation, especially for high-pressure fires, should be approached with the unique aspects of oxygen materials compatibility and ignition factors in view. Within enclosed chambers, where gaseous flow is minimal, fire propagation is strongly influenced by the material flammability characteristics and increased fire spread rates due to oxygen-enrichment and elevated pressure (Figure 5). The dominant mechanism of heat transfer is usually convection due to the buoyancy effects from the thermal energy evolved during the fire. Radiation is also a strong mechanism for direct line of sight with any point of intense burning. Due to natural buoyancy and strong thermal patterns, heat transfer effects and material flammability are generally considered to drive chamber fire development. The OI and ΔHc of the flammable materials provide the data necessary to assess the propagation development and damage potential under oxygen-enriched burning.

At high pressures, such as within the oxygen delivery system or manifold, fires can develop into an intense involvement of the structural metals through kindling chain mechanisms that start with ignition of contaminants and/or the system nonmetallic materials (i.e. seals, seats, etc.). Determination of the origin of burning (i.e. the initial point of ignition and first material ignited) is often the key to reconstructing the cause of these fires. Once the origin is determined, the hazard analysis process can be used to assess the probable cause(s) of the fire since the analysis process addresses both material compatibility/flammability and ignition influences. For instance, if the origin of a fire occurred at a sudden change in direction of gas flow, at a region of high gas velocity, then particle impact would rank high as a likely ignition mechanism. Further, if inspection of the evidence indicates that ignition developed at a flammable metallic target material (i.e. valve body), then the ignition energy may have been due to particle impact and the cause of the fire may have been due to ineffective filtration or particulate contamination during maintenance (or both). The hazard analysis process provides a methodology for assessing the active ignition mechanisms at the point of origin and comparing that data to the physical evidence and sequence provided by witnesses (if any).

Cause and Origin Analysis—Origin First

One of the first steps in a fire investigation is to establish the proximate point of origin of the fire's initiation and the first material ignited. Only when the origin is known can the active ignition mechanism be determined and compared to the vulnerability of the material(s) in that proximity. Further, the sequence of events leading to the fire must be assessed as they relate to the origin of ignition. This results from the fact that different ignition mechanisms exhibit varying strength/efficiency depending on where they are applied in the system. For instance, at a dead end, such as the seat of a closed valve, adiabatic compression is highly efficient if pressurization rates are rapid. Further, where ungrounded/unbonded human bodies are in contact with each other or with ungrounded insulating materials, then charging and ESD potentials are increased.

The origin of a fire in an oxygen delivery system is determined by examining the fire propagation patterns exhibited by the evidence. This determination often requires a detailed examination by someone experienced with oxygen-enriched fires who is trained to recognize the propagation patterns. The fire-damaged components may include valves, regulators, tubing, and other high-pressure components downstream of the point of origin. The detailed examination is often performed under high magnification to evaluate the melt/flow patterns, and chemical/metallurgical analysis may be utilized to assess the materials that were present as reactants during the fire at the origin.

The following summarizes some of the propagation indicators that help an investigator determine the point of origin.

- **Fire follows flow:** The general adage that "fire follows flow" holds true for oxygen-enriched fires just as it does for other fire investigation technologies. This behavior suggests that the point of origin is likely to be proximate to the site of the most upstream burning, if oxygen was flowing during the fire. One rule of thumb is that for flowing systems, such as in pipelines and valves, the point of origin is often near the site of burning located farthest upstream. At this point in the system, it is often possible to identify active ignition mechanisms and kindling chain probabilities consistent with the materials that have ignited and burned.

  Figure 10 depicts this principle and shows an aluminum-bodied medical regulator that ignited catastrophically and burned-through when the cylinder valve was initially opened. The pressure in the oxygen cylinder was reported to be approximately 1,800 PSI prior to the fire. Inspection and disassembly of the regulator and cylinder valve revealed that, in the direction of flow, burning began at the regulator's filter located at its immediate inlet. Upstream components, including the regulator yoke, inlet seal, and the cylinder valve did not exhibit evidence of ignition or combustion. The internal combustion patterns indicated an initial ignition mechanism that was active at the filter and spread from there to the regulator body and downstream components. The regulator body was constructed of aluminum and was not protected around the filter region, in this design, and is highly flammable at the elevated pressures.

  Assessment of the active ignition mechanisms in the proximity of the inlet filter, during the initial pressurization of the regulator, suggested that particle impact was highly probable (high gas velocity, particle targets at the filter, and exposure to flammable materials). Further investigation revealed that aluminum particulate debris was being ejected from the cylinder and cylinder valve during the initial high velocity flow transients while the regulator was pressurizing. This evidence suggested that particle impact was the probable ignition mechanism, and the particulate contamination inside the cylinder was the probable cause of the fire along with the unprotected nature of the aluminum in this regulator design.

While experience indicates that a fire will seldom propagate against the dominant gas flow, two notable exceptions have been observed. First, experience indicates that nonmetallic materials burning on their surface, such as the interior of a Teflon-lined flex hose, may propagate in an upstream direction if the flow is near static. Second, vapor-burning metals like aluminum have been observed to propagate in an upstream direction during momentary containment of the fire.

- **Melt/flow patterns:** The melt/flow patterns created by combustion gas flow and metal slag deposits during a fire provide evidence as to the fire's direction of travel and can be used to help establish the origin. These patterns comprise the melted areas on the surface of burned materials and the combustion deposits that cover the surfaces. The propagation of a fire can be followed by examining these melt/flow patterns and by documenting the materials that have burned (i.e. the kindling chain). Surface deposits will exhibit a directional pattern consistent with the local flow, especially on the edges, and flow impingement surfaces will often exhibit deep melting/burning where hot gases or slag was deposited. Examination under magnification is helpful to reveal flow patterns that are missed with the un-aided eye. In most oxygen-enriched fires, the location of greatest burning will be exhibited by the materials having the highest flammability (i.e. lowest promoted combustion thresholds [metals] and lowest oxygen index [nonmetals]). Experience also indicates that damage may increase downstream of the origin as more slag is produced and deposited on vulnerable surfaces.

- **Burn-through patterns:** Burn-through is a melt/flow pattern that is often mistaken for the point of origin. During a fire, the combustion residue will often sweep downstream and concentrate burning at a location where a change in the flow direction occurs or at any impediment to the flow, such as a flow restriction or elbow. A burn-through often occurs due to the impingement of hot gas/slag concentrated in this area. The materials in this proximity may also ignite/promote and burn or just melt through. An approach to identifying the origin is to examine the melt/flow patterns proximate to the burn-through, and work upstream looking for the point of first burning. This is often the actual origin and care should be exercised in looking for active ignition mechanisms in this proximity rather than at the burn-through location.

  It is often critical that the components upstream of the burn-through be inspected to ensure all of the important evidence is collected and examined. If only the area near the burn-through is collected, then the actual origin may be missed.

- **Kindling chain:** Many oxygen-enriched fires start as a kindling chain event and examining the evidence for kindling chain sequences (i.e., material A ignited material B which ignited material C) sometimes leads directly to identification of the origin and cause of the fire. The AIT, ΔHc, OI, and PC (for metals) behavior of the materials that have burned provide kindling chain information as to their relative ease of ignition and heat release (i.e.potential for kindling adjacent materials) once ignited. These parameters are crucial to assessing the kindling chain sequence. Examination of the evidence and documentation of the fire's propagation path provides the information necessary to track the kindling chain sequences.

  In many cases the kindling chain may start with the introduction of a material/contaminant material (i.e. oils or greases) that is flammable or could lead to ignition of components in the flow stream. Contamination of an oxygen system during maintenance or servicing due to improper handling is a common kindling chain ignition hazard. Even for an oxygen system that has operated without incident for several years, the introduction of a flammable contaminant may lead to ignition. For instance, the components upstream of the valve shown in Figure 11 exhibited internal contamination which was considered to contribute to the kindling chain but would not have been identified had the uninvolved components of the full system not been inspected.

- **Gas versus slag:** When evaluating kindling chain sequences, it is important to consider that metallic slag produced by metals combustion is more efficient at kindling fires in surrounding components than the gaseous combustion products produced by polymeric materials. Metal combustion generally produces coalescing liquid metal/metal oxides of high heat capacity at temperatures approaching the oxide boiling points. Metal combustion products may produce very little gaseous metal oxides since the oxides largely dissociate upon vaporization and generally don't exist as oxide vapors. In contrast, combustion of polymers produces gaseous products that tend to dissipate, rather than concentrate, the heat release. Furthermore, gaseous combustion products often compete with the oxidizing environment and can sometimes inhibit fire spread under static conditions.

Oxygen Fire Failure Analysis—Summary

For the hyperbaric chamber fire shown in Figure 9, each of these principles was applied leading to the conclusion that the fire's origin was inside the chamber rather than from the oxygen supply system. The oxygen flow system was carefully evaluated and evidence of fire in a delivery component was not identified, indicating that fire had not traveled into the chamber from an origin upstream. Based on analysis of the fire patterns inside the chamber, and testimony of witness observations after the fire was observed, initial development near the occupant backrest progressing into the mattress and foam followed by rapid flashover of the cotton linen was considered likely.

Most ignition mechanisms discussed herein were ruled out, with the exception of those that might be present inside the chamber (Table 1). Evidence of heating devices or electrical faults inside the chamber were also not observed. However, evidence that the clothing worn by the two occupants (also a violation of standards for monoplace chambers) were known to increase triboelectric charging hazards. Antistatic grounding/bonding for occupants required by standards was not utilized, which would have allowed charge accumulation of the occupants and discharge to a charge receptor in the area of origin. Therefore, ESD ignition of flammable materials in the pressurized chamber was considered the most likely ignition energy present, proximate to the area of origin, for the factors that were understood to exist.

To a great degree the hazard analysis approach discussed herein works hand in hand with the familiar techniques for origin and cause reconstruction. The hazard analysis approach allows one to critically evaluate the severity of the environment and the active ignition mechanisms, whether during the design phase or working backward from the evidence during a fire investigation. The materials analysis principles allow for ranking of the materials based on their relative flammability in oxygen with a view toward judging either the potential effect of a fire or the kindling chain sequences exhibited by a fire's propagation.

References and Endnotes

1. Werley BL (ed). TM Standards Technology Training Course. Fire Hazards in Oxygen Systems. Second Edition, Education Subcommittee of ASTM Committee G04 on Compatibility and Sensitivity of Materials in Oxygen-Enriched Atmospheres. Philadelphia, PA: ASTM; 1991.
2. Ibid.
3. WHA International, Inc, formerly Wendell Hull & Associates (WHA), is a private engineering consulting firm specializing in oxygen fire hazards analysis and forensic fire investigation located in Las Cruces, NM. Personnel who were formerly employed by NASA-WSTF staff the oxygen technology division of WHA.
4. ASTM D 2863: Standard test method for measuring the minimum oxygen concentration to support candle-like combustion of plastics (oxygen index). The oxygen index is the minimum oxygen concentration required to support flaming combustion in a flowing oxygen/diluent (usually nitrogen) mixture.
5. Benning MA. Measurement of Oxygen Index at Elevated Pressures. Flammability and sensitivity of materials in oxygen-enriched atmospheres. Philadelphia, PA: ASTM STP 812. 1983:68-83.
6. Ibid.

7. ASTM. ASTM G63-92: Standard guide for evaluating nonmetallic materials for oxygen service. Philadelphia, PA.
8. British Standard 3N-100. British Standard Aerospace Series: General design requirements for aircraft oxygen systems and equipment. London, United Kingdom; 1985.
9. Bryan CJ, Lowrie R. Comparative results of autogenous ignition temperature measurements by ASTM G 72 and pressurized scanning calorimetry in gaseous oxygen. Flammability and sensitivity of materials in oxygen-enriched atmospheres. ASTM STP 910. 108-117.
10. See reference #7.
11. Lowrie R, Werley BL (ed). Heat of combustion and oxygen compatibility. Flammability and sensitivity of materials in oxygen-enriched atmospheres. ASTM STP 812. ASTM. 1983:84-96.
12. See reference #7. Note also that materials must be chosen based on balancing the compatibility data, including heat of combustion, with the mechanical demands of the design on the material. Materials with higher heats of combustion may be used successfully as long as ignition energy is minimized and protection is provided for adjacent flammable materials.
13. ASTM. ASTM G 124-95: Standard test method for determining the combustion behavior of metallic materials in oxygen-enriched atmospheres.
14. Situationally flammable materials are those materials that are flammable based on standard test data under the conditions of use. A material that is nonflammable under one condition may be flammable when oxygen concentration or pressure is raised. For instance, Teflon® is nonflammable at 1 atm in less than 95% oxygen. However, as the pressure is raised to approximately 204 atm (~3000 PSI), it will support combustion in 21% oxygen. Hence, Teflon® becomes situationally flammable in high-pressure air.
15. Characteristic elements have been developed for each of the ignition mechanisms known to be active in oxygen systems. These elements are the unique factors that increase the severity of a particular ignition mechanism. For instance, for particle impact, the characteristic elements are a) high velocity gas flow; b) flammable particles likely in the flow stream; c) flammable targets subject to flow impingement; and d) sharp angles or changes in direction of flow. When each of these characteristic elements are present, and some are severe, such as higher gas velocity, then particle impact ignition probability increases. WHA personnel routinely provide a consulting service to industry and government in applying these principles and performing oxygen hazards analyses for oxygen designs. WHA also maintains a database of materials compatibility information and a test facility to perform oxygen flammability assessments.

16. Daniel JA, et.al. A hazards analysis method for oxygen systems including several case studies. Flammability and sensitivity of materials in oxygen-enriched atmospheres. ASTM STP 1197. P. 364.
17. Williams, RE, et. al. Ignition of steel alloys by impact of low-velocity iron/inert particles in gaseous oxygen. Flammability and sensitivity of materials in oxygen-enriched atmospheres. ASTM STP 986. 72-84.
18. Kindling chain ignition is akin to promoted ignition but usually starts with a contaminant (hydrocarbon grease or flammable particulate debris) that is easily ignited, promoting a more difficult material in the system. Kindling chain ignition of metals in high-pressure oxygen systems can also develop due to the initial ignition of system nonmetallic materials. The analogy of starting a fire with paper to ignite twigs (kindling) to ignite a log is an example of a common "kindling chain" event.
19. Materials such as thin wall stainless steel tubing has been used successfully up to 10,000 PSI (even though it is flammable at low pressures, less than 100 PSI) by maintaining scrupulous cleaning practices and using the hazard analysis process to identify the active ignition mechanisms and design limiting their influence. The approach must be used in total, however, and the flammability of the materials and the risk of ignition must be constantly guarded against.
20. ASTM G 93-96: Standard practice for cleaning methods and cleanliness levels for material and equipment used in oxygen-enriched environments.
21. ASTM G 128-95: Standard guide for control of hazards and risks in oxygen enriched systems.
22. Werley BL. An oxygen index update. Flammability and sensitivity of materials in oxygen-enriched atmospheres. ASTM STP 986. 248-261.
23. A detailed discussion of the common ignition mechanisms is provided in this chapter.
24. Cronk JO. Taming oxygen hazards: awareness must come first. ASTM Standardization News; September 1983.
25. CGA Pamphlet 4.4: Industrial practices for gaseous oxygen transmission and distribution.
26. The reconstruction of an unintended fire should start immediately after the event has concluded and the immediate safety requirements are addressed. Among the most urgent post-incident efforts is the preserving of the evidence so that a forensic analysis can be properly performed. Very often in an attempt to "do something," the evidence is destroyed by an overzealous response to the fire. It is strongly encouraged that thorough documentation be obtained before any change in the evidence is performed. Just moving fire-damaged equipment or disassembling the components may mask the fire patterns that are meaningful to a fire investigator. ASTM Standard Guide G 145-96: Standard guide for studying

fire incidents in oxygen systems provides a helpful discussion pertaining to failure analysis of oxygen-enriched fires.

27. Noon, Randall. Engineering analysis of fires and explosions. CRC Press; 1995.
28. DeHaan, JD. Kirk's fire investigation, 3rd Edition. Brady Division of Prentice-Hall Inc., 1991.

Appendix A. Selected Material Compatibility Data

Material	Chemical Name	AIT (oC)	HoC (cal/grm)	OI (%)	Ref.
	Plastics				
ABS	Acrylonitrile-butadiene-styrene	243	8500	18–39	1,3,9
Delrin, Acetal	Poly(acetyl)	178-195	4029	14.2–16.1	1,5,9
Halar	Ethylene-chlorotrifluoroethylene	171	3254-3900	52	1,9,11,13
Kel-F 81	PCTFE plastic	388	2300	DNP	14
Kynar	Polyvinylidene fluoride (PVDF)	268	3277	39-43.7	2,3, 11
Lexan	Polycarbonate	286	7407	27	3,5
Mylar	Polyethylene terephtalate	181	2300	22.7	3,5
Neoflon	PCTFE plastic (Daikin Japan)	382	1220	DNP	3, 8
Noryl	Polyphenylene oxide-polystyrene	348	6615	33.3	15
Nylon	Nylon 66, Polyamide	178-259	7400 - 7900	23.5 - 30.5	1,2,3,7
PEEK	Polyetheretherketone	305-325	7775	35	3,11,12
Plexiglas	Poly(methylmethacrylate)	230	6000	17-18.5	1.2,3,5
Polycarbonate, Generic	Polycarbonate, Generic	300-340	7400-9400	22.5 - 27.4	3,5
Polyester (Mylar)	Polyethylene terephthalate (PET)	181	5306	22.7	1
Polyethylene (PE)	Polyethylene plastic	176	11100	17.5	2,3,11
PPS	Polyphenylene sulfide	285	6853	43	3
Polypropylene (PP)	Polypropylene Plastic	174	11000	17-18	1,5,11
Polystyrene (PS)	Polystyrene, Hard Plastic	250	9900	17-23	2,3
PVC	Polyvinyl chloride	170-240	4300-5400	20-38	2,3
PVDC	Polyvinylidene chloride		5000	60	3
Rulon A, E, J, LD	Glass-filled TFE fluorocarbon	360-427	1400-2100	DNP	2,3
Teflon FEP	Fluoroethyl propylene	378	2500	77	1,11
Teflon PFA	Perfluoroalkoxytetrafluoroethylene	424	1250	100	1,11
Teflon TFE	Polytetrafluoroethylene	427+	1700	95-100	1,7,11
Tefzel	ETFE, copolymer of tetrafluoroethylene and ethylene	243	3538	30	1,3,11
Ultem	Polyetherimide	385	7026	47	3
Vespel SP21	Polyimide with 15% graphite	328-347	6002-6318	53-65	2,3

Material	Chemical Name	AIT (oC)	HoC (cal/grm)	OI (%)	Ref.
Lubricants and Sealants					
PTFE Pipe Tape (clean)	TFE-fluorocarbon tape thread sealant	427+	See TFE	83-100	2
Christo-Lube MCG111	Perfluoroalkyl polyether grease	470	1049	DNI	2
Everlube 811	MO S2 in sodium silicate	271			2
Fluorolube GR362	PCTFE/filler	427+	4994	67	2
Fluorolube LG160	PCTFE lube	382	2516		2
Fluorosilicone (Dow Corning)	Fluorosilicone (FS) Grease	292	3500	30	2,14
Fomblin RT15	Perfluoroalkyl polyether grease	427+	995	DNP	2
Halocarbon PCTFE Oil	PCTFE Oil (various grades)	385-410	1047-1994	75-DNP	2
Halocarbon PCTFE Grease	PCTFE Grease (various grades)	427+	1600-2366	67-DNP	2
Krytox 240 AC	Perfluoroalkyl polyether grease	427+	900-1000	DNP	2
Loctite pipe sealant	Anaerobic sealant (cured)	170-260	4204-7600	17-20	2
Molykote Z Powder	Pure MOS2	260	1709	45	2
Silicone Grease (Dow Corning)	Polysiloxane Grease	260-270	6200-7800	25-27	2,3
Gaskets					
Blue Gard 3000	Garlock Co., Arimid/Buna N Gasket		3047	30.5 ± 0.5	2
Durabla gasket	Asbestos in GRS binder		1600	28.0 ± .5	2
Gore-Tex	Expanded PTFE		1431	100	2
Grafoil GHE, GHR	flexible graphite, SS tong metal interlayer	400+			2
Gylon Fawn	Filled PTFE		1069		2
Elastomers					
Aflas	FKM coated with PTFE	254	4000		2
Buna-N (Nitrile Rubber)	Butadiene-acrylonitrile	173-200	5400-9911	18	2,3
Butyl Rubber	copolymer of isobutylene and small quantities of isoprene	208	10789	17.1	3
Disogren (Urethane Rubber)	Polyurethane Rubber	265-271	5850	28	3
EPR Rubber (EPR and EPDM)	ethylene-propylene rubber	153-206	8833-11287	21.9-25.5	3
Fluorel	FKM, Copolymer of vinylidene fluoride and hexafluoropropylene	297-302	3400-3992	73.9-93.5	3
Hycar	Nitrile Rubber Copolymer	180-310	8500		2
Hypalon Rubber	Chlorosulfonated polyethylene	25-27	6800	27	2,3

Material	Chemical Name	AIT (oC)	HoC (cal/grm)	OI (%)	Ref.
Kalrez	FPM elastomer, Generic	355	1565-2089	DNP	3
Neoprene	Polychloroprene	258	6532	26	1,2,3
Nitrile Rubber, Generic	Butadiene and acrylonitrile	142-173	9911	18-22	2,3
Nordel (EPDM)	Ethylene propylene rubber	170-190	9220	25.5	2
Silicone Rubber, Generic	Poly(methyl phenylsiloxane)	262	3300	21-33	2,3
Viton A	FKM, Fluorocarbon rubber	268-322	3600	57-58	2,3
Other Materials					
Cotton (untreated)	Cotton	325	4000	20-21	2,4
Epoxy/Graphite		258	7072		2,3
Nomex Nylon	Polyamide Fiber	300	6000	27-30	2,4
Notes					

NOTE: Data for all tests not available for some materials

DNI – Did not ignite; DNP – Did not propagate

Compatibility Data References:

1. ASTM G 63: Standard Guide for Evaluating Nonmetallic Materials for Oxygen Service.
2. WHA Materials Testing Database. www.wha-international.comcs.
3. ASTM Manual 36: Safe Use of Oxygen and Oxygen Systems, Handbook for Design, Operation, and Maintenance, 2nd Edition.
4. NFPA 53-1999, Table F-3.3.8.
5. Ikeda GK. Oxygen Index Tests to Evaluate the Suitability of a Given Material for Oxygen Service. ASTM STP 812; pps. 56-67.
6. Bryan C., Lowrie, R. Comparative Results of Autogenous Ignition Temperature Measurements by ASTM G72 and Pressurized Scanning Calorimetry in Gaseous Oxygen. ASTM STP 910; pps:108-117.
7. Chou TC, Fiedorowicz, A. Oxygen Compatibility of Polymers Including TFE-Teflon, Kel-F 81, Vespel SP-21, Viton A, Viton A-500, Fluorel, Neoprene, EPDM, Buna-N and Nylon 6,6"; STP 1319; p 325.
8. Waller JM, Haas JP, Beeson HD. Polymer-Oxygen Compatibility Testing: Effect of Oxygen Aging on Ignition and Combustion Properties. STP 1395: p. 83.
9. Union Carbide Research Report. Engineering Memorandum No. 5062-G.
10. ASRDI Oxygen Technology Survey, Volume IX, Oxygen Systems Engineering Review.
11. Hshieh FY, et.al. Autoignition Temperature of Selected Polymers at Elevated Oxygen Pressure and Their Heat of Combustion, Fire and Materials, Vol 20, 301-303. 1996.
12. Wendell Hull & Associates, Test Report.
13. Solvay Solexis Material Datasheet.
14. Lowri, R. Heat of Combustion and Oxygen Compatibility. ASTM STP-812: p. 89 (as KSC PCTFE).
15. Hirsch D, et.al. Issues Related to the Flammability Assessment of Polymers for Hazard Analyses of Oxygen Systems. ASTM STP 1454.
16. Currie J. The Ignition Behavior of Silicone Greases in Oxygen Atmospheres. ASTM STP 1040: pps: 125-141.

CHAPTER 5.5
How to Determine If a Material Is Safe for Use in the Hyperbaric Chamber

Richard C. Barry, MS, STS, CHT-A

Introduction

Within the hyperbaric industry, there is one element that affects every patient, staff, and piece of material or equipment utilized: a material's compatibility in the pressurized gas environment. The *NFPA 99 Health Care Facility Code* (*NFPA 99*) calls for the agreement of two individuals—the hyperbaric safety director and the lead physician (medical director/physician in charge)—before allowing an item into a chamber that would generally be prohibited. Furthermore, the code calls for the approval to use a normally prohibited item to be documented in writing. *NFPA 99* also states the safety director shall make recommendations regarding policies and procedures and have the authority to restrict or remove potentially hazardous items from entering the chamber, thus illustrating the importance of the designated safety director and the need to have in place an assessment process.[1]

This chapter intends to focus on a process for use by the safety director and medical director to follow when determining to approve or prohibit an item from entering a chamber. The term *material* will be used to describe an item to be evaluated, but the term *product* or *item* may be used synonymously. Evaluations of medical devices such as ventilators and infusion pumps are outside the scope of this chapter. Also, in the context of this chapter, the phrase safety director refers to the hyperbaric unit's designated hyperbaric safety director, and the term medical director refers to the hyperbaric medical director.

Most of the materials used in hyperbarics (excluding mechanical chamber parts) were designed and evaluated for use at normobaric pressure and temperature. As hyperbaric professionals, we are taking these same materials and placing them in an altered environment that includes but is not limited to the following:

- **Temperature changes:** Temperature increases during compression, stabilizes at treatment depth, and decreases during decompression.

- **Pressure changes:** Occurs when going from ambient pressure to a prescribed treatment pressure.
- **Variety of gas mixtures:** Compression gases of air or oxygen are most common, but other combinations are used depending on the application.
- **Enclosed space:** There is a limited amount of space in a monoplace chamber and smaller multiplace chambers.

Each hyperbaric program should design and follow a risk assessment process to do the following:

- Make informed decisions regarding the materials that will and will not be allowed in their chamber.
- Establish a list of approved and prohibited materials.
- Protect patients, staff, and equipment from injury or damage due to materials.
- Protect the hyperbaric industry from mishaps.
- Understand code requirements.
- Document reasoning for the use or nonuse of a material.

What Are Safe, Safety, and Hyperbaric Safety?

To be *safe*, to practice *safety*, and to implement *hyperbaric safety*, the hyperbaric program must first define what these terms mean to their given application of hyperbarics. The hyperbaric program leadership, e.g., medical director, program manager, clinical manager, technical director (if designated), and safety director should spend time defining what these terms mean to them. The programs that can define *safe, safety,* and *hyperbaric safety* are better positioned to implement the practice of these terms. Conversely, the program that is not able to define these terms is not able to achieve them effectively.

Below are example definitions by the author, but you are encouraged to define these terms at your facility for your application of hyperbaric utilization.

- **Safe:** Free from harm or risk; secure from the threat of danger, harm, or loss to patients, personnel, and equipment.
- **Safety:** The condition of avoiding danger, harm, or loss to patients, personnel, and equipment.
- **Hyperbaric safety:** Implementing safe acts, training, policies, and procedures in and around the altered environment of hyperbarics to include aspects of medical and technical choices.

While these terms may seem universal, it is essential to recognize that the application of hyperbarics is used in various ways, with the gas one uses to pressurize the chamber and the number of occupants entering the chamber constituting the main differences. Each one of the examples below requires a different approach to researching a material/product/item for use in the chamber. For example, the use of a product in an oxygen-filled monoplace chamber may be prohibited but in the air-filled environment of the multiplace chamber, the same product may be allowed.

Examples of delivery methods of hyperbarics (not all-encompassing) are as follows:

- Monoplace chamber pressurized with oxygen
- Monoplace chamber pressurized with air, with the patient breathing oxygen from a mask or hood
- Multiplace chamber pressurized with air, with the patient breathing oxygen from a mask or hood
- Presence of both monoplace and multiplace chambers at the same facility

Materials

Potential materials you can expect to evaluate include but are not limited to the following:

- Wound care dressing, bandages, and wraps
- Wound care gels, ointments, and powders
- Synthetic skin grafts
- Surgical closures (staples or sutures)
- Pillows, mattresses, and body-positioning pads
- Linen such as pillowcases, sheets, blankets, and patient garments
- External fixators used for stabilization and immobilization
- Fiberglass or plaster casting material
- Internal devices such as implantable cardioverter defibrillator, pacemakers, bone stimulators, and pain pumps
- External devices such as continuous glucose monitoring systems
- Patient belongings of a religious or cultural aspect such as wedding band/ring, patron saint necklaces, temple garments (undergarments), and head/face coverings (hijab, niqab, burka)

Process

The author's recommendation for evaluating a material may be viewed as a six-step process.

1. Data collection
2. Review of information
3. Determination
4. Document in writing

5. Dissemination of information
6. Document storage

In the following pages, each step will be explained in detail. The safety director is encouraged to review these steps with the medical director and edit to match the nuances of their hyperbaric facility.

STEP ONE – Data Collection

Once an item of question has been identified, the safety director will collect data and record information relevant to its use or nonuse in hyperbarics on an evaluation form.

Sources of data collection include but are not limited to the following:

- Searching through the World Wide Web
- Reviewing the product manufacturer's website
- Discussing the use of the product in hyperbarics with the manufacturer's technical support staff or engineers and ask if they have commissioned any laboratory testing of their product to include the following:
  - *Autogenous ignition temperature for hyperbaric testing:* This determines the minimum ignition temperature at which a material self-ignites in oxygen at hyperbaric conditions.[7]
  - *Heat of combustion testing:* This is the amount of combustion energy released per unit mass.[8]
  - *Oxygen index testing:* This shows the minimum concentration of oxygen that supports self-sustained burning at atmospheric pressure.[9]
  - *Oxygen exposure testing:* This subjects a sample to severe hyperbaric conditions and monitors for exothermic activity and mass loss.[10]
- Reading the product literature supplied with the product
- Review product information found on the U.S. Food and Drug Administration's website
- Review safety data sheets (formerly known as material safety data sheets)

In this chapter, the author is using a self-produced Material/Product Evaluation Form as an example of data collection and recording. The information below will be useful to those reviewing the material, both local reviewers and any external sources you may consult. The example is meant to establish an evaluation method, but there may be items not listed that one will want to include based on experience, education, and training.

Material/Product Evaluation Form
(Example - Blank)

Section One – General Information

Facility Name	
Patient Medical Record Number	
Date	
Item Manufacturer	
Item Name	
Item Description	
Item Martial(s)	
Purpose of Item	
Chamber Class	
Pressurizing Gas	
Data Collector(s)	

Section Two – Specific Information

	COMMENTS
Item provided by	In this section, for each line item answer with yes, no, not applicable, unavailable, unknown, or an informative note of explanation.
Is this a prescribed item?	
Is the item easily removable?	
Is a flammable gas or vapor present?	
Does the item produce heat?	
Alternative	
Concern	
Can the item trap gas?	
Is a strong odor present?	
Is the item electrically powered?	
Is ESD a concern?	
Does the item contain metal?	
Is the item made with rubber?	
Fabric blend or composition	
SDS Reviewed	
NFPA 99 Reviewed	
FDA Reviewed	
Manufacturer Information Reviewed	
Manufacturer Approved/Prohibited	
Depth, Time, or Gas Limitation by the Manufacturer	
List of Attachments	

Section Three – Finalize

Reason for approving or prohibiting this item for use in the hyperbaric chamber:
Stipulation or conditions for allowing this item in the hyperbaric chamber:

The use of this item is:
[ ] APPROVED AS-IS
[ ] APPROVED WITH STIPULATIONS
[ ] PROHIBITED
Hyperbaric Safety Director: Print, Sign, Date, Time
Hyperbaric Medical Director: Print, Sign, Date, Time

Explanatory Information for Each Line Item.

Section One – General Information

- Facility Name. Record the name of the facility or hospital and department.
- Patient Medical Record Number. Since this form is not part of the patient's medical record, note the patient's medical record number to allow for ease of patient identification.
- Date. Record the date of evaluation with a standardized method of showing the date; e.g., MM/DD/YYYY (month/day/year).
- Item Manufacturer. Maker of the item.
- Item Name. Note the name of the item as given by the manufacturer.
- Item Description. Describe the item as stated by the manufacturer. Include as much information as possible, such as model, serial number, batch number, lot number, size, and quantity.
- Item Material(s). Describe the materials as stated by the manufacturer. For example, description of the material and its characteristics, such as gel, liquid, ointment, wound care material, bandage, metal or nonmetal, fabric, strong odor, or electrical.
- Purpose of Item. Describe the purpose of the item as stated by the manufacturer.
- Chamber Class. Use the *NFPA 99* and *NFPA 99B* classifications for chamber type.[1,3]

    i. Class A. Human, multiple occupancy (hyperbaric)

    ii. Class B. Human, single occupancy (hyperbaric)

iii. Class C. Animal, no human occupancy (hyperbaric)

iv. Class D. Human-rated, air atmosphere not oxygen enriched (hypobaric)

v. Class E. Human-rated, oxygen-enriched atmosphere (partial pressure of oxygen is above 0.235 ATA) (hypobaric)

- Pressurizing gas. State the type of gas or gases used to pressurize the chamber.
- Data collector(s). The person(s) involved with researching the material.

Section Two – Specific Information

- Item provided by? State who provided the item. Was it provided by the wound care center or hyperbaric facility, the referring physician, the patient, or other entity? You will need to know this in case you have questions for the person who supplied the item.
- Is this a prescribed item? Is the material used for a prescriptive purpose? If prescribed, by whom? Consider implanted medical devices as prescriptive.
- Is the item easily removable? Describe if the material is easily removable or not. Caution: Just because an item is easily removable does not mean you should remove it. For example, a prescribed medication patch is easily removable, but you must consult with your medical director before removing a prescriptive item.
- Is a flammable gas or vapor present? For example, an alcohol prep pad releases flammable vapors and must be avoided in hyperbarics.
- Does the item produce heat? If yes, state how heat is produced, the expected maximum temperature, and can the heat be removed or stopped? Heat-producing items should be avoided in hyperbarics.
- Alternative. Describe if an already evaluated/approved material is available as an alternative.
- Concern. Describe the concern for use in hyperbarics. Some examples of concerns are whether the material is static or heat-producing, effects of pressure and temperature, are batteries or electrical wires present, and can the material cause damage to the chamber or chamber acrylic.
- Can the item trap gas? Perhaps the item itself is safe in hyperbarics, but the potential exists for gas to become trapped while under pressure. The concern is gas compressing during descent and expanding during ascent.
- Is a strong odor present? Perhaps the item itself is safe in hyperbarics, but the item presents with a strong odor such as a solution of sodium hypochlorite. In this case, the chamber ventilation should be increased.
- Is the item electrically powered? If yes, state power source. Determine if the power source is acceptable in your application of hyperbarics.

- Is electrostatic discharge (ESD) a concern? Do you believe electrostatic discharge to be possible?
- Does the item contain metal? If yes, state the type of metal. Are the edges sharp or dull? Does the metal pose a risk of sparking against other metal components? Can the metal scratch the acrylic? If yes, can you cover the metal to prevent sparking or scratching?
- Is the item made with rubber? If yes, neoprene and other rubber material could be compressible during descent. Determine if this is a concern or not. Items with compressible elements may become loose or dislocated while pressurized.
- Fabric blend or composition. State the blend or composition (e.g., 100% cotton, blend of cotton and poly of 60/40% respectively). Synthetics (e.g., 100% polyester or nylon) and wool are to be avoided in hyperbarics due to static potential.
- Safety Data Sheet (SDS) reviewed. State if SDS was available and if reviewed. If available, attach a copy or save an electronic copy with this form. When reviewing the SDS, if available, remember the formation of the information was under normal use conditions and not those of hyperbarics. Even so, a statement such as "extremely flammable liquid" should be concerning to the safety director. Also, not everything will have an SDS. For example, an external fixator most likely will not have a manufacturer-supplied SDS nor will many nonhazardous chemicals.
- *NFPA 99* reviewed. Review *NFPA 99*, the hyperbaric or hypobaric (NFPA 99B) sections to determine if the item is listed as prohibited by NFPA.[1,3]
- FDA (U.S. Food & Drug Administration) reviewed. Visit https://www.fda.gov and type in the item name in the search block to see if any adverse events have been reported to the FDA.[4] What you are looking for is any potential risk that may be associated with the item.
- Manufacturer information reviewed. Describe response from the manufacturer or any information related to hyperbarics or pressure changes as found in the product literature. Document any conversations or emails you have with the manufacturer.
- Manufacturer approved or prohibited. State if the manufacturer has approved or prohibited the item regarding hyperbarics. In situations where the manufacturer has recommended against the products use in hyperbarics, it is still within the safety director and medical director's discretion to approve or prohibit the item, but the organization's risk management department should be brought into the conversation.
- Depth, time, or gas limitation by manufacturer. State if the manufacturer has placed any depth or time limitations for use in hyperbarics.
- List of attachments. List the documents used during the evaluation, such as SDS, published reports, emails from the manufacturer, and abstracts.

Section Three – Finalize

- Reason for approving or prohibiting this item for use in the hyperbaric chamber. State your reasoning.
- Stipulation or conditions for allowing this item in the hyperbaric chamber. This is a place to document any stipulations or special instructions for allowance of the product. For example, allowing an item but covering it with a pillowcase to protect the acrylic from being scratched.
- Choose one of the blocks to indicate the use of this item.
- Signature blocks for the hyperbaric safety director and the hyperbaric medical director. The safety director and medical director should both acknowledge the decision in writing by printing and signing their names, along with the date and time.

STEP TWO – Review of Information

Upon completion of the Material/Product Evaluation Form, the safety director will review the information with the medical director. The questions to answer are the following: What is the concern(s)? and Are we able to mitigate or overcome the concern? You must define your concern to determine if you are going to approve or prohibit an item.

This is the safety director's opportunity to show and explain all of the information gathered during the evaluation. The safety director should approach the review from a nonmedical perspective and discuss the verifiable information whereas the medical director should review the potential medical risk associated with the material/item/product under review.

STEP THREE – Determination

After the review, the safety director and medical director will decide to approve the product as-is for use in the hyperbaric chamber, approve the product with stipulations, prohibit the product from use in the hyperbaric chamber, or solicit guidance from recognized experts in the field of hyperbaric safety. One example of support is found within the Undersea & Hyperbaric Medical Society's Safety Committee.[2] A second example may be within an organizational safety committee/department.

It should be recognized that *NFPA 99* calls for the safety director and medical director to review a product that would normally be prohibited, but it is the opinion of the author that these same two individuals should review any material/item/product the hyperbaric program is considering for use inside of the hyperbaric chamber. Understandably, situations may arise that necessitate a decision be made by the safety director only, such as the allowance of clothing worn by a patient or inside chamber operator at a multiplace facility, which is allowed by *NFPA 99*, but this should be viewed as the exception and not the standard.[1]

In cases of conflict, where one person wants to approve the product but the other person wants to prohibit the product, a third party should be consulted for guidance. In the interim, leave the item out of the chamber until both the safety director and the medical director agree with approval or approval with stipulations.

STEP FOUR – Document in Writing

Once a decision has been made, document as such on the Material/Product Evaluation Form by choosing the approved block, the approved-with-stipulations block, or the prohibited block and then print, sign, date and time by the safety director and medical director.

STEP FIVE – Dissemination of Information

Now that the form as been completed, the safety director must do the following:

1. Document the decision in the patient's medical record and note any stipulations or unique conditions. It is a best practice to instill a method of immediate staff communication to ensure all personnel involved with the care of a patient are made aware of any updates regarding approved or prohibited items. Also, implementation of a Pass-Down Logbook (passing down of information) is highly recommended as a means of logging day-to-day updates. The logbook should be review by the hyperbaric staff at the beginning of each working shift.

Example Pass-Down Logbook page:

Date:	Action Taken / Updates	Initials
12/12/18	XYZ gauze approved for use in hyperbarics	RCB
12/13/18	ICD by XYZ Company prohibited by the manufacturer for use in hyperbarics	RCB

2. Inform the other supervising hyperbaric physicians and nonphysician providers.
3. Inform the hyperbaric staff and nursing staff.
4. Add the item to the approved or prohibited list.
    - A listing of approved items is something the facility will need to develop and maintain on their own, but *NFPA 99* does give allowance for garments comprised of 100% cotton or a blend of cotton and polyester fabric, e.g., 70/30 or 60/40 cotton-poly blends as long as cotton is 50% or greater.[1]
    - A listing of prohibited items is also something the facility will need to develop on their own, but a starting list comes from *NFPA 99*, in which the following are prohibited[1]:
        - Smoking
        - Open flames
        - Hot objects
        - Personal warming devices (e.g., therapeutic chemical heating pads, hand warmers, pocket warmers)

- Cell phones and pagers
- Sparking toys
- Personal entertainment devices (e.g., MP3 players, electronic readers, music devices)
- Hearing aids

Upon adding an item to the approved list, there is no reason to repeat a new analysis unless the item undergoes a significant change, but it is a good practice for the safety director to review both the approved and the prohibited listing at least annually to ensure they are kept current.

STEP SIX – Documentation Storage

Once the form has been completed, the facility should have a known place to store the form and supporting documentation. Your research should be readily accessible if you have a need to review the same or revised material at a later date or you have a need to research a similar material. Storage may be in a paper form or electronic, but in either case, if protected health information is shown on the form, then the storage location must be secure.

Examples of Completed Material/Product Evaluation Forms

Material/Product Evaluation Form
(Example - One)

Section One – General Information

Facility Name	XYZ Regional Medical Center
Patient Medical Record Number	12345
Date	12/12/2018
Item Manufacturer	XYZ Medical
Item Name	Zap Insulin Pump and Sensor
Item Description	Small sensor enclosed in plastic that is used with Zap Insulin Pump
Item Martial(s)	1 cm x 1 cm electronic chip enclosed in plastic
Purpose of Item	Monitors blood glucose level and delivers insulin when attached to Zap Insulin Pump
Chamber Class	Class B
Pressurizing Gas	Oxygen
Data Collector(s)	XYZ Name – Hyperbaric Safety Director

Section Two – Specific Information

	COMMENTS
Item provided by	Endocrinologist Dr. XYZ Name (555) 555-5555
Is this a prescribed item?	Yes
Is the item easily removable?	In part
Is a flammable gas or vapor present?	No
Does the item produce heat?	Attached – yes; detached – no
Alternative	No
Concern	Heat while attached and unknown if the pump's communication/ sensors will be affected under pressure
Can the item trap gas?	Yes
Is a strong odor present?	No
Is the item electrically powered?	Yes – battery
Is ESD a concern?	No
Does the item contain metal?	No
Is the item made with rubber?	No
Fabric blend or composition	Not applicable
SDS Reviewed	Not applicable
NFPA 99 Reviewed	Yes – no contraindications from *NFPA 99*
FDA Reviewed	Yes – no reported event located.
Manufacturer Information Reviewed	Yes
Manufacturer Approved/Prohibited	Approved with stipulations. See below.
Depth/Time Limitation by Manufacturer	None
List of Attachments	Manufacturer's email Manufacturer's product information

Section Three – Finalize

Reason for approving or prohibiting this item for use in the hyperbaric chamber: Approving: The patient must keep part of the sensor attached, but the item does not pose a risk in hyperbarics when following manufacturer's recommendations.
Stipulation or conditions for allowing this item in the hyperbaric chamber: The sensor will be detached from the insulin pump before the day's hyperbaric treatment and reattached once the treatment is complete. Once the pump is detached, the sensor emits no heat and does not communicate with the pump. Information regarding sensors safety for treatment verified by XYZ Medical – XYZ Name of Tech Support; XYZ Name@XYZ Medical.com / (555) 555-5555.

The use of this item is:

[ ] APPROVED AS-IS

[X] APPROVED WITH STIPULATIONS

[ ] PROHIBITED

Hyperbaric Safety Director: XYZ Name, *XYZ signature*, 12/12/2018 – 1000

Hyperbaric Medical Director: Dr. XYZ Name, *XYZ signature*, 12/12/2018 – 1000

Material/Product Evaluation Form
(Example - Two)

Section One – General Information

Facility Name	XYZ Regional Medical Center
Patient Medical Record Number	54321
Date	12/18/2018
Item Manufacturer	XYZ Medical
Item Name	ICD 2000
Item Description	A fully implantable cardioverter defibrillator
Item Martial(s)	Metal container with wires
Purpose of Item	Used to continuously monitor and control life-threatening electrical problems with the heart.
Chamber Class	Class B
Pressurizing Gas	Oxygen
Data Collector(s)	XYZ Name – Hyperbaric Safety Director

Section Two – Specific Information

	COMMENTS
Item provided by	Cardiologist Dr. XYZ Name (555) 555-5555
Is this a prescribed item?	Yes
Is the item easily removable?	No
Is a flammable gas or vapor present?	No
Does the item produce heat?	Unknown
Alternative	No
Concern	Why does the patient have the ICD? What if the ICD delivers an electrical pulse to restore a normal heart rhythm?
Can the item trap gas?	No
Is a strong odor present?	No
Is the item electrically powered?	Yes – internal battery
Is ESD a concern?	Yes
Does the item contain metal?	Yes, but the device is entirely internal
Is the item made with rubber?	No
Fabric blend or composition	Not applicable
SDS Reviewed	Not applicable
NFPA 99 Reviewed	Yes – no contraindications from *NFPA 99*
FDA Reviewed	Yes – no reported event located
Manufacturer Information Reviewed	Yes

Manufacturer Approved/Prohibited	Approved, but limited
Depth/Time Limitation by Manufacturer	Limited to a depth of 1.5 ATM for no greater than 90 minutes
List of Attachments	Manufacturer literature

Section Three – Finalize

Reason for approving or prohibiting this item for use in the hyperbaric chamber: Prohibiting due to depth and time limitations stated by the manufacturer.
Stipulation or conditions for allowing this item in the hyperbaric chamber: Not applicable.

The use of this item is:

[ ] APPROVED AS-IS

[ ] APPROVED WITH STIPULATIONS

[X] PROHIBITED

Hyperbaric Safety Director: XYZ Name, *XYZ signature*, 12/18/2018 – 1400

Hyperbaric Medical Director: Dr. XYZ Name, *XYZ signature*, 12/18/2018 – 1400

Conclusion

To effectively research and evaluate materials for use in the oxygen-enriched atmosphere of a hyperbaric chamber, the safety director must adopt an attitude of continual learning. As time moves forward, so does new information, codes, and standards. Below is a list of recommended resources for the safety director to consult.

- *NFPA 99, 2018 Edition, Health Care Facilities Code.* Published by the National Fire Protection Association.[1]
- *NFPA 99B, 2018 Edition, Standard for Hypobaric Facilities.* Published by the National Fire Protection Association.[3]
- Food and Drug Administration (FDA). Through the FDA's website (FDA.gov), one can sign up for medical equipment and medication alerts, which are sent via email, to be informed of FDA actions such as product recalls and adverse reactions.[4]
- *Safe Use of Oxygen and Oxygen Systems: Handbook for Design, Operation, and Maintenance, 2nd Edition.* Published by ASTM International.[5]
- *NFPA 53, Recommend Practice on Materials, Equipment, and Systems Used in Oxygen-Enriched Atmosphere.* Published by the National Fire Protection Association.[6]

To make an informed decision, you must know the material and physical properties to understand the concern. Research takes time, but the more you go through the analysis process, the quicker and better you will be. With each evaluation, the investigators will gain new information that may be used for subsequent research projects.

References

1. National Fire Protection Association. NFPA 99, Health Care Facilities Code. 2018 ed. Quincy, MA: National Fire Protection Association; 2017.
2. Undersea & Hyperbaric Medical Society [Internet]. Resources. MEDFAQs. Safety/Technical: Question pertaining to safety and technical information [cited 2018 Nov 30]. Available from: https://uhms.org.
3. National Fire Protection Association. NFPA 99B, Standard for Hypobaric Facilities. 2018 ed. Quincy, MA: National Fire Protection Association; 2017.
4. U.S. Food and Drug Administration [Internet]. Search FDA. Update 2018 December 04. Available from: https://www.fda.gov.
5. Beeson HD, Smith SR, Stewart, WF. Safe Use of Oxygen and Oxygen Systems: Handbook for Design, Operation, and Maintenance. 2nd ed. West Conshohocken, PA: ASTM International; 2007.
6. National Fire Protection Association. NFPA 53, Recommended Practice on Materials, Equipment, and Systems Used in Oxygen-Enriched Atmospheres, 2016 ed. Quincy, MA: National Fire Protection Association; 2015.
7. ASTM G72. Standard Test Method for Autogenous Ignition Temperature of Liquids and Solids in a High-Pressure Oxygen-Enriched Environment [Internet]. Current Edition. Available from https://astm.org.
8. ASTM D4809. Standard Test Method for Heat of ombustion of Liquid Hydrocarbon Fuels [Internet]. Current Edition. Available from https://astm.org.
9. ASTM G125. Standard Test Method for Measuring Liquid and Solid Material Fire Limits in Gaseous Oxidants [Internet]. Current Edition. Available from https://astm.org.
10. WHA International Custom Test [Internet]. Retrieved from https://wha-international.com/.

References

PART 2
A Practical Approach to Hyperbaric Safety

CHAPTER 6
Safety in the Hyperbaric Facility

CHAPTER 6.1
How Accidents Happen

Stephen D. Reimers, PE and Ramesh K. Dixit, PE

Introduction

For some accidents there is a clear "smoking gun." However, most accidents are caused by a combination of factors, each of which contributes in some manner. Often these factors accumulate over some period of time preceding the accident. This chapter addresses the factors that foster conditions under which accidents are more likely to happen and discusses some of the steps to be taken to avoid them. Also included is a case history illustrating several of the factors.

Creating the Necessary Conditions

The factors that commonly contribute to situations favoring accidents can generally be divided into four groups:

- Personnel/management
- Design factors: facility and equipment
- Equipment failure
- Access/tampering

Each of these groups and their constituent factors are discussed in the following sections.

Personnel and Management

When one commences a task to reconstruct how an accident happened, personnel and management factors are often "at the head of the class." Some of the more commonly occurring factors are discussed in this section. It should be noted, however, that this list is not all-inclusive. The factors that can contribute to accidents are many and varied. As technology and operations become ever more complex, our ability to create new ways to "do ourselves in" are amazing.

Operator Fatigue

This factor is one of the more common ones. When people get tired, their level of attention to what they are doing decreases. Especially vulnerable is the level of appreciation for hazards that cannot be seen. Reflexes and fine motor control deteriorate and sloppiness increases. People become capable of doing stupid things that, when rested, they would never do. Necessary maintenance and other jobs that don't have immediate necessity also tend to get skipped over. Operator fatigue seems like such an obvious risk factor that everyone in a managerial position should be constantly on the watch for it. However, operator energy is also a limiting factor in the ever-present drive to cut costs and increase productivity. Many employees, as they are asked to do more, will try to keep up until finally they crack, quit, or do something foolish. This is an area where safety and economy are natural competitors, and managerial personnel need to be constantly on the alert for signs that operational personnel are being asked to do more than they can be reasonably expected to do without excessive fatigue or stress.

Boredom and Inattention

This risk factor is almost the opposite of operator fatigue. Operators on long watches at stations where there is little to do have a tendency to invent things to occupy their minds. This can create a situation where the early warning signs of an impending problem can go unnoticed until a situation has deteriorated to a point where recovery is difficult. Warning devices are helpful. A typical example of such a device is the washboard surface that is now commonly added to the shoulders on interstate highways. Whenever possible, a better approach is to design the mental workload for a given position so that the person's brain has enough to do to keep it alert. Requiring nonrepetitive voice communications is one remedy that is effective in this area. Students at a boring lecture often perk up smartly when asked to raise their hand in response to a question.

Inappropriate Operator Response to an Otherwise Manageable Problem

This factor is closely related to the following one. Many unexpected situations in the hyperbaric environment do not require an immediate response. The best response is often to DISTURB NOTHING, THINK, and then ACT. If one has a blowout while driving, often the worst possible thing to do is to brake strongly. The same is often true in hyperbarics. The best procedure is usually to stabilize the situation, determine the problem, assess possible corrective actions and their risks, and then proceed. In many situations, 50% or more of the solution to a problem is a correct determination of what the problem is.

Some years ago, two divers died of hyperthermia in a North Sea commercial saturation diving operation. The facility operator was monitoring a depth gauge that could be connected to any one of several compartments in the facility. The operator was somehow under the belief that the gauge was connected to the diving bell where the divers were when it was, in fact, connected to one of the deck chambers. The deck chamber developed a large leak. Thinking the bell was losing pressure, the operator added helium to the bell at an ever-higher rate. The comfort zone in a helium environment is very narrow due to its very high thermal conductivity. By the time the operator realized his error, the bell had been quickly pressurized several hundred feet of seawater and the resulting temperature increase in the bell proved lethal to both divers. There were several accident factors at work in this case. However, chief among them was an operator response that was inappropriate to the problem.

Failure to Practice Emergency Responses

This risk factor has two faces: personnel and equipment.

Personnel who have not practiced an emergency situation have a higher probability of an inappropriate response than those who have. Some unpracticed operators will freeze and do nothing until the time window for situation-saving action has passed. A useful example is a beginner automobile driver and a slippery road. Many drivers on their first loss-of-traction experience will either freeze and do nothing or brake. Both responses usually do a fine job of turning a modest sideslip of the rear wheels into a full-fledged spin. The driver who has practiced a few deliberate spins on a snow-covered parking lot has a much better chance of keeping the car on the road.

Using emergency equipment during practice drills has a twofold advantage. First, the operators get used to the "feel" of the equipment. Secondly, the equipment gets much needed "exercise." This is particularly true of hyperbaric fire suppression systems, which are high-performance equipment expected to work flawlessly after long periods of idleness. It is not surprising that as the length of idleness increases, the probability of flawless performance decreases.

Pressure to Meet Deadlines and Quotas

Deadlines and quotas are an unavoidable part of life. The pressure to meet them is generally proportional to the perceived cost of missing them. However, rarely is a deadline worth the price of an accident. The same can be said of quotas. In both cases, management personnel need to carefully monitor their staff for warning signs of fatigue and other risk factors. It is also important for management to create an environment where staff personnel feel safe reporting to superiors when they feel they are being asked to do more than they feel they can safely do.

Outright Operator Stupidity

Given enough operations by enough people, eventually someone will do something consummately dumb. Typical examples are a "gas king" on a saturation diving system sending pure inert gas to a diver and a pilot taking off with too much weight or too little fuel in the airplane. Sometimes, there are steps that can be taken ahead of time to mitigate the effects of these types of errors. In the early days of saturation diving, the inert gas supplies (usually helium) were kept as pure gas. Subsequently, operators have found that a much better practice is to make certain that their inert gas stores always contain a small amount of oxygen, typically about 2%. In that way, if a gas king makes a bad mistake, the results are embarrassing but not disastrous.

Disabled or Unused Safety Devices

Nearly everybody knows someone who doesn't use seat belts when driving their car. Most such people have never been in an accident. Safety devices cost money and sometimes get in the way. However, they always have a purpose. In the author's case, the use of a seat belt once made the difference between disaster and an exciting ride when he was run off a road at 50 mph and had to dodge a series of obstacles. To be effective, safety devices must be used, and that use often requires disciplined action. An atmosphere where the time and effort required to maintain and use safety devices is encouraged does not accidentally occur. It has to be nurtured by management.

Inadequate Training

Proper and sufficient training is one of the major contributors to a safe operation. Hyperbaric operations can appear deceptively simple. However, the consequences of a significant operational error can easily be disastrous. Keeping "cool" when things are going well is rarely difficult. When ugly surprises come along, a properly trained operator will have a much better chance of maintaining control. Training in this sense means having a fundamentally sound understanding of what is going on as well as simple action-reaction training.

Inadequate Staffing/Management Pressure to Cut Costs

The pressures to cut costs and increase revenues that are typical of today's health care environment can easily lead to many of the risk factors discussed in this chapter. What is safe and reasonable in any given situation is up to the judgment of the facility safety director and/or other persons in positions of responsibility. National Fire Protection Association, *NFPA 99, Health Care Facilities Code,* Chapter 14: Hyperbaric Facilities (section 14.3.1)[1] and its subsection describe the role of facility safety director in such situations.

Overcrowding

Loading any machine beyond its design capacity is rarely a good idea. Yet reports of accidents involving overloaded vehicles are commonplace. Exceeding the design population of a chamber is no different. Most chambers are designed to support a maximum number of persons, and this number should not be exceeded. Exceeding the design population means people will be present in the chamber in places the system designers did not expect them to be. This can sometimes lead to surprising consequences as the case study presented later in this chapter will illustrate. Exceeding the design population also creates air conditioning demands that the chamber air conditioning system may not be able to adequately support. Most chambers also have a fixed number of breathing devices for use by the chamber occupants in the event of a fouled atmosphere in the chamber. The number of occupants should *never* exceed the number of available breathing devices.

Failure to Respect Known Hazards

A popular phrase that is applicable here is, "Familiarity breeds contempt." This is particularly true in clinical hyperbarics where chamber pressures are expressed in terms of atmospheres (ATA) or pounds per square inch (PSIG). A pressure expressed as 2 ATA or its psig equivalent, 14.7 PSIG, does not seem like a large number, especially when compared to the 3,000 PSIG pressures typical of self-contained underwater breathing apparatus (SCUBA) cylinders. However, the total force exerted over any significant area can be enormous and must be respected. The following "Volkswagen Rule" can be helpful in fostering an understanding of the magnitude of the total forces involved at normal therapeutic pressures:

14.7 pounds per square inch (1 atm) times an area of 144 square inches (1 sq. foot) = 2,116 pounds force

or more simply:

1 atm x 1 square foot > 1 ton force

The concept of 1 ton of force is sometimes hard to grasp, especially by non-technical personnel. In such cases, the following paraphrase is often helpful:

1 atm differential equates to a force equal to the weight of approximately 1 Volkswagen Beetle per square foot.

The total area of a 30-inch diameter door is 4.91 square feet (706 square inches). Consequently, the effect of releasing the latches on an outward opening door with a pressure of only 1 PSIG still in the chamber is the same as releasing the latches on the door with an angry giant on the other side trying to throw the door open with a force of over 700 pounds. A sudden "loss of pressure" of 1 PSIG is rarely a risk for a person inside a chamber. However, a suddenly accelerating door can do a fine job of flinging a careless outside operator a considerable distance. The resulting landing is never graceful and nearly always painful.

Doors that open with pressure are required by most pressure vessel codes to be fitted with interlocks that prevent the following:

a) the vessel from being pressurized unless the door latches are fully engaged

b) the door latches from being released prior to the complete release of pressure from the vessel

The hardware required to implement the above two interlock requirements may be different for each of the two cases. The presence of such interlocks is of significant importance, and they need to be well maintained.

Contraband Smuggled by Patients

In recent years, this factor has been the leading cause of chamber fires and is the primary cause in at least six known fatal chamber fires. Usually, the "contraband" has been a pocket warmer, such as the conventional type (butane lighter inside a metal cage) or a more recent implementation (sealed pouch filled with iron filings). When the pouch is opened to allow oxygen and moisture to reach the iron, heat is produced as a result of oxidation of the iron. Both types, when taken into an oxygen-enriched atmosphere, can quickly produce sufficient heat to start the pocket they are residing in on fire. Another fatal fire was caused by a toy pistol with a spark-generating flint. The pistol was carried into a chamber by a small boy who later ignored pleas from the outside operators not to use it. Yet another was caused by a diver who was taken into a chamber unconscious from decompression sickness. The diver woke up at depth and decided he needed to light a cigarette that he still had in a pocket.

Chamber operators must explain the "do's and don'ts" of what can be safely carried into a chamber to all personnel. However, even with that, some form of confirmation is warranted. Some facilities require the wearing of chamber clothes that are nearly 100% cotton and pocketless. There are additional safety measures that can be put in place by the facility staff to enhance the safety of overall care, such as metal detectors, patient searches, etc.

Incapacitated or Absent Operators

The risk of an incapacitated chamber operator is a hazard that is always present but rarely happens. However, chamber operations should always be designed in such a way that there are other personnel immediately available who could take over should an operator become incapacitated.

More real is the risk of an operator that is distracted or absent from the room. Modern chambers can maintain pressure nicely for long periods of time without operator attention. Operators can sometimes develop a strong need to make a visit to the local bathroom. Procedures and personnel need to be in place for such situations and other events that may require the primary chamber operator to leave the room while the chamber is in use.

Design Factors: Facility and Equipment

The second largest group of factors that may contribute to an accident are design factors. These factors can be like bandits waiting for the right set of circumstances to come along. These factors are typically ones that promote operational mistakes or increase the potential severity of simple miscues such as a fall. The factors discussed in this section, as in the previous section, are not all-inclusive. Operational personnel need to be constantly on the lookout for conditions that appear capable of promoting an accident.

Controls/Indicators that Lie or Confuse

One group of "equipment factors" that are commonly found in accident reconstruction is controls or indicators that encourage an operator to make an error. These factors can appear in an endless variety of forms. Designers, operators, and safety directors should constantly be on the lookout for them and fix them when found. Too often, the presence of such factors is known, but personnel make the decision, either deliberately or by default due to inaction, to make allowances for them and proceed. Some of the more common forms of this factor are described below.

- **Switchable chamber pressure (depth) gauges:** The idea of a highly accurate master gauge that could be switched to any one of several chambers in a large saturation diving system was popular at one time. However, the presence of a switchable gauge carries with it the need for clear and unmistakable indication of the chamber to which it is connected.
- **Multiple or inconsistent gauge scales:** Many gauges, especially pressure gauges, come with dual scales. Scales of pounds per square inch (PSIG) and kilo-pascal (kPa) are a common pairing. Often the scales are different colors and one is clearly "dominant" over the other from a visual viewpoint. When such gauges are used, care should be taken to make sure that the scales in all gauges in the facility have the same general arrangement. Operators quickly get used to reading the scale that they prefer. If suddenly a gauge comes along that has the scales reversed, operators are highly likely to read the scale in the place on the gauge where they are accustomed to looking or in the color they are used to reading. Some years ago, a commercial airliner ran out of fuel at 37,000 feet over Canada because the fuel level in the tanks had been measured in liters and reported in gallons.
- **Multiple devices on chamber pressure (depth) gauges:** Chamber pressure gauges are highly accurate devices that are often at the end of a long, small, diameter tube. Under normal circumstances that arrangement works fine. However, if a leak develops near the gauge end of the line, the resulting flow through the line is often sufficient to generate a pressure drop in the line large enough to cause seriously erroneous gauge readings. *ASME PVHO-1-2016*, section 4-9.4.3[2] requires that chamber pressure gauge lines have a diameter of not less than 0.12 inches (3 mm) and that the lines to chamber pressure gauges are not shared by other devices.

Alarms with High Rate of Nuisance Alarms

Alarms that go off frequently without due cause are annoying. If the situation persists, the usual result is that the alarms are soon disabled and the supervision capability they were intended to provide is lost. To be effective, alarms must be set so that they have real meaning yet leave enough margin so that they do not require instantaneous or precipitous action. A common method of implementing this is to have two levels of alarm condition. The first one is a warning level requiring assessment of the situation but not necessarily corrective action. The second level, reached only after passing the first level, is an action level requiring some form of response by the facility operators.

Absence of Appropriate Safety Devices

This is a very good way to encourage an accident. Safety devices that are sometimes overlooked in hyperbaric facilities include the following:

- Appropriately sized relief valves downstream from pressure reducing regulators. Too often relief valves are sized on the basis of, "If the line size is one inch, then a one-inch relief valve should be okay." Instead, the relief valves located downstream of pressure-reducing regulators need to be sized for a full-open failure of the upstream regulator at maximum possible supply pressure. In many circumstances, this can result in a relief valve that is several sizes larger than the nominal size on the line it is installed on. Positive means of avoiding inadvertent mixing of outlet gases or the back-feeding of one supply gas into another in circuits where one outlet can be switched between multiple inlets should be taken.
- Reverse pressure relief on doors that can be dogged closed.
- Relief valves between every pair of stop valves on lines that may contain liquefied gases. Any segment of a piping systems where a cryogenic liquid can possibly become trapped must have a relief valve.

"Temporary" Hookups that Never Get Cleaned Up

While this is just good housekeeping, in older facilities, the number of "dead" lines can be surprising. Such lines lead to clutter and confusion, especially if they no longer appear on facility drawings, and should be removed. Unneeded equipment still in place was a contributing factor to the accident discussed in the case history at the end of this chapter.

Room Pressure Relief and the Effects of Gas Discharges

The need for attention to the possibility of overpressurizing or underpressurizing the room housing the chamber (room barotrauma) is discussed in Chapter 4.2: Piping Systems.

However, the effects on room gas composition of gas discharges from the facility also need to be considered. A typical portable liquid oxygen cylinder contains the equivalent of 4,500 standard cubic feet (scf) oxygen. That much oxygen released into a chamber room that is 20 ft wide by 40 ft long by 10 ft high (8,000 cubic ft total volume) would raise the oxygen fraction in the room to over 50% by volume, a very dangerous level. Such a discharge is unlikely when the facility is in operation because the noise would be noticed. However, an improperly tightened connection can easily discharge the entire contents of a liquid cylinder over a weekend or overnight. This is why oxygen cylinders are required by *NFPA 99*, Chapter 5 to be stored in vented rooms. *NFPA 99*, Chapter 14 (section 14.2.1.6)[1] requires the storage and handling of nonflammable gases in a hyperbaric facility to conform to *NFPA 99*, Chapter 5 and Chapter 11 rules. This requirement is located in the Administration and Maintenance section of *NFPA 99*, Chapter 14.

Similar care needs to be taken any time inert gases, such as nitrogen used for dilution purposes, are introduced into a hyperbaric facility. Here the risk is not one of fire but rather one of risk to personnel if significant quantities of the inert gas are accidentally released. For example, if nitrogen purging is employed in a chamber, consideration must be given to the effect on the oxygen level in the chamber should a purge line be left running overnight in an almost closed chamber.

Patient Handling Provisions

In many facilities, the biggest safety risk is not fire, high oxygen, structural failure, or any of the other well-known hazards of hyperbaric operations. It is the risk of back injuries to personnel from handling patients. A related risk is the risk of losing control of a patient. It is easily recognized that asking two 90-pound nurses to move a comatose 300-pound patient into a 60-inch diameter chamber where no one can stand erect is not a good idea unless a very effective patient handling system in place. The nature of patient handling operations is such that similar, although not so extreme, conditions can easily occur in many facilities given the right set of circumstances. Facility safety directors must be aware of the capabilities and limitations of their facility in this regard and be continually alert to avoid situations that place patients and/or staff at risk. Necessary guidelines may need to be established ahead of time in order to prevent personnel from being placed in situations with a high degree of risk.

Personnel Hazards

- **Head-crackers:** Fire suppression nozzles protruding from the ceiling in a small chamber can make business for the local emergency room physician. So can a variety of other devices. The author at one time observed a chamber fire suppression header where the nozzles had been turned to an ineffective orientation in order to reduce the risk to the attendants' heads. This situation was quickly corrected and the "head-cracker" hazard eliminated by making an acrylic shroud for the fire suppression header with appropriately placed holes for the nozzles. Head-cracker hazards are best eliminated at the design stage. However, if encountered in service, most such hazards can be mitigated by properly designed covers or guards.

- **Trip hazards:** Trip hazards are, as their name implies, things that can easily catch feet. Door sills are unavoidable in many chambers. However, uneven floors and other protrusions that can be eliminated should be corrected. If a trip hazard cannot be eliminated, it should be marked.
- **Impalement hazards:** Impalement hazards are items that can do bodily injury if someone should fall on them. Such hazards are not common, but do occur. If found, corrective action should be taken.
- **Grab hazards:** Any item in a chamber that is placed such that a person who has lost his balance could reach for it to steady himself should be strong enough to not pull loose under the load.

Excessively Noisy Environments

Excessive noise interferes with communications and contributes to fatigue. The hard, smooth surfaces typical of chamber interiors tend to make them highly reverberant enclosures. This can amplify any noise that is generated inside the chamber. The principal noise sources in most chambers are the pressurization and exhaust lines and the fans used for air conditioning. Effective mufflers are necessary on *both* supply and exhaust lines. Air conditioning fans and related equipment also need to be selected for minimum noise generation.

Maintenance Impediments

Maintenance is important. However, medical hyperbaric facilities are also expected to operate nearly continuously. Maintenance that cannot be done easily tends to be maintenance that doesn't get done. Some typical examples follow.

- **Fire systems that cannot be tested without deluging the chamber:** It is recommended that fire suppression systems (FSS) be exercised at full capacity at least once every six months. *NFPA 99,* (section 14.3.4.3.5)[1] now requires such a test at least semiannually. It has been shown repeatedly that FSS that are not exercised regularly may not work when called upon. However, if exercising the FSS means pouring large quantities of dirty, rusty water into a clean medical chamber that is difficult to restore to a clean state, it is not difficult to understand why operating personnel will try to find any reason possible to avoid such an event. *NFPA 99* (section 14.3.4.3.5.2)[1] specifically permits a deluge bypass test in lieu of wetted test if bypass system is installed. Bypass deluge test allows the maintenance test water to be discharged outside the chamber and therefore less time consuming. The use of such bypass provisions is encouraged. Another alternative for smaller chambers is the attachment of a hose leading out of the chamber to each nozzle or nozzle base.
- **Absence of access:** Filters and other devices requiring periodic maintenance must be accessible with reasonable effort. Effective service access for compressors

may require both personnel access and access for necessary lifting devices. Consoles need to be designed and positioned such that maintenance access to internal items is provided.

- **Redundancy and downtime limitations:** All compressors require periodic maintenance and sometimes emergency repairs. The same is true of many other components. However, downtime is expensive. Maintenance and repair functions are more easily and reliably carried out if the facility has been designed with sufficient redundancy so that necessary maintenance can be done without taking the facility out of service.

Controls Subject to Inadvertent Activation

Controls subject to accidental operation can easily contribute to an accident situation. If such controls are found, appropriate corrective action should be taken. Typical examples follow.

- **Fire suppression deluge controls:** Toggle style and push-button controls should be fitted with protective covers.
- **Controls for compressors and rotating machinery:** Start-stop controls should be placed where they are not subject to accidental operation. Local lockout switches at each machine are required by most occupational safety organizations so that personnel performing maintenance can be assured that the device cannot be started from remotely located control stations.

Equipment Failure

Serious failures in modern day equipment are not common. Equipment failure factors also are usually obvious once they have occurred. The key safety aspect of this group of factors is prevention. Some of the more common factors are discussed below.

Mechanical/Electrical Failures

Although rare, equipment items do sometimes break even when properly maintained and operated.

Fire

In the context of this discussion, a fire originating in chamber-related equipment is considered to be an equipment failure.

Omitted Maintenance

Nearly everyone knows someone who had to buy a new engine for their car because they forgot to check the oil level regularly or someone who spoiled a tire because they failed to maintain adequate tire pressure. Omitted maintenance is a leading cause of equipment failure. One of the best ways to encourage personnel to go to the time and trouble of performing necessary maintenance is to be able to provide a few examples of what has happened in situations where maintenance has been omitted. Typical examples follow.

- **Filters:** Filters are usually placed in systems because there is a realistic chance of contamination at the location of the filter. Filters not inspected regularly can load up with contamination. The result can be blockage of the line or collapse of the filter element or both.
- **Fire suppression systems:** Hyperbaric chamber FSS are high performance equipment expected to sit idle for long periods of time, then work perfectly when called upon. This will happen reliably only if necessary, maintenance is regularly performed. Following the fatal chamber fire in Italy in 1998 where the facility had a nonfunctional FSS, many other hyperbaric facilities took a closer look at their own systems. Two deluge systems were found to be nonfunctional. One had a line blocked with sludge. The other had a deluge control valve that was stuck.
- **Air compressors:** High-pressure compressors (2,000 PSIG and up) are almost all of an oil-lubricated design. If not adequately maintained, the internal temperatures can easily rise to the point where partial oxidation of the lubricating oil occurs and carbon monoxide gas is produced. Nearly all such machines are fitted with filter systems that include a Hopcalite catalyst that oxidizes carbon monoxide to carbon dioxide. The oxidation reaction is highly exothermic. Some such compressors have been known to *generate enough carbon monoxide to cause the downstream Hopcalite catalyst converter to melt.* In another case, a worn oil-free compressor with a closed distance piece design once passed enough oil to contaminate a large portion of a hospital medical air system. Local management, however, resisted replacing the compressor until it exploded during a test run subsequent to cleaning of the system

Wear and Simple Old Age

Hyperbaric facilities don't have many components where wear is a problem, but they do have some. The U.S. Navy Experimental Diving Unit (NEDU) once had a yoke-type clamp on a carbon dioxide scrubber housing fail during a test run prior to a dive. There were no injuries. However, the scrubber lid demolished an air conditioning duct and bent a major roof beam before coming to rest. The clamp had failed due to accumulated wear. Soft goods (O-rings, gaskets, etc.) do lose some of their vital properties as they age. Periodic inspections will usually detect wear and soft goods deterioration prior to an accident condition developing provided the inspections are thorough enough to look in all the necessary places. The problem one is watching for is rarely the one that causes an incident. The problems usually come from places that aren't being watched.

Contaminated Systems

Systems can become contaminated in a variety of ways. Some examples include the following:

- **Leftovers from initial construction:** This is a very common problem. The bigger the system, the more likely this situation is to occur.
- **Water and corrosion products accumulating in air systems:** Air, when compressed, cannot hold as much moisture as it can when uncompressed. The result is that in most climates, liquid water is a normal byproduct of air compression. If this water is not removed, it will collect in the downstream piping where it promotes corrosion. Over time, the accumulated water and corrosion products can damage the sensitive components and sometimes block lines.
- **Bottle exchanges:** Where systems use bottle exchanges, such as systems purchasing oxygen in standard high-pressure bottles, the system is opened every time a bottle is changed. Each opening provides an opportunity for contamination either from the local environment or from contamination carried in with the new bottle. Care should be taken to maintain a clean environment in the bottle change area. Care should also be taken to inspect each incoming bottle for contamination.
- **Oil in compressor discharge air:** This is a classic form of system contamination. It is especially dangerous in a medical air system since oil in medical air has been observed to cause some ventilators to fail without triggering their built-in alarms.

Access/Tampering

Prevention of Sabotage/Malicious Mischief

Facilities should be provided with sufficient access control so that unauthorized persons do not have access to vital facility controls either during operating hours or at other times. During off-hours, access to the entire facility should be controlled. Surveillance may be desirable for normally unoccupied, sensitive areas.

Segregation of Operator and Patient Areas.

Control areas should be segregated from patient traffic areas.This reduces the chances of operators being distracted by patients. It also reduces the opportunities for curious patients to do something they shouldn't.

The Antidote: Constant Vigilance

As our technology and operations get more sophisticated, we continually invent new ways to do ourselves in. What is the antidote?

- Adequate staffing
- Properly trained staff
- Facility layouts that manage traffic patterns well
- Well-designed equipment
- Maintenance done on a timely basis
- Practicing of emergency responses. Do not act in haste.
- All personnel constantly on the alert for that strange new condition/situation that just doesn't seem right.
- Well-identified responsibilities, including a safety director (required by *NFPA 99*, 14.3.1.3.2)[1] with adequate training and meaningful authority.

Case History: Blown Chamber Door and Suction Injury, Nedu, 1970

Background

During the summer of 1970, Mr. Stephen Reimers, a co-author of this chapter, was a young Lieutenant, Junior Grade at the U. S. Navy Experimental Diving Unit (NEDU) in Washington, DC. Not long before he had earned the designators of Salvage Diving Officer and Saturation Diving Officer. He wore his diver's insignia, a diving helmet cradled

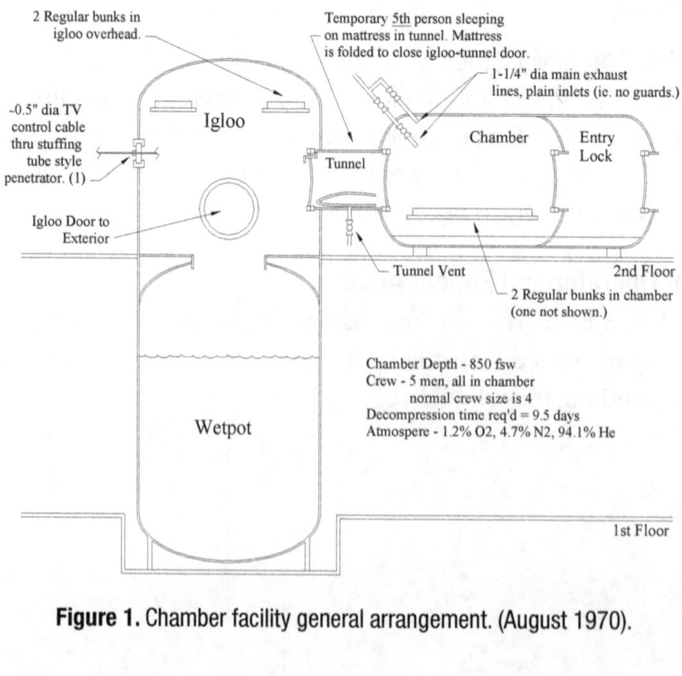

Figure 1. Chamber facility general arrangement. (August 1970).

by a pair of dolphins, with pride. NEDU had two saturation diving complexes called Complex 5 and Complex 6, both rated for saturation diving at depths up to 1,000 feet seawater (33 atmospheres). Both complexes were arranged approximately as shown in Figure 1. Both complexes had been originally built in 1942 and extensively updated. However, their original 1942 technology remained evident in many places and would become a contributing factor to this story. Complexes 1 through 4 were at the U. S. Navy School of Diving and Salvage, which shared the same building.

In 1967, NEDU experienced a disastrous fire in the chamber compartment of Complex 6 that resulted in the deaths of the two divers who happened to be in the chamber compartment at the time. Two other members of the four-men diving team were in the igloo at the time the fire broke out and escaped injury by jumping into the wet pot, which at the time was full of water. Complex 6 had been restored to service only shortly before Stephen's arrival in the fall of 1969. Memories of the 1967 fire were still fresh in the minds of many of the NEDU personnel, several of whom had been stationed there at that time of the fire. At the time, the U.S. Navy was pushing hard, as were many of the other navies of the world, to expand the depths at which divers could operate productively. Complex 5 was being used regularly for deep saturation dives. Complex 6 had been restored to service. However, it was being used primarily for surface-oriented dives, such as diving helmet evaluations and similar functions.

In early 1971, NEDU's parent command, the Naval Sea Systems Command, Office of the Supervisor of Diving and Salvage, tasked NEDU to conduct three saturation dives to 850 fsw in quick succession during the forthcoming summer months. The turnaround time between dives was to be only one week. Also, to permit more testing to be done, the dive crews were to be five persons instead of the usual four. The diving time was desperately needed to support several high priority equipment development programs. The first saturation dive was conducted in Complex 5 without incident. However, during the second saturation dive, both air conditioning system blower fans in the life support system in Complex 5 failed. The use of bootstrap methods of CO_2 removal (large pans of CO_2 absorbent placed wherever there was an available flat surface) permitted the dive to be completed safely without missing any of its assigned objectives. The only way to be ready to perform the third dive on schedule was to shift to Complex 6. The complex was fully operational but had not been used for a long-term saturation dive since the 1967 fire.

The Dive

This particular dive was scheduled for one day of compression time, seven days bottom time at 850 feet seawater, and approximately 9 1/2 days of decompression time. The dive was plagued from the beginning with a variety of minor technical problems, mostly related to the underwater breathing apparatus that was being tested and its supporting equipment. Several weeks of nearly continuous, round-the-clock operations had made the crew weary and forced the postponement of all but the most essential repairs. However, most of the objectives of the dive were being met.

The first problem directly related to this tale was a television cable that had been installed to support a video camera in the overhead of the igloo. See Figure 1. The video camera had been removed, but the supporting cable had been left in place. The cable was about 0.5 inches in diameter with many small wires in it. It was passed through the pressure boundary of the igloo via a "stuffing tube" style penetrator that had been installed in a steel blank located in a viewport housing. The stuffing tube employed a rubber insert that was compressed against the cable's outer jacket to make a seal and hold the cable against the hydrostatic force tending to eject the cable from the chamber. Early on a Sunday afternoon, the cable extruding out through the stuffing tube. About 10 inches had been forced out when the situation was first discovered, and the displacement was continuing at the rate of about $^{1}/_{16}{}^{th}$ inch per hour. This created a dangerous situation. Provisions were available to deal with a complete severance of the cable. However, if the cable were to shred, it would create a major leak that there would be no way to stop short of surfacing the igloo.

At that time, the NEDU wet pots had no water filtration system and no way to change the water with the chamber under pressure. Every third day, the igloo and wet pot were returned to surface pressure for a water change and replenishment of needed supplies. This necessitated moving the entire dive team into the chamber for the duration of the replenishment operation. The chamber made for cramped quarters for five persons, so the outside (topside) crew always tried to complete the replenishment operation as quickly as possible.

The wet pot was due for surfacing for a water change and replenishment that evening. The decision was made to terminate diving operations early to allow time to deal with the stuffing tube situation during the replenishment cycle. The repair was made by removing the entire stuffing tube/blank viewport assembly and replacing it with a glass viewport of the type that had been originally installed. However, that change represented a change to the structural integrity of the igloo. The practice in such a case was to require a pressure integrity/leak test prior to resuming manned operations.

To test the window replacement, it was decided to pressurize the igloo to 1,000 feet of seawater (fsw) using the usual procedure of pressurizing the first 200 ft with pure helium and the rest of the way with compressed air. This was a predive pressure integrity check commonly used at the time. It put enough helium content in the atmosphere to expose any significant helium leaks yet was economical regarding the amount of helium consumed. With the chamber at 850 fsw, pressurizing the igloo to 1,000 fsw would require the igloo pressure to "pass" the pressure level in the chamber. Since the tunnel had doors at both ends, this appeared to be a simple maneuver.

The chamber-tunnel door was already closed. With chamber pressure holding the chamber-tunnel door shut, the dogs (e.g., latches) for the door had been released. The dogs were designed such that the gravity pull on the handles would cause them to release automatically once a pressure differential was established across the door. As a pressure differential was established across a door, the door seal would compress and release the restraint load on the dogs. The heavily weighted handles would then rotate the dogs to their "released" position automatically. Usually this worked as intended. However, rotation of the dogs to the release position sometimes had required a manual assist, especially if the dogs had been tightly set to overcome a leaky door seal.

To begin the pressure test of the igloo, the igloo-tunnel door had to be closed as well. However, to close the igloo-tunnel door, it had been necessary to do something with the mattress for the fifth diver that had been normally residing in the tunnel. This was accomplished by folding the mattress over. (See Figure 1 for detail.) The seemingly innocent move completed the creation of the conditions necessary to produce the incident that occurred a few minutes later. Following closure of the igloo-tunnel door and other necessary preparations, pressurization of the igloo to 1,000 fsw commenced.

The tunnel, which was intended only for transit use, had no dedicated pressure gauge, but it did have a vent line, nominally ¼ in size. Further, the crew knew that getting doors on this complex with their 1942 seal designs to seal completely was difficult. The dogs on the igloo-tunnel door had been set as tightly as possible, since there would be no one in the igloo to adjust them if the door did not seal well. The crew monitored the gas flow out of the tunnel vent as the igloo was pressurized towards 1,000 fsw. Initially, there was a fair amount of gas flow, then it subsided to a negligible level as the igloo passed 200 fsw. Thinking a complete seal had been obtained on the igloo-tunnel door, the order was given to proceed to 1,000 fsw. What was not known was that the mattress in the tunnel had unfolded slightly, just enough to cover the opening to the vent line located on the bottom of the tunnel. The heavy vinyl cover of the mattress sealed the opening to the vent line. Meanwhile, a complete seal had *not* been achieved on the igloo-tunnel door. The pressure in the tunnel increased nearly as rapidly as did the pressure in the igloo with the topside crew comfortable in their belief that the tunnel was remaining steady at nearly atmospheric pressure.

A few minutes later, the pressurization of the igloo/wetpot was stopped at 900 fsw to check for leaks prior to proceeding to the final test pressure 1,000 fsw. While the igloo was 900 fsw, the leakage into the tunnel allowed the tunnel pressure to pass 850 fsw and the un-dogged chamber-tunnel door swung slightly open to looks of disbelief on the parts of the dive team and topside crew. No gas was coming out of the open tunnel vent, and there should have been *192 tons* of force holding the 36" diameter chamber-tunnel door shut. Yet it opened by itself. Was this some sort of divine intervention? What we were confident of, however, was that the gas on the tunnel side of the door wherever it had come from, was likely to be the same predominantly air mix that was in the igloo, and air is not a good choice for use as a breathing gas at 850 fsw (26.8 ATA). At this point, several actions were taken in quick succession.

- The order was given to commence a "vent" in the chamber with pure helium immediately. Venting the chamber was accomplished by opening the exhaust line and maintaining pressure with the supply line. In 1971, the NEDU chamber, like most military hyperbaric chambers at the time, did not have mufflers on the supply and exhaust lines. Consequently, venting the chamber produced enough noise (well over 100 decibels (dBA)) to make normal voice communications with the dive team impossible.

- The order was given to surface the igloo.
- One of the dive team members moved to push the chamber-tunnel door shut.

Meanwhile, as the diving officer, Stephen Reimers watched the oxygen monitor for the chamber, knowing it would tell him how much air had leaked into the chamber. The needle was heading upscale but not at a fast rate. About this time two more "events" occurred.

- A loud "boom," accompanied by a perceptible vibration in the building floor.
- One of the diver crew flopped on the chamber floor in what initially appeared to be convulsions.

Once again, everyone was bewildered. It seemed like things were progressing quickly from bad to worse. Was the entire dive team in serious danger? Everyone kept their composure and took the time to assess the situation before acting. Soon the situation began to stabilize.

1. A large black-blue blister was noticed on the left palm of the dive team member on the chamber floor, indicating physical injury as the cause of his situation, not an oxygen convulsion from an atmosphere heavily contaminated with air. Whatever was ailing the injured diver was unlikely to be a risk for the remainder of the dive team.
2. The indication on the chamber oxygen monitor was observed to be leveling off at about 0.5 ATA pO_2, and the vent was stopped. Stopping of the vent permitted normal voice communications with the dive team to resume. Given the effects of helium on normal speech (helium voice processors in 1971 weren't very good), normal voice communications were not great but better than nothing.
3. The topside crew realized the "boom" had to have been the igloo-tunnel door. The action taken to surface the igloo had reversed the pressure differential on the igloo-tunnel door, which had been securely dogged shut, and the doors were not fitted with reverse pressure relief. A door had "blown."
4. Once communications were restored with the dive team, it was learned the injured diver had managed to place his left hand over the opening to the chamber exhaust during the chamber vent. Given the confusion of the moment, the dive crew had not heard the "standby for vent" warning from topside. The injured diver had long hair and had been sitting directly under the opening to the chamber exhaust line. The flowing gas picked up his hair, and he reached up

> with is left hand to investigate. In the process, he somehow managed to make a nearly perfect seal over the inlet to the 1" diameter exhaust pipe with the palm of his left hand. Fortunately, the exhaust line being used was the 2-valve exhaust that had an internal stop valve. Another team member realized what had happened, closed the internal stop valve, and succeeded in removing the injured diver's hand. The diver had then fell to the chamber floor in intense pain.

Once the situation was stabilized, an assessment was made of the conditions of the dive team and the facility. The main points were as listed below:

1. The injured diver had what could be described as a gigantic blood blister on the palm of his left hand and impaired ability to move the corresponding third and fourth fingers. However, no body parts were found to be broken or missing. The wound was treated as needed and the diver's pain subsided.
2. Once the igloo was returned to surface pressure, the damage to the igloo-tunnel door was assessed. The two dogs farthest from the hinges had been sheared off completely. The two nearest the hinges had been bent. The two bolts fastening the bottom hinge to the chamber were also sheared off. The 2,000 lbs door hinge was being supported by only one of its two hinges! Fortunately, the remaining (upper) hinge had a very robust (over one-inch diameter) hinge pin. Analysis of the loads on the pin confirmed what mother nature had already demonstrated—the single hinge was capable of supporting the door by itself. The door was left as it was. Although the door was damaged, it was still usable in an emergency.

Based on the assessments made, it was determined safe to proceed normally with the remainder of the dive, given that the divers were obligated to 9½ days of decompression time, and there was no other way to get them out of the chamber. From that point on, however, the dive proceeded without incident. Following the conclusion of the dive, the chamber system was repaired and the injured diver eventually regained full use of his hand with no residual impairment.

Following the dive, several recommendations were made for potential hardware changes, notably the following:

- Depth gauges on ALL independently pressurizable compartments, regardless of size
- Suction injury preventers on the inlets to all lines where gas flows out of the chamber

Contributing Factors

Factors that contributed to this incident included the following:

- Operator fatigue from a heavy operations schedule
- Pressure to meeting deadlines and quotas from operational needs

- Overcrowding with five divers in a facility designed for four
- Controls/indicators that lie or confuse, i.e. no depth gauge on the tunnel
- Absence of appropriate safety devices
    - › no reverse pressure relief on the doors
    - › no suction injury preventers on the chamber exhaust lines
- Temporary hook-ups that never get cleaned up, like the leftover television cable
- Excessive noisy environments with the absence of mufflers on the chamber supply
- Exhaust lines
- Equipment failure/malfunction (the leaky igloo-tunnel door)
- Wear and old age (the aging television cable and the age of the door seals)

It is Stephen Reimers' belief this particular dive was the genesis of the currently widely accepted code requirement that all chamber exhaust lines be fitted with suction injury preventers.

Case Report Summary

Lesson learned from this case story is that often there are number of underlying clues indicating something wrong is going to happen. Big accidents or equipment failures are often not caused by a single event but a chain of them. Each one of them narrows your options down to point where failure or accident becomes inevitable. There were a number of contributing factors involved that led to the accident. It is important not to ignore the telltales that often help you understand the nature of accident or equipment failure but follow them to get to the root cause of the problem in order to avoid something bigger from happening.

Acknowledgment

Gratitude is expressed to the U.S. Navy for its permission to make the story of this incident available to the hyperbaric community.

References

1. National Fire Protection Association. NFPA 99 health care facilities code, 2018 ed. Quincy, MA: NFPA; 2018;Chapter 14:99-108 to 99-121.
2. American Society of Mechanical Engineers. ASME PVHO-1-2016 safety standard for pressure vessels for human occupancy, 2016 ed. New York, NY: ASME; 2016.

CHAPTER 6.2
Role of the Hyperbaric Safety Director

Kevin I. "Kip" Posey, CHT and John Posey, CHT

Disclaimer: One of the authors is a member of the National Fire Protection Association's (NFPA) Technical Committee on Hyperbaric and Hypobaric Facilities. The content of this chapter solely reflects the personal opinions of the authors and does not necessarily represent the official position of the NFPA.

The safety director plays a critical role in the operation of a hyperbaric facility, ensuring the facility provides care compliant with national, state, and local safety standards. The first step in your development as the hyperbaric safety director should be to understand your role. The safety director should not be a scapegoat, superhero, know-it-all, or roadblock. The safety director should be an organizer, educator, coach, mentor, and leader of the safety team.

The NFPA, specifically *NFPA 99, Health Care Facilities Code, 2018 Edition,* (Chapter 14: Hyperbaric Facilities)[1] is an excellent resource to set the framework for your facility safety program. NFPA mandates that each hyperbaric facility designates an onsite hyperbaric safety director but does not cite any qualifications for the job. The Undersea and Hyperbaric Medical Society (UHMS), however, offers guidance on safety director qualifications. A comprehensive list of qualifications is included in this chapter and in the *UHMS Guidelines for Hyperbaric Facility Operations 2nd Edition.*[3] The NFPA and UHMS outline specific responsibilities of the safety director and most are addressed in this text. Understanding what is expected of you, your attitude toward your duties, and how you conduct yourself will have a significant impact on your success as safety director.

The title of safety director should not be considered equivalent to a hospital department director position. It is intended as an additional set of safety responsibilities assigned to a technician, nurse, administrator, or physician in the hyperbaric department. The NFPA currently recommends the medical director not serve as the safety director, as it is considered a conflict of responsibilities.[1]

The NFPA lists directly defined responsibilities for the safety director including recognition of hazards, policy development, oversight, maintenance, and documentation. There are also implied responsibilities, including implementation and conformance with applicable sections of *NFPA 99*, Chapter 14.

The NFPA has defined interrelationships between the safety director, hyperbaric medical director, other hyperbaric physicians, and facility management. Specifically, the NFPA requires the safety director and medical director to jointly develop the minimum staff qualifications, experience, and complement based on number and types of chambers, maximum treatment capacity, and the type of therapy normally provided.[1] Staff composition can vary greatly based on the above-mentioned factors. How do we comply with this requirement? You can use the following questions and answers to help you decide the staff qualifications. Are you using multiplace or monoplace chambers? Multiplace chambers have nurses or technicians inside the chamber with the patient(s) and provide direct access to the patient during the hyperbaric treatment. This, in turn, could mean we are able to treat more acutely ill patients. Is your facility an on-call (7 day/24 hour) service available to treat critically ill patients? If yes, you would expect the staff makeup to include critical care nurses, physicians, and other specialized staff such as respiratory therapists. Nonlicensed staff should also have more extensive training and experience in critical-care hyperbarics. On the other hand, if your facility only treats outpatients or is limited to treatment of low-acuity cases, you should not need the same level of staff qualifications to meet your patients' needs. You must, however, be prepared to handle any patient complication or coincidental medical event. Emergency procedures or contingency plans are an integral part of the department's policies and procedures. They should be tailored to fit the specific needs of each department and exercised regularly. Practicing mock patient emergencies is an excellent way to prepare your staff to handle any type of patient complication. Conducting emergency drills is required by the NFPA and the UHMS and must be part of your training and competency programs.

NFPA 99 states the organized medical staff has the responsibility to adopt and enforce regulations with respect to the use of hyperbaric departments located in health care facilities.[1] The medical director of the hyperbaric facility is the obvious choice to lead this effort. The safety director must assist the medical director by making recommendations for safety policies and procedures and by participating in the development of these regulations.

The safety director's relationship with the physician on duty is also discussed in the NFPA standards. The safety director shall have the authority to restrict or remove any potentially hazardous supply or equipment items from the chamber.[1] This authority given to the safety director is one of the most important safety director responsibilities. Creating a go/no-go list of items allowed and prohibited inside the chamber is an ideal way to begin addressing this task. The go/no-go list should include all wound dressings employed in the wound center, linens, patient care items (air-break masks, oxygen hood, etc.), and any other item that might be used inside the chamber. Two important notes: 1) This list will often need to be updated due to the development of new dressings, medication patches, and implantable devices used on patients; 2) Exceptions to the list are allowed. The physician in charge, with the concurrence of the safety director, may use certain prohibited items in the chamber.[1] Chapter 5: How to Determine If a Material Is Safe for Use in the Hyperbaric Chamber in this book is a great resource for addressing and deciding the items on your go/no-go list. The chapter also covers exceptions for use of prohibited items (normally found on the no-go list) inside the chamber. The approval to use prohibited items inside the chamber must be stated in writing and signed by both the physician and safety director. File the exception document in the patient's medical record and put a copy in the operational chamber log. You may also want to file a copy in your safety book. Consider maintaining a master list of reviewed items at the beginning of the safety book to reduce research time. If the exception is going to be permanent, then it should be added to the allowed items in the go/no-go policy. Otherwise, state a specific time the exception expires.

The safety director shall ensure that electrical, monitoring, life-support, protection, and ventilation arrangement in the hyperbaric chamber are inspected and tested as part of the routine maintenance program of the facility.[1] This does not require the safety director to conduct all of these inspections and tests, only ensure they are conducted and documented.

Antistatic procedures, as directed by the safety director, shall be employed whenever atmospheres containing more than 23.5% oxygen by volume are used.[1] These procedures include connecting the chamber occupant(s) to the chamber with a high-impedance conductive pathway in contact with the skin.[1] This device, commonly referred to as the grounding strap, should be tested for continuity prior to each patient treatment. These requirements are generally considered to be specific to static control inside oxygen-pressurized monoplace hyperbaric chambers; however, if a multiplace chamber employs an atmosphere of greater than 23.5% by volume,[1] this requirement would also apply. All chambers are required to be grounded to the building common ground with less than one (1) ohm[1] of resistance between the chamber and the building. This ground should be tested periodically, and some monoplace chamber users test it as often as daily.

The safety director also participates with facility management personnel and the hyperbaric physician(s) to develop procedures for the operation and maintenance of the facility.[1] Documentation of the involvement of all parties can be challenging. Minutes from meetings and signatures verifying review and coordination by each party may be sufficient. Each time a procedure is changed significantly, there should be documentation of involvement by each party.

The safety director should also consider developing relationships with the state/local pressure vessel inspector, local fire marshal, fire department, and emergency medical services providers for your facility. Each individual or group can help the safety director in a number of ways. Depending upon the jurisdiction you are in, pressure vessel inspectors may be required to conduct periodic inspections of your hyperbaric chambers and other pressure vessels. The safety director must be familiar with the code requirements in your jurisdiction. The fire marshall is most involved during the planning, building, and certification of new or renovated facilities. However, he or she may visit your facility at any time. If you develop and cultivate a positive relationship with the fire marshall, you may avoid costly delays with fire code compliance. The fire department and emergency services personnel will respond to any emergency within the department and may be of assistance as you develop your emergency procedures.

The UHMS provides valuable guidance on the role of the safety director. According to the UHMS, the safety director should ensure department compliance with *NFPA 99*, Health Care Facilities, Chapter 14 and with department safety policies and procedures. The safety director should perform the following:

- Review all department safety incidents, collect information regarding equipment and patient safety, report relevant incidents to the staff, and periodically provide in-service training on accident prevention and other safety-related topics.
- Work closely with the medical, nursing, and technical (if assigned) directors to develop and annually review/revise department policies and procedures and operational and maintenance documents.
- Work closely with the program manager to coordinate and approve all hyperbaric chamber upgrades, modifications, and repairs to the hyperbaric system, including interaction with hospital maintenance personnel and outside contractors, to ensure that all maintenance activities are done in accordance with appropriate safety standards.
- Evaluate, test, and sign off any modification or maintenance action before the next patient treatment.
- Evaluate equipment and supplies to ensure they meet all safety requirements before they are permitted inside the chamber.
- Ensure a safe environment in the hyperbaric facility for patients and staff and use approved and recognized decompression procedures for all persons with a hyperbaric exposure to inert gases. The *US Navy Diving Manual* would be one example of an approved and recognized source for decompression procedures.
- Inform personnel of any special work conditions, such as infection control precautions and unique hazards in and around the chamber.
- Serve as one of the hyperbaric facility's technical trainers and provide in-service training related to the various aspects of hyperbaric physiology, decompression requirements, equipment operations, safety, and treatment protocols.
- Validate in-chamber safety training of new staff before their initial entry into the hyperbaric chamber (multiplace only).
- Develop and supervise hyperbaric chamber safety drills.
- Conduct annual review of safety related events to identify trends and monitor improvements.

The safety director and the medical director review and document all safety-related events and present lessons learned to the appropriate staff. Most of these tasks are self-explanatory but require diligence, discipline, organizational and administrative skills to accomplish. The safety director should look to current staff to assist with these duties. Remember, the safety director can delegate authority to accomplish a task but the responsibility for the safety program remains with the safety director.

Safety Director Education and Training

Education and training is an ongoing process and should be a high priority. Start this process by reading and frequently referring to *NFPA 99, Health Care Facilities Code.* There are eighteen specific references in Chapter 14 of the *NFPA 99* related to the safety director. The safety director must be well-versed in the content of Chapter 14 and both Annex A and B. The safety director should be familiar with all the chapters, especially Chapters 3 (Definitions), 5 (Gas and Vacuum Systems), and 11 (Gas Equipment). Consider acquiring the *Health Care Facilities Code Handbook* that accompanies each new edition of the code. The *Handbook* contains the entire code but also has additional commentary not included in the basic code. These comments are written by the Technical Committee on Hyperbaric and Hypobaric Facilities and are included to help in understanding the rationale of a code item or why certain code requirements were added, changed, or deleted. Understanding why code requirements exist should help develop a more global perspective and improve risk management skills. In addition to attending formal training, the safety director should develop a comprehensive library comprised of the books and other documents listed below. This library is not just for good looks but should be read and referenced regularly. The library of a working safety director should be worn, dog-eared, and contain highlights and sticky notes identifying critical chapter and sections.

The safety director will find some useful tools in the annexes of *NFPA 99.* Chapter 14: Annex A, for example, contains a risk assessment process for hyperbaric wound dressings and textiles (A.14.3.1.6.4.3). The flowsheet and detailed explanation give a process to evaluate the risks of using a wound dressing and other new or unknown textiles in the hyperbaric chamber. Annex A also suggests the safety director review other safety, operational, and maintenance criteria of organizations such as the UHMS and Compressed Gas Association (CGA) (A.14.3.1.3.2). Annex B outlines the nature of hazards (B.14.1) and contains suggested procedures for fire inside and outside monoplace and multiplace chambers (B.14.2, B.14.3). Always customize any procedures to fit your specific needs, but these suggested procedures can be useful when developing procedures or comparing them to those in the NFPA code.

Other valuable references include *NFPA 53 Recommended Practice on Materials, Equipment, and Systems Used in Oxygen-Enriched Atmospheres.*[4] This document contains technically complex concepts that can be daunting to even the most experienced hyperbaric personnel. However, it also contains details of fires and explosions from oxygen-enriched environments reported to the NFPA and charts of burning rates and flame spread data of various materials. Learning from mishaps and understanding fire behavior helps the safety director assess the risks within his or her department.

The *Risk Assessment Guide for Installation and Operation of Clinical Hyperbaric Facilities, 5th Edition*[5] is another reference to have on your bookshelf and refer to often. It is the first place to check when questions arise regarding the risks involved in clinical hyperbaric facilities. It addresses the various types of hazards associated with hyperbaric facilities and measures to contain identified risks. It is a user-friendly tool and very helpful to both new and experienced safety directors.

The safety director should also be familiar with the UHMS *Guidelines for Hyperbaric Facility Operations 2nd Edition*[3] and the most current *Hyperbaric Facility Accreditation Manual.*[6] The *UHMS Guidelines for Hyperbaric Facility Operations* is a must-have reference for the safety director and program manager. Guidance on staff qualifications, training, suggested elements of a safety program, a physician credentialing checklist, and job descriptions that can be used as a framework for your documentation are provided. The UHMS expects the safety director to complete at least a 40-credit-hour introductory hyperbaric medicine course approved by the UHMS or National Board of Diving and Hyperbaric Medical Technology (NBDHMT) and a UHMS or NBDHMT-approved hyperbaric safety course. The hyperbaric safety director should be certified by the NBDHMT within one year of assuming the responsibilities of safety director. The safety director should have at least 12 months experience in clinical hyperbaric chamber operations and a working knowledge of all applicable hyperbaric safety codes and decompression procedures before assuming the role as safety director. The UHMS further suggests the safety director attend courses specifically related to operational hyperbaric safety issues. The safety director should also have training and/or experience in hyperbaric chamber maintenance. Consider expanding safety knowledge by including other safety books and training not specifically related to hyperbaric medicine. The hospital safety officer should have resources to help identify additional safety subjects of benefit. *NFPA 101, Life Safety Code* is one such reference the safety director should consider that is not specific to hyperbaric medicine.

What if the entire hyperbaric staff is new with no prior experience? You still need to assign someone the hyperbaric safety director title, then provide this individual with resources and training to fulfill the responsibilities. Ideally, the entire clinical staff is involved in the safety process. It is never one person's responsibility, no matter the title or credential. However, in the case of all new staff, you would be more restrictive about what is allowed inside the hyperbaric chamber until you understand why something is safe. Learning what is allowed or not allowed into the hyperbaric chamber is an unending task because as previously mentioned, there are always new products developed for health care.

The *UHMS Facility Accreditation Manual* is a free download and can be found on the UHMS website in the section titled Hyperbaric Facility Accreditation Program. Even if you are not currently seeking accreditation, you will find this document useful. It contains all the elements UHMS surveyors would use to assess a facility. You can use this information to evaluate your department's compliance with internationally recognized standards or to prepare for an accreditation survey. A number of the items in the accreditation manual directly reference NFPA code. However, other subjects including staff qualifications, training, experience, physician supervision requirements, and much more are covered in the *Guidelines for Hyperbaric Facility Operation* and in the accreditation manual in an organized and functional format.

Guidelines for the care and maintenance of your acrylic windows are available in *PVHO 2 Safety Standard for Pressure Vessels for Human Occupancy: In-Service PVHO Acrylic Windows,*[2] published by the American Society of Mechanical Engineers (ASME). This document has information to protect and prolong the use of your acrylic windows beyond their design life and should be in your reference library.

In 2002, The Joint Commission (TJC) established its National Patient Safety Goals (NPSGs) program. The NPSGs were established to help accredited organizations address specific areas of concern in regard to patient safety. This guidance contains the most up-to-date information on patient safety within health care facilities and should be included in your safety program.

The safety director should also be highly educated in the handling of pressurized gases. Training staff on the proper handling of all pressurized gas systems and the potential for serious injury associated with these systems is a must. The authors strongly believe this is an under-addressed area of safety training. You may refer to the CGA guidance for specific information on safe handling of gases, specifications, and other medical gas information. If the facility has a respiratory care department, it may provide gas safety training. Also, the hospital facilities or maintenance departments may have the responsibility to replace empty high-pressure air and oxygen cylinders. However hyperbaric department staff should also have the proper training to perform these duties. The liquid oxygen system (LOX) also requires attention and the safety director should be familiar with the system. Although the liquid oxygen contractor fills and maintains the system, and the hospital facilities' manager may have overall responsibility for the hospital LOX system, the hyperbaric department is likely the largest single user of oxygen within the hospital. Oxygen, under hyperbaric conditions, is our primary drug. The safety director or designee should inspect the LOX system regularly. Some facilities are equipped with separate LOX systems to serve the hyperbaric facility. In those cases, the safety director should maintain documentation regarding maintenance and repair activities conducted on the system (provided by the hospital facilities' manager) in addition to purity analysis documentation provided by the vendor with each fill of the LOX tank.

Education and professional development are ongoing processes and should include different avenues to help reach goals. Joining professional societies like the UHMS or its counterparts in other countries, such as the European Underwater and Baromedical Society, the South Pacific Undersea Medicine Society, the Southern African Undersea and Hyperbaric Medical Association, and any local chapters of these organizations provides opportunities to access knowledge and experiences of hyperbaric colleagues.

As safety director, you should participate in the hospital safety committee, if possible. Find a mentor such as the hospital safety officer, your program manager, or the corporate safety director if you are part of a corporation to help you develop your skills. You should also be a mentor and work to increase safety awareness in your staff. You may also find yourself mentoring other individuals who have worked for you in the past and moved on to other positions. As you advance in your career, you may want to serve on committees in organizations like the NFPA or the ASME.

More than just safety training is needed to be a successful safety director. You will need to expand your administrative, management, and speaking skills as you may find yourself developing and presenting training materials. More and more documentation is being handled electronically and you will need to stay abreast of the latest technology. Many opportunities exist for you to develop your skill set. Remember, you are not alone. This is a team effort and there are resources available to help you meet your goals.

One of your most important roles as the safety director is staff training. According to the NFPA, it is a responsibility of the governing board of a hospital to ensure rules and regulations exist regarding the practice and conduct in the hyperbaric facility (relative to safety of patients and personnel) and the qualifications and training of personnel. The safety director will be involved in the development of these rules, normally with the assistance of the program manager and medical director. Documentation of these rules will form the basis of the department safety program and policies.

The NFPA offers specific guidance on training department staff. There are also requirements to train maintenance personnel and housekeeping staff. Although not specifically required by code, the safety director should familiarize security and maintenance personnel with special conditions within the hyperbaric department and provide the facility operator an after-hour contact plan. Properly executed contingency plans and rapid notification of department personnel help mitigate the impact of incidents that occur after normal business hours.

Your primary training responsibility is your immediate staff, including physicians, nurses, technicians, administrators, and part-time staff. To paraphrase the NFPA, hazards can only be mitigated when all hazards are fully recognized by all personnel. This is the goal we must strive to meet, and training is the best way to achieve it. Thorough training of all staff is an absolute must, with special consideration to part-time staff. Since part-time staff is typically used as a cost-control measure on an as-needed basis, they may receive less recurring training and therefore be less familiar with the hyperbaric system and emergency procedures. It is obvious we must pay close attention to new staff members when conducting training, but even experienced staff needs refresher training.

Hyperbaric treatments are generally safe with few serious complications. The low incidence of complications can lower staff awareness of potential safety hazards. The safety director should take measures to prevent employees from becoming complacent. Conducting and discussing a variety of mock patient emergency drills and daily safety briefings to staff are two ways to keep staff prepared for all contingencies.

Specific NFPA training requirements include training staff to safely decompress the chamber when powered equipment is inoperative. Multiplace users should drill using backup systems such as manual valves to control the chamber if power or control is lost on the primary system. In the majority of monoplace chambers, the chamber is pressurized with, and the control system is dependent upon, oxygen pressure. If oxygen supply or pressure is lost, you normally have limited or no control of the chamber. You must know how your system will behave and how much control you have if the chamber supply gas is interrupted. Every chamber operator should know the location of every shutoff valve in the chamber gas supply piping system. Most systems will have at least three shutoff valves in the oxygen plumbing. Normally, there will be one near the LOX supply (after it is converted to gas), a zone valve immediately outside the hyperbaric department, and another shutoff valve at the foot of the chamber. During training sessions, you should turn off the supply gas at each shutoff valve (with the other valves open) to determine how the chamber controls are affected. Of course, never close any oxygen valve during training that may affect another department. You may consider adding this skill and troubleshooting to your annual staff competencies.

The NFPA states all personnel must be trained on emergency procedures, with emergency procedures and fire training drills conducted at least annually and documented by the safety director. Consider conducting drills more frequently, especially if you have a new facility or high staff turnover. Conduct and document drills on each one of your emergency procedures at least annually.

What value do we gain from emergency procedure drills other than complying with NFPA code? If drills are realistic and taken seriously, you will gain valuable information about your ability to handle a real emergency. This information can be used to adjust emergency plans and focus your training. Preparation is the key to a calm and accurate response to a real emergency. Drills can be a team-building exercise. Finally, the UHMS accreditation program lists the lack of documented emergency drills as a stand-alone reason to defer a department's accreditation. This is another example of the importance of conducting and documenting emergency drills. You never want to miss a training opportunity. Occasionally you might be able to conduct unplanned training with your staff. Consider the following scenarios. One example is a multiplace hyperbaric facility that rarely has emergent patients yet is on call to treat emergencies. The call team has to respond, but other staff could be asked to also come in, if possible. This will afford more staff the experience of treating the one-off type of patient and retrain or renew skills not often exercised. Any time a treatment is aborted, we must review why it was terminated early, discuss ways to prevent a recurrence, and evaluate the staff response to the event. This is also true for an equipment malfunction that may or may not cause a treatment to be aborted. Routine maintenance and incorporating new equipment into the department are other examples of training opportunities not necessarily on the training schedule. If we have a new device we plan to employ within the wound center and specifically in or around the hyperbaric chamber, consider having the equipment vendor provide as much information as possible about the use and safety of the device. The medical director and safety director obviously must decide if the device is safe to use in or around the chamber(s). More information should result in better decisions and safer practices.

The safety director and medical director should work together to develop department emergency procedures. Refer to Chapter 7: Emergency Procedures for more information and guidance on how to develop them. All staff members who operate the chamber must be trained to handle patient complications. Stopping the chamber during pressurization or depressurization (commonly known as "level off") is the first step during a patient complication or chamber malfunction. Every chamber operator should be able to accomplish this task without delay. All chamber operators should have clear guidance on managing patient complications. Difficulty equalizing pressure in the middle ear is the most common patient complication. Chamber operators should know how to manage this complication and be authorized to take appropriate action to alleviate the condition. Nonlicensed operators should be given specific guidance on how and when to manage this patient complication, and when to halt the treatment and contact the physician or nurse. Annual emergency drills are mandatory, but chamber operator knowledge of the system and understanding of how and when to act are key to proper handling or prevention of patient complications.

The NFPA states all personnel, including those involved in maintenance and repair of the hyperbaric facility, shall be trained on the purpose, application, operation, and limitations of emergency equipment. The safety director is the obvious choice to plan and conduct this training, but what does it entail? You may include the location of personal protective equipment, oxygen and medical air zone valves, electrical breaker boxes, fire extinguishers, and fire pull stations. How much you train your hospital support staff is up to you, but you must consider staff turnover and have a plan to efficiently train new staff. This often requires the safety director to develop a one-one-one relationship with managers of other departments to be kept aware of changes and train these personnel before they come in contact with your department. Initial and recurrent training also includes personnel who work nights, weekends, and contractors such as workers who strip and wax floors quarterly or semiannually. Consider including the hospital security staff in this training. Document all support staff training in your safety book and consider having a copy in the employee's personnel file.

There is a section in *NFPA 99* that mandates training of housekeeping personnel working in the hyperbaric department. Document all training given to housekeeping staff. Housekeepers may work after normal business hours without hyperbaric staff present and have a greater than normal turnover rate. The safety director should develop a close relationship with the manager of the housekeeping staff and ensure housekeeping staff is aware of the special conditions and potential hazards within the hyperbaric department to prevent injury or damage to equipment. Housekeeping personnel must be trained to avoid potential damage to equipment from cleaning procedures, including (at minimum) the chamber itself, supply and exhaust piping, and ancillary equipment like medical air cylinders. If you allow housekeeping personnel around the chamber, you must ensure they understand specific cleaning procedures and the potential for personal injury from chamber systems. The safety director must make sure housekeepers understand what equipment is not to be cleaned.

The role of safety director is always going to be challenging. This is true for those new to the position and those who have been doing it for a long time. The safety director's evolution is going to consist of many obstacles and/or opportunities for improvement. The primary challenge is deciding what is and what is not allowed inside the chamber during treatment. When we are new to the field of hyperbaric medicine, we must strictly limit what is allowed inside the chamber. As we gain more understanding, we may decide to allow more items inside the chamber because we have learned and understand **why** it is safe to allow something previously prohibited. Additional challenges include but are not limited to the following: introduction of new wound care products, medication patches and implantable devices; staff turnover; staff complacency; fiscal constraints that limit training opportunities; regulatory changes; and electronic health records and documentation requirements.

This chapter, and to a much greater extent this textbook, describes detailed concepts to address these challenges. If you have a positive attitude, commit to a lifetime of learning, and work as a team, you will establish the foundation to excel in your role as a hyperbaric safety director.

References

1. National Fire Protection Association. NFPA 99: Health Care Facilities Code. Quincy, MA: National Fire Protection Association; 2018.
2. American Society of Mechanical Engineers. ANSI/ASME PVHO-2-2012 Safety Standard for Pressure Vessels for Human Occupancy: In-Service Guidelines. New York: American Society of Mechanical Engineers; 2012.
3. Workman, WT. Undersea and Hyperbaric Medical Society Guidelines for Hyperbaric Facility Operations, 2nd Edition. North Palm Beach, FL: Best Publishing Company; 2015.
4. National Fire Protection Association. NFPA 53: Recommended Practice on Materials, Equipment, and Systems in Oxygen Enriched Atmospheres. Quincy, MA: National Fire Protection Association; 2011.
5. Burman F. Risk Assessment Guide for Installation and Operation of Clinical Hyperbaric Facilities, 5th Edition. San Antonio, TX: International ATMO, Inc.;2016.
6. Undersea and Hyperbaric Medical Society. Undersea and Hyperbaric Medical Society Clinical Hyperbaric Facility Accreditation Manual, 4th Edition. Retrieved from https://www.uhms.org/images/Accreditation-Documents/Fourth_Edition_UHMS_Accreditation_Manual_Final_6-4-2018.pdf. 2018.

CHAPTER 6.3
How Administration Affects Facility Safety

Noel A. Jett, DHA, MPH, CHT-A, CWS

Since the printing of the first edition of this textbook in 1999, much has evolved and matured in the field of hyperbaric medicine. Driven by advances in medical science, economics, and today's regulatory environment, there is little doubt that those trends will continue at an exponential rate.

A prime example of that dynamic process is exemplified in the (previously known as) Joint Commission on Accreditation of Healthcare Organizations (JCAHO) undergoing a significant rebranding process in 2007 and adopting the simplified name, The Joint Commission (TJC). This included name, logo, and tag line change to "Helping Health Care Organizations Help Patients." Beginning in 2001, the Undersea and Hyperbaric Medical Society (UHMS) initiated an accreditation program for hyperbaric facilities that was modeled on TJC hospital accreditation process. In 2010, the UHMS Hyperbaric Facility Accreditation program was recognized by TJC as meeting their requirements as a "complementary accreditation body."[1] Additionally, the UHMS accreditation program is ISO 9001:2015 certified by International Certifications, Inc.

Another organization recognized by the Centers for Medicare and Medicaid Services (CMS) that has been granted authority to perform accreditation for hospitals in the United States since 2008 is DNV GL Health Care (DNV GL HC), which is an operating company of Det Norske Veritas Germanischer Lloyd (DNV GL). Although currently not as widespread across the United States, this may well be the agency your facility works with or will work with in the future regarding standards for facility accreditation. The DNV GL HC utilizes NIAHO® (National Integrated Accreditation for Healthcare Organizations) standards that combine CMS Conditions of Participation and the ISO 9001 Standard regarding quality management. DNV GL HC, as of 2018, is the accrediting agency for approximately 500 U.S. hospitals.[2]

Accrediting agencies establish a wide range of standards which apply to health care facilities. Under TJC standards, responsibilities for health care institution leaders and the role of safety are specifically addressed under the Elements of Performance section.

The segue to safety as it applies to health care (specifically hyperbaric facilities) and administration places considerable reliance on TJC standards in the area of the environment of care (EC). Life safety code (LSC) is another area that has received significant attention in recent adoptions and changes mandated by CMS (see discussion later in this section). Since the majority of state governments recognize TJC accreditation as a condition of licensure, and the receipt of Medicaid reimbursement as well as Medicare reimbursement under what is called "deeming" authority for which TJC currently qualifies,[3] health care administrators recognize the important role compliance with these standards plays in their organizations, especially from the fiscal perspective.

Other regulatory bodies and consensus standards agencies in addition to TJC that directly interface at some level with the administrator's role in hyperbaric facility safety include the National Fire Protection Association (NFPA), International Organization for Standardization (ISO), American National Standards Institute/American Society of Mechanical Engineers (ANSI/ASME), FDA (Food and Drug Administration), CFR (Code of Federal Regulations), Compressed Gas Association (CGA), American Society for Testing and Materials (ASTM), Occupational Safety and Health Administration (OSHA), and the local or state "authority having jurisdiction" (AHJ, i.e. fire marshal, fire engineering, fire department, building and construction planning department, etc.).

The 2018 edition of *NFPA 99* Chapter 14: Hyperbaric Facilities specifically speaks to the responsibility of administration in the health care setting. The following is used with permission from *NFPA 99-2018, Health Care Facilities Code,* Copyright© 2017, National Fire Protection Association. This reprinted material is not the complete and official position of the NFPA on the referenced subject, which is represented only by the standard in its entirety. It may be obtained at www.nfpa.org.

14.3.1.3 Responsibility

14.3.1.3.1 Personnel having responsibility for the hyperbaric facility, and those responsible for licensing, accrediting, or approving institutions or other facilities in which hyperbaric installations are employed, shall establish and enforce programs to fulfill the provisions of this chapter.

14.3.1.3.2 Each hyperbaric facility shall designate an on-site hyperbaric safety director to be in charge of all hyperbaric equipment and the operational safety requirements of this chapter.

> *14.3.1.3.2.1* The safety director shall participate with facility management personnel and the hyperbaric physician(s) in developing procedures for operation and maintenance of the hyperbaric facility.
>
> *14.3.1.3.2.2* The safety director shall make recommendations for departmental safety policies and procedures.

14.3.1.3.2.3 The safety director shall have the authority to restrict or remove any potentially hazardous supply or equipment items from the chamber.

14.3.1.3.3 The governing board shall be responsible for the care and safety of patients and personnel.

14.3.1.3.4 By virtue of its responsibility for the professional conduct of members of the medical staff of the health care facility, the organized medical staff shall adopt and enforce regulations with respect to the use of hyperbaric facilities located in health care facilities.

Administration clearly has a responsibility in assuring that safety compliance in facilities housing hyperbaric operations is met in a comprehensive way. The "buck stops here" for top administration is reinforced in 14.3.1.3.1, 14.3.1.3.3, and 14.3.1.3.4.

What Comprises the Hyperbaric Facility "Administration"?

Titles may vary from institution to institution but they can include the following:

Upper Management Level

Chief Executive Officer (CEO), Chief Operations Officer (COO), Chief Financial Officer (CFO), Chief Medical Officer (CMO), Chief Nursing Officer (CNO), Chief Information Officer (CIO), Chief Compliance Officer (CCO)

Mid-Management Level

Medical Director, Program Director, Facility Safety Director/Officer, Contract Service Provider

Direct Management/Department Level

Hyperbaric Nurse Director, Hyperbaric Technical Director, Hyperbaric Safety Director

Each has a function that either directly or indirectly interfaces with hyperbaric facility safety from the top to the bottom. At the department level, the administrative team must ensure a safety program that is integrated in to the overall facility safety program. The goals of this program can touch on a myriad of areas including the following:

- Safety policy development, review, and implementation
- Clearly outlined personnel responsibilities
- Infection control
- Hazardous waste
- Disaster planning and mitigation

- Fire prevention and protection program
- Compressed gas safety and handling
- Equipment repair and maintenance
- Electrical/electronic safety
- Medical emergency management and mitigation
- Personal protective equipment (PPE)
- Operational and patient safety checkoff procedures
- Hyperbaric specific guidelines for housekeeping
- Emergency procedure and contingency guidelines
- Data management and reporting systems
- Records management and retention
- Staff education and development
- Strategic planning
- Patient education and satisfaction
- Quality assurance and quality improvement
- Cost control and management of budget
- Revenue cycle management

At the mid-management level, the medical director and hyperbaric safety director need the ability to interact with the facility safety officer to integrate overall institutional safety initiatives along with those specific to the hyperbaric unit, such as quality improvement, sentinel event monitoring and reporting, and facility fire drills and evacuation.

At the upper management level, chief administrators and those dealing with facility governance have the authority over and provide direction for overall facility risk management, compliance, and fiscal responsibility. Top administration must be supportive of safety related initiatives for them to be successfully developed and integrated throughout the organizational culture of the institution.

Top level administrators also deal with *NFPA 101 Life Safety Code*[5] issues as applied to the overall health care entity. The *LSC* is a compilation of fire safety requirements for new and existing buildings and is updated and published every three years by the NFPA. Medicare and Medicaid regulations have historically incorporated these requirements by reference for the following: a final rule (CMS-3277-F)[6] was published to update fire safety requirements for hospitals; long-term care (LTC) facilities; critical access hospitals (CAHs); inpatient hospice facilities; programs for all inclusive care for the elderly (PACE); religious non-medical health care institutions (RNHCI); ambulatory surgical centers (ASCs); and intermediate care facilities for individuals with intellectual disabilities (ICF-IID). This final rule adopts provisions of the NFPA 2012 edition of the *LSC* as well as provisions of the NFPA's 2012 edition of the *Health Care Facilities Code*. This rule was effective July 5, 2016.

Administration is charged with the integration of TJC's *Statement of Conditions and LSC*.

Risk Management

Risk management issues permeate every level of the modern health care organization. High on the administrators' list of priorities is the need for functional methodologies to address that risk. Many forward-looking administrators in today's health care industry are successfully employing such concepts as Six Sigma,[7] Lean Six Sigma, and Design for Six Sigma processes to make cultural changes and improve quality. The methodology is a combination of traditional tools with recent breakthroughs in conjunction with statistics organized in a disciplined structure. Six Sigma strives to do the following:

- understand and reduce variation
- improve performance
- improve customer satisfaction

These factors can be readily adapted to safety processes managed via identification of risk variables, controlling for those variables, and applying processes and procedures to keep this loop continuous. Executive leadership sets the vision and allocates resources to achieve the desired outcomes utilizing these tools. Conceptually, Six Sigma strives to reduce defects or errors to a near-perfect number (equates to 3.4 per million opportunities) and to statistically control associated processes to minimize variability. Many hospitals today are developing quality improvement programs using similar methodology as a cultural change throughout their organizations. While this is a useful tool for performance and quality improvement, in the health care facility—especially the hyperbaric unit—one "error" can be catastrophic, so it alone is not enough.

Interaction with the hyperbaric administration team includes working with facility risk managers, compliance officers, information systems, and security. Much has changed in the world since the 9/11/2001 World Trade Towers and subsequent events. Health care institutions may now be on the list of potential targets, and integration of security and the role it plays in safety sensitive areas such as a hyperbaric department cannot be ignored. Planning and preparation must include contingencies that take into account the potential hazards the hyperbaric unit may present to the housing facility in the face of an overt act by unauthorized intruders.

The potential exists for computer virus or system hackers to gain access to equipment designed to control medical devices. Hyperbaric chambers, infusion pumps, cardiac monitors, and blood glucose monitors may have computer interfaces and connectivity capability. Anything that is connected to a network has operating systems and subsequently control software that has the potential for unauthorized access. Assurance that safeguards are in place to prevent this from happening must be coordinated via administration to the involved parties to include the hyperbaric safety director, the medical director, health information systems, systems information management, network engineers, and the device manufacturers.

Data Collection and Management

The collection, assimilation, and analysis of data are critical to any process improvement task. Safety in the hyperbaric facility is no different. A methodology to collect, aggregate, and act on this data is very important. Several tools exist to accomplish this data management. The primary tool with major impetus and driving force is the electronic medical record (EMR)/electronic health record (EHR). Why should administration be concerned with the EMR/EHR?

President Barack Obama signed into legislation the American Recovery and Reinvestment Act of 2009 (ARRA), (Stimulus Bill) on Feb. 17, 2009. A component of this bill, the Health Information Technology for Economic and Clinical Health Act (HITECH) was created. This bill also made permanent the Office of the National Coordinator for Health Care Information Technology (ONC) whose function was to establish standards and policy, direct, oversee, and measure success of the implementation of EHRs. This position was originally created in 2004 under the Bush administration via Executive Order.

Late in 2009, ONC established the first set of policies and standards for these systems, defining mandated Meaningful Use criteria and certified EHR requirements (HITECH phrases). Strict conditions for sharing of data, data documentation, data management, and clinical decision support were set. CMS has the goal to create lifetime individual medical records that are accessible by any provider, anywhere. The expectation is that utilization and quality reports would be submitted from provider EHR systems directly to CMS. CMS is also expecting EHRs to help decrease health care costs, and since CMS reimburses significant dollars to these entities, acute care hospitals and physicians' offices are the first-round targets of EHR system mandates.

ARRA funding expired in 2015. Different levels of compensation were based on the percentage of Medicare patients served, facility designation, and the timeliness of implementation and are components of this plan. Meeting certified EHR and Meaningful Use requirements are a prerequisite to any of this funding, and compensation decreases with delays in EHR installation. Failure to implement EHRs not only means the loss of payment for installation of EHRs, but also penalty via decreased Medicare reimbursement for patient care. Acute care hospitals and physician offices must have EHR systems in place, which meet Meaningful Use Stage 1 and 2 criteria to avoid Medicare reimbursement penalties.

It is projected that the potential growth in the health care services and technology market has the potential to increase from $35 billion in 2016 to close to $50 billion in

2021.[9] Some of the major global companies currently engaged in hospital EHR development include the following:

- Allscripts Healthcare Solutions
- Cerner Corporation
- Epic Systems Corporation
- Fujitsu
- McKesson
- Medical Information Technology
- Siemens Healthcare

In addition to the hospital/health care system-wide companies mentioned above, there are a limited number of wound care/hyperbaric medicine specific niche companies who have systems tailored specifically for that area.

Administration is keenly aware of the potential impacts regarding the electronic medical record, especially on the "bottom line" regarding reimbursement. The direct correlation is, without adequate funding, service expansion and attention to details such as safety initiatives, equipment upgrades, and staffing may become lower on the list of priorities. Subsequent reduction in staffing, aging equipment, and inadequate facilities leads to potential decrease in the ability to ensure a safe work environment.

With the mandate for the EHR as a backdrop, just how can the EHR help the administrator with safety in the hyperbaric setting?

Examples include the following:

- Real-time access to information
- Report generation
- Monitoring frequency of adverse events
- Eliminate medication errors
- MSDS consolidation
- Diagnostic assistance
- Treatment outcome
- Medical equipment management
- Preventive maintenance
- Staff training
- Hazard alerts
- Recall notification
- Root cause determination

- Quality improvement
- Benchmarking and performance
- Integration into other hospital systems
- TJC compliance
- Patient information confidentiality
- Group notification (on-site and off-site)

Conclusion

Administration has a multifaceted role that touches every area of the hyperbaric unit as well as the overall health care facility where it resides. Administration's role is critical to the acceptance and overall integration of the unit into the institution. It must establish the framework for the leadership, support, and foundation of the program. This will enable everyone involved in the chain of service delivery to provide a well-balanced hyperbaric program inclusive of positive patient outcomes and efficient use of limited health care dollars in a safe and effective manner.

References

1. Undersea and Hyperbaric Medical Society. Clinical Hyperbaric Facility Accreditation Manual, 4th Edition. North Palm Beach, FL: UHMS; 2018.
2. DNV GL HC. Det Norske Veritas Germanischer Lloyd (DNV GL). Accessed [2018]. https://www.dnvglhealthcare.com/accreditations/hospital-accreditation.
3. The Joint Commission. Accessed [2018]. https://www.jointcommission.org/facts_about_federal_deemed_status_and_state_recognition/.
4. National Fire Protection Association. NFPA 99-2018, Health Care Facilities Code. Quincy, MA: NFPA; 2017. www.nfpa.org.
5. National Fire Protection Association. NFPA: Life Safety Code, 2012 Edition. Quincy, MA: NFPA; 2012.
6. Federal Register (Nov. 4, 2016) https://www.gpo.gov/fdsys/pkg/FR-2016-11-04/pdf/2016-26583.pdf.
7. Motorola. Six Sigma. 1993.
8. Federal Register (Oct. 16, 2015) https://www.gpo.gov/fdsys/pkg/FR-2015-10-16/pdf/2015-25595.pdf.
9. Singhal S, et. Al. McKinsey white paper: The future of health care: finding the opportunities that lie beneath the uncertainty. January 2018.

CHAPTER 6.4
How to Manage Your Hyperbaric Facility Safety Program

Wilbur T. Workman, MS, CAsP, CHT-A, FAsMA, FUHM and James Bell, CHT, EMT, CFPS

Webster defines safety as: 1: the condition of being safe from undergoing or causing hurt, injury, or loss. 2: a device (as on a weapon or a machine) designed to prevent inadvertent or hazardous operation.[1]

Key components of any successful hyperbaric safety program are active development of a "culture of safety" and a strong safety program with a well-defined and implemented plan. Such a program is multifaceted, incorporating a variety of important complementing program elements, such as the following: carefully controlled operational procedures; attention to detail; practice; competency assessment; preventive maintenance; vigilance; training; and equipment knowledge. It is not sufficient to just have policies and procedures. Staff members must fully understand their responsibilities in maintaining the highest level of safety. Maintaining a safe environment for patients and staff is not automatic; it results from actively promoting and developing a culture of safety.

Culture of Safety

The term "culture of safety" is widely used and often misunderstood. For the purposes of this chapter, we will use The Joint Commission's (TJC's) definition: *"Safety culture is the sum of what an organization is and does in the pursuit of safety. The Patient Safety Systems (PS) chapter of the Joint Commission accreditation manuals defines safety culture as the product of individual and group beliefs, values, attitudes, perceptions, competencies, and patterns of behavior that determine the organization's commitment to quality and patient safety."*[2]

Key components of a culture of safety include the following:

- An open, nonthreatening approach to reporting and learning for adverse events, near misses, unsafe conditions, and sentinel events.
- Risk-based processes for recognizing and identifying human errors and system errors from unsafe and fault-worthy actions.

- Facility leadership adopts, champions, and demonstrates the behaviors and efforts to eliminate intimidation.
- Policy and procedures support a culture of safety and reporting of adverse events. These policy and procedures are enforced and communicated to and for all.
- Recognize and support team members who report and identify unsafe conditions, near misses, and make suggestions for safety improvements.
- Develop a safety report for the facility to measure and keep track of the culture of safety performance.
- Analyze the culture of safety reports on a regular basis to determine opportunities for improvement. These reports are used as lessons to the team.
- Use the information from the assessments to develop safety and quality improvement projects.
- Include team training on a culture of safety and quality improvement to strengthen the safety systems.
- Constantly assess the systems strengths and weakness; work on improvement as a process.

Practical examples of these components include the following:

- **Daily huddle:** There are several practical ways a facility can work on a culture of safety. One of the easiest is to have a daily huddle. The daily huddle is not a new concept and has been embraced by the military, as well as large and small corporations. Sometimes called a safety meeting, the daily huddle happens at the beginning of the shift and covers safety events, equipment concerns, plan for the day, and staffing and care plan for the patients that will be seen that day. Time is given for new information to be brought forward and to recognize and honor team members.
- **Monthly/annual reports:** The daily huddle should be documented and used as the basis for monthly and annual reports. The reports can then be used at staff meetings as education and saved and analyzed for opportunities for improvement. The information included in the reports should be de-identified so that there is no fear of reporting a safety event. The exception from de-identification would be for recognition of a team member; these should to be brought forward and encouraged.
- **Accountability:** Developing a nonthreatening environment, where anyone feels comfortable to bring information to the group, stop process if necessary, and even go outside the "chain of command" without fear of repercussion. However, all members of the team are held accountable for their actions. Equal and fair consequences for actions is important.

Multifaceted Program

A safety program is multifaceted. Although there can be a variety of program elements depending on the specific setting and need, there are several common aspects elementary in program design and execution. These basic elements are as follows:

- **Operational policy and procedures:** Management, medical directors, and safety directors should develop a comprehensive set of operational policies and procedures that cover the complete spectrum of issues based upon the type of patients treated and equipment employed by a given facility.
  - *Policy:* Policy is an umbrella statement developed by administration that covers a broad course or principle of action.
  - *Procedure:* Procedure is the detailed practice developed by the management, medical director, and safety director of the hyperbaric facility. Not only should these procedures cover all items of medical equipment to include the chamber or chamber system, they should also address patient care activities as well.
- **Attention to detail:** Procedures should address every aspect, no matter how mundane, of operating and maintaining a given type of chamber system, medical device, or patient treatment processes. The level of detail should be sufficient to ensure no critical process or procedure has been omitted. Being thorough is a time-consuming process and one that some can easily justify not completing; however, thoroughness is necessary.
- **Vigilance:** An organization may have the most comprehensive safety plan possible, but if the staff is not constantly aware of their surroundings and the consequence of their actions or the actions of others, it means little. As noted in Chapter 6.1: How Accidents Happen, mishaps are rarely the result of a single event but from a chain of events that lead to an accident. Maintaining constant awareness of one's situation may help break a link in this chain.
- **Checklists:** Checklists are an invaluable tool in a safety program. Conducting frequent workplace safety, pre- and post-chamber operations, preventive maintenance, and environment of care inspections using checklists is one of the most widely accepted means of identifying hazards and unsafe behavior. Regular self-inspection using safety checklists is an essential component in every proactive safety program.
- **Risk assessments:** Documented risk assessments are becoming more commonplace. The safety director should have training in how to conduct risk assessments. These can be complex or simple assessments depending on the issue at hand. It may be a piece of equipment required for patient care that is not approved by the manufacturer for hyperbaric conditions or a wound dressing that the facility has not encountered. The ability to complete an adequate risk assessment and accompanying documentation is a skill the hyperbaric safety director should have.

- **Preventive maintenance:** Keeping all equipment in peak working order depends directly on a comprehensive preventive maintenance program. In general, hyperbaric equipment is well designed and highly reliable, requiring relatively little maintenance (except perhaps for large multiplace hyperbaric complexes). As a result, in times of fiscal restraint, preventive maintenance may be relegated to a lower priority. Such management decisions usually prove to be costly in the long run. Senior management must fully support routine maintenance expenditures, since it is generally cheaper to keep equipment in good working order than to face the higher cost of repairing a component after a major failure.
- **Proper training:** The importance of this element cannot be overly stressed. Safety awareness begins in the classroom and is applied in the facility. Mishap data clearly points to the dominance of operator errors in hyperbaric accidents. Proper initial instruction, timely continuing education, and regular competency assessments can help mitigate these tragic findings in the future. Minimum training standards must be developed, adopted, and enforced throughout the international hyperbaric community. Training outcomes should be focused at providing all staff members with sufficient information for them to know when to question an action or situation. It is neither practical nor desired to educate every staff member to be an expert on every aspect of hyperbaric operations. However, if a person notes that something does not seem right, stops, and investigates the situation, then a major training objective has been met. This person may have broken the chain of events leading to an accident. The team member(s) that should cause concern are those whose knowledge level is not high enough to recognize something is not right and who may continue to allow the situation to exist, perhaps ending in a tragic mishap.
- **Practice, practice, practice:** The proper response to an emergency should be calculated and immediate. Although it is not practical for each staff member to memorize every emergency procedure, it is important for them to routinely practice planned reactions to a range of emergency situations. Everyone should be familiar enough with all department or equipment emergency procedures to allow them, with the aid of emergency checklists, to deal with any quick response situation. Being aware of others' responsibilities is crucial. Anyone can be in a position of having to respond to an incident when the staff member normally responsible for that function is not immediately available. Practicing as a group helps the staff to better appreciate the responsibilities of others and fosters development of the hyperbaric team. As difficult as it is, time should be set aside on a recurring basis for focused unit safety training. Although monthly staff safety training is recommended, the minimal interval should be no more than quarterly. An example of this is the timed evacuation drill required at least annually by *NFPA 99, Health Care Facilities Code*, Chapter 14: Hyperbaric Facilities.[3] The first time a staff member conducts an emergency drill should NOT be in response to an actual event!

- **Safety mindset:** Attention to the above elements helps cultivate a culture of safety mindset for the entire hyperbaric facility staff. This obvious safety attitude becomes evident to the patient, helping to instill confidence and easing any fears. Safety must be an overriding philosophy that guides the attitudes and actions of the entire staff.

Codes and Standards (Equipment)

Thanks to the hard work done over the years by many people representing a variety of engineering and safety disciplines, there are codes and standards in place to ensure the safety of the equipment installed in hyperbaric facilities. These various codes and standards exert their influence before the doors of the hyperbaric facility are open for business.

The first organization coming into contact with the basic equipment for a hyperbaric facility is the American Society of Mechanical Engineers (ASME) and the standards developed by its Pressure Vessel for Human Occupancy Committee (PVHO). *ASME PVHO* establishes the design and fabrication rules for hyperbaric chambers. Although not recognized throughout the world as the internationally accepted standard, it is considered by many as the premier guidance governing this issue. A pressure vessel intended for human occupancy must be designed and fabricated in accordance with some sort of recognized safety standard.

A second organization having tremendous influence on the safe design of a hyperbaric system is the National Fire Protection Association (NFPA). The chapter on hyperbaric facilities in *NFPA 99 Health Care Facilities Code* (various editions) establishes minimum criteria for the chamber(s), room housing the chamber(s), ancillary hyperbaric support equipment, and systems such as the fire suppression system, intercommunications system, air quality monitoring, electrical requirements, etc. Though *ASME PVHO* as a stand-alone code is not mandatory in all 50 American states, *NFPA 101 Life Safety Code* is. *NFPA 101* invokes by reference compliance to the *NFPA 99* chapter for hyperbaric facilities.[4] *NFPA 99* requires any hyperbaric chamber installed in a health care facility to be in compliance with *ASME PVHO*. Therefore, by reference in *NFPA 101*, compliance to *ASME PVHO* is a nationwide mandate. As of this writing, in the United States, the Centers for Medicare & Medicaid Services (CMS) has adopted *NFPA 101* and *99* (2012 editions) as the basis for reimbursement. The Joint Commission has followed CMS in this requirement for accreditation.

A third organization is the Food and Drug Administration (FDA). The FDA classifies hyperbaric chambers as Class II medical devices and requires that manufacturers comply with 510(k) Pre-market Notification Requirements before a specific chamber design can be legally placed into commercial sales. Any health care organization considering purchase of a hyperbaric chamber or hyperbaric system should require the manufacturer to produce evidence of premarket clearance. Such documentation verifies that the manufacturer surpassed a rigorous third-party review of design and fabrication adequacy and that the system complied with recognized industry standards. If a hyperbaric system under consideration for purchase does not have a cleared 510(k) or is not "grandfathered" (few are), it is suggested that other equipment alternatives be considered. Similar requirements, such as CE Marking in Europe, are being established in other world regions that will ultimately raise the level of quality of hyperbaric systems. Improved quality leads directly to improved safety.

Guidelines developed by the American Society for Testing and Materials (ASTM) are used extensively to direct designers of oxygen equipment and oxygen system components to proper material selection, design, and maintenance. These guidelines help ensure that consideration is given to these elements to minimize the risk of fire due to improper materials, inadequate design, or suboptimal maintenance.

The Compressed Gas Association (CGA) develops guides for the installation of primary and secondary gas delivery systems and gas purity. The CGA has set standards for color coding of the various gases and specific threads so that gases are not able to be incorrectly connected to a regulators or manifold. Compliance with these standards gives the new operator assurance that the necessary steps have been taken to ensure delivery of high-quality gas supplies to either the patient or the chamber.

The Undersea and Hyperbaric Medical Society (UHMS) has produced numerous companion safety guidelines for both monoplace and multiplace hyperbaric chamber systems. Two of the most current are *Compressed Gas (Air) Supply System* and the *Safe Design and Operation of Hyperbaric Chambers.*[6] These documents are intended to provide a hyperbaric facility with a better understanding of the issues that should be understood when contemplating installation of a hyperbaric system. They have now become valuable resource documents for users and engineers alike. The UHMS hyperbaric facility accreditation manual is an excellent source document for installation and operation of a hyperbaric facility. We are aware of facilities that have used the accreditation manual as a template for their facility. Referring to these documents in the early stages of facility planning has proven to be a valuable effort by many.

The *Facilities Institute Guidelines,*[7] published by the American Society for Healthcare Engineering, includes a chapter on hyperbaric suites. It is intended for architects to use as minimum standards for health care facilities with hyperbaric chambers.

Hyperbaric medicine is poised for rapid expansion into developing areas of the world. Comprehensive safety standards like those mentioned above are not in place in many of these countries to help establish and support the growth of the specialty. Aggressive efforts are underway to promote adoption of comprehensive safety standards throughout the world.

Codes and Standards (Facilities)

Not only are there codes and standards that govern the design and fabrication of hyperbaric chambers and their affiliated component systems, there are also standards in the United

States and a few other countries that establish minimum facility requirements that must be met before the hyperbaric chamber can be installed. At present, the building requirements as set forth in *NFPA 101* and *NFPA 99* are for any occupancy housing a hyperbaric chamber. The UHMS monoplace and multiplace safety guidelines, the society's hyperbaric facility accreditation manual, and the *Facilities Institute Guidelines* address general facility issues to be considered. The type of building into which a hyperbaric chamber is installed is immaterial. There are basic facility standards that should be met to ensure continued safe operation regardless of the building occupancy classification.

Guidelines (Staff Training)

The elements that frame equipment and facility requirements generally work and are conducted behind the operational scene. Hyperbaric staff should have at least a baseline understanding of many of the details of the codes and standards related to hyperbaric medicine. The initial training the staff receives before beginning hyperbaric chamber operations should include this information in the syllabus. Although these aspects of a viable hyperbaric safety program are important, training is a critical element.

As in any discipline, training is central to successful outcomes. The operator must acquire the knowledge to understand the *what, why, when, where,* and *how.* Raising the knowledge level of each hyperbaric operator high enough to know when to ask a question when something does not seem right has already been stressed. Experience also contributes to this higher order awareness. We encourage the readers support in adopting the philosophy to obtain a thorough education about our practice and to expand it through experience. More basic, however, is the need to have a minimum skill and knowledge level in place before hyperbaric operations even begin. Training after the fact, although better than no training at all, leaves an organization open to potential legal pitfalls should an accident occur involving a person who has not been properly trained.

More directly, training is one of the links in the accident chain of events over which the management of any hyperbaric facility has direct control. At present, there are no mandatory requirements in the United States for minimum training standards for all hyperbaric staff. Though there are efforts underway to establish these minimums, there is much work that needs to be done.

Core Program Elements

The basic elements of any comprehensive hyperbaric facility safety program should include at least the following:

- Defined responsibilities
- Documented safety procedures based on the type and size of the facility
- Documented in-service training
- Documented maintenance
- Documented measurement and validation

Responsibilities

One of the first individual responsibilities is to ensure that each person directly involved in hyperbaric operations is knowledgeable of all potential hazard sources. If there is ever doubt about a situation or procedure, then stop and ask for clarification. Do not continue blindly down what may be the beginning of the accident chain of events.

Each organization should develop a program that includes four major checkpoints. It is important to do all that is practically possible to indoctrinate everyone from the most senior hospital executive to the most junior technician on the hyperbaric staff. The more they understand about what hyperbaric medicine is, what its limitations are, and what the requirements are to provide high quality care safely, the better they can serve as an advocate for the program. The four checks are as follows:

- The governing body (hospital board of directors, etc.) should set a firm hyperbaric safety policy.
- The hyperbaric facility management should develop comprehensive safety procedures.
- The technical staff of the hyperbaric facility should implement the procedures.
- Accrediting agencies (such as TJC and Det Norske Veritas-Germannischer Lloyd [DNV-GL] in the United States and similar organizations in other countries) should survey for compliance. UHMS hyperbaric facility accreditation in areas where this is available is strongly encouraged.

The institutional governing body should establish a firm hyperbaric safety policy. Ultimate responsibility for safety resides with this senior management group. They must work closely with the hyperbaric safety director (SD) to ensure that these policies are developed and rigidly adhered to. Adherence implies there is an ongoing dialog between the governing body and the hyperbaric facility. This should be encouraged. Developing a close working relationship between the governing body and the SD is extremely important as it establishes credibility of the SD with senior institutional management. Again, the more institutional management understands your program, the better they can serve as your spokesman and knowledgeable advocate.

Continuing down the hierarchy, the administration of the host institution plays an important role as well. Specifically, the institution's administration should adopt and correlate regulations and standard operating procedures to ensure that both the physical qualities and operating maintenance methods pertaining to the hyperbaric facility meet the standards required of other departments of the institution. Administration must have an appreciation of the unique compliance issues cited by various codes and standards pertaining to hyperbaric facilities. The more administration understands the requirements, the better they can offer support and funding for major department expenditures such as periodic maintenance, etc.

As this hierarchy becomes more functional, the hyperbaric medical staff is not exempt from responsibility. The hyperbaric medical director should work closely with the SD to develop department specific regulations and procedures. Other medical personnel should also make themselves available to the SD to assist in this effort. Finally, the hyperbaric medical director should adopt and ensure that all staff adhere to the procedures developed.

Perhaps the most visible position of a comprehensive hyperbaric safety program is that of the designated safety director. This is the only position directed by the *NFPA 99 Health Care Facilities Code.*[3] In the United States, every facility, regardless of size or the type or number of chambers employed, shall have a SD. This individual has a tremendous responsibility to ensure the safe order and discipline among the staff and patients. Specific responsibilities of the SD are covered later in this chapter and elsewhere in this textbook.

Documented Safety Procedures

There are a variety of issues that should be documented in your safety program. It is not the intent of this text to provide a specific list for your use. Instead, you are encouraged to think through each process, procedure, concern, activity, etc., and conduct a step-by-step analysis of each. Construct a set of guidelines for each action that is appropriate for your facility. There will be many procedures that you will have in common with all other hyperbaric facilities, but there may also be those that are unique to your department.

There are general and specific areas mentioned in *NFPA 99* that are recommended for inclusion in your documentation.

General Facility Safety

- **Conduct of personnel**: This area should address such issues as staff performance and evaluation, conduct around patients, etc.
- **Apparel**: Based on documented mishap data, this is also an area of great concern. Apparel is one aspect over which any hyperbaric department has direct control. The Sheffield and Desautel analysis of hyperbaric/hypobaric mishaps indicates a high percentage of accidents where contraband or unauthorized items and synthetic materials were allowed into the chamber interior.[8] *NFPA 99* requires that the hyperbaric facility reclothe the patients with apparel approved by the facility.[3] Street clothes are not allowed unless specifically approved by the onsite safety director. Contraband can also more easily be managed by having the patient wear only garments provided by the facility. Personal clothing may have numerous pockets where items such as a cell phone, personal electronic devices, cigarette lighters, matches, fuel or chemical warmers, etc., may go unnoticed. If the patient is given a garment to wear that has had the pockets sewn closed, or better yet, no pockets at all, then the likelihood that contraband could be brought into the chamber is greatly minimized.
- **Safety time-out/pause (STOP)**: A documented safety stop prior to chamber operations is best practice and required by *NFPA 99.*[3] The UHMS has posted a position statement on a safety time-out: "*. . . For the safety of patients and staff, we strongly encourage documentation of a STOP verifying the "Right patient,*

Right Treatment and Right Safety." The STOP should include checking the patient ground (monoplace) and that all prohibited items are removed from the chamber (both monoplace and multiplace). The treatment profile and staffing plan should be confirmed and the completed STOP checklist dated and signed or initialed by two staff members prior to closing the door of the chamber . . ."[5]

- **Posting of procedures:** Although it is not recommended to post all emergency procedures throughout the facility for the patients and others to see, there are key procedures that should be posted in public view. Procedures such as building evacuation routes fall into this category. Any chamber operator, whether monoplace or multiplace, should have immediate access to a complete series of emergency procedures for use in any emergency. Consider posting emergency procedures at each control station in a quick-reading flipchart folder for ready access.
- **Staff familiarity with procedures:** The operative words here are practice, practice, practice! Though each person has their specific responsibilities within the unit, each should be aware enough of the duties of others to be able to respond to any emergency that might happen when they may be the only one around. Frequent practicing, playing the role of other staff members, etc., will help develop an esprit de corps and a sense of being a member of the hyperbaric team that will be advantageous in the event of an accident. During mishaps, things may happen quickly, leaving little time to contemplate your next action. Practice helps minimize this hesitation and facilitates one's confidence in dealing with the adverse situation regardless of how drastic.

In an organization that has adopted the concept of a culture of safety and incorporates recurring in-service safety training, response to an emergency becomes second nature and part of the routine. For those organizations that seldom or never devote the time necessary to practice staff safety skills, there is, in our opinion, higher risk for a mishap.

Specific Facility Safety

- There should be specific procedures developed, based on the unique characteristics of your hyperbaric chamber or system, that cover situations such as fire in the chamber, patient egress, contaminated air, equipment component failure, fire in the building, etc. Failure to develop these specific response actions will add to the confusion that generally accompanies a mishap situation and will certainly increase one's response time necessary to interrupt the accident chain of events. As noted earlier, these procedures should also be posted at auxiliary control stations for multiplace hyperbaric chamber systems.
- In addition to developing a comprehensive response posture to mechanical or operational emergency situations, a companion list should also be developed to address physiological emergencies such as ear/sinus pain, confinement

anxiety, oxygen toxicity, etc. Refer to Chapter 7: Emergency Procedures for more detailed information on developing these crucial operational safety aides.

Documented In-Service Training

The familiar theme of **practice, practice, and more practice** cannot be stressed too strongly. However, we recognize it may be easier said than done. Time must be routinely set aside; otherwise, in-service training will often take the back seat to other important activities. Ideally, an organization should devote time to monthly safety training. However, if this is not feasible, it is recommended to establish the frequency best suited to your needs but no less than quarterly. Use unexpected events or mishaps as opportunities to review the departmental procedures, and document the events as drills. The important thing is that training be routinely done. Safety must be given priority in the ongoing business of a hyperbaric facility. We find that even with an experienced staff that have completed the drills many times, we learn from each drill. It is easy to become complacent and the drills also help serve to remind us to be aware.

Examples of training topics are as varied as the mind is creative. It is not possible to include all scenarios. Several suggestions are offered below to stimulate thinking:

- Fire drills: Not only should your fire suppression system (FSS) be exercised periodically (for multiplace chambers so equipped), the local fire department should be frequently involved.

  The FSS may sit idle for months and then be expected to perform flawlessly when needed. The FSS must be routinely activated to maintain peak efficiency. There have been several mishaps in which a faulty FSS has been implicated in the accident chain of events. Activating of the FSS every six months for a functional test and an annual full test of the FSS is required by *NFPA 99*.[3] Staff participation in the activation of the FSS will help instill operator confidence in the system and assure proper function when needed.

  We encourage organizations to invite the local fire department personnel into their facility. The patient egress requirements for a hyperbaric environment are different from those of a regular health care facility setting. This is true in multiplace and monoplace hyperbaric chamber facilities, Fire department personnel need to understand the unique requirements of the hyperbaric facility and be given the opportunity to practice them. Otherwise, they will be unable to provide the quality support necessary during any mishap situation. An excellent opportunity to foster this mutually beneficial relationship is to have local first responders to participate in a worse-case scenario drill that is now required by *NFPA 99* to be conducted and documented at least annually.[3]

- Mock patient emergencies: The staff must be capable of responding to the complete spectrum of patient emergencies such as confinement anxiety, ear/sinus pain, oxygen toxicity reactions, etc. Practice helps the staff develop those reflexive actions necessary to deal with a patient emergency in a timely fashion.

- **Simulated equipment failure:** Although hyperbaric equipment is generally reliable, they are mechanical devices and are subject to failure. A good example for multiplace chamber operations is to practice the steps necessary to deal with a leaking door seal. A good example for monoplace chamber operations is the operator's response to loss of pressure control. There are numerous other equipment failures for any type of chamber that can be simulated for practice.
- **Contaminated air:** The quality of the air produced for hyperbaric chamber operations depends on the quality of the air used for compression and the proper function of the compressor. Fortunately for the human, one of the most sophisticated alarms for air contamination is the nose. Hydrocarbon-based contaminates can easily be detected. Of concern, of course, is carbon monoxide, which is odorless. Dealing with contaminated air should be routinely practiced.
- **Updates on codes and standards:** Fortunately for the in-service trainer, change in this area is very slow, making it easy for the trainer to stay current. Change does occur, however, and hyperbaric personnel are encouraged to maintain currency. We encourage the hyperbaric staff to be involved as much as possible with the codes and standards. *NFPA 99*, for example, is a consensus standard and anyone with internet access can participate in developing the code. Emphasizing the codes and standards in your training program helps broaden your staff's knowledge base for factors that influence the everyday world of hyperbaric medicine.

Vital to an effective on-going hyperbaric training program are those sessions for which continuing education credits are offered. This is especially crucial for technical personnel. Generally, there is no problem with professional medical staff personnel in satisfying continuing medical educational credits. Unfortunately, technical staff do not often have the administrative support to routinely participate in these ongoing educational activities. They can rarely afford to attend these functions at their own expense, and as a result, they usually do not attend. This situation needs to change. As an alternative, larger clinical hyperbaric medicine programs are encouraged to apply to organizations such as the National Board of Diving and Hyperbaric Medical Technology (NBDHMT) for continuing education credits for their on-going in-service training program. This approach will help ensure staff members have the opportunity to maintain currency for minimal cost and less time away from the facility. Further, it is highly recommended that technical personnel attend courses related to fire safety, oxygen systems, hyperbaric safety director, hyperbaric team training, chamber maintenance, etc. If a good working relationship has been established with the institution's administrative management, it is easier for the director of hyperbaric medicine to advocate on the technician's behalf to help justify funding the educational need.

Membership in professional hyperbaric organizations is vital. Participation and membership in these organizations is one of the best ways to stay current. Attendance and participation in international and local hyperbaric scientific meetings are encouraged, not only to obtain education but to collaborate with your peers and share knowledge and experience. If we are to grow as a medical specialty, we need to support and encourage participation in the practice of hyperbaric medicine at large. The value of presenting abstracts and research cannot be discarded. We will not grow without continued research and participation in the various hyperbaric organizations. A network of peers you can call on is invaluable, and many attend the meetings to grow their network.

Board certification in hyperbaric technology is becoming increasingly important. This is a valuable tool to recognize staff competence and should be a priority for every hyperbaric facility. Developing a comprehensive in-service training program assists those technicians not yet certified to achieve the background preparation necessary to successfully complete the certification exam.

Acting as a surveyor for the UHMS hyperbaric facility accreditation program, where available, is an excellent way to increase your knowledge of hyperbaric medicine and related operations. Being a surveyor provides the unique opportunity to see first-hand how other facilities operate. We encourage participation in the program.

Consider training in safety issues outside of hyperbaric medicine. There are several safety-related certifications, licensures, or registrations, such as certified health care facility manager (CHFM), certified health care safety professional (CHSP), health care environmental manager (HEM), certified industrial hygienist (CIH), certified safety professional (CSP), and certified fire protection specialist (CFPS).

Finally, there is an old military saying that goes something like, "If you did not write it down, you did not do it!" It is very important for you to document what you do. A program's development and execution tend to be more organized when documentation is required.

Documented Maintenance

Preventive and responsive maintenance on all components of a hyperbaric chamber or system is required. Considering the total number of hyperbaric facilities in the United States, few are fortunate enough to maintain sufficient technical expertise on staff to handle most of maintenance needs in-house. Generally, third-party contractors or the chamber manufacturer are relied upon. Regardless of your situation, all aspects of maintenance ranging from daily inspections to major component overhauls should be documented in detail. Failure to maintain detailed maintenance records often makes future repairs more expensive since historical system actions cannot be validated. There is also liability that comes with missing or incomplete documentation in the event of a mishap.

Documented Measurement and Validation

In setting up any program for which outcomes are important, the processes developed to achieve those outcomes must be measurable. If not, there is no mechanism for feedback to determine if the process is needed, if it is achieving the desired result, or if it is as efficient as it can be. It is relatively easy to measure outcomes in an industrial setting where a product is produced. You can measure machining tolerances, component rejection rates, etc. It is more difficult to measure management outcomes, yet this is still attainable. If an organization has no tool by which they can assess performance, regardless of the measurement area, then they are omitting an important tool that management can use to ascertain the success of a given program. This is equally true with the need to assess outcomes of a hyperbaric safety program. Compliance organizations such as TJC traditionally review such interdepartmental documentation to assist with their survey of a particular department or patient service.

Safety Director

One of the key positions of every hyperbaric facility is that of the safety director. Every hyperbaric facility, regardless of type, shall have a designated SD.[3] The term safety director is for convenience. Depending on your facilities' human resources rules, the actual title may be different. Someone is assigned the responsibility for facility safety and accepts that responsibility in writing. Due to the extensive nature of responsibilities of the SD, no attempt will be made to provide a detailed discussion of each. Instead, these responsibilities are provided in list form.

Knowledge and Experience

- Completion of a recognized course in hyperbaric medicine (UHMS, ACHM, NBDHMT or similar nation-specific requirements)
- Training or experience in hyperbaric chamber maintenance and operations (primarily for multiplace hyperbaric facilities)
- Working knowledge of safety codes and decompression requirements (multiplace operations)
- Certification in hyperbaric technology (**highly desired**)

General Responsibilities

- In charge of all hyperbaric equipment in the absence of a technical director. (Note: There is no requirement in *NFPA 99* for a designated technical director as there is for the SD.[3] Monoplace hyperbaric facilities do not have a technical director whereas multiplace hyperbaric facilities do, in part because of the increased complexity of multiplace systems.) Responsible for the safe/effective operation and maintenance of the hyperbaric chamber and related support systems and ancillary components

- Reviews maintenance/repair activities and authorizes return to service following completion of those activities
- Works closely with facility management and hyperbaric physician(s)
- Recommends and implements safety procedures as appropriate
- Serves on institutional safety committee (strongly encouraged)
- Has authority to restrict or remove potentially hazardous items or supplies from inside the chamber
- Provides training and leadership
- Maintains all safety related codes and standards as required by various licensing and regulatory agencies

Specific Responsibilities

- Ensures compliance with the hyperbaric facility specific requirements found in *NFPA 99* (or other country-equivalent requirements as appropriate) and unit safety policies and procedures
- Reviews safety incidents, collects information on equipment/patient safety, reports relevant incidents, and provides periodic in-service training on accident prevention
- Works closely with the medical, nursing, and technical directors to develop and annually review and revise documents pertaining to policies, procedures, operations, and maintenance
- Fosters positive relationships between department personnel and local regulators, such as the local fire marshal, director of emergency services, pressure vessel inspector, etc.
- Works with the technical director (if designated) to coordinate/approve all routine maintenance, upgrades, modifications, and repairs to the hyperbaric chamber or hyperbaric system
- Interacts with hospital maintenance personnel and outside contractors to ensure all maintenance is performed in accordance with applicable codes and standards
- Ensures that all system modifications are tested prior to manned chamber operations and approves equipment for return to service
- In consultation with the medical director, evaluates equipment and supplies before they are used inside the chamber
- Maintains a safe environment for the staff and patients alike
- Monitors to ensure that appropriate decompression procedures are used for all persons with hyperbaric exposure to inert gases
- Informs personnel of any special work condition such as infection control, hazard control, etc.

- Serves as technical trainer for full-time and part-time staff
- Provides in-service training on aspects of hyperbaric physiology, equipment operations, safety, decompression requirements, and treatment protocols
- Validates in-chamber safety training of new staff and ancillary support personnel before their initial entry into the hyperbaric chamber (multiplace)
- Generates and supervises safety drills which are tailored to the special needs of the facility
- Conducts annual review of safety related events to identify trends and monitor improvements
- Sets up procedures to assist the medial director in reviewing, documenting, and reporting safety related events to the staff to facilitate learning

Summary

A well-structured safety plan consists of a variety of components, each with its relative importance. Proper training serves as the foundation for continued safety.

To maintain a safe operational hyperbaric environment, everyone must realize it is a team effort. Though a particular aspect of daily operation may not be a specific person's responsibility, each must appreciate the role of another. Each person must do his or her part by developing a culture of safety to strengthen the chain of mishap avoidance.

The safety director is a key figure in any hyperbaric medicine department's safety program and has wide-ranging responsibilities to ensure that the functions of hyperbaric safety are properly planned, executed, documented, and validated.

For additional guidance on staffing, training, safety program development and management, see the UHMS publication *Guidelines for Hyperbaric Facilities Operations, 2nd Edition.*

References

1. Merriam-Webster Dictionary. Definition of Safe. https://www.merriam-webster.com. Accessed: Sept 13, 2018.
2. Joint Commission. Accreditation and certification: survey improvements made for how Joint Commission assesses safety culture. Joint Commission June 13, 2018. https://www.jointcommission.org. Accessed: Aug 25, 2018.
3. National Fire Protection Association. NFPA 99, Health Care Facilities Code. Quincy, MA: National Fire Protection Association. https://www.nfpa.org/. Accessed: Aug 25, 2018.
4. National Fire Protection Association. NFPA 101 Life Safety Code. Quincy, MA: National Fire Protection Association. https://www.nfpa.org. Accessed: Aug 25, 2018.

5. UHMS. Safety time out/pause-STOP, UHMS Position Statement. https://www.uhms.org/about/position-statements.html. Accessed: Aug 25, 2018.
6. UHMS. Various position statements and safety articles. www.uhms.org. Accessed: Sept 27, 2018.
7. Guidelines for Design and Construction, Facility Guidelines Institute. https://fgi.madcad.com. Accessed: Aug 25, 2018.
8. Sheffield PJ, Desautels, DA. Hyperbaric and hypobaric chamber fires: a 73-year analysis. *Undersea Hyper Med.* 1997; 24(3):153-164. http://rubicon-foundation.org.

Bibliography

1. ASTM International. West Conshohocken, PA. www.astm.org.
2. CGA G-7.1-2018: Commodity Specification for Air, Seventh Edition. Compressed Gas Association, Inc. Chantilly, VA: Compressed Gas Association, Inc. https://blog.ansi.org.
3. Clinical Hyperbaric Facility Accreditation Manual, 4th edition. North Palm Beach, FL: UHMS. http://uhms.org.
4. Risk Assessment Guide for Installation and Operation of Clinical Hyperbaric Facilities 5th edition revised by F Burman. International ATMO. https://hyperbaricmedicine.com/risk-assessment-guide/.
5. Safety Standard for Pressure Vessels for Human Occupancy (ANSI/ASME PVHO-1: 2016). New York: American Society of Mechanical Engineers. http://www.asme.org.
6. UHMS Guidelines for Hyperbaric Facility Operations 2nd Edition. North Palm Beach, FL: UHMS. https://www.bestpub.com.

CHAPTER 6.5
The Medical Director's Responsibility to Hyperbaric Facility Safety

Marc Robins, DO, MPH, FUHM, FAAFP

Introduction

Whether in a stand-alone hyperbaric facility or a combined wound care and hyperbaric facility, hospital-based or private institution, a knowledgeable and well-trained physician plays a very important leadership role, which is paramount for the success of that unit. Ultimately the medical director has the direct responsibility to ensure timely and accurate diagnosis along with safe utilization and management of the most effective treatment available for the patients seeking care within his/her clinic. In addition to the medical knowledge and training required of the medical director and provider staff to achieve this goal, the medical director must also have a well-rounded understanding of the safety policies and procedures, maintenance of equipment and materials, and training of personnel involved with the treatment process.

Knowledge and application of quality-based programs may improve efficient functioning of the unit, but when these strategies are used to stratify risk through data collection of meaningful parameters, a well-designed safety program will determine not only the quality of care provided but the underlying safe application of care individualized for each patient. Ultimately this is best achieved through a close working relationship between the hyperbaric medical director and the hyperbaric safety director.

Medical Director

The position of medical director should be filled by a medical doctor/osteopathic doctor (MD/DO) who is considered a subject matter expert in hyperbaric medicine with experience and expertise commensurate with the responsibility to not only attend and supervise HBO_2 treatments but also supervise and lead other providers in the department. The minimum training standard preferred for a medical director is primary residency training with board eligibility or board certification in a primary specialty with further training beyond an approved introductory course in undersea and hyperbaric medicine (UHM) such as the Program for Advanced Training in Hyperbarics (PATH) provided by the UHMS. It is highly recommended that a medical director is board-eligible or board-certified in UHM through an accredited source administered by the American Board of Medical Specialties (ABMS)[1] or the osteopathic certificate of added qualifications (CAQ) in UHM administered by the American Osteopathic Association (AOA) Board of Specialties.[2] Additionally, this provider should have a minimum of 12 months' experience as a provider supervising hyperbaric treatments prior to assuming the role of medical director.[3]

The medical director has responsible oversight of all staffing and training for the facility. The provider mix should be determined to safely manage and supervise all treatments according to the number and acuity of patients treated. For our purposes, the term provider includes all trained physicians (MD/DO/DPM), and qualified advanced practice providers (APPs), also known as advanced practice clinicians (APCs). Both terms include nurse practitioners (NP) and physician's assistants (PA). Additional auxiliary medical and administrative staff is determined according to type and number of chambers, population served, and productive flow of the clinic.

Providers attending HBO_2 treatments fall into one of three functional classifications:

1. **Independent supervisors of HBO_2** are MD/DOs who meet the criteria to independently attend HBO_2 treatments and supervise or proctor other providers attending HBO_2 treatments. These physicians hold a valid unrestricted medical license to practice within their state jurisdiction and have completed an approved introductory course in hyperbaric medicine. It is highly recommended that these courses meet the accreditation standard of the Undersea and Hyperbaric Medical Society (UHMS). To be credentialed, they must have additionally been proctored by a physician experienced in hyperbaric medicine until determined to be reliably trained and ready to independently supervise HBO_2 treatments. To maintain their status as an independent supervisor of HBO_2, they are required to maintain a minimum of 12 continuing medical education credits in hyperbaric related topics per year.[3] The UHMS recommends this new minimum credentialing standard for all independent supervision after June 30, 2022.[3] After that time, completion of hyperbaric-based education beyond the approved introductory course in hyperbaric medicine may become a requirement for facility accreditation. Hyperbaric physicians not ABMS or AOA board-certified in the subspecialty of UHM must complete an ACGME-approved fellowship in hyperbaric medicine or obtain a CAQ in hyperbaric medicine such as PATH or another approved program within two years of being granted privileges in hyperbaric medicine.
2. **Providers** are MD/DOs and APPs who meet criteria for attending HBO_2 independently but do not possess the appropriate training and/or experience to supervise other providers (as determined by the hospital or health care facility credentialing policies).

3. **Providers who are undergoing their period of privileging proctorship** with immediate availability of a medical director or independent supervisor of HBO_2 (as defined above) throughout the entirety of each and every HBO_2 treatment until such time as they satisfy credentialing criteria to independently attend HBO_2 treatments. Typically, this includes the following: MD/DOs new to the field of UHM; experienced MD/DO UHM physicians transferring from another HBO_2 practice but within their period of privileging proctorship; APPs; limited license DPM providers; MD/DO fellows; and other medical trainees.

Many facilities rely on PRN and or part-time providers for coverage of shifts. Initial education, training, and proctoring requirements are the same as described above to attain one of the three levels described. Annual CME requirements are the same and it should be expected that these individual practitioners will pursue a higher level of training and certification. It is up to the medical director, in association with the facility credentialing committee, to determine the minimum work hours or number of patients treated that may be necessary to maintain adequate experiential knowledge.

APPs attending HBO_2 part-time may require immediate in-person availability of an independent supervisor of HBO_2 during treatments.

Doctors of podiatric medicine (DPM) are licensed with a scope of practice limited to musculoskeletal injuries and diseases below the knee. At the time of this writing, some facilities credential DPMs to supervise HBO_2 treatment of patients with indications for treatment below the knee only. Application of this credentialing standard depends on specific state legal statutes. The medical education and clinical training required to appropriately assess patients being considered for HBO_2 or to attend complications resulting from, or associated with, HBO_2 treatment limits their ability to be an independent supervisor of HBO_2. For this reason, DPMs should also not serve as medical directors for hyperbaric clinics. Appropriately educated, trained, and proctored DPMs who are credentialed and privileged by the facility may attend routine HBO_2 treatments of stable patients with wounds below the knee when there is oversight by an independent supervisor of HBO_2.

In the United States, the Centers for Medicare and Medicaid Services (CMS) do not dictate credentialing requirements or training for providers treating HBO_2, but many regional Medicare administrative contract (MAC) providers recommend that all providers supervising hyperbaric treatments must be certified in advanced cardiac life support (ACLS) and are trained in life-saving procedures for the worst possible complications associated with HBO_2 treatment, such as chest tubes placement or needle thoracostomy for tension pneumothorax, or management of seizures. Some have written such requirements into local coverage determinations (LCD) to dictate requirements they believe necessary prior to reimbursement. It's important to know what, if any additional requirements such as these, is required by the jurisdiction MAC whether it is written in an LCD or not.

Additional Training

The medical director has responsibility to ensure that all staff members are adequately trained and maintain competency to ensure the safety and proper treatment of patients. All supervising providers should be trained and comfortable in possible emergency scenarios involved with HBO_2 treatment. This may include but is not limited to treatment of tension pneumothorax or pulmonary barotrauma, cardiac arrhythmias or arrest, oxygen seizures, and hypoglycemic reactions. They should also be well versed in nonemergent problems and concerns like ear and/or sinus squeeze (barotrauma), changes in vision, and pulmonary oxygen toxicity. Many facilities do not treat critical-care hyperbaric patients, but if they do and even if it's in the scope of the provider's practice and credentialing, they may require additional training in utilization of myringotomy, intubation and management of ventilators, management of intravascular lines, and medication dosing in hyperbaric conditions. Some facilities include portions of critical-care management, such as IV fluid and medication administration and patient-monitoring modalities, which require an elevated knowledge and understanding not only of equipment and pass-through devices but how pressure changes delivery. Initial training includes hands-on management of chamber and all equipment, including fire suppression equipment. All supervising providers should have a basic operational knowledge of the chambers that they supervise treatment in. The medical director should not only be comfortable with operational knowledge but have a clear understanding of required maintenance and related safety protocols associated with the chamber or chambers. This knowledge should be sufficient to maintain an effective working relationship with the safety director.

Awareness of the standard training requirements for all nurses, techs, and even nonclinical managers is important in order to provide the careful coordination and oversight of training, certification, and maintenance of competency. It is recommended that the medical director keeps an up-to-date tracking file of all staff training and continuing education. The specific requirements for all nonprovider staff are discussed in related chapters.

Proctoring Providers

Mentoring providers new to the knowledge, discipline, and responsibilities relevant to hyperbaric medicine is one of the most important roles of the medical director. The proctorship process represents only the first steps in a carefully planned mentorship. It should be designed to bring the individual to competency, but mentorship continues beyond the period of proctoring to encourage an attitude of continuous learning to attain expertise. Skillful medical directors, while seeking the same personal attainment of expertise, will broaden their understanding and the understanding of staff through individually tailored hands-on training, case reviews and "open door" availability for immediate "real time" review of cases. During the proctorship period, a qualified independent supervisor of HBO_2 must be immediately available physically, on campus, or in close enough proximity to be considered a safe response time to the facility where HBO_2 treatments are conducted.

The medical director has a responsibility to determine the proper training that will ensure competency in the provider, within parameters that follow the standard of care. The number of HBO_2 specific consultations and dual-supervised HBO_2 treatment sessions may be determined by previous experience of the provider in question, but a general suggested guideline is a minimum of five (5) proctored consultations and attending more than twenty-five (25) HBO_2 sessions with direct, one-on-one immediate oversight by an independent supervisor of HBO_2 or preferably the medical director, followed by an additional indirect oversight of at least 100 sessions. This indirect oversight can be accomplished through chart review, and the specific cases or notes from the review should be available for credentialing oversight, peer-to-peer review and/or other audit reviews. The Joint Commission and the UHMS accreditation program recommend that facilities develop a routine focused professional practice evaluation process (FPPE) for ongoing practice oversight. Every US hospital with a CMS certification number must collect data for FPPE related to provider's performance within their hospital or system.[4] Most hospital credentialing offices will have a template or information on how to set up an FPPE if one is not already in place.

Proctoring requirements may be modified as needed for providers transferring from another hyperbaric facility or those otherwise with previous experience. If prior work experience can be verified to meet the proctoring requirements and the individual has satisfactorily demonstrated a safe and competent working knowledge of hyperbaric medicine over the previous two years, the proctoring requirements may be modified or waived as appropriate.

Use of APPs may vary depending on individual state law or facility licensing and credentialing practices. The use of clinical nurse practitioners and physician assistants in both wound care and hyperbaric practice as a physician extender is becoming more commonplace as a standard of care. The efficient use of APPs mixed with physician providers is determined by the medical director.

Documentation of all staff training, proctoring, and recredentialing is the responsibility of the medical director. Maintaining a file to record all training documentation is an accreditation standard and highly recommended best practice.

Setting Up a Clinic

In an ideal situation, the medical director will be involved with the initial set up of the clinic, allowing evaluation for the most efficient layout according to patient flow patterns around a central work area with proximity to the chambers. Different clinical floor plans can be observed, mapping out walking traffic patterns as staff members perform tasks during a normal workday to evaluate for inefficient, time-consuming steps or choke points. A typical choke point might be found if a path from the waiting area to the exam room intersects with staff or provider work areas allowing potential for unnecessary interruptions. It may be more efficient to arrange placement of providers' offices to keep the provider free from such distractions. Patterns that minimize extra steps and maximize efficiency should be determined for efficient placement of treatment rooms, offices, supply centers, and utility rooms. For the safety of both patients and staff, clinic design must take into account the quickest, most efficient egress routes determined for all possible emergency scenarios.

It is also important to staff a clinic efficiently enough to keep overhead low while maximizing throughput. Staffing the clinic with a mix of registered nurses and medical attendants may help contain overhead costs. However, an insufficient number of staff available may increase patient wait times and frustration, but more importantly, it may reduce overall safety of the unit. Too many staff may drive costs up inappropriately but not enough to manage the typical higher acuity patients seen in most hyperbaric facilities. This may impact the overall safe management of all patients. Managing a higher clinic mix of elderly patients with multiple comorbidities may require a higher staff-to-patient ratio than is seen in most primary care clinic settings.

Utilization of medical assistants (MAs) varies from state to state. Some allow a certified medical attendant (CMA) to administer both topical and parental medications, change dressings, apply total contact casting, and other specialty dressings, while other states only allow this within the nurse's scope of practice. Some MA/CMAs may also attain credentialing as certified hyperbaric technologists (CHT). Having intimate knowledge of your local regional differences for nursing and medical technician utilization is an important function for the medical director.

Documentation of care is coordinated either through written or electronic health records to ensure that all important data is recorded. It is highly recommended to include documentation of safety checklists and instructions, given in the patient's primary language with verbal repeat back to show their understanding. The record should also clearly state the medical necessity requiring hyperbaric treatment, the type and dosing of treatment to include number of treatments, atmospheric pressure involved, and percentage of oxygen the body will be exposed to. Utilization reviews will document either the continued need for or the ineffectiveness of treatment necessitating discontinuation. The treatment plan should include goals that are discussed between the patient and provider. Progress toward the expected outcome should be clearly documented.

Policies

In addition to providing patient care, the medical director plays a leadership role in policy development. Through consultation with the clinic manager, the medical director helps determine policies for governance and efficient management of the clinic. With the safety director, they determine policies and procedures to help execute safe treatment of patients, minimizing risk and mitigating all potential safety hazards with well-prepared procedures and protocols to be implemented in case of emergencies. These policies should be reviewed annually, with staff awareness and training implemented on a regular schedule.

Procedures should include a process of patient education, with allowance for informed decision-making by the patient and/or family. Appropriate educational materials and handouts should be regularly reviewed by the medical director for accuracy and up-to-date information. These materials will not only explain the medical reasons for treatment in patient-friendly language but will also outline risks, treatment side effects, and safety measures utilized to mitigate these risks for appropriate patient knowledge for informed consent.

Continuity of care requires close coordination between all provider, nursing, and technical staff to ensure treatment plans are well-timed and that patients receive the best care available. Periodic patient review and coordination should be organized to ensure any updates to the care plan are communicated with all members of this team as well as the patient. Periodic utilization review should be conducted, with analysis of documentation to ensure that hyperbaric treatment is effective and not overutilized, and this, too, should be documented in the medical record.

Procedures should be in place to organize plans for evaluation and mitigation of adverse events. A system for root-cause analysis should be designed, with a stepwise approach that can be implemented on an emergency basis as needed, with the ability to remove, control, or contain any hazard immediately. Included in this policy should be a schedule for review, practice, and drills of all procedures and protocols. It is best to include all local community resources, such as fire department and other rescue personnel that may be involved in emergency procedures. A fire drill can highlight best evacuation and escape routes, positioning of fire trucks in relation to hydrant access, and areas of extra concern as determined by the fire marshal. Rehearsals will include execution of these protocols and allow assessment of staff knowledge of the escape routes, location of oxygen shutoff valves, and location and use of available protection equipment. Drills also allow staff from other areas of the facility who may be required to respond to an emergency within the hyperbaric facility to become familiar with the layout and operations of the facility.

Policies should include periodic inspection and maintenance schedules, the prohibited materials checklist, approved cleaning supplies and materials, and specific instructions and precautions listed for housekeeping personnel. Additional policies should be provided for any deviations from standard procedures, for ensuring gas purity, and even policies for opening and closing procedures.

In collaboration with the safety director, the medical director must ensure that any devices to be used within or in conjunction with hyperbaric treatments has documentation on file, showing pressure testing to the maximum pressure of their chambers with safety approval. Devices and materials not included in the standard-approved list must undergo a separate evaluation process by the safety director and medical director that is documented in the patient record. These devices may include, but are not limited to, respiratory ventilators, intravenous infusion pumps, cardiovascular monitoring devices including implantable cardiac monitoring with or without defibrillation devices, electrocardiogram or blood pressure monitoring devices, and medication delivery devices both external and implantable. Any hospital- or clinic-provided devices will also need approval from their prospective bioengineer department. One resource for questions related to devices or materials that may not have this testing or documentation available is the UHMS Safety Committee publications that include updated safety and equipment articles, manufacturer notices, and other safety references.[5] Policies and procedures must be developed for the use of these devices along with application of any external attachments or chamber pass-through penetrators, and what trained personnel provides care, including the administration of any medications, wound care treatments, and appropriate follow-up schedules. Any limitations of the chamber and or staff should also be documented.

Providing an Environment of Safety

In a well-run clinic, the leadership chain of command is well defined and should ultimately end with the medical director. Maintain open lines of communication with all staff members, emphasizing discussions related to safe practices in the workplace. Keep a cooperative, working rapport with the safety director and use frequent huddles or meetings to go over daily or weekly actions that produced good safe results, as well as those that may have had a negative outcome. Provide a nonretribution means of reporting near-miss episodes or unsafe incidents or mishaps, then utilize a team approach to develop a preventive plan of action. A wise medical director will know how to listen and analyze information obtained and delegate as needed. Continue to refine these steps while promoting a daily mindset focused on providing both the staff and patients with an environment of safety. While not required, a recommended best practice is for the medical director, as well as the safety director, to attend a hyperbaric safety course.

Personnel exposed to environmental risk, such as the inside observers for a multiplace chamber, should have periodic health assessments to determine fitness for the duties required. These are typically performed every three to five years of employment by a qualified provider. A qualified provider should be one who has intimate knowledge of the requirements for the duties involved. This may be an occupational medicine specialist, another hyperbaric or dive medicine trained physician, or the medical director of the hyperbaric unit. To avoid possible conflict of interest, it may be preferred to avoid performing fitness for duty evaluations on personnel who work for the medical director. Initial screening of past medical history should be evaluated, and as indicated, additional screening tests may include chest X-ray (CXR), pulmonary function tests (PFTs), hearing testing, and possibly additional lab screening as deemed necessary by the medical director. The medical director should also publish policies that spell out physical requirements necessary for the duties as well as health or physical attributes that may increase risk and thus disqualify an employee for specific duties.

Careful preparation of policies related to known hazards or possible unsafe practices requires an intimate knowledge of each step within the treatment process. Remember, common things happen commonly. Prevention is always the best practice but often protection of patient and staff requires utilization of administrative controls, personal protective equipment (PPE), and/or engineered controls.

Examples:

Administrative Controls (not all inclusive):

1. Shift scheduling to ensure adequate rest for staff
2. Appropriate time intervals between hyperbaric treatments for patient safety
3. Adequate staffing:
   - One CHT operator for no more than two monoplace chambers
   - Three CHT operators (two outside and one inside observer) for multi-place chambers
   - Adequate monitoring of inside observer risk for decompression illness (DCI) with appropriate surface intervals and prevention of heavy exercise tasking in the recovery period
4. STOP (Safety Time-out/Pause) procedures[6-7] (patient safety checks)
   - Check patient grounding (monoplace)
   - All prohibited items removed from the chamber (monoplace and multiplace)
   - Treatment profile and staffing plan confirmed
   - The completed STOP checklist dated and signed or initialed by two staff members prior to closing the door of the chamber
5. Medical screening of patients and pressure exposed staff (initial and prior to each treatment)
6. Air breaks (duration and timing)

PPE:

1. Patient clothing (100% cotton or 60/40 blend = 60% cotton / 40% polyester)
2. Grounding straps for monoplace chambers
3. Hood and appropriately fit neck dam (multiplace)
4. Smoke hoods and emergency air supplies

Engineering Controls:

1. Pressure regulated pop-off valves
2. Periodic inspections of acrylics, valves, electronic components, and all moving parts
3. Routine required maintenance
4. Fire suppression systems, including regular operational testing
5. Air-break systems

Summary

The role of medical director is the most important leadership role for any medical clinic because of the breadth of medical knowledge needed to keep all clinical, administrative, and safety issues relevant to medically focused patient care. Keeping current with all issues within the specialty has been emphasized throughout this chapter, including evidence-based indications, knowledge of research initiatives, reimbursement related changes, and the safe application of all treatments to protect the welfare of both patients and staff. Involvement in professional societies related to the specialty is an important avenue to maintain current knowledge and develop a network of resources with other medical directors and/or individuals with similar education, experience, and interests. The following professional hyperbaric societies are currently available to the medical director and involvement, with one or more highly recommended to help promote continuing education as well as advancement of scientific knowledge and professional awareness among peers and associates in the field of hyperbaric medicine:

1. The Undersea and Hyperbaric Medical Society (UHMS)
    - Regional Chapters:
        - Pacific Chapter
        - Gulf Coast Chapter
        - Midwest Chapter
        - Northeast Chapter
    - National and International Affiliates:
        - Aerospace Medical Association (AsMA)
        - European Underwater and Baromedical Society (EUBS)
        - South Pacific Underwater Medicine Society (SPUMS)
        - Canadian Undersea and Hyperbaric Medical Association (CUHMA)
        - Sociedade Brasileira De Medicina Hiperbárica (SBMH)
        - Gesellschaft Für Tauch-und Über-druck-medizin e.V (GTUM)
        - Japanese Society for Hyperbaric Medicine (JSHM)
        - Société de Médicine et de Physiologie Subaquatiques de Langue Française (MEDSUBHYP)
        - Southern African Underwater and Hyperbaric Association (SAUHMA)
2. American College of Hyperbaric Medicine (ACHM)
3. International Hyperbaric Medical Association (IHMA)

4. International Hyperbarics Association (IHAUSA)

5. Veterinary Hyperbaric Medical Society (VHMS)

6. National Hyperbaric Association (NHA)

7. National Board of Diving and Hyperbaric Medical Technology (NBDHMT)

8. British Hyperbaric Association (BHA)

References

1. ABMS. Value of Board Certification to Health Care. Retrieved from American Board of Medical Specialties: https://www.abms.org/board-certification/value-of-board-certification-to-health-care/. Jan 2019.
2. American Osteopathic Association. American Osteopathic Undersea & Hyperbaric Medicine Examination Committee. https://certification.osteopathic.org/undersea-hyperbaric-medicine/. 2017.
3. The Joint Commission. Standards Interpretation Frequently Asked Questions (FAQs) . https://www.jointcommission.org/standards_information/jcfaq.aspx?ProgramId=5&ChapterId=74&IsFeatured=False&IsNew=False&Keyword=FPPE&print=y. 2019.
4. The Joint Commission. The Joint Commission, Standards, National Patient Safety Goal, Universal Protocol. http://www.jointcommission.org/standards_information/up.aspx. 2019.
5. UHMS Safety Committee. Undersea & Hyperbaric Medical Society Resources. www.uhms.org/resources/medfaqs-frequently-asked-questions-faq/53-safety-technical.html. 2019.
6. Undersea & Hyperbaric Medical Society. News & Announcements, Safety Time Out/Pause - "STOP." https://www.uhms.org/resources/news-announcements/106-safety-time-out-pause-stop-posted-7-31-2014.html. 2019.
7. Undersea and Hyperbaric Medical Society. UHMS Guidelines for Credentialing, Privileging and Supervision of Hyperbaric Oxygen Therapy in the U.S.A. https://www.uhms.org/images/Position-Statements/UHMS_Cred_and_Priv_Guide_Jan_31_2018.pdf. 2019.

CHAPTER 6.6
The Role of the Nurse in Promoting Hyperbaric Facility Safety

Connie Hutson, CHSP, STS, ACHRN, CHWS, CWCN, RN, MS

Introduction

Hyperbaric medicine has a 100+ year history, with nurses playing an integral role in the past 60 years of the century of practice.[1-2] Hyperbaric nursing developed in Europe in the 1950s before coming to North America in the 1960s when the field became more clinically-focused with an increase in the number of clinical conditions treated with hyperbaric oxygen (HBO_2). The need for a professional hyperbaric nursing organization was evident, resulting in the formation of the Baromedical Nurses Association (BNA) in 1985.[3] From the beginning, the mission of the BNA was to provide nurses with a professional organization to maintain and promote the status and standards of practice in hyperbaric nursing, and this same mission continues today.

The founding nurses of the BNA, and those pioneering nurses before them, paved the way for nurses to contribute to the operation of hyperbaric facilities, working collaboratively with the hyperbaric health care team developing, implementing, assessing, and monitoring the safety program. The nurse must understand the codes and standards applicable to the operation and safety of the hyperbaric program, along with possessing a clear understanding of the clinical application and reimbursement criteria necessary for hyperbaric oxygen therapy.[4]

The nurse is involved all aspects of the hyperbaric facility safety program; however, the nurse plays a more active role in certain aspects which affect the direct delivery of patient care, including the following: patient assessment and reassessment; patient/family teaching/education; and staff competencies, ensuring there are appropriate staffing levels to meet patient needs while also considering budgetary parameters. The nurse also plays an important role in ensuring standardized policies and procedures are followed, along with ensuring quality improvement processes are in place. The most critical role of the hyperbaric nurse is to provide safe patient care at all times.

Nursing Scope of Practice

The nursing profession offers various levels of practice, including the certified nursing assistant (CNA), the licensed practical/vocational nurse (LPN/LVN), the registered nurse (RN), the graduate nurse, and the advanced practice nurse (APN), with each of these levels having a different scope of practice based on their educational preparation and experience.[5] Each state is responsible for regulating and establishing standards for nursing practice. The nursing scope of practice helps ensure safe practice by legally defining the actions and procedures the nurse is permitted to perform. Nurses working in the hyperbaric facility must know their own scope of practice, along with the other health care team member's scope of practice to ensure safe patient care is being delivered.

Certified Nursing Assistant (CNA)

The certified nursing assistant (CNA), sometimes called a nursing aide, assists patients with their basic health care needs, which includes activities of daily living. They typically work in hospitals or long-term care facilities. The CNA works under the direct supervision of the RN or LPN/LVN, and each state determines the certified nursing assistant (CNA) scope of practice.[6-7]

Licensed Practical Nurse/Vocational Nurse (LPN/LVN)

The licensed practical nurse (LPN) is the term used in all states, except Texas and California, where the term licensed vocational nurse (LVN) is used for entry level nursing.[8] The LPN/LVN has successfully completed a LPN/LVN-approved training program and received a certificate or diploma. There are many different programs and educational tracks available to the individual wanting to pursue a practical or vocational nursing profession. The program is typically nine months to one year in length and is offered by vocational, technical, community, junior, or nursing colleges. After graduation, the successful candidate is then required to pass the national council licensure examination for practical nurses (NCLEX-PN) before being licensed in that state as a LPN/LVN.[9]

The LPN/LVN is vital to the nursing profession as the LPN/LVN serves as a valuable health care team member in many capacities. The LPN/LVN nurse provides patient care in the hyperbaric facility under the supervision of a registered nurse (RN), advanced practice nurse (APN), or physician.[10] The care responsibilities of the LPN/LVN may vary from state to state, and it is the responsibility of the LPN/LVN to know the specific state-delineated scope of practice (along with other federal, state, or local practice mandates) in order to promote safe working environment by practicing within the scope of practice.

The LPN/LVN educational curriculum consists of learning the disease processes along with receiving clinical training in a health care setting. The LPN/LVN provides basic patient care, monitors the patient's condition, and reports changes or adverse reactions to the supervising RN, APN, or physician. The LPN/LVN works collaboratively with the supervising RN, APN, or physician in contributing patient data collected from the patient assessment and helping to formulate and guide the patient's plan of care.[9-10] The LPN/LVN also participates in quality improvement initiatives and provides input on policy development/changes.

The LPN/LVN's role in the hyperbaric facility would focus on providing safe patient care and promoting a safe working environment whether in the clinician role of delivering the prescribed dose of hyperbaric oxygen to the patient while closely monitoring patients during their treatment and/or serving as the safety director of the facility. In some facilities the LPN/LVN may serve several roles, which only adds to their value in the hyperbaric facility as they can also serve as a wound care clinician if the HBO_2 facility offers wound care services. Successful hyperbaric facilities utilize all staff skill sets, education, and training to the optimum level.

Registered Nurse (RN)

Though there are different educational paths or tracks to choose from, there is a diploma, associate degree, or bachelor's of science in nursing programs, in which all of these programs prepare the future nurse to sit for the National Council Licensure Examination (NCLEX-RN), a standardized exam that each state board of nursing uses to see if the nurse meets their standards to practice nursing in that state. Each of the training tracks offer a different educational curriculum to include the following:

Nursing diploma: The nursing diploma program is the oldest type of nursing educational training in the United States. The nursing diploma programs are typically two to three years in length and are usually hospital-based with the bulk of training focused on clinical nursing.[11]

The individual receives general education and support courses in health care. With the rise in university-based training programs, diploma programs are dwindling in numbers across the United States.

Associate degree: The associate degree program is a popular path in achieving a RN degree because it is typically two years in length, which prepares the successful graduate to sit for the NCLEX-RN exam in a shorter amount of time than the other educational programs.[12] Eligibility to sit for an exam in two years is attractive to many in the current economy.

Associate degree programs vary, but typically an associate degree program offers courses in medical-surgical, maternal/child health, pediatrics, and mental health nursing, along with a clinical component to prepare the nurse for entry level nursing. The associate degree program does focus on the nurse achieving technical skills.

Bachelor's of science in nursing degree (BSN): The bachelor's of science in nursing degree program is a four-year program and includes liberal arts education plus social and behavioral science, along with extensive amount of nursing courses. The BSN program offers additional instruction in community nursing, leadership, and management.

The BSN prepares the nurse for a professional role away from the bedside if the nurse desires this career path. The Bureau of Labor Statistics reports the nurse with a BSN degree will have better job prospects than those without one.[13]

The RN role offers flexibility to the hyperbaric facility clinical operations. The RN may serve as a staff nurse to provide patient care, provide education to patients and their families about the various disease states, provide case management services for the higher acuity patients, and develop the patient care plan to include the patient's short- and long-term nursing goals. The RN also assesses and reassesses the patient and their care plan to see if the nursing goals have been met. The RN makes changes to the care plan if the goals have not been met. The staff RN may also supervise the LPN/LVN nurse and nursing assistant working in the hyperbaric facility as part of the RN duties.

The RN may work in the hyperbaric facility in a more administrative role as the nurse manager. The managing RN's role would be to oversee the clinical aspects of the hyperbaric facility and work collaboratively with the other hyperbaric health care team members.

Advanced practice nurse (APN): The advanced practice nurse is a registered nurse who has a master's degree in nursing and has gained advanced preparation in extended clinical practice. There are four recognized specialized areas in advanced practice nursing: nurse anesthetists, nurse midwives, clinical nurse specialists (CNS), and nurse practitioners (NP).[14] The nurse anesthetist delivers anesthesia, the nurse midwife provides care to women during pregnancy and birth, the CNS is an expert clinician who works in a specialty area, and the NP focuses on providing primary care to patients.

The APN is trained to work in a variety of health care settings. However, the NP or the CNS may choose to work in a hyperbaric facility as a practicing clinician or in a more advanced role to serve as consultant, educator, researcher, or supervise hyperbaric oxygen therapy (HBOT) as a health care provider. However, supervising HBOT would depend on government regulations, APN scope of practice, the facility's credentialing guidelines, reimbursement, and a contract with a physician, if not an independent practitioner.

Nursing Process

The nursing process, first introduced in 1958, typically consists of five phases: assessment, diagnosis, planning, implementing, and evaluation. Depending on the state where the nurse practices there may be a sixth phase—outcome setting.[15] The APNs and RNs utilize data collected from the nursing process to develop the patient's care plan. The nursing care plan guides individualized patient nursing care and includes the nursing diagnosis, nursing interventions, and patient-centered goals to achieve expected or desired outcomes.

All the phases of the nursing process combined produce a framework in which nurses provide care in a systematic and organized manner. APN or RNs are responsible for directing the nursing process with LPN/LVN's contribution, according to their state's nursing practice parameters. The APN or RN oversees the patient's care but may delegate duties to another trained responsible person, providing the facility has policies in place to address such delegation.

Assessment

The APN or RN completes an initial comprehensive history and thorough physical assessment according to the facility guidelines. Assessment usually includes a health history, general medical condition, physical review of body systems, list of medications (prescription and over the counter [OTC]), hospitalizations/surgeries, social and psychological status, allergies, physical capabilities, nutrition, fall risk, and learning needs. The history and physical of a hyperbaric patient can be time-consuming as there are many things to consider, including the following:

- history of cancer, received chemotherapy, currently receiving chemotherapy, received radiation, or currently receiving radiation therapy
- any barotrauma risks
- any ophthalmic risk to include glaucoma or ocular surgery
- any pulmonary dysfunction
- any medications administered subcutaneously, intramuscularly, or transdermally through a patch, as HBOT has vasoconstrictive qualities which could delay absorption of the medication and also has vasodilation qualities which could also affect the rate of medication delivery
- any medications to slow the heart rate/rhythm, as HBOT could contribute to bradycardic effects
- history of hypertension and taking oral blood pressure medications to reduce the blood pressure, as careful attention is needed to monitor the blood pressure since HBOT could contribute to hypertension
- monitor toxicity if patient is taking digitalis
- any diuretic medications (what diuretic medication, dose, schedule of the medication, any parameters given for taking the diuretic medication, and when the last dose was taken)
- any insulin, oral hypoglycemic medication (or both), or on an insulin pump, as the patient may need to have medication adjusted since HBOT may lower the blood glucose reading. Also, if on an insulin pump (nonimplantable), may need to be switched to an insulin sliding scale during the time the patient is receiving HBOT (implantable pumps discussed at the end of this section).
- seizures or history of seizures and is currently taking anticonvulsant medication for prevention of seizures, as lab values would need to ordered by the

provider to ensure the patient was in therapeutic range of that particular anticonvulsant medication

- narcotics, as patient would need further assessment since narcotic medications can decrease the respiratory drive and put the patient at risk for oxygen toxicity seizures
- using marijuana, as the provider would need to consider the state laws, along with hospital policies, to consider the CNS effects of THC (tetrahydrocannabinol) and how the patient presents themselves for their HBOT treatment
- if smoking or using vaporless smoking, the provider may instruct patient to reduce or stop smoking during the time the patient is receiving HBOT, as nicotine possesses vasoconstrictive effects
- high doses of steroids, which could increase the risk of oxygen toxicity seizures
- any absolute or relative contraindications to receiving HBOT
- medically unstable or requires mechanical ventilatory support
- existing tubes, such as chest tubes, intravenous lines to maintain or change to receive HBOT. If the intravenous lines had caps with alcohol inside the cap, this may pose a problem inside a 100% oxygen environment.
- gastrointestinal tubes (GI or percutaneous endoscopic gastrostomy [PEG] tubes to be open/capped, checked for patency, and secured prior to receiving HBOT)
- existing drains to address prior to receiving HBOT
- any wound care dressings in place to address prior to receiving HBOT, to see if the dressings would be approved/prohibited
- any implantable device to be verified with the manufacturer for safe use inside a hyperbaric chamber

The above list is not intended to be all inclusive.[16-19]

Depending on the hyperbaric facility, the APN or RN may document the findings of the history and physical into an electronic medical record (EMR) utilizing a desktop computer, laptop, iPad, or mobile device at the point of care while in the patient's room. If the facility does not have computerized documentation available or there is no interfacing of software, the APN or RN writes the findings on paper documentation while at the bedside. The paper documentation becomes part of the patient's medical record and is stored in a secure place, according to the facility guidelines, whereas the computerized method of documenting stores the data electronically in the patient's EMR or electronic health record (EHR) for easy access.

Hyperbaric facilities are at various stages of utilizing an EMR, as the systems can be complex and costly to implement, but once in place, EMR systems can improve care, communications, and reduce health care costs. EMR can enhance patient privacy by limiting access to medical records and patient information to those health care professionals authorized to care for the patient. Computerized documentation has the potential to decrease medical errors, improve patient safety, and increase staff productivity.

Diagnosis

After the hyperbaric patient is thoroughly assessed, the next step involves utilizing the nursing diagnosis to help identify the patient's actual or perceived problem(s). Nurses do not make medical decisions, as this is outside their scope of practice. Medical decisions are made by the physician/provider.

The nursing diagnosis differs from the medical diagnosis as the medical diagnosis deals with the disease process while the nursing diagnosis deals with the patient's response to stimuli. Nursing diagnoses are developed in accordance with the North America Nursing Diagnosis Association (NANDA) International. NANDA was founded in 1982, added "International" in 2002 to represent the growing number of members, and became NANDA International, Inc. in 2011, due to the increase of growth of members outside North America. The nurse makes clinical decisions by using the nursing diagnosis from the NANDA International, Inc. list.[20]

In part, NANDA International, Inc. was formed to provide standard nomenclature for use in the patient's medical record for better understanding among health care team members. NANDA International, Inc. promotes patient safety by using their evidence-based nursing diagnoses into clinical practice and decision making.[21]

Planning

The third step in the nursing process involves developing the patient's plan of care. The APN or RN collects data from the patient assessment to identify problems. After the problems are identified, the nurse develops the care plan by choosing the nursing diagnosis, defining the patient-centered goals, and choosing the nursing interventions best suited for the patient to achieve the desired or expected goals. The APN or RN also develops an appropriate teaching plan for the patient and their family or significant others, as there is much education before receiving HBOT.[22-23]

Effective communication skills are vital to all members of the health care team. Information about HBOT can be highly technical which may be difficult for patients and family to understand. Communication must be clear and focused. The nurse must be able to communicate complex terminology using language that is appropriate to the patient's education and comprehension level.

Developing the hyperbaric patient care plan is made easier by using the newly revised *2018 BNA Guidelines of Care* for the patient receiving HBOT. These guidelines have been in existence for many years and are referenced in many hyperbaric textbooks with the latest revision (2018) being posted on the BNA website.[24]

The *BNA Guidelines of Care* for the patient receiving HBOT list the problems the hyperbaric patient may experience while receiving HBOT. These standards of care include the problems, goals, and interventions along with the necessary rationale needed to develop the patient plan of care. One of goals of the BNA is to provide education to all HBOT nurses and not just to their members. The guidelines are easy to download and print by clicking on a "Nursing Guideline" link on the BNA website.

Implementation

After the care plan is completed, the APN or RN uses the information from the care plan to implement the patient care. The APN or RN may be the person performing the care or task, but the APN or RN may also choose to delegate the care or task to another staff member who may be licensed or unlicensed. The APN or RN must evaluate the staff member prior to delegating care or task to ensure the staff member has had the educational preparation, is competent to perform the assigned care or task, and within their job description. However, the APN or RN delegating to another staff member remains accountable for carrying out the care or performing the task.

Nurse delegation can be confusing, as different states have different perspectives regarding whether delegation is allowed or not allowed. The APN or RN must follow all regulatory guidelines regarding delegation and must practice within their scope of practice in order to provide safe care. The National Council of State Boards of Nursing addresses delegation in their position paper to provide a resource to state boards of nursing, employers, and nurses to provide a framework wherein safe care is being delivered.[25]

Evaluation

Evaluation of the patient's care plan is ongoing throughout the HBOT course. The evaluation involves the RN reassessing the patient's response to HBOT in order to determine the appropriateness and effectiveness of the therapy. The RN evaluates the patient's progress to see if there are any identifiable or potential problems hindering the patient from reaching the desired goals. The patient reassessment may be multidisciplinary to include input from the LPN/LVN. The patient care plan may change as a result from data collected during the reassessment process.

Nursing Documentation

The nurse documents in the patient's medical record (or oversees the proper documentation) of HBOT, as documentation is an essential element of safe, quality, and evidence-based nursing practice.[26] However, nursing documentation is also used for reimbursement purposes which is essential for HBO_2 operations. Centers for Medicare & Medicaid Services (CMS) requires the treatment details to include treatment number, date, patient demographics, diagnosis, descent time, ascent time, air-break times (if done in clock time), vital signs, treatment response or complications, how tolerated, and the person performing the treatment.

Staffing

It is vital for the hyperbaric facility to employ skilled staff to provide consistent, safe and high-quality care. However, for this to occur, there must be appropriate staffing to meet these expectations. Arranging staffing can be a daunting task for the nurse manager, as there are many factors to consider before staffing schedules are created. Hospitals use a variety of productivity tools to help the inpatient nurse manager determine staffing levels, and there has been research conducted on staffing levels for inpatient hospital settings which produced productivity tools. However, the majority of HBO_2 facilities are in an outpatient setting where productivity tool research is limited. Therefore, the nurse manager has limited accessibility to productivity tools to utilize due to this limited amount of research and publication of a tool on staffing productivity, which consider patient acuity, hyperbaric treatments, along with wound care and other ancillary care. Common practice for staffing for monoplace HBO_2 facilities is 1:2 ratio (one chamber operator per two chambers).[27]

Staffing in a hyperbaric facility depends on the number of patients receiving HBOT, the type and number of hyperbaric chambers in the facility, and acuity level of the hyperbaric patients. Staffing may include the treating physician/provider, the hyperbaric technician, RN/APN, respiratory therapist, LPN/LVN, and unlicensed assistive personnel.

The nurse manager considers staff qualifications along with the patient's acuity to ensure the patient receives safe care. Providing safe care is the most important consideration when arranging staffing. The nurse manager for a multiplace hyperbaric facility would need to arrange more staff, depending on the patient census and acuity as the multiplace chamber requires more staff to operate. The nurse manager for the multiplace facility also considers health issues of the inside attendant, such as age, extreme fatigue, dehydration, colds, and pregnancy.[28-29]

Competent Staff

The nurse manager working in the hyperbaric facility works collaboratively with the medical director, the safety director, and other members of management to hire competent staff. After the staff are hired, the nurse manager must ensure the staff receive hyperbaric specific training. There are 40-hour introductory courses recommended and approved by the National Board of Diving and Hyperbaric Medical Technology (NBDHMT) or Undersea Hyperbaric Medical Society (UHMS) but not statutory. However, the 40-hour NBDHMT or UHMS-approved courses are a requirement for UHMS facility accreditation.

When the staff completes their hyperbaric specific training, there is additional comprehensive orientation provided. The orientation period is designed to assess staff's performance and each facility has its own orientation period/process specifically designed for their facility. Staff are also required to complete initial, yearly, and ongoing competencies as required. Another duty of the nurse manager is to verify certifications and licensure.

Initially, the hyperbaric staff are trained by attending an introductory 40-hour hyperbaric medicine course approved by the NBDHMT, UHMS, and now, American College of Hyperbaric Medicine (ACHM), which includes online portions of the training.[30] However, currently, neither the UHMS or NBDHMT supports online introductory training in hyperbaric medicine but rather recognizes the course to be 40 hours of face-to-face instruction, including practical chamber-side environment.[31] UHMS accreditation standards address the need for the safety director to receive additional training by attending a UHMS or NBDHMT-approved hyperbaric safety director course.[32] The online training does not allow the HBO_2-trained person to sit for NBDHMT certification, which is recommended for UHMS accredited facilities.

Clinical competencies can be performed by different methods but must be pertinent to the particular needs for the staff's assignment.[33] Hospital or facility competencies could include a myriad of different topics, including training in CPR, ACLS, patient privacy, lifting, disaster training, adverse event reporting, exposure control, and infection prevention. The hyperbaric staff would also need to complete other competencies related to working in the hyperbaric environment, as there are many competencies related to safety. In addition to staff completing the important competencies, it is highly recommended for staff to receive monthly in-services containing hyperbaric topics.[34]

A major safety function of the nurse manager related to hyperbaric safety is to manage all aspects of the competency requirements, which entails staff to successfully complete and pass the competencies within the time frame allowed, attend all mandatory in-service training, and maintain the necessary certification and licensure required. The nurse manager is also responsible for observing staffs' skills/performance and developing educational or performance action plans for improvement if needed.

Policies and Procedures

Policies and procedures are required by The Joint Commission (TJC) and other regulatory bodies for health care facilities as policies are intended to guide the facility. The procedures explain the series of steps needed to complete a particular action. As more facilities have electronic accessible policies and procedures, hard copies are not as readily available. However, a set of the hard copies is available in the chief nurse executive or director of nurse's office in case there was a power outage.

The policies and procedures address all aspects of care provided in the hyperbaric facility and cover all scopes of practice in accordance with all applicable regulatory guidelines. Policies and procedures are reviewed annually and more frequently, if needed. Safe patient policies establish certain expectations that staff will practice the safest techniques to accomplish patient handling tasks.[35]

All staff need to understand policy and procedures and recommend/make changes when needed. To be a contributing member of the policy and procedure development team, the hyperbaric nurse must be knowledgeable about research in the industry, attend hyperbaric conference seminars, pursue/maintain certification in the hyperbaric field, and belong to professional organizations.

Quality/Patient Safety

There continues to be heightened focus on the ever-increasing cost of health care and the demand for health care facilities to reduce their cost. While health care facilities are tasked with the burden of reducing these skyrocketing costs, they must also address improving quality and safety initiatives.[36] With all the financial challenges placed on health care facilities, it is imperative for health care facilities to develop and maintain strong quality and patient safety initiatives.

Hospital safety has been a concern for many years. In 1999, a landmark publication by the Institute of Medicine (IOM), "To Err Is Human: Building a Safer Health System," focused attention on safety in hospitals.[37] Efforts to improve safety have mostly focused on the inpatient hospital setting, but in the last 30 years the delivery of care has transitioned from the inpatient hospital setting to the outpatient or ambulatory care setting.[38] With the increased growth of patient care taking place in the outpatient or ambulatory care settings, research is expanding to provide a better understanding of emerging safety trends in the ambulatory care setting.[39]

With all of the attention and intense focus on providing quality care and patient safety, nursing is put in a position to drive these indicators, as nursing is the largest profession in health care. Because nurses have continuous interactions with patients and families, they are in a position to positively influence experiences of care and other significant health outcomes. They can leverage that power to their advantage.[40] Health care literature takes this idea further to discuss the importance of having nurses in leadership roles for quality improvement, as they have knowledge of what works and what doesn't work.[41]

Conclusion

The hyperbaric nurse has a duty to provide safe patient care while providing a safe environment for the patient to receive and staff to deliver care.The hyperbaric nurse serves a multifaceted role in the hyperbaric facility, and this role will become more involved as the hyperbaric field continues to grow and evolve with the ever-changing demands of the health care field. The hyperbaric field has new nurses joining the ranks to learn all they can using the resources available, while the field maintains the experienced nurses who share their knowledge and field experiences to coach the new recruits.

The hyperbaric nurse makes valuable contributions to the hyperbaric safety arena and should make themselves available to professional hyperbaric organizational and educational opportunities in order to serve as a resource to others. The hyperbaric nurse can also use these resources to provide leadership in attaining/maintaining UHMS clinical hyperbaric facility accreditation to ensure the highest quality and safest care is being offered.

References

1. Messina V. Hyperbaric nursing. In: Whelan, HT, Kindwall, EP, editors. Hyperbaric Medicine Practice, 4th Ed. North Palm Beach, FL: Best Publishing Co.; 2017;11-129.
2. Handley S, Clarke D. Hyperbaric history and the nursing evolution. In: Larson-Lohr V, editor, Norvell H, Josefsen L, Wilcox JR, co-editors. Hyperbaric Nursing and Wound Care. Flagstaff, AZ: Best Publishing Co; 2010;1-12.
3. http://hyperbaricnurses.org/AboutBNA.htm. Accessed: [Nov 22, 2018].
4. Workman WT. Accreditation and regulation in hyperbaric and wound centers. In: Larson-Lohr V, Norvell H. (Eds.), Hyperbaric nursing and wound care. Flagstaff, AZ: Best Publishing Co.; 2010;65-74.
5. American Nurses Association. Scope and Standards of Practice, 3rd Ed. Silver Spring, MD; 2016.
6. https://www.bls.gov/ooh/healthcare/print/nursing-assistants.htm. Accessed: [Nov 22, 2018].
7. McMullen TL, Resnick B, Chin-Hansen J, Geiger-Brown JM, Miller N. Certified nurse aide scope of practice: State-by- state differences in allowable delegated activities. Rubenstein R. Journal of the American Medical Directors Association. 2015;20-24.
8. Dahlkemper TR. Nursing Leadership, Management, and Professional Practice for the LPN/LVN. Philadelphia, PA: F A Davis Co.; 2013.
9. www.nursing.ohio.gov. Accessed: [Nov 30, 2018].
10. Spector N. National Council of State Boards of Nursing, Inc. Practical Nurse Scope of Practice White Paper, August 2005.
11. https://www.nursingschool.org/nursing-programs/program-types/diploma/#context/api/listings/prefilter. Accessed: [Nov 30, 2018].
12. https://www.registerednursing.org/degree/adn/. Accessed: [Nov 30, 2018].
13. https://www.bls.gov/ooh/healthcare/registered-nurses.htm#tab-6. Accessed: [Nov 30, 2018].
14. https://nursejournal.org/advanced-practice/advanced-practice-nursing-fact-sheet/. Accessed: [Dec 1, 2018].
15. Wilkinson JM. Nursing Process and Critical Thinking, 5th Ed. Upper Saddle River, NJ: Pearson: 2017.
16. Neuman TS, Thom SR. Physiology and Medicine of Hyperbaric Oxygen Therapy. Philadelphia, PA: Saunders Elsevier; 2008.
17. Lohr-Larson V, Norvell HC. Hyperbaric Nursing. Flagstaff, AZ: Best Publishing Co.; 2002.
18. Garcia J. Management of the critically ill patient in a hyperbaric setting: Nursing considerations and preventions. In: Larson-Lohr V, editor, Norvell HC, Josefsen L, Wilcox JR, co-editors. Hyperbaric Nursing and Wound Care. Flagstaff, AZ; 2010;83-108.

19. Kindwall EP, Whelan HT. Hyperbaric Medicine Practice, 4th Ed. North Palm Beach, FL: Best Publishing Co.; 2017.
20. Herdman TH, Kamitsuru S. Nursing Diagnoses Definitions and Classification 2018-2020, 11th Ed. New York, NY: Thieme; 2018.
21. http://www.nanda.org. Accessed: [Dec 1, 2018].
22. Norvell HC, Lohr-Larson V, Fabus S, Josefsen L. Patient Education. In: Larson-Lohr V, Norvel HC, Hyperbaric Nursing. Flagstaff, AZ: Best Publishing Co.; 2002;243-258.
23. Scarban M. Patient Education. In: Larson-Lohr V, editor, Norvel, H, Josefsen L, Wilcox JR, co-editors. Hyperbaric nursing and wound care. Flagstaff, AZ: Best Publishing Co; 2010;175-190.
24. http://hyperbaricnurses.org/nursing-guidelines/. Accessed: [Dec 1, 2018].
25. Russell KA. Nurse practice acts guide and govern: update 2017. *Journal of Nursing Regulation*. 2017;18-25.
26. American Nurses Association. Principles for Nursing Documentation Guidance for Registered Nurses. Silver Spring, MD; 2010.
27. Barry R. Operational and safety: Common elements shared by hyperbaric facilities. In: Larson-Lohr V, & Norvell H. (Eds.), Hyperbaric nursing and wound care. Flagstaff, AZ: Best Publishing Co.; 2010;75-82.
28. Fife CE, St. Leger M. Women and pressure diving and altitude. Flagstaff, AZ: Best Publishing, Co; 2010.
29. The Joint Commission Sentinel Alert. Issue 48. December 14th, 2011. Addendum: May 14, 2018;2-3.
30. https://s3.amazonaws.com/webcme-courses/HBO103/marketing/Hybrid+Hyperbaric+Course+Brochure.pdf. Accessed: [Dec 1, 2018].
31. http://www.nbdhmt.org/position_statements.asp. Accessed: [Dec 2, 2018].
32. https://www.uhms.org/images/Accreditation-documents/Fourth_Edition_UHMS_Accreditation_Manual_Final_6-4-2018.pdf. Accessed: Dec 2, 2018].
33. https://www.jointcommission.org/standards_information/jcfaqdetails.aspx?StandardsFaqId=900&ProgramId=46. Accessed: [Dec 2, 2018].
34. Miller L, Josefsen L. Staff competencies and training. In: Larson-Lohr V, editor, Norvell H, Josefsen L, Wilcox JR, co-editors. Hyperbaric nursing and wound care. Flagstaff, AZ: Best Publishing Co; 2010;191-198.
35. https://www.osha.gov/dsg/hospitals/program_development.html. Accessed: [Dec 2, 2018].
36. Milton CL. An ethical exploration of quality and safety initiatives in nurse practice. Nursing Science Quarterly. 2011;107-110.
37. Kohn LT, Corrigan JM, Donaldson MS (Eds.) To err is human: Building a safer health system. Washington, DC: National Academy Press, Institute of Medicine; 1999.

38. Mitchell PH. Defining patient safety and quality care. In: Patient Safety and Quality: An Evidence-Based Handbook for Nurses. Rockville, MD: Agency for Healthcare Research and Quality (US); 2008;1-5.
39. Mastal M, Matlock AM, Start R. Ambulatory care nurse-sensitive indicators series: capturing the role of nursing in ambulatory care-the case for meaningful nurse sensitive measurement. Nursing Economics. 2016;92-95.
40. https://psnet.ahrq.gov/primer/16/Ambulatory-Care-Safety/q=ambulatory+nurse+led+patient+safety. Last updated 2018. Accessed: [Dec 2, 2018].
41. Duffy J. Nursing and health systems. In: Quality Caring in Nursing and Health Systems. 2nd ed. New York, NY: Springer Publishing Co., LLC; 2013.
42. McKinney M. Nurses in charge. Modern Healthcare.2010;28-30. Revised 2015.

CHAPTER 6.7
The Responsibilities of the Technologist to Hyperbaric Facility Safety

Richard (Dick) Sample, BSPH, RCP, RRT, CHT

Introduction

Technologists play a critically important role in hyperbaric facility safety, operating the hyperbaric chamber and often being the final step in the process of ensuring the highest degree of safety for the patient as well as the surrounding environment. They must be highly trained and able to recognize and identify potential hazards with both the patient and chamber that could result in tragedy. They are relied upon by patients and co-workers to minimize risk and react appropriately to adverse circumstances.

Responsibilities

Depending on technologists' specific job description, they are often responsible for preparing the chamber(s) for each day's use by completing the chamber manufacturer's recommended daily checklist. This requires the complete and thorough inspection of a chamber and its components to ensure operational safety. All acrylic surfaces need to be inspected for crazing, scratches, and other imperfections, which may require the attention of the safety director and/or chamber manufacturer. Patient treatments should begin only after a chamber is deemed operationally safe. It is beyond the scope of this chapter to deal with the unique differences between monoplace and multiplace chambers; however, technologists in each environment must be familiar with the individual safety requirements.

Safety should be paramount in a technologist's mind at all times. He or she should vigilantly guard against becoming complacent when things operate smoothly. They must constantly be on high alert to visual and/or audible changes in a chamber's operation which may indicate a potential problem. Audible changes are particularly important. If a chamber begins to sound different and no changes have been made to account for it, the technologist must look for the cause and attempt to correct it before further problems develop. The technologist may need assistance from a more knowledgeable technologist and also may require contacting the chamber manufacturer to consult with a service representative. If the problem cannot be resolved internally or by a phone call, an on-site service call by a chamber manufacture service technologist may be needed. Never risk the safety of a patient or the hyperbaric facility staff. If in doubt, shut the chamber down and resolve the problem prior to continuing its use.

Preparing a patient for treatment is one of the most important safety elements a technologist may be involved with. A pretreatment safety checklist should be completed prior to treating each, regardless of how many prior treatments a patient has received. This checklist should include asking the patient specific questions to determine if all safety requirements have been met and if it is safe to proceed with the treatment. Failure to do this can have catastrophic results, as historically evidenced by tragic events worldwide. The safety checklist can easily become ritualistic and lose its effectiveness when treating the same patients day after day. The technologist must guard against this. Patients should be informed in their pretreatment education what is expected of them, what they will be allowed/not allowed to wear, and what products will not be permitted either on their body or in the chamber. Signs and/or posters displayed in high-visibility areas of the treatment room are useful reminders to the patients. They should also be informed of what the technologist will do prior to each treatment to help ensure their safety. Examples of items not permitted to go into a hyperbaric oxygen chamber (particularly Class B) include electronic devices, petroleum-based products (i.e. deodorant, make-up, hair care products, perfume/cologne, lotions, skin care products), exposed metal, noncured acrylic nails and/or nail polish, noncured casts, books/magazines, spark-emitting devices, butane hand warmers, chemically activated skin warmers, matches, lighters, or any other potential ignition sources. Although generally not needed, a body search may be necessary if there is any doubt that your patient is not honestly answering your questions or is trying to hide something.

Implanted electronic devices, such as cardiac pacemakers, cardioverter defibrillators, nerve stimulators, drug delivery pumps, pain relief/management devices, etc., can be problematic in a pressurized hyperbaric environment. All such devices must be tested under hyperbaric conditions to determine their functionality, reliability, and safety. Prior to treating a patient with such a device, the manufacturer of the device must be contacted and provide written documentation of the testing done on each specific device and model number. It is this author's experience that the testing of many implanted devices, particularly cardiac pacemakers, has been limited to 3-4 atmospheres absolute (ATA), thus restricting their treatment depth in chambers capable of pressures greater than this.

With advancements in modern medical technology have come the development of nonelectronic devices which must be critically evaluated prior to treating a patient. Examples include penile implants and external ventricular drains. These devices may contain air and need to be evaluated to determine if the air will change in volume during compression/decompression and if the volume change could become a patient safety issue.

Petroleum-based dressings can also present a challenge in a hyperbaric environment. Although petroleum products are generally not allowed in a hyperbaric chamber, dressings impregnated with petroleum may be difficult or even detrimental to remove.

In such cases, the safety director must confer with the medical director or supervising physician to determine the safest and most efficacious option for treatment.

It is advisable to have signs or posters patients can easily see to remind them of what is allowed in the hyperbaric chamber. These are available from companies specializing in hyperbaric education or you can create your own specific to your individual unit and needs. In the United States they are commercially available in full color with photo illustrations and are also in English and Spanish.

As mandated by the National Fire Protection Association (NFPA), all hyperbaric facilities regardless of size or type of chambers must have a designated safety director.[1] In many facilities, this individual is also a technologist or is very familiar with the duties and responsibilities of the technologist. As such, the technologist must work closely with the safety director and follow all the safety guidelines established for their facility. Additionally, if the hyperbaric facility is accredited by the Undersea and Hyperbaric Medical Society (UHMS), a certified hyperbaric technologist (CHT) should be present whenever patients are receiving hyperbaric oxygen therapy.

Training

Every hyperbaric technologist should strive to become a CHT through the National Board of Diving and Hyperbaric Medical Technology (NBDHMT). Although this certification is not mandatory to be a technologist and operate a hyperbaric chamber, it ensures the technologist has the necessary education and knowledge to pass the exam and obtained the required continuing education units (CEUs) every two years to maintain their CHT certification. An exception to this currently exists in Ohio, where the chamber operator must be a CHT or a licensed health care provider, such as RCP, RN, etc.

Conclusion

Technologists are vital members of the hyperbaric facility staff and relied upon to ensure the safety of the patients, staff, equipment, and surrounding environment. They must work closely with the safety director and fellow staff members to foster a culture of safety within the hyperbaric facility. We are all familiar with the American proverb, "It is better to be safe than sorry," but first and foremost technologists need to develop a safety mindset. Safety should be deeply ingrained in the thinking process as they interact with and treat patients. Safety also doesn't happen without concerted effort. It is not enough to simply know safety, it must be practiced.

SAFETY

S Search for hazards
A Analyze the risk
F Find the cause
E Eliminate the cause
T Tell others
Y You are safe

Excellent words of advice for all hyperbaric technologists to put into practice!

References

1. National Fire Protection Association. Hyperbaric Facilities, Chapter 14. NFPA 99 Health Care Facilities Code, 2018 Edition. National Fire Protection Association, Quincy, MA: NFPA; 2018:121.
2. Baker PC. Staffing and Training. In: Workman, WT, editor. Hyperbaric Facility Safety: A Practical Guide, 1st Ed. Flagstaff, AZ: Best Publishing Co.; 1999.

CHAPTER 6.8
The Responsibilities of the Patient to Hyperbaric Facility Safety

Laura Josefsen, RN, ACHRN and Becky Evenson, RN, BSN, MBA, ACHRN, CWS

Patients' responsibilities are emerging as a way to enhance patient activation and involvement in today's ever-changing health care system with the goals of increasing patient understanding, having a voice in their plan of care, knowing what to expect, being involved in decision making, and being an advocate in their care. This process is evolving as legal, ethical, accountability, role responsibility, and moral issues are being evaluated. It is important for the health care team to recognize that this process is still in the early stages of development. It is also vital that comprehensive documentation is in place regarding patient and family level of understanding and involvement of responsibility.

Patients have increased access to extensive internet information including patient rights and responsibilities. The goals of patient responsibilities are expanding to involve patient awareness and involvement in expanding areas of the health care system. This includes, but is not limited to, knowing, understanding, and participating in safety measures, quality improvement guidelines, compliance, utilization of resources, and financial obligations. Patient safety responsibility includes providing complete and accurate medical history, up-to-date medication list, notification of any changes regarding their health condition, and notifying staff if it is felt that the plan of care needs revision.

Patient Activation

The Joint Commission is "encouraging patient activation. To achieve the best outcomes, patients and families must be more actively engaged in decisions about their health care and must have broader access to information and support. Patient activation is inextricably intertwined with patient safety."[1]

The Joint Commission states, "A patient-centered approach to care can help organizations assess and enhance patient activation. Achieving this requires leadership engagement in the effort to establish patient-centered care as a top priority throughout the organization. This includes adopting the following principles:

1. Patient safety guides all decision making; patients and families are partners at every level of care.
2. Patient- and family-centered care is verifiable, rewarded, and celebrated.
3. The licensed independent practitioner responsible for the patient's care, or his or her designee, discloses to the patient and family any unanticipated outcomes of care, treatment, and services.
4. Staff and licensed independent practitioners must be fully engaged in patient- and family-centered care as demonstrated by their skills, knowledge, and competence in compassionate communication.
5. Standard RI.02.01.01 states, 'Inform the patient about his or her responsibilities related to his or her care, treatment, and services.'"[2]

Reprinted with permission.

The Team Approach

A recommended way to achieve patient activation is to use the team approach. The team approach utilizes a patient-centered model of health care to enhance patient involvement and responsibility to include identifying patient-specific goals. These goals include patient-specific outcomes as well as areas of a greater understanding of their previous and current health condition to be able to make informed decisions going forward in their care, to have increased support, to be listened to, to understand enough to ask questions, and to feel actively involved in the process.

A successful health care team takes time to develop as patient responsibilities are evaluated.[3] This includes developing good listening skills for the patient/family and all staff members to develop trust and to determine the patient's ability and willingness participate.[4]

The Agency for Healthcare Research and Quality (AHRQ) provides a model and a collection of tools and training to support the implement of shared decision making in practice that can be assessed at the AHRQ website at **www.ahrq.gov/shareddecisionmaking**.

The SHARE Approach model includes 5 steps:

Seek your patient's permission

Help your patient explore & compare treatment options

Assess your patient's values and preferences

Reach a decision with your patient

Evaluate your patient's decision[5]

Reprinted with permission.

Hyperbaric safety is based on a patient-centered focused multidisciplinary team concept under the leadership of the physician, with each member of the team having defined roles and responsibilities. The practice of safety in hyperbaric facilities includes comprehensive education and teamwork to increase patient and family knowledge on safety, medical, and risk factors when receiving hyperbaric oxygen therapy. Hyperbaric safety standards are in place and are continuously monitored and updated. Patient and family involvement in the hyperbaric setting has been an intricate part of this process from the beginning. This concept is supported by the *UHMS Clinical Facility Accreditation Manual.*[6]

Quality Improvement

Patient understanding of quality improvement measures are vital to this process. Let's take one example: patient compliance. It was noted in one facility that patients were not showing up for hyperbaric treatments at a fairly significant rate which impacted time, clinical operations, and costs. The hyperbaric team evaluated the factors and with increased education and communication with the staff and patients, were able to reduce missed visits. With everyone working together as a team, patient and staff satisfaction increased and stress levels decreased.[7]

Evolving Role of Patient Responsibility

As the role of patient responsibility is evolving, it is again important for the health care team to recognize that this process is still in the early stages of development. The current general acceptable guidelines are the beginning steps in this process. The guidelines listed below are an overview of the current responsibilities accepted by several states, facilities, and organizations.

This list of patient responsibility guidelines for the patient to hyperbaric safety includes the following:

A. Health care staff responsibilities

B. Patient responsibilities

C. Implementation ideas to consider

I. Provide comprehensive information regarding your health status [8-21]

A. Health care staff responsibilities:

1. Complete physician and nursing assessment
2. Determine patient/family ability and willingness to cooperate
3. Awareness of cultural differences
4. Assess family/social support
5. Identify coping skills

6. Identify barriers to learning
7. Encourage patient/family involvement
8. Identify patient expectations and goals

B. Patient responsibilities:

1. Provide your current and past medical history
2. Include any history of seizures, confinement anxiety, ear difficulties, pulmonary and cardiac issues, pain management, mobility issues, history of falls, comorbidities, current and previous treatments, and other matters relating to your health

C. Implementation ideas to consider:

1. Provide patient with health history and medication form prior to visit so he/she can fill out at home, allowing the patient more time to think about answers.

II. Be involved in learning the concepts of safety for hyperbaric treatments [8-21]

A. Health care staff responsibilities:

1. Provide initial and ongoing education regarding safety issues in simple, understandable terms
2. Review the procedure and number of treatments and explain why consistent, complete therapy is required
3. Perform patient assessment as well as review prohibited items in the hyperbaric chamber prior to every hyperbaric treatment
4. Assess patient/family level of understanding

B. Patient responsibilities:

1. Ask questions until there is understanding regarding the treatment plan, procedures, prohibited items in the chamber, risks and benefits of hyperbaric treatments, alternative treatments, and other resources as needed
2. Understand and adhere to and reasons for the daily safety protocols for hyperbaric treatments

C. Implementation ideas to consider:

1. Patients absorb information in different ways and at different times.
2. Recommend providing multiple education resources including pamphlets, take-home materials, DVD, videos, picture books—even can create YouTube video.
3. Share with patients and family members

III. Clarify instruction[8-21]

A. Health care staff responsibilities:

1. Provide information regarding treatments, expectations, and desired outcomes
2. Provide education regarding the initial and ongoing plan of care

B. Patient responsibilities:

1. Understand the plan of care, expectations, and recommended treatment schedule
2. Know and understand the risks involved
3. Ask if more information is needed
4. Ask the staff to explain medical terminology

C. Implementation ideas to consider:

1. Provide patient with written treatment plan, including type of treatment, start and stop date, and when their progress will be reviewed
2. Explain the treatment plan may need to change and patient and family will be consulted to review changes
3. Patients are more likely to be compliant if they understand the treatment process and know that there is a defined time frame for care

IV. Participate in mutually accepted course of treatment plan[8-21]

A. Health care staff responsibilities:

1. Reinforce the importance of following treatment recommendations and instructions
2. Review the initial and ongoing treatment plan regularly
3. Monitor patient adherence to treatment plan to ensure it is continuing to be appropriate
4. May need to consider alternative treatment plan

B. Patient responsibilities:

1. If unable or refusing to follow the treatment plan, notify the hyperbaric staff so the treatment plan can be reviewed and or modified to better accommodate the patient needs
2. Understand that health consequences may occur if treatment plan is not followed

C. Implementation ideas to consider:

1. Consider having patient sign a "treatment commitment," "confirmation of instruction," or "compliance agreement" outlining patient responsibilities

V. Keep appointments as scheduled [8-21]

A. Health care staff responsibilities:

1. Schedule treatments to accommodate patient schedule as much as possible
2. Review the importance of showing up for scheduled treatments on time
3. Review the importance of coming for all scheduled treatments
4. Identify issues that may interfere with patient being able to get to the facility (lack of transportation, illness, other appointments, etc.)

B. Patient responsibilities:

1. Keep scheduled appointments
2. If unable to keep scheduled appointment, notify hyperbaric staff as soon as possible
3. Notify hyperbaric staff when patient is ill, has a cold, flu-like symptoms, ear pain, or other condition

C. Implementation ideas to consider:

1. Once treatment schedule is determined, print out month view of plain calendar and enter treatment dates and times
2. These calendars should be reviewed with patient at each visit and altered if patient has conflicting commitments
3. Print out a copy of the calendar for the patient
4. Keep log of missed appointments detailing why patient was unable to make the appointment
5. This information should be reviewed with each patient and also can be used to see if there are any recurring issues with multiple patients, such as transportation issues, that can be addressed

VI. Pursue healthy lifestyle [8-21]

A. Health care staff responsibilities:

1. Assist the patient to understand the importance and benefits of a healthy lifestyle

B. Patient responsibilities:

1. Follow the no-smoking policy guidelines of the facility

2. Follow nutrition, medication, and exercise recommendations
3. Monitor blood glucose levels
4. Notify hyperbaric staff of events of flu symptoms, colds, or any contagious event

C. Implementation ideas to consider:

1. Provide patient with educational materials on why smoking should be avoided
2. Provide patient with educational materials on why it is important to maintain appropriate glucose levels.
3. Offer wound healing and diet recommendations
4. Explain rationale for avoiding hyperbaric treatment if they have an upper respiratory infection

VII. Be respectful and considerate of the rights of others [8-21]

A. Health care staff responsibilities:

1. Respect of patient and family
2. Open communication
3. Respect for confidentiality

B. Patient responsibilities:

1. Be considerate of the rights of others
2. Be aware of noise levels
3. Be respectful of property of others and the facility
4. Respect the confidentiality of other patients
5. Respect the time of staff and other patients

C. Implementation ideas to consider:

1. Include consideration of these responsibilities in HBO_2 education materials and or compliance agreement or other type of agreement outlying patient responsibilities

VIII. The patient's financial obligations [8-21]

A. Health care staff responsibilities:

1. Inform the patient of the co-pay for each visit
2. Inform the patient of fees for hyperbaric treatment services, including facility and physician fees

3. Provide a referral to social service or financial counseling, if required
4. Hyperbaric staff will get pre-authorization, if available, for hyperbaric treatments

B. Patient responsibilities:

1. Patient should be knowledgeable about health plan coverage
2. Patient to make arrangements for bill payment

C. Implementation ideas to consider:

1. Provide patient with a statement of expected fees
2. Explain that more than one physician may submit bills if a physician panel model is used in the center

IX. Patient to state and/or provide a copy of advanced directive, if available [8-21]

A. Health care staff responsibilities:

1. Ask patient if advanced directive is in place and available

B. Patient responsibilities:

1. Patient to state if advanced directive is available

C. Implementation ideas to consider:

1. Many states have a process to provide advanced directive without requiring a lawyer.
2. The American Hospital Association has links to each state's information, as well as good educational materials for patients. Search: Putitinwriting[22]

X. Patients are to report if they are unhappy with their care [8-21]

A. Health care staff responsibilities:

1. Provide the patient with information regarding the process for notification of dissatisfaction both within the facility and the contact referral for outside the facility
2. Provide the patient with after-hours contact information

B. Patient responsibilities:

1. Patient to have the information and understanding for the reporting processes

C. Implementation ideas to consider:

1. Instruct patient to speak up if they are unhappy with any service

2. Provide patient with satisfaction survey, hospital process for reporting complaint, and the complaint hot line number

Conclusion

As health care is transitioning to accommodate increased regulations from governmental and other agencies, the safety of the patient continues to remain the top priority in hyperbaric medicine. The patient responsibility guidelines are to assist the health care staff and patient team to evaluate the optimal and safest way to achieve patient-specific goals together to increase safety and outcomes for the patient.

The entire health care team has the increased responsibility of providing professional, accurate, comprehensive education, information, and guidance to promote patient and family involvement and understanding, specifically regarding safety in the hyperbaric setting.

"It is important to recognize that a patient's outcome may be linked to the information that was given to them."[23]

References

1. The Joint Commission. Comprehensive Accreditation Manual for Ambulatory Care. Patient Safety Systems (PS)-Joint Commission. https://www.jointcommission.org/assets/1/6/PS_chapter_AHC_2019.pdf PS – 17-18 CAMAC.
2. The Joint Commission. Comprehensive Accreditation Manual for Ambulatory Care. Patient Safety Systems (PS)-Joint Commission. https://www.jointcommission.org/assets/1/6/PS_chapter_AHC_2019.pdf PS – 17-18 CAMAC. January 2019.
3. Smith C, Balatbat C, Corbridge S, Dopp A, Fried J, Harter R, Landefeld S, Martin C, Opelka F, Sandy L, Sato L, Sinsky C. Implementing optimal team based care to reduce clinician burnout. NAM Perspectives. Discussion paper, National Academy of Medicine. Washington, DC. https://nam.edu/implementing-optimal-team-based-care-to-reduce-clinician-burnout. doi:10.31478/201809 c. 2018.
4. Schilling D. 10 Steps to Effective Listening. https://www.forbes.com/sites/womensmedia/2012/11/09/10-steps-to- effective-listening. 2012.
5. Agency for Healthcare Research and Quality. The SHARE Approach. Content last reviewed August 2018. Rockville, MD. https://www.ahrq.gov/professionals/education/curriculum-tools/shareddecisionmaking/index.html.
6. UHMS. Clinical Hyperbaric Facility Accreditation Program. Undersea and Hyperbaric Medical Society 2018 at UHMS.org, HBOPR 1.5, 1.5.1.

7. Hirsch M, Wells-Landry K, Walters L, Driskill B, Rome C. Improving patient adherence to HBO treatment schedule-a Performance improvement experience. WCHM: 2015;4(1).
8. English DC. Moral obligations of patients: a clinical view. J Med Philos. 2005 Apr30((2):139-52. DOI:10.1080/03605310590926821.
9. Evans HM. Do patients have duties? J Med Ethics. 2007 Dec;33(12):689-94. p689-694. DOI:10.1136/jme.2007.021188.
10. Gauther C. The virtue of moral responsibility and the obligations of patients. Journal of Medicine and Philosophy. 2005;30(2):153-166.
11. NIH Clinical Center.Patient Responsibilities. https://cc.nih.gov/participate/patientinfo/legal/responsibilities.html . 2017.
12. Mayo Clinic. Rights and Responsibilities of Patients. Rights and Responsibilities of Patients. https://www.mayoclinic.org/documents/mcj6256-pdf/doc-20079237.
13. Natchitoches Regional Medical Center. Patient Rights and Responsibilities. nrmcdev.longevitydesign.com/patients-visitors/patient-right s-and-responsibilities/.
14. UCSF Medical Center. Patient Rights and Responsibilities. https://www.ucsfhealth.org/pdf/patient_rights_and_responsibilities.pdf.
15. Orlando Orthopaedic Center. Patient's Bill of Rights and Responsibilities. https://www.orlandoortho.com/wp-content/uploads/2016/.../Florida-Patient-Rights.pdf.
16. National Health Council. Principles of Patients' Rights and Responsibilities. www.nationalhealthcouncil.org/.../nhc.../principles-patients-rights-and-responsibilities.
17. University Health. Patient Rights and Responsibilities. www.uhsystem.com/Conway/patient-rights-and- responsibilities.
18. American Medical Association. Code of Medical Ethics: Patient Responsibilities. https://www.ama-assn.org/delivering-care/patient-responsibilities.
19. UCSF Medical Center. Patient Rights and Responsibilities. https://www.ucsfhealth.org/pdf/patient_rights_and_responsibilities.pdf.
20. Mapua Health Centre. Hyperbaric Oxygen Therapy: Patient Rights and Responsibilities. www.mapuahealth.com/wp-content/uploads/Patient_Information_Booklet.
21. RWJF. Engaging patients in improving ambulatory care. https://www.rwjf.org/en/.../03/engaging-patients-in-improving-ambulatory-care.html.
22. AHA. Put It In Writing. https://www.aha.org/2017-12-11-put-it-writing.
23. Skarban M. Patient Education, In: Hyperbaric Nursing and Wound Care, Larson-Lohr V, editor. Flagstaff AZ: Best Publishing Co; 2010;176,184.

CHAPTER 6.9
The Impact of Quality Improvement on Facility Safety

Tina Ziemba-Diehl, RN, ACHRN, CHT

Introduction

"It may seem a strange principle to enunciate as the very first requirement in a hospital that it should ***do the sick no harm.****" —Florence Nightingale*

The concepts of quality improvement (QI) and performance improvement (PI) in health care are not new and have been around in some form for many years. Implementing best practices and establishing quality and safety standards ensures that a hyperbaric department attains a high level of safe patient care. The patient safety program must be integrated with all quality or performance improvement activities. In today's world measurement, proof and evidence are more valued and even demanded by more payers as a condition of contracting. Therefore, it is sensible and ethical for health care professionals to develop measures that evaluate performance in increasing desired outcomes.[1]

QI and PI both take a systems view of improvement rather than focusing on individual performance, negative or positive. They are both data driven since they rely on measurement to come to decisions and evaluate any changes made. Both seek to understand how processes work and generate improvements by making understandable changes to processes. QI and PI view poor performance as a reflection of problems inherent in the system of delivering care and show that individuals are seldom the root cause of poor performance. The primary difference between QI and PI is more emphasis placed on human factors in PI and more emphasis on systems performance in QI. Most organizations use the terms PI and QI interchangeably. The term quality improvement will be used throughout this chapter.[2]

Many available methods provide tools to help achieve improved patient outcomes and reduce safety risks. This chapter will explore realistic processes the hyperbaric department may put into practice to substantiate that QI safety goals and processes are reached and documented. QI is not a static process. The plan must be flexible enough to accommodate significant service changes, structure changes, and unusual events. The patient safety program should be integrated with all QI activities.

As always, the goals of the QI program must mesh with the goals of the health care facility and/or the hyperbaric management company. Examples of goals may be the following:

- To identify the structure for defining quality and performance improvement actions
- To facilitate communication in reporting and documenting all quality and performance improvement activities
- To focus and coordinate organization-wide QI and patient safety activities
- To promote teamwork and group responsibility in identifying and implementing opportunities for improvement
- To establish an environment that supports safety, encourages blame-free reporting, addresses maintenance, and improves patient safety issues.[3]

History of Quality Improvement

In 1924, Walter Shewhart created a method for quality control for production using statistical methods, which became the foundation for his ongoing work on statistical quality control. Later, W. Edward Demming applied this statistical process control during World War II to successfully improve the quality in the manufacturing of munitions and other strategically important products. After World War II, Japan decided to make QI a national imperative as part of their economic rebuilding and sought the help of Shewhart, Demming, and others. Demming championed Shewhart's ideas in Japan from 1950 onward and is best known for his management philosophy establishing quality, productivity, and competitive position. Japanese products from the 1950s were known for cheapness and low quality. By the 1970s, Japan achieved very high levels of quality in their products by using Demming's principles. During this time, Japan also developed many highly successful quality initiatives which provided techniques for process improvement as well as addressing the people factor (culture). Many of these methods are now adopted by western countries.[4] Through the years, the health care industry has adopted and adapted these quality initiatives resulting in improved patient outcomes and satisfaction as well as increasing safety awareness.

Terms and Defintions

Understanding QI or PI ideas requires a basic knowledge of terms and definitions used throughout the chapter. Included below are important terms and definitions.

- Analysis: Examination of facts and data that helps identify gaps in desired organizational performance.

- **Aspects of care:** Key functions, procedures, processes, interventions, services, or other activities that affect consumers; activities or processes identified as high volume, high risk, or problem-prone for consumer or service providers.
- **Assess:** Measure, appraise, estimate, or judge the characteristics, qualities, or attributes of a problem, issue, or condition. Helps to identify the practices, attitudes, culture, and activities that enhance or hinder the achievement of continuous QI.
- **Benchmark:** Goal used to measure the rate of progress toward a larger goal; answers the question of where an organization should be; historically, "best in class."
- **Benchmarking:** Continuous practice of comparing service practices with others; a point of reference by which others may be measured and continually improved.
- **Best practice:** A superior method or practice that contributes to the improved performance of an organization; usually recognized as best by other peer organizations.
- **Continuous quality improvement:** A philosophy for capabilities and processes and improving them repeatedly to achieve customer satisfaction.
- **Culture:** A common set of values, beliefs, attitudes, perceptions, and accepted behaviors shared by individuals within an organization.
- **Data:** Facts or figures from which conclusions are drawn.
- **Evaluation:** Determination after data collection to see what processes work well and which do not work.
- **Goal:** The desired end toward which activities are directed.
- **Indicator:** Measures of specific, measurable, objective events, occurrences; key performance indicators are certain aspects of care that show an organization that it is improving its processes and quality.
- **Monitoring:** Planned, systematic, and ongoing collection, compilation, and organization of data about an indicator or the quality or appropriateness of an important aspect of care.
- **Objective:** A statement assisting in determining if there is movement away or toward a goal.
- **Outcome:** The results, products, or effects of a process.
- **Performance improvement:** Primary result of efforts to improve a situation or process; continuous assessment of functions and processes of an organization to increase the probability of achieving desired outcomes and to better meet the needs of the customers and users of services; a process for achieving desired institutional and individual results; goal of PI is the provision of high quality, sustainable health services.
- **Process:** Series of steps to a desired outcome; continuing activity or function that gradually leads to a particular result.

- **Quality assurance:** Distinguishing characteristics that determine the value or degree of excellence and the mechanisms to efficiently and effectively monitor and improve customer care/service delivery provided by competent providers with appropriate resources; tends to unveil the fact of flaw, not the cause.
- **Quality improvement:** All actions taken throughout the organization to increase the effectiveness and efficiency of the activities and processes in order to provide added benefits to both the organization and its customers; focuses on organizational systems rather than individual performance.
- **Risk:** Potential hazard or quality deficiency associated with a product, service, or process.
- **Root-cause analysis:** Tool used to distinguish the source of a defect or problem; structured approach focusing on the original cause of a problem or condition.
- **Threshold:** Predetermined intervention/event or pre-established level of performance for staff, process, or organization related to a specific indicator; attainment or nonattainment triggers a review.

Basic Principles of Quality Improvement

It is imperative not to underestimate the human factor

Any improvement takes time to implement and to gain acceptance, in addition to stabilizing it as accepted practice. Once the staff has decided that a practice or process is worthy, the chances of successfully implementing it increase substantially. Often real change works best when a crisis happens and changes must be made and implemented quickly for patient and staff safety.

Meet or exceed the expectations of your patients and staff members

Hyperbaric medicine units depend on patients (customers). Staff members need to understand current and future customer needs and plan to meet these needs. Any organization with this as the primary goal will have more success.

Develop and maintain strong leadership

Leaders of an organization establish direction and unity of purpose.[5] An environment needs to be created and maintained where staff and patients are fully involved.

Encourage involvement of people in the organization

It is essential that people of all levels of an organization buy into the goals and objectives of the organization. Complete involvement enables the organization to use their abilities and talents for its benefit.

Choose a workable quality improvement method

Developing the right metrics, which are valid, reliable, feasible, meaningful, and action-oriented is critical to the success of a QI program.[6] Choosing a QI process which is time-consuming, irritating to physicians and staff, inconvenient, too involved, and wasteful will most certainly fall short and possibly fail. Become familiar with several processes and decide on one that meets needs of the unit, hospital, management, and leadership.

Performance and quality do not exist in the absence of measurement

These concepts are embedded in the idea of evaluation or assessment, which can take the form of a patient's subjective view of services rendered or an intricately constructed model. Measurement gives tools to focus on effective improvement rather than wasting time on ineffective measures.[7]

Utilize The Joint Commission's (TJC) National Patient Safety Goals (NPSG)

This set of standards provides an in-depth look at preventing life or limb-threatening problems or potential injury. The goals are updated and revised annually and are extracted from sentinel alerts and events. The NPSGs will help direct the unit to safe practices.

The Importance of Quality Improvement in a Hyperbaric Department

It is critically important to practice QI in the hyperbaric setting. Patients (i.e. customers) are becoming more aware of quality issues in health care and are demanding higher quality and accountability. Media coverage of adverse events such as medication errors and wrong-site surgery also brings attention to the significance of QI issues. The Joint Commission says that at some point, everything drills down to safety, therefore, safety issues should be at the forefront of QI endeavors. The Undersea and Hyperbaric Medical Society's accreditation process, the National Committee for Quality Assurance and other accrediting bodies, organizations, and agencies share a great interest in quality improvement. Groups with purchasing power, such as health maintenance organizations (HMOs) or insurance companies, also want to work with organizations whose focus is a commitment to improved outcomes. It should also be part of a staff member's personal ethics to do the best job possible while meeting the organization's goals.

Developing a Quality Improvement Program

What does it take to develop and implement a strong QI program? It begins with leadership. The leadership is responsible for developing strategies and processes for the care and safety of patients and personnel.[8] The leadership assigns a safety director whose primary focus is to provide a safe environment and seek ways to improve the safety of the environment. This is accomplished by playing a significant role in implementing and developing successful QI projects.

Resistance to change is the most common barrier to QI. The safety director must recognize this and help to eventually overcome resistance by encouraging a constant commitment to safety. The safety director has a key role in creating a culture of safety by continually putting into practice safety related QI initiatives within the organization. Big changes can be disruptive. It is easier to work within existing cultural boundaries and make small improvements.[9] Backlash from employees is reduced and commitment to improvement is more likely when the process is fully understood and staff understand that improvement is a work in progress. Looking closely at hyperbaric unit activities will give all staff members a clear picture of how important QI is as it relates to safety. Many of these safety issues and potential QI initiatives can be addressed in monthly staff meetings, which in turn will increase staff awareness.

After discerning leadership objectives and considering regulatory requirements, opportunities for improvement need to be identified. Leadership objectives include the following: acknowledgment of high-risk and error-prone activities; seeking solutions to vulnerabilities; and willingness to direct organizational resources to this process. The first step is to recognize that this activity is a team effort including patients, families, caregivers, and staff members. Often a QI team is formed to address potential issues and monitor the processes. The second step is to review reliable and practiced approaches and determine the unit's goals in QI. Drawing on hyperbaric safe practice principles is one way to start the process, since many procedures relevant to improvement are already in place. In the quality plan, the customers (staff, patients, etc.) are identified, the scope of service is clarified, and the important aspects of care determined.

Selecting a Quality Improvement Process

Developing a plan means designing a systematic approach for monitoring and evaluating care and services. Evaluating data allows for the clear identification of patterns and trends. Included in this systematic approach are all safety procedures and actions. Important aspects of care should be explored, including procedures, processes, interventions, services, or other activities that affect customers. Examples of aspects of care are maintenance records, checklists, chart audits, hyperbaric treatments, patient education, and fire prevention. From these aspects of care, indicators (i.e. activities or processes identified as high volume, high risk, or problem prone) can be distinguished. These are specific elements that can be monitored. In a small department, a service performed three or four times daily may be high volume. A high-risk process may be a clinical procedure or safety activity. Problem prone may mean that a process fails once a week or even daily, such as omitting a predive blood glucose in patients at risk for substantial glucose changes.

Other indicators which may be monitored and assessed are ear barotrauma, fire drill responses, patient satisfaction, and appropriate referrals to hyperbaric oxygen therapy. There are many other areas which provide worthwhile indicators. After using a chosen method of monitoring and determining that the indicator has met the established threshold, the indicator may be dropped and revisited at a later date. During the course of monitoring a specific item, benchmarking is an excellent tool for use in comparing the monitored indicators to many others performing the same activity. An example could be ear barotrauma. If the national rate of ear barotraumas is less than 5%, and if a department's rate is 10%, benchmarking provides a reference that tells improvement is needed. Sometimes a deeper assessment of a problem is needed and root-cause analysis required. The root-cause analysis is used to distinguish the source of a defect or problem. Once this has been determined, the quality plan or process can begin. The Joint Commission requires root-cause analyses for all sentinel events. Root-cause analysis is useful and very effective in the near-miss scenario. With root-cause analysis, the focus is on the what (the event) and the why (the system), not the who.[10]

There are many QI approaches that have been developed and refined for the health care industry. The safety director must be aware of organizational, hospital/management goals, and have the support of leadership in order to become an integral part of developing an appropriate QI plan for the department. It is important to note that a QI program depends entirely upon documentation. Once care is given, the only evidence of that service is the documentation.[11]

The Most Common Approaches to Quality Improvement Processes

Problem list: The start of a QI program may be as simple as making a list of problems and employing problem solving techniques. The steps taken to solve the problem are documented and can be included in monthly staff meeting minutes.

Plan Do Study Act (PDSA)

Plan: Plan the test or observation, including a plan for collecting data.
Do: Try out the test on a small scale.
Study: Set aside time to analyze the data and study the results. Look at the data before and after the change and reflect on what was learned.
Act: Refine the change, based on what was learned from the test. This process is supported by the Agency for Healthcare Research and Quality (AHRQ), part of the Department of Health and Human Resources. The PDSA cycle is shorthand for testing a change, implemented by planning it, trying it, observing the results, and acting on what is learned. This is the scientific method, which is used for action-oriented learning. The PDSA is a never-ending cycle repeated over and over again.

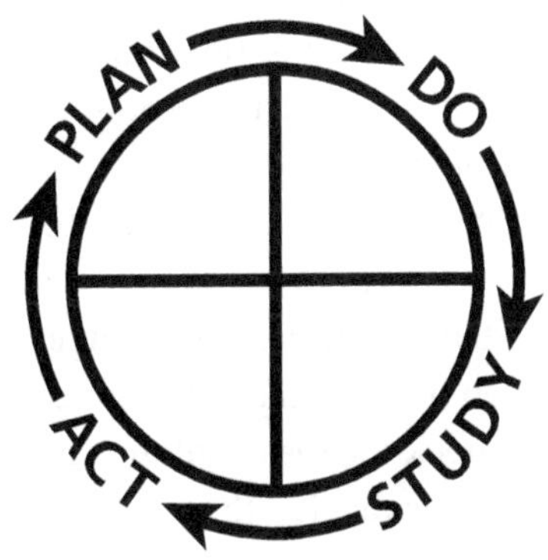

Figure 1. PDSA cycle.

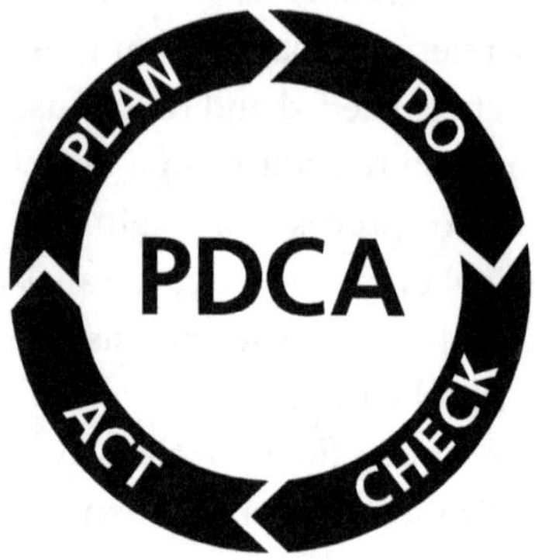

Figure 2. PDCA cycle.

Plan Do Check Act (PDCA)

Plan: Plan changes after identification of the problem; consider which aspects of care (potential safety problems) are involved.
Do: Put the changes in place.
Check: Check that the changes are actually working and meeting the goals set.
Act: Make the changes permanent. An example of this is a department that provides water bottles for each dive. The water bottle always spilled or the patient drank too much and needed to be removed from the chamber. The problem identified was the method of providing water (the water bottle). The plan (P) was to change the way water was provided. This was done (D) by providing small "sippy cups" for several patients to test. Several days after the plan was instigated, it was reviewed and checked (C) and found to work well. This action (A) was put into place and became procedure. PDCA is a repetitive cycle.

FOCUS PDCA

This method identifies topics that require more extensive and problem-solving efforts.
F: Find the problem that needs improvement. Look at high-volume, high-cost, and problem-prone areas.
O: Organize a multidisciplinary team that knows the process.
C: Clarify the current knowledge of the process.
U: Understand the process variations.
S: Select solution to the problem/improvement opportunities. Choose a portion of the process to improve, which will have the best likelihood of success.
P: Plan recommended changes.
D: Do put the changes in place.
C: Check the results of the changes.
A: Act by making the workable changes permanent.

PDMAI Plan Design Measure Assess Implement (PDMAI)

This process was developed by the The Joint Commission.
Plan and prioritize improvement needed.
Design the strategy by which the activities within a process highlights an opportunity for improvement.
Measure by comparing results with requirements via indicators and thresholds.
Assess and interpret the results.
Implement by putting into place the action and track the effectiveness of the improvement. For example, a busy monoplace chamber unit was practicing a quarterly fire drill

involving lateral evacuation with little success. Because of new employees and lack of practical experience, it was very important to quickly get them comfortable and able to perform well. The unit manager identified the problem (P) as new employees with no experience. He planned and designed (D) a new lesson plan and method of practicing fire drills. After practicing several times, he found there were areas which needed refinement to be effective. He eventually decided that it should take employees two minutes to do a successful evacuation. He then tested all employees against the two-minute threshold (M) and after assessing the staff's ability to fulfill this threshold safely (A), he made this policy but continued to monitor the staff's progress periodically (I).

Other helpful tools

Pareto Chart ranks problems or causes from most significant to least significant based on the Pareto Principle, which suggest most effects come from relatively few causes. Eighty-percent (80%) of the trouble comes from 20% of the problems. This principle may help decide which problem to solve first.

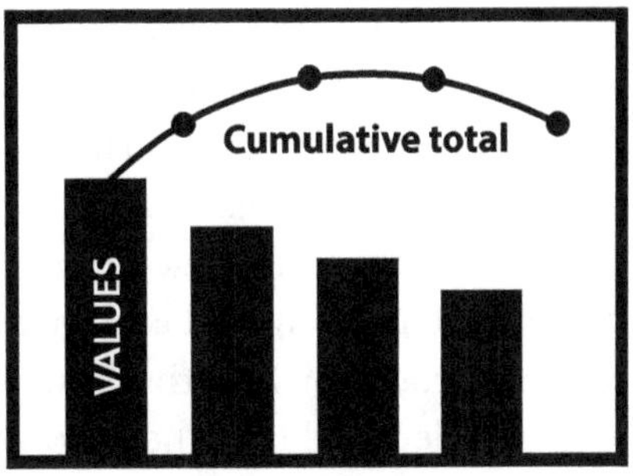

Figure 3. Pareto chart.

Cause and effect diagram (fishbone) is a diagram that identifies and organizes possible causes of problems (or factors needed to ensure success of an effort). The problem or event is listed on the right, and branches off the central arrows indicate main categories of items. The diagram allows people to see the relationship between factors. This can be used as a starting point when a problem is identified and can be an effective tool for root-cause analysis.

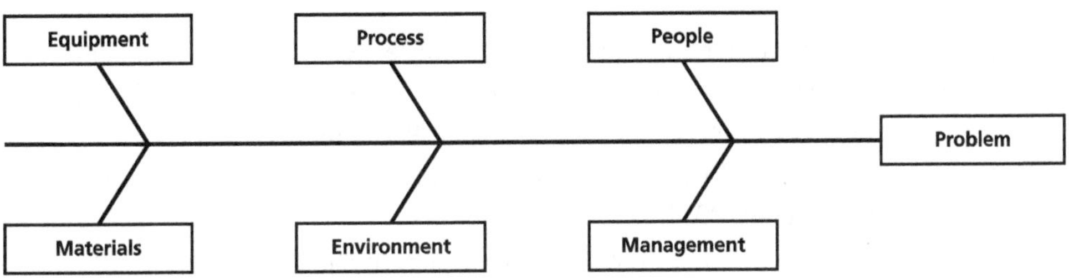

Figure 4. Example of cause and effect diagram (fishbone).

Flowchart is used to visually represent or illustrate a process; helps in understanding the process steps and identifying areas that are problem prone.

Run chart plots data over time in the order the data happened; helps identify variations and trends.

Histograms are graphic depictions of observations, useful to identify the distribution of data, and help visualize data.

Summary

It is important to remember that an organization is exhibiting quality if it is doing what is necessary to achieve its goals, and a quality audit (quality improvement plan) checks an organization's effectiveness in achieving those goals. The Joint Commission says every facility must have organized, systematic, and ongoing methods, which focus on safety and quality.[11] Often simply setting patient satisfaction as the goal of the QI program will be helpful in prioritizing projects and areas of needed improvement. QI in health care is always evolving. QI in health care makes sure the organization complements and supports the following: customers, knowledge, roles, and responsibilities within itself. Every core principle of the QI process needs to be fully understood. Every core activity needs to be examined and challenged to find the necessary steps for improvement. It is important for hyperbaric staff to grasp the basic principles and concepts of QI and to understand how these principles and concepts are part of everyday procedure. Staff members should continuously be alert to ways of improving patient outcomes and reducing the risks associated with providing hyperbaric oxygen therapy.

Good people improve things every day by identifying and fixing problems. We just don't always take credit for it. In reality, everything we do can be put in the context of QI. The key is to create an organized process that encourages and documents our intrinsic ethics to do what is right for our patients and staff.

References

1. Performance Improvement: A Change for the Better. San Diego, CA. RN.com.
2. Performance Improvement: A Change for the Better. San Diego, CA. RN.com.
3. University Medical Center. University of Toledo Performance Improvement Safety Plan. University of Toledo. 2011. utmc.utoledo.edu/depts/quality/docs/Quality and Patient Safety Plan. P3.
4. University Medical Center. University of Toledo Performance Improvement Safety Plan 2011. utmc.utoledo.edu/depts/quality/docs/Quality and Patient Safety Plan. P3.
5. Hoskins EJ, Sayger SA, Westman JS. Quality improvement in patient distribution at a major university student health center. J Am Coll Health. 2002 May; 50(6):303-8.

6. Quality Measurement, Monitoring and Analysis. Briefings in Patient Safety: 10:9 (Sept 2009):p8.
7. Quality Measurement, Monitoring and Analysis. Briefings in Patient Safety: 10:9 (Sept 2009):p8.
8. NFPA. NFPA 99 2012 edition. Quincy, MA: National Fire Protection Association. Para 14.3.1.3.3.9. University Medical Center; University of Toledo Performance Improvement Safety Plan FY07.P2.
9. Quality Measurement, Monitoring and Analysis. Briefings in Patient Safety: 10:9 (Sept 2009):p8.
10. Woodhouse D. Quality improvement through quality audit, quality in higher education. Jul 2003;9(2):133.
11. Dunn D. Five keys to performance improvement. The Joint Commission Ambulatory Buzz, Mar 25, 2014.

Bibliography

1. Institute for Healthcare improvement: http://www.ihi.org
2. The Joint Commission: http://www.jointcommission.org
3. National Association for Healthcare Quality: http://www.nahq.org
4. Institute for Health Care Research and Quality: http://www.ahrq.gov

CHAPTER 6.10
Online Resources Related to Hyperbaric Facility Safety

Jeff Mize, RRT, CHT, CWCA

The development and continuation of a safety program for a hyperbaric facility can be arduous. The task(s) of initiating safety procedures, employing equipment maintenance policies, and implementing employee competency standards can leave the hyperbaric safety director buried in stacks of reference books, manuals, and files.

Advances in technology have brought us smartphones, social networking, and real-time correspondence. Like it or not, they have made their way into the area of hyperbaric safety. The industry demand for instant access to the safety regulations, codes, and requirements has arrived! This chapter will provide an overview of the online resources available that can help you optimize your safety program.

Undersea and Hyperbaric Medical Society (UHMS)

While only members have total access to society's website (www.uhms.org), there is a wealth of information available to nonmembers. The site offers a wide range of information that should serve as a useful tool for the hyperbaric practitioner when seeking references or resources in the development and enhancement of the hyperbaric safety program. Sections on the UHMS site are briefly described to provide an overview of the content. The UHMS website includes information about the history of UHMS, committees, the society's constitution and bylaws, position statements, corporate partnerships, chapters of the UHMS, scheduled symposia, and educational opportunities as well as news and announcements.

Publications: The UHMS produces a number of publications, ranging from books to peer-reviewed journals (e.g., the *UHM Journal*) and newsletters. Information about purchase, subscription, and the availability to view online content is readily available, including *UHMS Guidelines for Hyperbaric Facilities 2nd Edition.*[1] While originally published as the *UHMS Operations Committee Report* in 2000, it was later revised and published as the *UHMS Guidelines for Hyperbaric Facility Operations*. It provides written guidance for operations, staffing, training, and safety within the hyperbaric facility.[2] The references stated as recommendation for the development of hyperbaric facility operations in this publication will be an area of focus for review of online resources in this chapter. In addition, society members may access downloadable safety documents, safety articles, equipment articles, manufacturer notices, and other safety references.

Accreditation: A vital component to the accreditation process is the evaluation of the hyperbaric safety program. Hyperbaric facilities seeking accreditation will find necessary accreditation documents, specifically the accreditation application, presurvey questionnaire, and the most current accreditation manual. Hyperbaric centers that have received hyperbaric facility accreditation by the UHMS are listed by state or country.

Resources: As the name would imply, active UHMS members are able to access resources such as archived publications, news, announcements, links, and a frequently asked question section titled MEDFAQ. MEDFAQ is an invaluable tool that allows members to submit questions pertaining to safety/technical issues. There is a disclaimer stating that questions submitted will not be answered for 48 to 72 hours.

National Board of Diving and Hyperbaric Medical Technology (NBDHMT)

The NBDHMT is a nonprofit, certifying organization designed to meet the clinical, technical, and safety needs of the discipline of UHM.[3] The NBDHMT website (www.nbdhmt.org) should be in all hyperbaric safety and management team members' toolbar. The NBDHMT website does not require membership and provides information about initial certification for diver medic (DMT), hyperbaric technologist (CHT), hyperbaric nurse (CHRN), and veterinary hyperbaric technologist (CHVT). NBDHMT position statements, continuing education requirements, certification confirmation, and a monthly briefing from the NBDHMT board president are available to all that access the site.

Baromedical Nurses Association (BNA)

The BNA is a nonprofit organization that was established in 1985 as forum for hyperbaric nurses to connect, share information, and provide professional support.[4] The BNA website (www.hyperbaricnurses.org) is well organized and contains information that hyperbaric nurses, allied health, and anyone involved in daily hyperbaric operations will find useful. Membership is limited to nurses. However, nonmembers have access to most, if not all, of the site content.

The site content includes the most recently published nursing guidelines, upcoming webinars, meetings, and continuing nursing education (CNE) offerings. Information about certified hyperbaric registered nurse (CHRN) qualification, eligibility, and renewal is available to members or nonmembers. In addition, job postings, safety articles, and archived newsletters are available to members and nonmembers.

National Fire Protection Association (NFPA)

The NFPA website (www.nfpa.org) has information available to both nonpaying and paying subscribers. The site includes content regarding codes and standards, safety, training opportunities, research, and public awareness. Articles and content can be conveniently located by way of word search. Handbooks and other resource materials are available for purchase on the website. Some publications (*NFPA 99, Health Care Facilities Code*) are available for download in pdf format. Currently, there is limited access content on the website with registration. Access to all content does require a paid membership. Considering that *NFPA 99* is the primary guidance for hyperbaric operation and safety in hyperbaric facilities, registering for (free) access to their site is worthwhile.

Compressed Gas Association (CGA)

The CGA addresses safety and technical information related to the manufacture, transportation, storage, transfilling, and disposal of gases and the containers and valve which hold compressed gases.[5] The CGA's website states that CGA maintains over 300 publications, safety alerts, safety bulletins, technical bulletins, technical reports, videos, and the CGA position statements. A subscription is required to access the CGA publications.

The Joint Commission (TJC)

Founded in 1951, TJC is the largest and most noted organization for standards setting and accrediting of health care facilities in the United States. TJC website (www.joint-commision.org) contains a lot of information to assist you. Access to the entire site does require a password. However, an impressive amount of information is available without a subscription. Information is organized by accreditation, certification, standards, measurement, topics, and daily updates. TJC can be also be followed on Twitter and Facebook. The amount of information available is more than can be outlined and discussed in this chapter. This website will prove to be a valuable resource for the development or enhancement of the hyperbaric safety program.

DNV-GL Healthcare

Det Norske Veritas (DNV) Healthcare, Inc. was approved, in 2008 by the Centers for Medicare and Medicaid (CMS) to deem hospitals in compliance with the CMS Conditions of Participation for hospitals. In 2013, DNV-GL was created as a result of a merger between Det Norske Veritas (Norway) and Germanischer Lloyd (Germany). DNV-GL is an international accredited registrar and classification society headquartered in Høvik, Norway. Its approach to accreditation utilizes the National Integrated Accreditation for Healthcare Organizations requirements. The DNV-GL healthcare website (https://www.dnvglhealthcare.com) is for members only. The website does provide limited access to articles and webinars. Registration is required to view the content.

General Safety Resources

Understanding the process "culture of safety" ironically became the foundation for identifying the online resources available for hyperbaric safety. Safety in the hyperbaric facility, whether monoplace or multiplace, is unique, as hyperbaric operations provide atypical challenges not seen in other work environments. The development and implementation of the hyperbaric safety program must begin and include "general" safety elements that are the cornerstone of safe, daily, operational procedures.

The Agency for Healthcare Research and Quality Patient Safety Network (AHRQ)

The AHRQ (https://psnet.ahrq.gov) provides an excellent background about the concept of safety culture, which originated outside of health care. The AHRQ website is well organized and contains information about patient safety. This site is recommended as a resource for ongoing safety training.

The National Safety Council (NSC)

The NSC is a nonprofit organization focused on the safety in the workplace, homes, and communities.[6] The NSC website (https://www.nsc.org) contains a vast amount of content including safety posters, safety talks, checklists, weekly safety updates, monthly safety newsletters, webinars, and podcasts. Access to content is available following free registration. The NSC website's information can be utilized as a resource in developing the culture of safety within the hyperbaric medicine program.

Social Media

Newsletters, blogs, LinkedIn, Facebook, and Twitter can be more than just another way of filling your inbox. Utilizing social media as a manner of networking with colleagues is invaluable.

Newsletters and blogs from many of our industry's organizations and leaders are posted online on a daily, weekly, or monthly basis. In most cases, subscribing to a newsletter or blog is free following registration.

LinkedIn.com is a business networking platform that allows members to connect with other members, direct message, and share or post articles, opinions, or announcements. LinkedIn is an effective way to stay connected with colleagues and industry leaders. Membership is free (paid membership is also available) and is worthy of sign-up.

International Certifications

Established in 1994, The International Organization for Standardization (ISO) offers more than thirty certifications. The UHMS accreditation program is an ISO 9001 certified program. ISO 9001 is an internationally recognized standard that has been designed to ensure organizations meet the needs of customers and other stakeholders while meeting statutory and regulatory requirements related to the company's products and services. ISO 9001 was developed and published by ISO, an independent, non-governmental membership organization, and the world's largest developer of voluntary international standards.[7] The ISO website (www.intlcert.com) offers information about public training courses and recent "news" and is a useful resource.

Wound Reference

WoundReference is a wound care and hyperbaric oxygen therapy knowledge base and clinical decision platform that provides optimal wound care and hyperbaric oxygen therapy treatment with evidence-based, graded recommendations.[8] Providers have an ever-increasing knowledge base of medicine to master and receive little formal training in wound care and hyperbaric medicine. The WoundReference knowledge base and clinical decision support platform is available to clinicians during a patient encounter at the point-of-care with reliable clinical and operational support with evidence-based treatment protocols, orders, safety guidelines, coding, reimbursement, and documentation (medical necessity checklists, initial consultation, and daily treatment notes guidelines).

Recommended Resources

The following websites are recommended as resource for the development of the hyperbaric safety program.

Organization	Website URL	Content Type
Undersea & Hyperbaric Medical Society	www.uhms.org	Hyperbaric operations, safety articles, position statements
Compressed Gas Association	www.cganet.com	Gas-handling safety and regulation
National Safety Council	www.nsc.org	Safety in the workplace
Agency for Health Care Research and Quality – Patient Safety Network	www.psnet.ahrq.gov/	Patient safety
Baromedical Nurses Association	www.hyperbaricnurses.org	Organization for hyperbaric nurses' website
National Board of Diving and Hyperbaric Medical Technology	www.nbdhmt.org	Hyperbaric certification, training, and continuing education
Wound Reference	www.woundreference.com	Hyperbaric knowledge base, safety, and operational topics

Summary

The importance of a culture of safety within the hyperbaric medicine environment requires an ongoing commitment to continuing education, skills maintenance, and ensuring a culture of safety is paramount to the delivery of patient care.

All of the resources mentioned in this chapter have been discussed to provide guidance and insight into the information available online for the development, continuation, and/or enhancement of a hyperbaric safety program. Advances in technology and the impact of social media are well chronicled and should prove to be the next steps in advancing our ability to ensure safe hyperbaric operations.

References

1. Workman, WT, MS, CAsP, CHT-A, FAsMA. Guidelines for Hyperbaric Facility Operations 2nd edition. North Palm Beach, Florida: Best Publishing Co; 2015.
2. https://www.bestpub.com/books/new-book-titles/product/421-uhms-guidelines-for-hyperbaric-facility-operation-2nd-edition.html.
3. National Board of Diving and Hyperbaric Medical Technology. http://www.nbdhmt.org.
4. Baromedical Nurses Association. http://hyperbaricnurses.org/about-us/.
5. http://www.cganet.com/publications.php.
6. https://www.nsc.org.
7. International Certification. http://intlcert.com.
8. https://woundreference.com/app/.
9. https://psnet.ahrq.gov/primers/primer/5/culture-of-safety.
10. Weick KE, Sutcliffe KM. Managing the Unexpected: Sustained Performance in Complex World, 3rd edition. San Francisco, CA: John Wiley & Sons; 2015. ISBN: 9781118862414.

CHAPTER 6.11
The Role of Professional Medical Societies' Subspecialty Accreditation in Improving Patient Safety & Effectiveness

John Peters, FACHE, with invited foreword by Derall Garrett, CHT

Foreword: The Role of Hyperbaric Specialty Societies in Improving Patient Safety

Promoting patient safety should be the top priority for all professional medical societies and associations. Fortunately, many professional medical societies and associations are currently engaged in efforts to improve patient safety through continuous process improvement efforts, creation and/or promotion of standards (which include guidelines, best practices, etc.), and subspecialty accreditation.[1]

A recent questionnaire sent out by the Undersea and Hyperbaric Medical Society (UHMS) as part of an effort to assess the international status of hyperbaric medicine safety for the 2nd edition of the *Hyperbaric Facility Safety* book showed surprising results. Almost half of the professional hyperbaric medical society responses reported they did not have mandatory standards on training, staffing, fire safety, or regulation of their hyperbaric chambers as medical devices, even though the UHMS and other professional societies and associations like the NFPA, ASME, etc., create and promote standards to address these important areas of practice that directly impact patient safety.

The results of the survey demonstrate that it's not just enough to create standards for a relatively unregulated practice field; there must be a carrot or stick for these standards to be adopted into practice, measured, and improved upon. An external validation process like accreditation can be both the carrot and the stick.

As with other professional medical societies and associations, hyperbaric societies and associations should be leading the patient safety effort for the field of UHM. This involves creating relationships with existing regulatory bodies and developing a strong network that can collaborate on important initiatives like the over 30 changes that were adopted by the *NFPA 99* based on lessons learned from the UHMS hyperbaric facility accreditation process.

Standards creation and hyperbaric facility accreditation are ideal mechanisms to address the major challenges the field faces today, and hyperbaric facility accreditation is the most effective risk management tool that a health care organization can employ.

In Search for Transparency

In today's health care environment, performance expectations by the public, payers, and regulators are higher than ever, and the talk of complete quality and price transparency in the health care transaction has gained significant momentum.[2-6]

These expectations are being driven in part by identified gaps in safety and quality and the unsustainable increases in US National Health Care Expenditures (NHE) as a percentage of the US gross domestic product (GDP).

The value of transparency is enhanced, according to the authors of *Fostering Transparency in Outcomes, Quality, Safety and Costs,* by engaging providers about their performance and informing the public about provider performance.[7]

Engaging providers about their experience and outcomes should create a more accountable relationship, while public reporting of provider experience provides stakeholders, including patients, payers, and regulators, information on outcomes and cost, to make decisions about purchasing, or contracting health care services.

Achieving transparency will lead to an improved clinical experience for the provider and outcome for the patient and will bring down the cost of health care.[5]

However, complete transparency has been elusive and arguably most efforts to create transparency have fallen short of their goal. One reason for this is that transparency is a moving target, and there is still little evidence that public reporting is currently influencing purchasing or referral patterns.[2, 8-9]

The earliest public attempts at transparency began nearly 30 years ago with the publishing of Best Hospitals by the for-profit magazine company US News and World Report. Since then, other companies entered the hospital ratings market and published their own versions of top hospitals, including the United State's largest single insurer, the Centers for Medicare and Medicaid Services (CMS), which publishes its *Star Ratings on Hospital Compare.*[10]

The effectiveness of these ratings has been subject to debate due to their lack of reproducible scoring, consistency with what is being measured, and how the measures that are available are being weighted amongst the numerous ratings companies. The published results are a major concern for providers who believe they are unfairly represented and powerless to address deficiencies that aren't publicly available.[3,11]

According to the American Hospital Association (AHA),[12] in the case of CMS, its Star Ratings are potentially inaccurate and may not be useful to patients who seek care for a specific illness. Basically, the AHA is telling the public to not trust the ratings. Their reasoning is that a hospital's Star Rating on Hospital Compare depends on a few select measures with disproportionate weights and the data is extremely aged, up to three years, by the time the star ratings are published.

Hospital ratings in their current state are therefore an ineffective or incomplete gauge for measuring the performance of health care organizations and their clinical departments and do not contribute to making health care more transparent or accountable.

What does promote both transparency and accountability at the patient level is health care accreditation. Validation surveys of clinical service lines by recognized specialty-specific accrediting organizations are the key to achieving breakthrough in making performance improvement continuous.[13]

Providers and stakeholders should value accreditation above other transparency methods because it saves lives. In one study involving nearly 2,000 hospitals, researchers compared patient mortality during The Joint Commission (TJC) accreditation survey weeks to nonsurvey weeks. Patients who were admitted during TJC weeks had significantly lower mortality, particularly in major teaching hospitals.[14]

This should resonate with those who argue voluntary accreditation is too expensive and strains resources in preparation for a survey. Operating at a high level of attention, as if a survey team were on-site, saves lives and it's this author's opinion that it is not acceptable for an organization to have to ramp up and let down based on an accreditation or state agency survey cycle.

While the author references United States (US) health care policy in this chapter, readers should note that triggers driving the US's policy changes are systemic to the global health care system and therefore make the case that accreditation's benefits are universally applicable.[15-17]

Additionally, this chapter is meant to complement the previously authored and comprehensive chapter, Accreditation and Regulation in Hyperbaric and Wound Care Centers, authored by Tom Workman, one of the editors of this book, in *Hyperbaric Nursing and Wound Care.*[18]

The author did an excellent job in describing the regulatory environment and climate for clinical hyperbaric medicine (HBO_2), the history of the UHMS Hyperbaric Facility Accreditation program, and very specifically, the details of how the UHMS HFA program is administered.

The UHMS has gained significantly more experience with accreditation since *Hyperbaric Nursing and Wound Care* was published 2010. To date, the UHMS HFA program has surveyed and accredited 267 hyperbaric facilities.

The UHMS has also made a significant investment in the HFA program with a focus on improving the experience of both the hyperbaric facility being surveyed and the survey team.

The UHMS recently released a new web-based software application for the HFA program and provides iPads for all UHMS surveyors. This new application allows data capture regardless of WiFi connectivity.

Additionally, the UHMS Hyperbaric Facility Accreditation program has been ISO 9001-2008 and now 9001-2015 certified.

The Triggers for Transformation

The gaps in safety, quality, and cost in health care are the triggers for change.

US health care's moment of pause as it relates to safety and quality came with the 1999 report from the Institute of Medicine (IOM), *To Err is Human*, which claimed as many as 98,000 patients die annually of preventable medical errors.[19]

To Err is Human was impactful, a real turning point for US health care because arguably for the first time, the public, regulators, insurers, and others became true stakeholders and not just bystanders. These new stakeholders were now involved in the conversation about quality because of transparency and this helped reenergize the performance improvement movement.[20]

This is supported by a follow-up study in 2006 by the same authors of *To Err is Human*, demonstrating an increase in patient safety-related publications and research grants awarded after the IOM's report was published.[21]

It also marked a shift in thinking about how care is delivered and making health care organizations and providers accountable for preventable harm as exampled by CMS refusing to pay hospitals after October 2008 for eight preventable medical errors.[22]

With advancements in the science of quality improvement, clinical knowledge, medicine, and technology, as well as the guiding hands of regulators and insurers, surely the US health care system would be able to right itself and experience near-zero preventable deaths, but that was not the case.

In 2013, a more stunning revelation was presented that pegged the number of preventable deaths at 210,000 and preventable harm to more than 400,000 people. This was reinforced by a study published in 2016 in the *British Medical Journal* (*BMJ*), listing preventable deaths at 250,000 and defining medical errors as the third leading cause of death in the United States.[23-24]

The costs of preventable harm are included in the overall national health expenditures (NHE) statistic and fall under the definition of waste, according to former Centers for Medicare and Medicaid Services (CMS) administrator, Dr. Don Berwick.

Shortly after leaving his post at CMS, Dr. Berwick authored the paper *Eliminating Waste in US Health Care.*[25] He defined waste in six categories, including failures in care delivery, failures in care coordination, overtreatment, administrative complexity, pricing failures and fraud, and abuse.

He estimated the cost of waste to be between 21% and 34% of *total* US NHE. In today's dollars, with the US NHE at 18.2% of GDP,[26] the cost is $3.7 trillion dollars. Applying Dr. Berwick's multiplier, waste can be estimated to be greater than $700 billion to over $1 trillion. US health care spending growth is expected to increase 5.5% over the next decade with NHE making up 19.4% of GDP.[27] This is unsustainable without significant and costly reform.[28]

One area that contributes to unsustainability is that in 2026, the US Hospital Improvement (HI) Trust Fund, also known as Medicare A-benefits, are projected to be liquidated. At that point for several years out, the HI trust fund will only be able to pay

$0.91 per $1 of Medicare A spending. That number fluctuates over future years; however, that fluctuation is irrelevant for this chapter.[29-30]

In 2008, US President Barak Obama took office with an eye on health care spending. In September 2009, he addressed Congress and stated that in order to have a viable health care system, *unnecessary* spending had to be eliminated.[31]

President Obama singled out health care fraud and abuse as a top priority, and with Congress's support, passed the Fraud Enforcement and Recovery Act (FERA) in May 2009, which strengthened the False Claims Act (FCA) of 1986 by increasing the burden of proof for the provider as well as increasing financial penalties. In March of 2010, Congress passed the Patient Protection and Affordable Care Act (ACA), which increased funding for health care antifraud efforts by hundreds of millions of dollars.[2, 32]

While this might seem "big picture" and not relevant to the individual HBO_2 provider, these laws spurred the creation of programs like Medicare Prior Authorization (mPA), Recovery Audit Contracting (RAC), Prepayment Review, and Targeted Probe and Educate (TPE), which are affecting providers because of identified overtreatment, fraud, and abuse.[33-35]

The first HHS Office of Inspector General (OIG) report on HBO_2 in 2000, the same report referenced in *Hyperbaric Nursing and Wound Care*, as a nidus to create the UHMS hyperbaric facility accreditation program, reported 38% of provider claims were paid improperly, either for inappropriate or excessive treatment and raised concerns about the quality of care and lack of physician involvement. Since then, the OIG has published additional audit reports looking specifically at Medicare Administrative Contractors (MACs) beginning with Wisconsin Physician Services (WPS) and First Coast Service Options (FCSO), who paid the largest amounts for HBO_2 outpatient services.[36-37] The published results of the OIG audits were hardly believable with payment error rates in the 90% range for FCSO and 60% for WPS.

Physicians and their documentation are at the center of the discussion because of the issues detailed in both reports about the medical records and lack of documented medical necessity.

However, this is not just a physician problem because for hospital outpatient departments (HOPD) HBO_2 is "incident to" physician supervision services and the hospital is on the hook for these errors.[38]

At the OIG's recommendation, WPS and FCSO have been sending letters to hospital providers in their geographic regions requiring audits and repayments. The question is how many HBO_2 facilities will survive after their hospital leadership teams have to write checks for hundreds of thousands of dollars in repayments back to the MACs/CMS.

Regardless of where HBO_2 services are rendered, providers should embrace transparency and external validation through accreditation in order to improve care and lower their risk of deficiencies, payment denials, and fines.[39-41]

One program mandated by CMS to contain costs and reduce waste, fraud, and abuse was the mPA for nonemergent hyperbaric medicine. This three-year program began March 1, 2015, and ended February 2018, and required providers in three states with the highest average number of HBO_2 treatments per beneficiary to request prior authorization for six covered conditions.[42-44]

One of those conditions, preparation and preservation of skin grafts, was later removed from the list due to the condition requiring urgent or emergent treatment, leaving five conditions requiring prior authorization. There was an additional wrinkle for HBO_2 providers during that same year, when ICD-10 was implemented on October 1, 2015. Overnight, some conditions historically accepted and treated in HBO_2 were unmasked when providers attempted to crosswalk them from ICD-9 to ICD-10, and there were not corresponding ICD-10 codes for those conditions.[45]

Conditions such as failing "flap" and chronic radiation proctitis (CRP) were stricken from the list of treated indications, although they were never listed specifically in the Medicare NCD 20.29 for hyperbaric oxygen therapy (HBOT).[46]

The financial savings from the mPA program for nonemergent HBO_2 and ICD-10 implementation was $27.3 million over the three-year period. On average, PA and ICD-10, saved the Medicare program $780,000 per month in the affected states.[47]

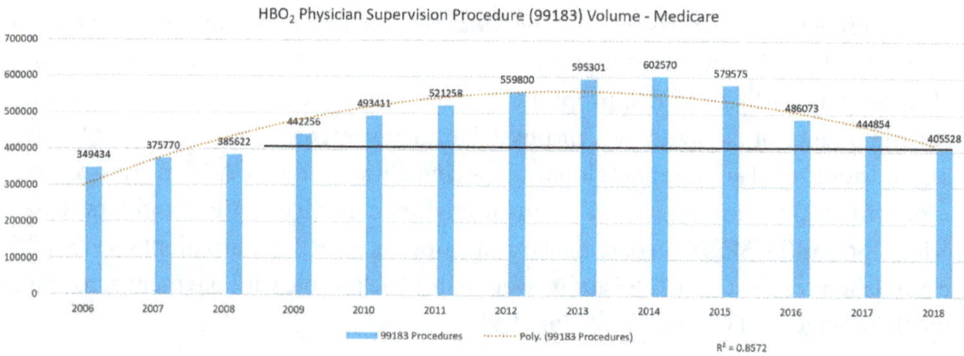

Figure 1.

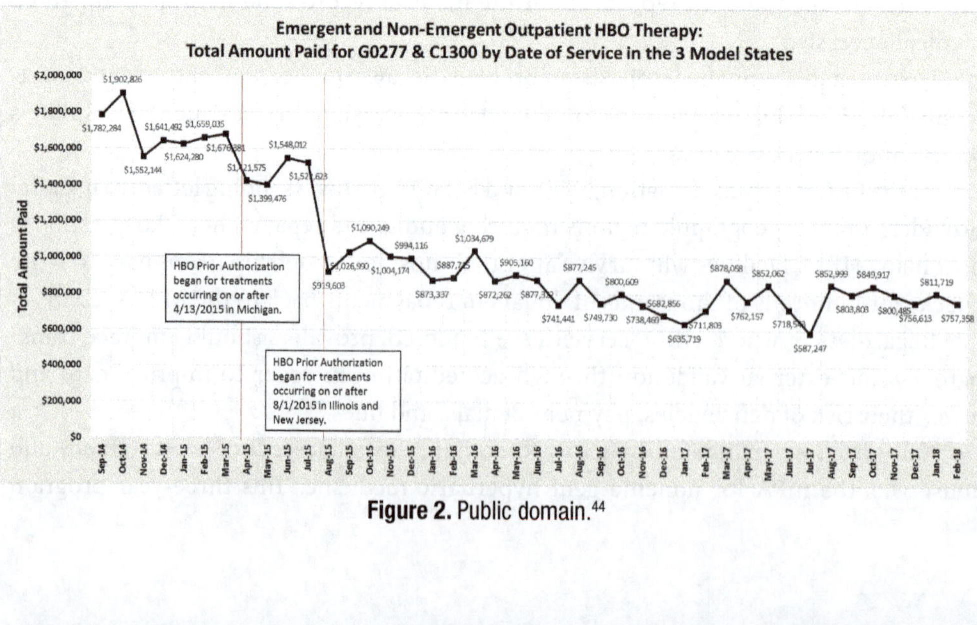

Figure 2. Public domain.[44]

mPA and ICD-10 are believed to have contributed to the overall decline in Medicare claims for CPT 99183 as seen in Figure 1. Through 2018, CPT 99183 volume declined by 33%, from their peak in 2014. That decline is statistically significant.

Despite the savings seen in Figure 2, CMS chose not to continue the mPA project. The decrease on total Medicare expenditures as a result of the program were not statistically significant according to Mathematica Policy Research, who authored the interim report to CMS. While the mPA program met its overall goals, there were challenges with delay in care and provider satisfaction with mPA. CMS noted that if needed, "other strategies can be considered in the future to achieve similar or greater results, and that these strategies can account for burden and the needs of different populations." CMS said it was keeping its options open and that mPA could be considered again.[43]

Providers of hyperbaric medicine should take note that CMS was very effective at bending both the volume and cost curves quickly and rather than waiting for the next version of cost containment to affect them, providers should seek external validation of their care processes, guidelines adherence, and process improvement strategy.[48]

Validation through Accreditation

Accreditation is key to reducing variation and increasing transparency-of-care processes at the patient level while building a sustainable culture of safety.[49-51]

When an organization subscribes to service line or subspecialty accreditation, they are committing themselves to adhering to evidence-based standards, which translates to better and safer care.[52]

Accreditation standards should be *viewed as a floor.*[53] It is unacceptable in this author's opinion for providers to not meet published standards and accepted guidelines and if providers do not follow them, then they do so at their own risk and to the risk of their organizations.

There is overwhelming evidence in the published literature that subspecialty accreditation including nuclear cardiology, stroke care, sleep care, radiation oncology, and venous care results in greater compliance to nationally and internationally based standards and guidelines, policies, and processes.[54-60]

These results should translate to the value of subspecialty accreditation for HBO_2 services.

When providers adhere to best practices, evidence-based standards, and guidelines, patients win. Patient outcomes are improved, and morbidity and mortality are reduced, when providers are accredited and certified.[61-63] In a robust systematic review of the impact of accreditation on health care services, clinical outcomes were improved significantly across different subspecialties.[64]

In another systematic review of bariatric surgery outcomes involving 1.5 million patients, there was a preponderance of evidence that supports accreditation in bariatric surgery, including a reduction in mortality in accredited bariatric programs. Additional benefits included reduced costs and complications.[65]

These examples reinforce that without accreditation, practice and patient outcomes will be substandard, regardless of who the providers are. If their performance is not measured, it's assumed to be less than the best.

Embracing continuous performance improvement married with subspecialty accreditation will build a culture of accountability, make health care transparent, reducing overtreatment, fraud and abuse, and reduce the cost of care.

Professional hyperbaric medical societies and associations play a key role in patient safety. Creation and promotion of standards and subspecialty accreditation are the most important tools available to improve the safety and efficacy of hyperbaric medicine, while reducing waste and overall costs.[13]

References

1. National Fire Protection Association. The value of standards development organizations. What are SDOs. https://www.nfpa.org/codes-and-standards/standards-development-process/the-value-of-standards-development-organizations.
2. Institute for Healthcare Improvement. NPSF call to action: preventable health care harm is a public health crisis. March 2017. https://www.npsf.org/page/public_health_crisis.
3. Semigran HL, Gourevitch R, Sinaiko AD, Cowling D, Mehrotra A. Patients' views on price shopping and price transparency. *American Journal of Managed Care.* 2017 Jun 1;23(6):e186-e192.
4. Durand DJ, Narayan AK, Rybicki FJ, Burleson J, Nagy P, McGinty G, Duszak R Jr. The healthcare value transparency movement and its implications for radiology. *J Am Coll Radiol.* 2015 Jan;12(1):51-8. doi: 10.1016/j.jacr.2014.08.015. Epub 2014 Oct 25.
5. Emery DW, De Brantes F. Curing an ill health care system: transparent multilateral benefits, cost, and quality. Healthcare Finance Management. 2015 Feb;69(2):80-3.
6. Sullivan T. CMS turns focus to transparency. Policy & Medicine. April 3, 2019. https://www.policymed.com/2019/04/cms-turns-focus-to-transparency.html.
7. National Academy of Medicine. Vital directions for health & health care. 2017;269-287.
8. Shaller D, Kanouse DE, Schlesinger M. Context-based strategies for engaging consumers with public reports about health care providers. *Medical Care Research & Review.* 2014 Oct;71(5 Suppl):17S-37S. doi: 10.1177/1077558713493118. Epub 2013 Jul 1.
9. Brown DL, Epstein AM, Schneider EC. Influence of cardiac surgeon report cards on patient referral by cardiologists in New York state after 20 years of public reporting. Circulation. Cardiovascular Quality & Outcomes. 2013 Nov;6(6):643-8. doi: 10.1161/CIRCOUTCOMES.113.000506. Epub 2013 Nov 12.

10. Centers for Medicare & Medicaid Services. CMS roadmaps for the traditional fee-for-service (FFS) program: overview. https://www.cms.gov/Medicare/Quality-Initiatives-Patient-Assessment-Instruments/QualityInitiativesGenInfo/downloads/RoadmapOverview_OEA_1-16.pdf.
11. Austin JM, Jha AK, Romano PS, Singer SJ, Vogus TJ, Wachter RM, Pronovost PJ. National hospital ratings systems share few common scores and may generate confusion instead of clarity. *Health Affairs.* 2015;34(3):423–430. doi: 10.1377/hlthaff.2014.0201.
12. American Hospital Association. Letter to Kate Goodrich, MD, Chief Medical Officer CMS. Overall hospital quality star ratings on hospital compare public input request. February 2019. https://www.aha.org/system/files/media/file/2019/03/190327-star-ratings.pdf.
13. Nicklin W, et al. Leveraging the full value and impact of accreditation. *International Journal for Quality in Health Care.* 2017;29(2):310-312. doi: 10.1093/intqhc/mzx010.
14. Barnett M, et al. Patient mortality during unannounced accreditation surveys at US hospitals. *JAMA Internal Medicine.* 2017:177(5);693-700. March 20, 2017. Doi:10.1001/jamainternalmed.2016.9685.
15. Deloitte. Analysis: 2019 global health care outlook. Shaping the future. https://www2.deloitte.com/global/en/pages/life-sciences-and-healthcare/articles/global-health-care-sector-outlook.html.
16. Shammari M, et al. Impact of hospital accreditation on patient safety in hail city, Saudi Arabia: nurses' perspective. *IOSR Journal of Nursing and Health Science.* 2015;4(1):1-5.
17. Salmon JW, Heavens J, Lombard C, Tavrow P. The impact of accreditation on the quality of hospital care: KwaZulu-Natal province, Republic of South Africa. Bethesda, MD: University Research Company, Quality Assurance Project; 2003 Oct. Operations Research Results; USAID Contract No. GPH-C-00-02-00004-00. P. 2003. https://www.popline.org/node/276015.
18. Workman T. In Larson-Lohr V, et al. Hyperbaric nursing and wound care. Accreditation and regulation in hperbaric and wound centers. Flagstaff, AZ: Best Publishing Company; 2010;65-73.
19. Institute of Medicine. To err is human: building a safer health system. 1999.
20. Marjoua Y, Bozic K. Brief history of quality movement in US health care. *Current Reviews in Musculoskeletal Medicine.* 2012;5:265–273. DOI 10.1007/s12178-012-9137-8.
21. Stelfox S, Palmisani C, Scurlock E, et al. The "To Err is Human" report and the patient safety literature. *Quality Safety Health Care.* 2006 Jun;15(3):174–178. doi: 10.1136/qshc.2006.017947.
22. Brooks J. US Medicare will stop paying for preventable errors. *Canadian Medical Association Journal.* 2007 Oct 9;177(8):841–842. doi: 10.1503/cmaj.071347.

23. James. A new, evidence-based estimate of patient harms associated with hospital care. *Journal of Patient Safety*. 2013;9:122Y128.
24. Makary M, Daniel M. Medical error – the third leading cause of death in the US. *BMJ* 2016;353:i2139.
25. Berwick DM, Hackbarth AD. Eliminating waste in US health care. *JAMA*. 2012;307(14):1513–1516. doi:10.1001/jama.2012.362.
26. Statista. U.S. national health expenditure as percent of GDP from 1960 to 2019. https://www.statista.com/statistics/184968/us-health-expenditure-as-percent-of-gdp-since-1960/.
27. Sisko A, Keehan S et al. National health expenditure projections, 2018–27: economic and demographic trends drive spending and enrollment growth. Health Affairs. Feb 20, 2019. https://doi.org/10.1377/hlthaff.2018.05499.
28. Organisation for Economic Co-operation and Development. Health care costs unsustainable in advanced economies without reform. September 24, 2015. http://www.oecd.org/health/healthcarecostsunsustainableinadvancedeconomieswithoutreform.htm.
29. Social Security Administration. A summary of the 2018 annual reports. https://www.ssa.gov/OACT/TRSUM/index.html.
30. The Hill. Medicare trust fund to be depleted years earlier than expected, trustees project. June 5, 2018. https://thehill.com/policy/healthcare/390801-medicare-trust-fund-to-be-depleted-in-2026-trustees-project.
31. Nolan Auerbach & White. President Obama vows to eliminate health care fraud and reduce waste. http://medicare-fraud.net/president-obama-vows-to-eliminate-healthcare-fraud-and-reduce-waste/.
32. Sullivan T. HHS turning up the HEAT on health care fraud charges. Policy & Medicine. May 5, 2019. https://www.policymed.com/2010/12/hhs-turning-up-the-heat-on-healthcare-fraud-charges.html.
33. Performant. Hyperbaric oxygen therapy (HBOT) for diabetic wounds. Recovery Audit Contractor. Issue_0129. January 29, 2019. https://performantrac.com/audit-regions/region-1/page/2/.
34. CMS Targeted Probe and Educate (TPE) program. https://www.cms.gov/Research-Statistics-Data-and-Systems/Monitoring-Programs/Medicare-FFS-Compliance-Programs/Medical-Review/Targeted-Probe-and-EducateTPE.html.
35. Novitas-Solutions. Targeted probe and educate topics and schedule of review. https://www.novitas-solutions.com/webcenter/portal/MedicareJH/pagebyid?contentId=00184116.
36. HHS OIG. Wisconsin physicians service paid providers for hyperbaric oxygen therapy services that did not comply with Medicare requirements. February 2018. https://www.oig.hhs.gov/oas/reports/region1/11500515.pdf.

37. HHS OIG. First Coast Service Options, Inc., paid providers for hyperbaric oxygen therapy services that did not comply with Medicare requirements. December 2018. https://oig.hhs.gov/oas/reports/region4/41606196.pdf.
38. CMS.gov. National coverage determination (NCD) for hyperbaric oxygen therapy (20.29). https://www.cms.gov/medicare-coverage-database/details/ncd-details.aspx?ncdid=12.
39. Urman RD, et al. Patient safety and office-based anesthesia. *Current Opinion in Anaesthesiology.* 2012 Dec;25(6):648-53. doi: 10.1097/ACO.0b013e3283593094.
40. Fogh, SE, et al. American College of Radiology (ACR) radiation oncology practice accreditation: a pattern of change. *Practical Radiation Oncology.* 2016 Sep-Oct;6(5):e171-e177. doi: 10.1016/j.prro.2016.01.010.
41. Williams SC, et al. Comparing public quality ratings for accredited and nonaccredited nursing homes. *Journal of the American Medical Directors Association.* 2017 Jan;18(1):24-29. doi: 10.1016/j.jamda.2016.07.025. Epub 2016 Sep 3.
42. CMS.gov. Prior authorization of non-emergent hyperbaric oxygen. https://www.cms.gov/Research-Statistics-Data-and-Systems/Monitoring-Programs/Medicare-FFS-Compliance-Programs/Prior-Authorization-Initiatives/Prior-Authorization-of-Non-Emergent-Hyperbaric-Oxygen.html.
43. Federal Register. Prior authorization of non-emergent hyperbaric oxygen (HBO) therapy. Vol. 79. No 225. Fri. Nov 21, 2014. Notices. CMS-6064-N. Medicare Program. https://www.govinfo.gov/content/pkg/FR-2014-11-21/pdf/2014-27578.pdf
44. Centers for Medicare and Medicaid Services. Medicare prior authorization of non-emergent hyperbaric oxygen (HBO) therapy modelstatus update (Posted 10-26-2018). https://www.cms.gov/Research-Statistics-Data-and-Systems/Monitoring-Programs/Medicare-FFS-Compliance-Programs/Prior-Authorization-Initiatives/Downloads/HBOPriorAuth_StatusUpdate_10262018.pdf.
45. CMS. Medicare prior Aathorization of non-emergent hyperbaric oxygen (HBO) therapy model status update. Posted 10-26-2018. https://www.cms.gov/Research-Statistics-Data-and-Systems/Monitoring-Programs/Medicare-FFS-Compliance-Programs/Prior-Authorization-Initiatives/Downloads/HBOPriorAuth_StatusUpdate_10262018.pdf.
46. Bozzuto T. The Case of the Disappearing Indication. https://www.uhms.org/resources/news-announcements/809-uhms-member-alerts-the-societ y-on-problems-with-cms-coverage-of-radiation-proctitis.html.
47. Asher A, et al. Interim report for the evaluation of Medicare prior authorization model for non-emergent hyperbaric oxygen (HBO). Mathematica Policy Research. June 2018. HHSM-500-2014-00034. https://innovation.cms.gov/Files/reports/interimevalrpt-mpa-hbo.pdf.

48. Falstie-Jensen AM, et al. Compliance with accreditation and recommended hospital care-a Danish nationwide population-based study. *International Journal for Quality in Health Care.* 2017 Oct 1;29(5):625-633. doi: 10.1093/intqhc/mzx104.
49. Wagner LM, et al. Impact of voluntary accreditation on deficiency citations in U.S. nursing homes. *The Gerontologist.* 2012 Aug;52(4):561-70. doi: 10.1093/geront/gnr136. Epub 2012 Mar 5.
50. Dotta A, et al. Accreditation of birth centres: advantages for newborns. *Journal of Maternal-Fetal & Neonatal Medicine.* 2013 Mar;26(4):417-8.
51. Wagne, LM, et al. Relationship between nursing home safety culture and Joint Commission accreditation. *Joint Commission Journal on Quality Patient Safety.* 2012 May;38(5):207-15.
52. Knuston A, et al. The role of the American College of Surgeons' cancer program accreditation in influencing oncologic outcomes. *Journal of Surgical Oncology.* 2014;110:611-615.
53. Warburton R. Quality accreditation and regulation: can they help improve patient safety? US Department of Health and Human Services. Agency for Healthcare Research and Quality. PSNet. Apr 2009. https://psnet.ahrq.gov/perspectives/perspective/74/accreditation-and-regulation-can-they-help-improve-patient-safety#figure2.
54. Maddux PT, et al. Improved compliance with reporting standards: a retrospective analysis of Intersocietal Accreditation Commission Nuclear Cardiology Laboratories. *Journal of Nuclear Cardiology.* 2018 Jun;25(3):986-994. doi: 10.1007/s12350-016-0713-y.
55. Johnson A, et al. Compliance with acute stroke care quality measures in hospitals with and without primary stroke care certification: the North Carolina stroke care collaborative. *Journal of the American Heart Association.* 2014 Apr;3(2):e000423.
56. Tain-Junn C, et al. Nationwide "Hospital Emergent Capability Accreditation by Level-Stroke" improves stroke treatment in Taiwan. *Journal of Stroke.* 2017 May; 19(2):205-212. Doi: 10.5853.jos.2016.01655.
57. Parthasarathy S, et al. A multicenter prospective comparative effectiveness study of the effect of physician certification and center accreditation on patient-centered outcomes in obstructive sleep apnea. Journal of Clinical Sleep Medicine. 2014; 10(3):243-249. http://dx.doi.org/10.5664/jcsm.3518.
58. Mikami M, et al. Impact of institutional accreditation by the Japan Society of Gynecologic Oncology on the treatment and survival of women with cervical cancer. *Journal of Gynecologic Oncology.* 2018 Mar;29(2):e23. doi: 10.3802/jgo.2018.29.e23.
59. Berger ER, et al. National accreditation program for breast centers demonstrates improved compliance with post-mastectomy radiation therapy quality measure. *Journal of the American College of Surgeons.* 2017 Mar;224(3):236-244. doi: 10.1016/j.jamcollsurg.2016.11.006.

60. Kabnick LS, et al. Exploring the value of vein center accreditation to the venous specialist. *Journal of Vascular Surgery.* 2016;4(1):doi: 10.1016/j.jvsv.2015.06.005.
61. Gray B, et al. Associations between American board of internal medicine maintenance of certification status and performance on a set of health care effectiveness data and information set (HEDIS) process measures. *Annals of Internal Medicine.* 2018 Jul 17;169(2):97-105. doi: 10.7326/M16-2643. Epub 2018 Jun 12.
62. Otsubo T, et al.Safety-related outcomes of the Japanese Society of hepato-biliary-pancreatic surgery board certification system for expert surgeons. *Journal of Hepato-Biliary Pancreatic Sciences.* 2017 May;24(5):252-261. doi: 10.1002/jhbp.444. Epub 2017 Apr 26.
63. Fleischut PM, et al. Provider board certification status and practice patterns in total knee arthroplasty. *Academic Medicine.* 2016 Jan;91(1):79-86. doi: 10.1097/ACM.0000000000000808.
64. Alkhenizan A, Shaw C. Impact of accreditation on the quality of health care services: a systematic review of the literature. *Annals of Saudi Medicine.* 2011 Jul-Aug;31(4):407-16. doi: 10.4103/0256-4947.83204.
65. Azagury D, Morton, JM. Bariatric surgery outcomes in US accredited vs non-accredited centers: a systematic review. *Journal of the American College of Surgeons.* 2016 Sep;223(3):469-77. doi: 10.1016/j.jamcollsurg.2016.06.014.

CHAPTER 6.12
Mobile and Relocatable Hyperbaric Systems

J. Steven Wood

Traditional hyperbaric chamber systems are fixed to specific locations. Some mission requirements dictate that the chamber must have the flexibility to be moved. In this chapter, we will provide a brief overview of the unique demands of the movable hyperbaric facility.

Movable chamber systems may be divided into two general categories: mobile and relocatable. Each style has unique system and environmental requirements. For purposes of brevity, we will refer to them generally as "mobile" systems.

Mobile systems are not new. The first mobile chambers were pulled by horse teams to hospitals in Paris in the late 1800s (see Chapter 1: History of Hyperbaric Chambers). Mobile chamber systems are designed to be placed on-site and into service within a short period of time (hours). A true mobile system will be fully self-contained with internal power generation, gas storage, climate control, and sanitary systems requiring only a site to support the system. Some mobile systems may require connection to utility services, necessitating some degree of site preparation. Housing for the chamber ranges from semi-truck trailers to modified recreational vehicles to shipping containers. Typical applications for mobile systems include the following:

- Providing short-term treatment at remote locations, including military operations and disasters
- Supporting diving or caisson operations
- Providing treatment for athletes at arenas or stadiums
- Veterinary treatment
- Temporary backup when fixed-base chamber systems are out of service
- Providing shared services at multiple nearby hospitals or other health care locations

Due to their need to be rapidly deployed, mobile systems are, by nature, small, generally limited to over-the-road vehicle width, length, and weight limitations. The small footprint (particularly width) of the carrier vehicle will limit the size of chamber allowed. Unless the carrier is designed with extendable side walls (similar to the slide-outs of recreational vehicles), multiplace chambers are limited to a maximum width of around two meters. Monoplace-based mobile systems are typically limited to two chambers maximum.

Relocatable systems are designed to be moved but may only be moved infrequently. These systems are commonly used as semi-permanent units when there is no space available within a building or if modification of an existing building is economically unviable. Some relocatable systems may stay in place for years, becoming de facto permanent facilities. A relocatable system may be constructed from a standard over-the-road trailer, a modular building, or shipping containers. These systems are usually not designed for rapid deployment. Most relocatable systems will require extensive site preparation and fixed utility connections (electricity, water, sewer, medical gases, telecommunications). Typical applications for relocatable systems include the following:

- Proof of concept for facilities planning to establish fixed-base hyperbaric services
- Temporary backup when fixed-base chamber systems are out of service

Regulatory Considerations

Mobile chamber systems fall into a regulatory black hole. The chambers contained in the facility are still subject to locally applicable boiler and pressure vessel codes (typically *American Society of Mechanical Engineers Pressure Vessels for Human Occupancy* [*ASME PVHO*]), but there are few, if any, regulations specific to these systems. Regardless of the presence or absence of regulations, it is incumbent upon the operator to ensure that the facility is designed for safe operation. For those units that are part of an accredited health care facility, the design and operational aspects of the unit must take into account inspection standards imposed by the accrediting organization ranging from safety to infection control to patient privacy. Before establishing any type of movable system, the operator should conduct extensive due diligence to determine which codes and standards the facility will be subject to. A mobile hyperbaric system meant for safely treating patents needs to be built to a recognized safety code or standard, no matter the jurisdiction or country in which used. The mobile system operator should know the codes to be applied and be diligent in ensuring the hyperbaric systems meet the local code. American and European Union codes are widely accepted throughout the world. One can often be used in lieu of the other in a jurisdiction lacking their own special codes. At a minimum, in the United States, the *Life Safety Code*, *National Electric Code*, *ASME PVHO*, and *National Fire Protection Association: 99 (NFPA 99)* standards should be followed.

Design Considerations

Both multiplace and monoplace must be housed in a structure that provides physical protection for the chamber, its occupants, and support staff. A mobile hyperbaric system need not meet the same building requirements as a permanent hyperbaric facility, especially if it is not connected to a permanent structure.

Planning

Once a need has been defined, the class of chamber (multiplace, monoplace, or animal) and the expected number and type of patients (critical care, ambulatory, etc.) has been determined, the chamber and its support systems can be designed or customized to fit the need.

Site geography and weather conditions are important considerations. The type of ground or surface the mobile system is set upon (asphalt, concrete, dirt, grass, shell, or underlying utilities) must be assessed. Will the surface support the chamber system and now allow sinkage and tilting of the chamber system? If not, plans for dispersing the mobile system weight must be developed during site design.

Local weather conditions may vary from freezing to sweltering. Mobile treatment facilities have been successfully employed in areas where hurricanes, snowstorms, heat waves, or strong winds are expected. The heating, ventilation, and air conditioning (HVAC) system must maintain the interior environment consonant with occupant comfort and also ensure support systems can be utilized no matter the outside temperature. Fire protection systems won't work if they are frozen.

The confines of a trailer or RV may make it hard to access important chamber hull valves (pressure safety relief valve, fire suppression system (FSS) bypass, hull-stop valves, etc.) Access to the valves must be made possible. Valve access can be achieved by using reach rods connected to the important valves or by installing access doors or panels on the outside of the trailer.

Pressure, building, and fire and safety codes need to be factored into both the chamber and its shelter's design or modification. Early interface with the fire marshal, code inspectors, and site facility engineering is important because many local regulatory authorities may not understand hyperbaric therapy and the existing design codes. *A fire marshal may not understand the hyperbaric patients in a multiplace chamber are protected from fire by an interior FSS.* Taking the time to educate these important others about hyperbaric therapy and its equipment will pay off in ease of installation and occupancy permits.

Other questions to answer before construction include the following: Will there be a need for exam rooms, medical gases, patient ramps or lifts, bathrooms, an office, waiting room, power, signal, water, drain? Where will the chamber operator's station be?

All of these questions need to be factored into the installation site plan. Preplanning by an experienced design team can save time and money during program development and enhance operational efficiency and safety once treatment operations begin.

Construction: Chamber

The hyperbaric chamber itself must meet local or national pressure vessel and safety codes. A chamber can be custom-built to fit a trailer or RV. However, it is more common to adapt the transport/housing unit to accommodate a standard chamber design.

Simply moving the mobile facility can affect the chamber, and these imposed stresses must be considered in developing an operational plan for relocation and setup. The chamber windows and their seals must be designed to accommodate the expected temperature ranges and stresses that will occur. In moving from site to site, the chamber system will experience many thousands—perhaps millions—of vibration cycles that can adversely impact devices, calibrations, and cause pipe or tubing leaks. The chamber must be securely fixed to the RV or trailer so it does not slide, jump, or move during transport. Instruments such as pressure gauges and analyzers must be protected against vibration during travel. This protection is often best achieved by removing the devices from the chamber and transporting them in cushioned containers. Gas and fluid piping may need flexible connections to avoid leaks from the vibration cycles.

The width of most over-the-road trailers limits the chamber dimensions to eight feet wide or less, depending upon the amount of insulation needed to keep the interior occupants comfortable. Chamber-mounted control and monitoring consoles are only possible on chambers of five-and-a-half feet or less. A remote console may be needed for larger chambers or if the geometry of the housing area does not allow easy access to a chamber-mounted console.

Hyperbaric chambers are heavy. Designers must take the loads imposed by the chamber(s) to ensure that the truck, trailer, or container that houses the chambers has the structural integrity to support and secure the chamber(s). Placement of the chamber(s) within the vehicle or trailer and providing secure anchorage must also be considered, as an ill-placed or shifted load may result in loss of control by the transport vehicle. The chamber doors will need a means to be kept in the closed position during travel; a 200 to 1200-pound steel door banging into the hull and door-sealing surface can destroy the chamber's ability to hold pressure. Ensure the chamber doors can be securely closed when traveling. Bungee cords are not reliable for this use.

Construction: Housing/Trailer

Mobile facilities are typically constructed with metal structural frames, engineered to accommodate loads imposed by the chambers. Trailer-based facilities are constructed of metal, typically aluminum. Relocatable facilities are commonly based on mobile home or modular building designs which closely resemble fixed operations (wooden wall framing, shingle, or metal roofing).

Insulation of the trailer is important for patient and staff comfort. Walls, ceiling, and floors need to be insulated to protect against temperature extremes. It seems a trailer is always colder during the winter and hotter in the summer.

A special room may be needed for chamber subsystems (built-in breathing systems [BIBS], supplies, air compressors, generators, environmental conditioning units, fire suppression tanks and spare air tanks). These systems are often inside and/or under the trailer, sometimes in a special purpose portable room.

Compressors and pumps add noise and vibration. Consider rubber shock dampeners for this type of equipment or locating these components in a separate portable housing.

A toilet and changing facility must be available for patients and staff. Any fluid (water supply, FSS tanks, etc.) line that is outside of the trailer (e.g., underneath) should be protected against cold by heat tape. The area under the trailer can be a major source of heat loss during the winter and a heat gain in the summer. Consider installation of fans, heaters, and enclosing the area with insulated panels, including louvered ducts that can be opened in the summer and closed in the winter. If enclosing this area, ensure there are access doors to permit inspection and servicing.

With a mobile facility, ensure that each corner of the system can be raised or lowered independently to achieve a level state. Many RVs have a built-in capacity for leveling. Relocatable buildings are stabilized and leveled with concrete piers or stanchions.

Ensure there are attachments for trailer tie-downs to fix the trailer securely to the ground even in the event of hurricane-force winds. Even if not required by local code, tie-downs may also be prudent in areas with regular seismic activity.

There must be a means of emergency exit. Trailers typically have doors that open from the outside. In an emergency, the staff and patients at the hyperbaric facility will need to exit by doors that open from the inside so they will not become trapped. Doors must be modified in some fashion to permit egress in the event of hazard such as fire. This may mean inserting a standard sized door into the existing trailer door, modifying the latching mechanisms to permit door opening from the inside, or removing the outside doors and replacing with sliding doors.

Installation Site

The installation site should be reasonably level and its surface compacted sufficiently to not permit any of the trailer leveling jacks or supports to sink. Ensure there are ties-downs to permit the anchoring of the trailer to the earth. A reliable earth ground is needed for the electrical system and to protect against lightning. Points of connection for power, medical gases, water, drain, or signal may be needed. Signs may need to be posted to direct patients and visitors to the hyperbaric facility. Ramp systems to provide access by nonambulatory patients must be provided that is compliant with accessibility standards such as the Americans with Disabilities Act.

Operations

Once the chamber system is set up, chamber treatment operations are no different than those inside of a building.

The chamber system must be level during operation. If not level, a number of chamber systems may be come unsafe.

- The chamber doors may not stay open, may not permit a pressure seal, or even complicate intracompartment transfers due to an interior door not staying in position.
- Instruments such as pressure gauges can become inaccurate if not used in their designed orientation, e.g., vertical or horizontal.
- Air compressors may not operate correctly if their fluid levels are askew.
- FSS level indicators may be in error.

Once the mobile system is in place, check its level with a spirit or bubble level, even by rolling marbles on the floor. Conduct pressure and operational tests on all chamber systems after each move and document appropriately.

Maintenance

A mobile system also requires a defined and published maintenance program or schedule that has been tailored to both the mobile system and its installation site. The number of checks and the interval between should vary depending upon how often the mobile system is moved. A mobile system that has been in place for five years need not be pressure or function tested as regularly as one that is moved on a weekly basis.

The trailer itself should be reflected in the maintenance program. Door hinges, sliding door track, and locks exposed to weather should be routinely lubricated. Louvered vents must be kept free of blockage (dust, snow, and ice). Units that are moved regularly should have scheduled inspections of tires, brakes, and other rolling gear to ensure proper and safe function.

Subsystems mounted under the trailer (heaters, fans, and spare air tanks) also must be maintained. Performing required annual visual inspections of spare air or FSS tanks can be difficult if they are suspended under a trailer or placed in a tight corner. A video borescope is a big help in performing the inspections; even a child's toy periscope can be used to accomplish these inspections.

Training

In addition to staff training common to all hyperbaric facilities, the mobile facility operator must develop a specific initial and continuing education plan that is specific to the mobile facility. All staff should be trained in the idiosyncrasies of the facility, particularly for the custom or purpose-built systems utilized.

As noted earlier, the design of the facility might make access to certain critical valves and components not intuitive, so emergency procedures training is vital to safe facility operation. It may be prudent to conduct operational emergency and evacuation drills on a more intensive schedule than that for a fixed facility, particularly for the mobile facility that is relocated regularly. These drills should not be limited to the facility staff but should also include participation by local first responders.

Conclusion

Mobile hyperbaric facilities provide a critical, often life-saving means of extending the reach of hyperbaric therapy to underserved locations. It is vital that all personnel associated with the design, construction, installation, and operation of these facilities are well-versed in the unique challenges that face mobile operations. Ideally, there should be no difference in the care provided by a mobile or a traditional fixed-site facility.

References

There is limited reference material specific to mobile/relocatable hyperbaric systems. This chapter would not have been possible without the contributions from David Heaney, who has extensive experience in mobile hyperbaric systems design and operation.

Conclusion

CHAPTER 7
Emergency Procedures

Jolene Cormier, BSN, RN, CHT, CHRN, Robert Sheffield, BA, CHT,
and Francois Burman, BSc Eng, PE, MSc

Introduction

Hyperbaric emergency procedures usually address a variety of problems ranging from mechanical malfunction to medical complications—important events that do not seem to share a common trait but cover a wide range of situations. Such a variable group of events must be discussed in a broad context. This chapter will discuss emergency procedures within the framework of the entire hyperbaric safety program. In this broader context, events that may or may not be emergencies belong together. That is why this discussion will replace the term "emergency procedure" with the term "contingency plan."

The term "risk" expresses the potential for an undesirable event. The risks associated with hyperbaric oxygen therapy (HBOT) are byproducts of the interactions between the environment, equipment, and people. The goal of the hyperbaric safety program is to mitigate risk by placing a variety of loss prevention and loss reduction measures (i.e. controls) over the environment, equipment, and people. Some controls are designed into the equipment or the facility; others are operational in nature. Operational controls include standard operating procedures and contingency plans. In a perfect world we would be able to exercise total control over our environment, use equipment that is fail-safe, possess perfect information about the nature of risks, design and implement perfect controls, and we would precisely follow procedures to operate the equipment properly. Because we do not live in a perfect world, incidents (e.g., unsafe conditions, unsafe acts) will occur. Incidents occur when controls are not in place, not adequate, or not used. Some hyperbaric incidents are fairly innocuous and others are mishaps associated with serious injury or death. Because not all incidents can be prevented, there must be post-loss measures such as contingency plans to control the situation and minimize losses (e.g., injuries, equipment damage, downtime) that occur.

The existence of different types of facilities with various staffing levels, patient populations, and equipment necessitates any contingency plan discussion to be expansive enough to cover a multitude of different hyperbaric operations. The safety challenges and needs of each hyperbaric facility will be different. Because it is not possible to cover every foreseeable risk and contingency plan, the goal of this chapter is to illustrate a process by which any hyperbaric safety issue can be analyzed and addressed. The steps involved in the development of safety practices and contingency plans are as follows:

1. Identify the hazards
2. Determine the potential losses these hazards represent, including who or what this will affect (i.e. risk assessment)
3. Determine what controls can be put into place to mitigate the risks
4. Implement these controls
5. Develop a contingency plan in the event the controls are not used or ineffective
6. Practice contingency plans on a regular basis
7. Develop a plan for post-incident analysis, a process also referred to as a retrospective risk analysis or after-action review (AAR)

Analyzing Risks

Analysis of hyperbaric facility risks is a difficult process. It begins with identifying the hazards in a hyperbaric facility. These hazards could be from a variety of sources: equipment related (e.g., loss of power, loss of gas supply, control system malfunction); operational (e.g., untrained or unprepared staff); medical (e.g., pressure injuries, medical complications); and environmental (e.g., contaminants, external disaster). The actual risks associated with a hazard depend on the probability, frequency, and severity of the potential losses.

At the simplest level, interventions in health care involve the interaction of patient and health care provider. The use of equipment adds complexity to this interaction but is merely an extension of the health care provider's capabilities. Like all other equipment, the hyperbaric systems required to accomplish HBOT add complexity. However, when HBOT is performed, the pressure of the physical environment is changed. This pressure change has effects on the patient, the health care provider, and the other equipment. Another dimension has been added to the interaction. Understanding this multidimensional interaction between environment, equipment, and people is central to risk assessment and to hyperbaric safety. It is also the reason why hyperbaric safety covers such a broad range of issues.

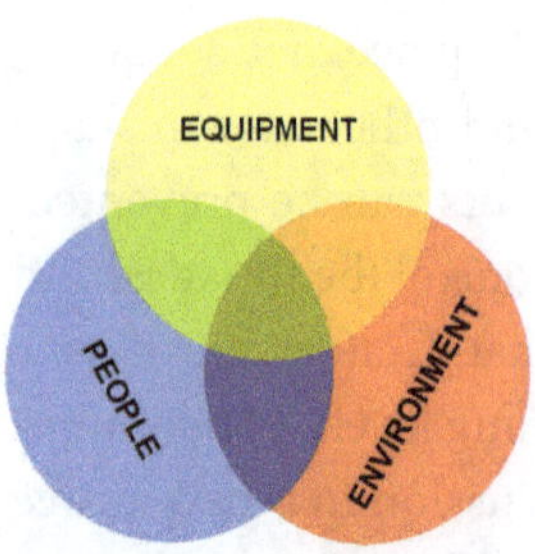

The interaction of environment, equipment, and people has numerous and varied effects. It is essential to understand how pressure and increased density of gas affect the human body and equipment. It is also essential to understand the nature of fire in a hyperbaric environment and how fire risk is changed in a hyperbaric chamber. Finally, one must be aware of potential medical complications of hyperbaric exposure and understand how the hyperbaric environment affects our ability to provide medical interventions.

Hazard—Pressure Change on the Body

Any hyperbaric exposure entails an increase and subsequent decrease of pressure. This will affect any gas containing space in the human body that cannot ventilate adequately. This is a mechanical effect of pressure change explained by Boyle's Law. The most frequently encountered incident is difficulty equalizing pressure in the middle ear.[1-2] The laws of physics cannot be changed; however, there are techniques that can facilitate equalization. Consequently, one necessary control is education of chamber attendants and patients about these techniques. The efficacy of these techniques depends on eustachian tube function. Some people have difficulty equalizing because of eustachian tube dysfunction or temporary congestion. Therefore, another necessary control is the screening of potential chamber occupants for these problems. The result of this screening may obviate the need for prophylactic medication or pressure equalization tubes. Even if one knows how to equalize and has functioning eustachian tubes, the rate of pressure change must be appropriate to allow time for the equalization technique to be used.[3] Another necessary control is the ability to manage the rate of pressure change. Faster compression rates have been associated with an increased incidence of barotrauma.[3-4] The ability to equalize is variable from person to person and from day to day. It is necessary to monitor and communicate with chamber occupants so that the rate of pressure change can be adjusted according to individual needs.

The above analysis identifies a variety of controls that involve equipment design, operating procedures, patient and staff education, medical screening, and prophylactic measures. All of these are intended to prevent the specific incident of difficulty equalizing pressure in the middle ear. If this incident does occur, the potential injury (i.e. risk) is middle ear barotrauma. The probability and frequency of this risk is high, but we try to minimize both by the controls mentioned above. The severity of this risk is generally low; but there must be a contingency plan to minimize injury from the barotrauma. The key elements of this plan are to stop pressure change and reverse pressure change slightly to relieve the pressure differential on the affected tissues. Along with one of the equalization techniques, this may be enough to resolve the incident. If the incident is not resolved, the patient's ability to equalize must be reassessed. This may result in a decision to terminate the current pressure exposure. Regardless of that decision, there should be a reassessment of the risk-benefit for future pressure exposure. Finally, the affected person needs medical attention appropriate to the injury.

Other gas containing spaces that could be affected are sinuses, teeth, gastrointestinal (GI) tract, and lungs. For the risks of barotrauma to the sinuses or teeth, the analysis and controls are the same as for the middle ear with minor differences. Eustachian tube function does not affect the sinuses or teeth, and pressure equalization tubes are not an appropriate control. Some equalization techniques are effective for the sinuses, but none are effective for the teeth. The contingency plan to manage the potential injuries of sinus barotrauma or tooth barotrauma is the same as for the middle ear. Barotrauma of the middle ear, sinuses, and teeth will usually occur during compression. It is unusual to have the first presentation of difficulty occur during decompression. If it does occur during decompression, further decompression will increase the injury. Ultimately, decompression back to normal atmospheric pressure must be achieved, but it should be done no faster than the affected person can tolerate.

In the intact GI tract, reducing gas volume during compression is of no concern. However, gas that is either swallowed or created by digestion during the pressure exposure can overexpand during decompression. Although there have been no reports of this type of injury in hyperbaric chambers, there is a report of a scuba diver with stomach rupture from overexpansion of swallowed air immediately prior to a rapid ascent.[5] Appropriate controls involve the rate of pressure change, monitoring, and communication with chamber occupants. An additional control is to prohibit consumption of gas-producing foods prior to pressure exposure. If overexpansion of gas does occur, the potential incident is GI discomfort. The contingency plan should include stopping decompression and allowing the chamber occupant to expel the gas.

There are reports of pulmonary overpressure from rapid decompression. These reports include cases in which the subject was observed breathholding and cases in which the subject was not breathholding but pulmonary air-trapping lesions were later detected.[6-7] One necessary control is medical screening of potential chamber occupants for pulmonary air trapping. This screening may determine that another control of prophylactic medication is necessary. Other controls involve the rate of pressure change, and monitoring and communication with chamber occupants. If pulmonary overpressure does occur, air from the lungs can go into a variety of places including the pleural space (pneumothorax) and the arterial system (arterial gas embolism). Either one can be fatal. The contingency plan must include stopping decompression and allowing physician assessment of the affected person. From that point, the plan will vary depending on the findings of the assessment and the capabilities of the hyperbaric facility. Regardless, the plan is focused on appropriate medical management. If arterial gas embolism has occurred, further decompression will make the problem worse. The definitive treatment is immediate recompression therapy. If a pneumothorax has occurred, recompression therapy will not resolve it; and the subsequent decompression may create a tension pneumothorax. The treatment for a pneumothorax is insertion of a chest tube. In either case, it may be necessary to continue decompression back to normal atmospheric pressure in order to provide appropriate interventions. The interventions provided will depend on the capabilities of the hyperbaric facility. The key piece of the contingency plan is to stop decompression until assessment is made and appropriate interventions are performed or made ready.

Sample List: Contingency Plans for Barotrauma (not all-inclusive)
• Difficulty equalizing ear(s) • Difficulty equalizing sinus(es) • Pain (tooth, head, stomach, chest, other) during pressure change • Shortness of breath and/or difficulty breathing during decompression (potential pulmonary barotrauma)

Hazard—Medical Complications

Medical complications in the hyperbaric environment include side effects of HBOT and coincidental medical events. Even if a medical event is not caused by the therapy, the management of that event may need to be altered because of the hyperbaric environment. In the analysis of medical complications, each complication is an incident that controls are intended to prevent. Before the contingency plans for these incidents can be designed, the following facility specific questions must be answered. What access to chamber occupants is available? What interventions can be performed?

In the hyperbaric environment, a variety of different factors contribute to confinement anxiety: size of the chamber; proximity of the chamber wall; view (or lack of view) to the outside; noise; temperature change; entrapment; breathing apparatus covering face or head; and feeling a loss of control. These factors can contribute to confinement anxiety in patients or inside chamber attendants. All potential chamber occupants must be screened for a history of confinement anxiety. This screening may identify an additional control of prophylactic medication. Because the use of anti-anxiety medication is inappropriate for inside chamber attendants, confinement anxiety may be a disqualification for work inside a chamber. An appropriate control for all chamber occupants is education and orientation specific to the hyperbaric environment. For patients, some type of entertainment or distraction technique can be helpful. The potential injury involved is psychological trauma. Physical trauma is also possible if panic leads to flailing. If the patient becomes combative in a multiplace environment, other patients and the inside attendant may be at risk of sustaining an injury. For confinement anxiety in inside chamber attendants, the contingency plan should be to replace the attendant. The inside attendant is responsible for the safety of other chamber occupants and cannot fulfill this responsibility if impaired by anxiety. In patients where HBOT is adjunctive, terminating the current pressure exposure is based on the patient's tolerance. Anti-anxiety medication may help the patient tolerate future treatments; however, the propensity for these drugs to cause drowsiness needs to be taken into consideration. If the facility is an outpatient facility, this side effect may affect the patient's ability to safely transport themselves. Where HBOT is the definitive treatment (decompression sickness, for example), the decision to terminate the current pressure exposure is a risk-benefit decision made by the hyperbaric physician. The patient always has the right to refuse treatment.

The occurrence of seizures in the hyperbaric environment has decreased in the past few decades, possibly due to changes in treatment protocols or patient screening and selection techniques. A review of current literature places the incident rate of seizure activity anywhere from 0.0024% to 0.06%, with increased pressure and duration of exposure associated with an increased rate of seizures due to oxygen toxicity.[8-10] Central nervous system toxicity can develop during hyperbaric treatments and manifest as seizure activity; however, seizures can occur due to a number of different factors including epilepsy, hypoglycemia, or carbon monoxide poisoning. Irrespective of the cause, if the patient is in the chamber when the seizure activity occurs, the contingency plan should include leveling a chamber that is pressurizing or depressurizing. Another step in the plan would be to remove the patient from oxygen. In a multiplace chamber this is accomplished by the inside attendant removing the hood or mask. In a monoplace chamber this is accomplished by the patient donning a mask (either demand or free-flow) supplied with breathing air, switching the chamber gas supply from oxygen to air and increasing the ventilation rate, or by decompression. To prevent a pneumothorax, it is important to ensure that tonic activity has ceased and the patient is breathing before decompressing the chamber. Medical management of the patient can occur after a safe depressurization is completed.

Side effects of HBOT are thoroughly discussed in other texts. With respect to the safety program, the controls that result from analysis of side effects are medical screenings and monitoring and communication with chamber occupants. For a known side effect of HBOT, there are certain predisposing factors that contribute to the risk of that side effect. Medical screening must identify those risk factors in the individual and trigger a risk-benefit decision about pressure exposure. One example is the inside chamber attendant who has a history of more than one event of decompression sickness from an unremarkable hyperbaric exposure. The risk of injury from decompression sickness may be too great to justify any future hyperbaric exposures. Another example is the prospective hyperbaric patient who has a history of congestive heart failure. The systemic vascular resistance caused by HBO_2 may precipitate this failure. The risk may be too great to justify HBOT for a chronic wound. If a side effect does occur, there are various potential injuries; however, the contingency plan to minimize the injury is the appropriate medical management of that incident. The hyperbaric environment only changes medical management if the incident occurs during pressure exposure because patient access and the capabilities of the facility may alter the way that medical management is performed. At a minimum, the hyperbaric facility must be able to provide supportive medical care and have access to definitive medical care for the potential side effects of HBO_2 treatment. The clinics' ability to provided supportive medical care and access to more definitive care is also true for management of a coincidental medical event. If the clinic is hospital-based, definitive care may involve transferring the patient to the emergency room or another hospital department. Stand-alone clinics will need to have other arrangements included in their contingency plans. It is important to consider the communication required between the hyperbaric facility and the accepting definitive care facility whose familiarity with the hyperbaric environment may be limited. The plans for definitive care should be included in the contingency plan.

A cardiac arrest may qualify as a coincidental medical event; however, the interaction between treatment equipment and the environment poses additional risks and warrants a more in-depth discussion. In the event of a cardiac arrest most facilities will have treatment protocols in place that conform to guidelines established by the American Heart Association; however, adjustments will need to be made if the arrest occurs in the chamber. The multiplace environment allows for interventions like CPR and airway control to begin almost immediately. It also permits additional staff to pressurize into the chamber for assistance. Defibrillation of a patient in a multiplace chamber can be performed safely if the oxygen concentration is normal (i.e. no more than 23.5%).

A monoplace environment presents different challenges due to restricted patient access and the introduction of a possible ignition source (the defibrillator) into a high oxygen environment. There will be a higher concentration of oxygen surrounding the patient when they are removed from the chamber. This is a result of oxygen dumping from the chamber when the door opens and the cell structure of fabrics (clothing and bedding) holding on to oxygen for a period of time after removal from the chamber. The risk of fire due to electrical arcs created during defibrillation is greater when defibrillator paddles rather than adhesive pads are used.[11] This appears to be due to inadequate pressure or poor contact with defibrillation paddles.[12-14] To mitigate the risk of fire, both multiplace and monoplace facilities should use a defibrillator with adhesive pads instead of paddles. To date, there have been no fires caused in an oxygen-enriched atmosphere when defibrillator pads instead of paddles are used for defibrillation.[11] The American Heart Association (AHA) recommends reducing the oxygen concentration around the patient's chest.[11] When oxygen levels were measured in the room after emergently decompressing and opening a monoplace chamber, Dr. Eric Kindwall and his team found the oxygen dissipated to the floor in about 30 seconds.[15] This coincides with the ECRI Institute's guidance which states oxygen concentration will return to ambient levels when the source of enrichment is turned off or removed.[12] The placement of defibrillator pads necessitates the removal of linens from the patient's upper body. The AHA also recommends ensuring adequate adhesive pad/paddle placement and skin contact when defibrillating to minimize sparking.[11] In his *Risk Assessment Guide,* Francois Burman recommends a minimum distance of six feet from the monoplace chamber door.[16] However, there is no definitive recommendation regarding either removal of fabrics or safe distance from the monoplace chamber for defibrillation. It is important to weigh the benefits of early defibrillation against any added time delay involved when considering removing fabrics and moving the patient away from the chamber.

Sample List: Contingency Plans for Medical Events (not all-inclusive)
• Confinement anxiety • Seizure • Cardiac arrest • Respiratory arrest • Unresponsive patient
Because of limited access for patient assessment in monoplace chambers, the contingency plan for cardiac arrest, respiratory arrest, and unresponsive patient may be combined into one plan.

One risk encountered by multiplace chamber attendants is decompression sickness. This is usually not a risk for hyperbaric patients; however, it is possible whenever air is available as a patient breathing gas. Chamber attendants breath air during treatments and depending on the treatment profile, may accrue decompression obligations that must be managed through decompression stops and breathing of 100% oxygen during decompression. See Chapter 9: Decompression Sickness in Inside Attendants. Both a working knowledge of decompression procedures and the availability of decompression tables are necessary to mitigate this risk and to design an appropriate contingency plan.

Hazard—Equipment Malfunction

To prevent equipment malfunction of any piece of equipment, there are several important controls: the equipment must be appropriate for the intended use; people must have specific training to use the equipment properly; the equipment must be in good working condition; and it must be maintained properly. In the United States, the American Society of Mechanical Engineers (ASME) has developed a set of safety codes for hyperbaric chamber manufacturers.[17-18] Along with National Fire Protection Association (NFPA) codes, these controls help ensure that chambers are designed and fabricated to be safe for HBOT.[19] Other types of equipment such as mechanical ventilators, infusion pumps, electrocardiogram (ECG) monitors, and blood pressure monitors are typically used with hyperbaric chambers, but there is a very limited selection of equipment that is designed for this application. NFPA codes address equipment from a fire safety standpoint, but no codes address the appropriateness of a particular piece of equipment. This decision is in the hands of the user. The effects of pressure change and elevated oxygen on the function and safe operation of the equipment must be considered. The hyperbaric environment affects the operation or use of most equipment. Therefore, people need equipment-specific training that highlights the unique aspects of operating the equipment safely in the hyperbaric environment. Operational readiness of equipment is usually established with some type of checklist. It may be a simple check of all equipment to ensure that it is intact and properly set up for use, but the elaborateness of the checklist increases with the complexity of the equipment used. The hyperbaric environment may also affect the reliability of equipment. Therefore, the equipment must be kept operationally ready through a maintenance program.

In general, equipment malfunctions fall into two categories: critical and noncritical. The defining point of a critical equipment malfunction is one that causes immediate harm or impairs the ability to continue the current pressure exposure. Some examples of critical equipment are chamber pressurization gas system, chamber breathing gas system, chamber control system, and life support equipment. One control is to have a redundant system in place for all critical equipment. As a minimum, the hyperbaric facility must identify a procedure for the loss of each critical system.

Sample List: Contingency Plans for Equipment Malfunction (not all-inclusive)
• Loss of electrical power • Loss of communication • Loss of pressurization gas supply • Loss of breathing gas supply • Uncontrolled pressure change • Ventilator malfunction • Patient monitor malfunction • Accidental activation of fire suppression system

Hazard—Inadequately Trained Staff

A discussion of staff education and training is essential. Considering the multidimensional interactions discussed at the beginning of the chapter, hyperbaric staff constitute a significant portion of the "people" part of this equation. Inadequately trained staff members pose a risk to the patients, themselves, and other staff. They can cause a minor incident to evolve into a life-threatening event. According to data from the Hyperbaric Incident Monitoring Study from Australia, the main contributing factor to incidents is the failure of staff to use or follow policies and procedures.[20] If the patient starts to seize in a monoplace environment, will the operator remain calm or immediately decompress the chamber? If something happens to the operator, does anyone else in the room know what to do in an emergency? In a monoplace environment, will anyone notice if the chamber operator becomes incapacitated? Each chamber type and facility pose different challenges including patient access, access to emergency medical services, and staff available to assist. Trained staff available to assist may present a greater logistical challenge for smaller clinics with monoplace chambers. These clinics typically have fewer trained chamber operators on staff. Under these circumstances, it may be prudent to cross-train other staff members, including doctors, so they are able to operate the chamber in an emergency situation. The basic steps involved in ceasing pressurization, normal depressurization, and how to depressurize in an emergency may be all that is deemed necessary.

Mitigating risks through engineering, maintenance, controls, and education are the primary methods for preventing an incident. When this fails, and the chain of events leads to a mishap, the ability of the staff to follow the contingency plan will determine the final outcome. The hyperbaric field has an admirable safety record, but this achievement can also be our downfall if it allows for complacency in detailing, discussing, practicing, and reviewing our contingency plans. According to *NFPA 99*, all hyperbaric emergency procedures should be drilled and documented at least annually.[19] The number of drills a facility will need to conduct depends on the needs of each facility; some are universal (e.g., fire drills) while others will be site and equipment specific. The importance of practicing contingency plans must be considered an essential part of any emergency procedure discussion and safety program.

Sample List: Contingency Plans for Operational Events (not all-inclusive)
• Wrong breathing gas • Inadequate decompression procedure • Missed decompression stop

Policies dealing with staff continuing education and training should address a number of points, including the following:

1. The frequency with which all staff members should perform a routine procedure in order to remain competent. For example, it may be policy that each chamber operator must perform at least one hyperbaric treatment per month. This could also apply to other functions such as being the inside attendant. Each hyperbaric facility should determine the appropriate frequency for itself.
2. If certain staff members (or physicians) are trained to operate the chamber only in an emergency, the frequency with which they will need to refresh these skills by participating in drills.
3. Depending on the number of emergency procedures that need to be drilled, time may need to be set aside on a monthly basis. This should also be outlined in policy.
4. The steps necessary to deal with any staff member who is unable to meet the training/competency requirements. For example, if a staff member has not operated the chamber within the specified time frame, a refresher course may be necessary, which includes chamber operator-specific drills.

Fire Risk

Fire risk in a hyperbaric environment is a function of several overlapping hazards, including elevated oxygen partial pressure, elevated oxygen percentage, presence of electrical sources, and the presence of combustible materials. The frequency is high (exposure to the potential risk every day), the probability is variable (depending on the specifics of the hazards listed above), and the severity is high (because of rapid flame spread rate and delayed egress). The analysis of fire risk in the hyperbaric environment has already been done by the NFPA.[19] This analysis produced a set of controls that addresses design of hyperbaric systems, facility design, and facility operations (i.e. *NFPA 99*). The contingency plan to minimize injury from a fire incident will vary from one facility to another.

The popular acronym RACE is used in many hospitals to teach the procedure for managing a fire. The acronym stands for Rescue individuals to a safe location, Alert the facility or fire department, Contain the fire, and Extinguish the fire and/or Evacuate. If a fire occurs in the area of the hyperbaric chamber (not inside of it), the principles are applied in the same order. The only consideration is the time it takes to decompress the hyperbaric chamber in order to rescue chamber occupants. If a fire occurs inside the hyperbaric chamber, the contingency plan becomes more complicated and the order of the steps must change.

The higher partial pressure and/or higher percentage of oxygen inside the hyperbaric chamber as well as the confined space of the chamber contribute to a rapid flame spread. Immediate egress from the hyperbaric chamber is not possible because the chamber must be decompressed first. Therefore, dealing with the fire must be addressed urgently. This is achieved in multiplace chambers by activating the fire suppression system (handheld or deluge). Because a monoplace chamber is not required to have a fire extinguishing system, it is necessary to decompress the monoplace chamber in order to extinguish a fire.[19] Regardless of chamber type, quickly stopping oxygen flow into the chamber is a critical first step. *NFPA 99*, Annex B contains recommended procedures in the event of fire for both monoplace and multiplace chambers.[19]

In addition to the in-chamber and department fire drills, a hyperbaric clinic located in a larger facility may require a separate contingency plan dealing with a fire alarm in the building. This plan should detail the person responsible for investigating the location of the fire and its proximity to the department that will necessitate evacuation of the hyperbaric chambers. This determination should be made in advance and may involve input and cooperation from numerous people throughout the facility, including the facility fire chief, emergency operations officer, the safety director, and the hyperbaric medical director.

When considering fire evacuation, it is important to understand that hospitals in the United States should be designed with "defend in place" architecture while business occupancies (including medical office buildings) are usually not. In the event of fire in a hospital, you are meant to stay in your unaffected area or evacuate horizontally to the next unaffected area and close the barrier doors. The smoke/fire barrier doors and smoke barriers inside the ventilation system protect hospital staff and patients without egress from the building. In the event of fire in a business occupancy, everyone is meant to egress the building. These differences in building design should be taken into consideration when designing contingency plans for fire events.

Sample List: Contingency Plans for Fire Events (not all-inclusive)
• Fire in hyperbaric chamber • Smoke or fire in hyperbaric area • Prohibited item (potential igniter) discovered in chamber during treatment • Building fire alarm

Creating the Contingency Plan

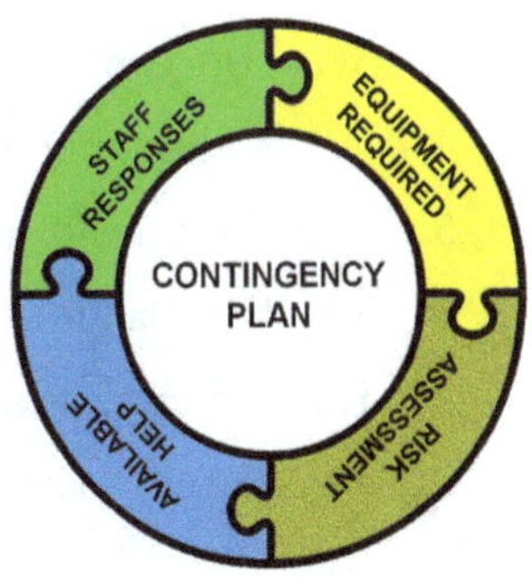

Analysis of hazards and risk assessment allows us to understand the true nature of the potential incident we are attempting to manage. This is an important first step in designing a contingency plan. There are several other important considerations that affect the design of the plan. Realizing the potential damage or injury helps us to identify appropriate staff responses. These responses should minimize the impact of the incident. It is important to consider what personnel are available to help (e.g., additional staff members, code team, and emergency responders) and how these individuals are capable of participating in the plan. Designing contingency plans with available personnel in mind drives minimum facility staffing decisions. It is also important to consider what equipment is available (e.g., personal protection, patient transportation, fire-fighting, and crash cart). All the considerations discussed above are likely to vary among different hyperbaric facilities.

The objective is to identify a series of steps (i.e. procedure) that will manage the incident and minimize any negative effects. In most cases, the appropriate steps can not all be performed simultaneously. In some cases, the design of the equipment or facility dictates certain steps come before others (e.g., the chamber must be decompressed before an occupant can be evacuated from the facility). In some cases, the sequence of steps is dictated by the urgency of staff actions (e.g., if a person is experiencing pain during pressure change, the first step is to immediately stop the pressure change).

A sample contingency plan is included to illustrate the process of putting the appropriate steps in the appropriate order (see Figure 1). The incident of smoke or flame inside a multiplace chamber was chosen because it contains many of the elements discussed above, including urgent actions, actions of at least two staff members, activation of emergency responders, chamber equipment, fire-fighting equipment, and personal protective equipment. It also contains a decision point where, after the urgent actions are taken, an assessment is made. If the incident is under control, a different set of actions are taken than if the incident is not yet under control.

Drills

Contingency plans must be rehearsed. By design, an incident should be a rare occurrence; therefore, it is necessary to perform routine drills and tests to ensure competence of the staff and adequate performance of equipment. Practice drills should be as realistic as possible in order to truly test the adequacy of the plan.

When an incident occurs, it is an opportunity to improve the safety program. Each incident should trigger an AAR. The following questions should be asked:

1. What controls were in place?
2. Were the controls used? If not, why?
3. Were the controls effective? If not, why?
4. What additional or different controls are necessary?
5. Was there a contingency plan in place?
6. Was this plan followed? If not, why?
7. How effective was the contingency plan?
8. What needs to be added or changed in the contingency plan?

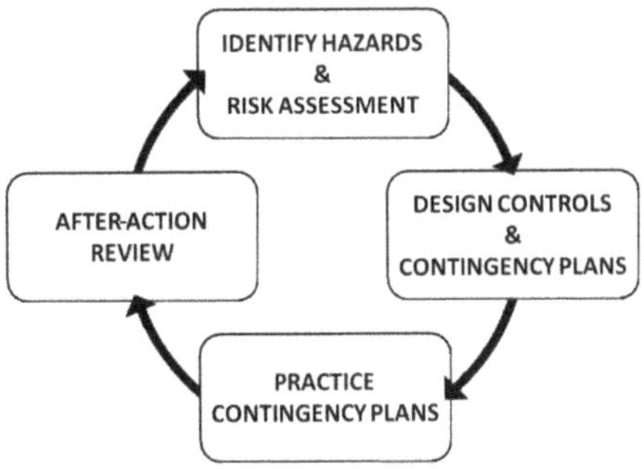
IDENTIFY HAZARDS
&
RISK ASSESSMENT
DESIGN CONTROLS
&
CONTINGENCY PLANS
PRACTICE
CONTINGENCY PLANS
AFTER-ACTION
REVIEW

The AAR helps identify previously unrecognized hazards, facilitates a reassessment of risk, and helps identify appropriate modifications to controls and contingency plans. The AAR should be performed whenever a contingency plan is used, either in a real incident or a practice drill.

Practicing contingency plans, followed by AAR, triggers a performance improvement cycle. This circular process from identifying hazards to AAR and back again makes the safety program dynamic.

Conclusion

In the grand scheme of a hyperbaric safety program, the overwhelming majority of the program focuses on preventing incidents. Contingency plans are a small but critical component.

Information is central to the process described in this chapter. Not only is it important to the analysis of risks, but staff and/or patient education is one of the controls for all types of risks in the hyperbaric environment. Below is a list of references that can be useful in analyzing risks, educating hyperbaric personnel, and developing contingency plans.

- *Characteristics and Safe Handling of Medical Gases*[21]
- *Guidelines for Clinical Multiplace Hyperbaric Facilities*[22]
- *Hyperbaric Medicine Practice*[15]
- *Monoplace Hyperbaric Chamber Safety Guidelines*[23]
- *NFPA 53: Guide on Fire Hazards in Oxygen-Enriched Atmospheres*[24]
- *NFPA 99: Health Care Facilities Code*[19]
- *Physiology and Medicine of Hyperbaric Oxygen Therapy*[25]
- *Risk Assessment Guide for Installation and Operation of Clinical Hyperbaric Facilities*[16]
- *US Navy Diving Manual*[26]
- *UHMS Guidelines for Hyperbaric Facility Operations, 2nd Edition*[27]

Figure 1. Sample contingency plan.[28]
Reprinted with permission.

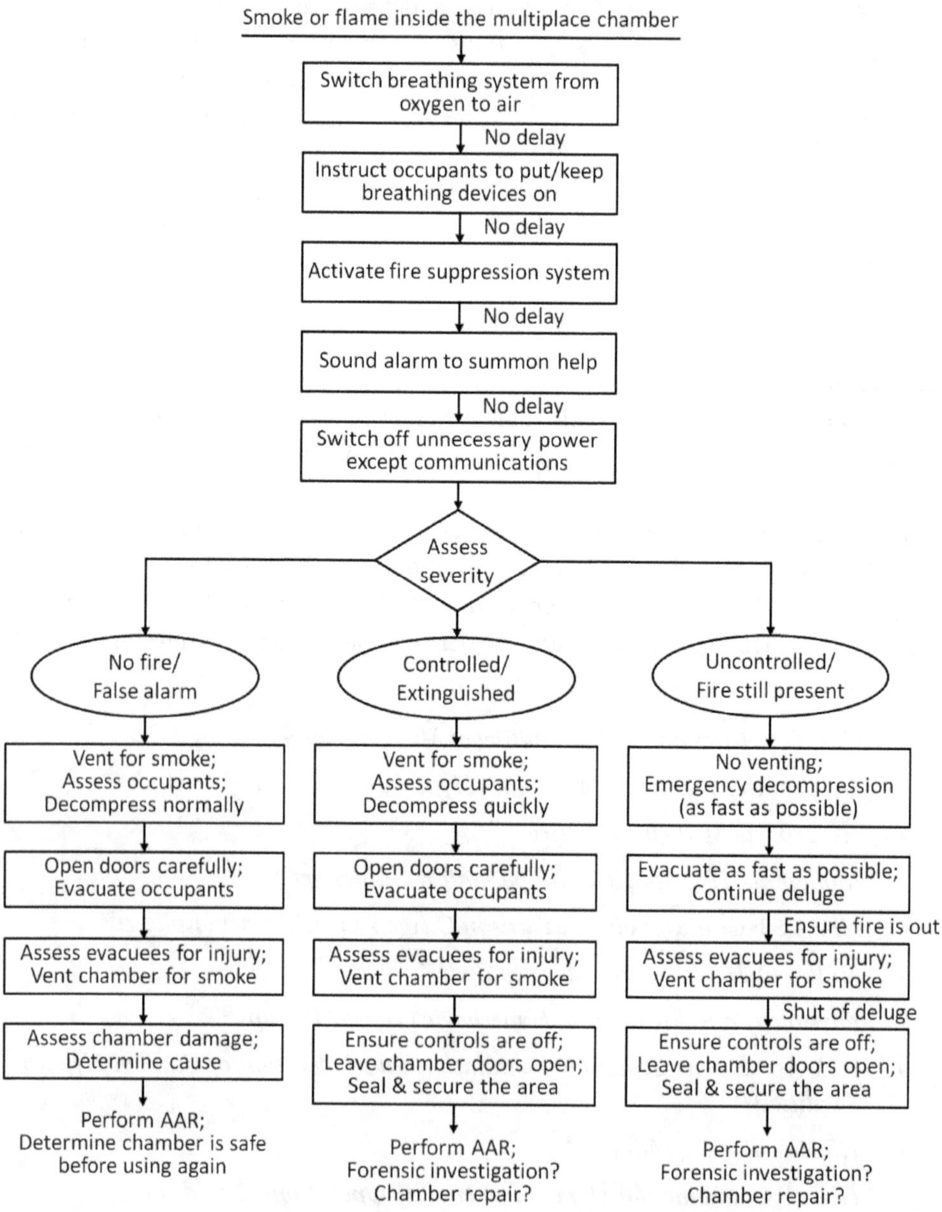

References

1. Davis JC. Hyperbaric medicine: patient selection, treatment procedures, and side effects. In: Davis JC, Hunt TK, editors. Problem wounds: the role of oxygen. New York: Elsevier Publishing; 1988. P. 232.
2. Hadanny A, Meir O, Bechor Y, Fishlev G, Bergan J, Efrati S. The safety of hyperbaric oxygen treatment - retrospective analysis in 2,334 patients. *Undersea and Hyperbaric Medicine.* 43(2):113-122.
3. Heyboer M, Wojcik S, Grant W, Chambers P, Jennings S, Adcock P. Middle ear barotrauma in hyperbaric oxygen therapy. *Undersea and Hyperbaric Medicine.* 41(5):393-397.
4. Vahidova D, Sen P, Papesch M, Zein-Sanchez M, Mueller P. Does the slow compression technique of hyperbaric oxygen therapy decrease the incidence of middleear barotrauma? *The Journal of Laryngology & Otology.* 2006; 120(06);446-449.
5. Sheffield PJ. Barotrauma lecture. In: Hyperbaric medicine team training. San Antonio, TX: International ATMO; 2018.
6. Bond GF. Arterial gas embolism. In: Davis JC, Hunt TK, editors. *Hyperbaric Oxygen Therapy.* Bethesda, MD: UHMS; 1977. P:147-152.
7. Cakmak T, Battal B, Kara K, Metin S, Demirbas S, Uzun G. A case of tension pneumothorax during hyperbaric oxygen therapy in an earthquake survivor with crush injury complicated by ARDS (adult respiratory distress syndrome). *Undersea and Hyperbaric Medicine Journal.* 2015;42(1);9-13.
8. Yildiz S, Aktas S, Cimsit M, Ay H, Togrol E. Seizure incidence in 80,000 patient treatments with hyperbaric oxygen. *Aviation, Space and Environmental Medicine.* 2004;75(11);992-994.
9. Banham ND. Oxygen toxicity seizures: 20 years' experience from a single hyperbaric unit. *Diving and Hyperbaric Medicine.* 2011;41(4);202-210.
10. Hampson N, Atik D. Central nervous system toxicity during routine hyperbaric oxygen therapy. *Undersea and Hyperbaric Medicine Journal.* 2003;30(2);147-153.
11. Sunde K, Jacobs I, Deakin CD, Hazinski MF, Kerber RE, Koster RW, Morrison LJ, Nolan JP, Sayre MR; on behalf of defibrillation chapter collaborators. Part 6: defibrillation: 2010 International Consensus on Cardiopulmonary Resuscitation and Emergency Cardiovascular Care Science with Treatment Recommendations. Resuscitation 2010;81:e71–e85. DOI: 10.1016/j.resuscitation.2010.08.025.
12. ECRI Institute. (2005 December). Guidance article: Investigating device-related "burns." *Health Devices.* 2005;34(12). Retrieved from: https://www.sfda.gov.sa/en/medicaldevices/gcc/Workshops/Documents/BurnsInvestigationProcedure_HealthDevices2005_3412.pdf.
13. ECRI Institute. (1994 July). Fires from defibrillation during oxygen administration. *Health Devices.* 1994;23(7):307-8. Retrieved from: http://www.mdsr.ecri.org/summary/detail.aspx?doc_id=8128.

14. ECRI Institute. (1987 March-April). Defibrillation in oxygen-enriched environments. *Health Devices*. 1987;16(3-4):113. Retrieved from: http://www.mdsr.ecri.org/summary/detail.aspx?doc_id=8126
15. Whelan HT, Kindwall EP. Hyperbaric medicine practice. 4th edition. North Palm Beach, FL: Best Publishing Company; 2014.
16. Burman F. Risk assessment guide for installation and operation of clinical hyperbaric facilities, 5th Ed. revised. San Antonio, Texas: International ATMO; 2016.
17. American Society of Mechanical Engineers. ASME boiler and pressure vessel code (BPVC), section VIII: Rules for construction of pressure vessels, Division 1. NY, NY: ASME Standard: BPVC-VIII-1-2017.
18. American Society of Mechanical Engineers. Safety standard for pressure vessels for human occupancy (ASME-PVHO-1). NY, NY: ASME Standard: PVHO-1- 2016.
19. National Fire Protection Association. NFPA 99: health care facilities code. Quincy, MA: NFPA; 2018.
20. Pirone CJ, Goble S. The hyperbaric incident monitoring study (HIMS): A new approach to patient safety. *Hyperbaric Medicine Today.* 2002;1(6):23-24.
21. Compressed Gas Association. Characteristics and safe handling of medical gases. Chantilly, VA: CGA Standard: CGA P-2; 2006.
22. Desautels D, Workman WT, Kindwall E, Van Meter, K, McCarthy J. Hyperbaric Chamber Safety Committee. Guidelines for clinical multiplace hyperbaric facilities. Kensington, MD: UHMS; 1994.
23. Weaver L, Strauss M. Hyperbaric Chamber Safety Committee. Monoplace hyperbaric chamber safety guidelines. Bethesda, MD: UHMS; 1991.
24. National Fire Protection Association. NFPA 53: recommended practice on materials, equipment, and systems used in oxygen-enriched atmospheres. Quincy, MA: NFPA; 2016.
25. Neumann TS, Thom SR. Physiology and medicine of hyperbaric oxygen therapy. New York, NY: Elsevier; 2008.
26. United States Navy. US Navy diving manual (SS521-AG-PRO-010) revision 7. Naval Sea Systems Command. Accessed: [2016]. Retrieved from: https://www.navsea.navy.mil/Portals/103/Documents/SUPSALV/Diving/Dive%20Manual%20Rev%207%20Change%20A.pdf.
27. Workman WT. UHMS guidelines for hyperbaric facility operations, 2nd ed. North Palm Beach, Florida: Best Publishing Company; 2017.
28. Burman F. Emergency planning: when things go wrong. Safety & Technical Training Course: October, 2017, Cozumel, Mexico. Divers Alert Network: Recompression Chamber Assistance Program. 2017.

CHAPTER 8
How to Establish a Hyperbaric Facility Maintenance Program

William J. Davison, CHT

Introduction

The importance of a quality, well-thought-out maintenance program cannot be overstated. It should be considered a vital part of your hyperbaric facility's safety program first with the added benefits of efficiency, cost savings, customer, and user satisfaction. By focusing on both routine and preventive maintenance, one can avoid equipment breakdown and the need for repair. The distinction between routine and preventive maintenance is that one uses periodic inspections to ensure that the equipment is constantly ready to provide service, while the other is designed to avoid major breakdowns in equipment by examining a system for defects and replacing parts before a major problem occurs.[1]

This chapter will focus on developing a new maintenance program, but the principles can be utilized for an existing program as well. As you read through this chapter, remember that your center is unique and the information herein will need to be tailored to your specific facility layout, region of the country, equipment, regulatory requirements, vendor support, staff resources, etc. The needs of a hospital-based program with multiple chamber configurations will be very different than a freestanding center with one chamber. However, the overall goals and program structure will be very similar.

Realize this endeavor is going to take time, so being organized from the start is crucial. Do your research! Along with books and manuals, there are plenty of people within the hyperbaric industry who will be glad to share their experiences and expertise with you. Networking is a valuable tool and goes beyond maintenance. If you are new to the industry, consider joining a hyperbaric medical society. An internet-accessible hyperbaric facility directory, such as the one on HyperbaricLink,[2] can also be a useful tool for connecting with experienced people locally as well as nationally. Look for established centers similar to your own. Politely ask pointed questions to set a baseline of trust: Are they accredited? How long have they been in operation? What is the background of their maintenance supervisor? Remember to reciprocate when you get that call from someone else.

It will take several drafts before you are satisfied with the final product, so start out with the big picture and work your way to the small stuff. Having a development team to spread the workload is a big help. Only you and your team can decide how comprehensive the program will be. There will be opportunity to make minor detail changes, up or down, at the next scheduled program review. If you as the team leader are not also the financial decision maker, make sure that person is part of the development team from the start. There are going to be plenty of budget decisions to make (i.e. human resource scheduling, software, equipment, parts inventory, maintenance contracts, training classes, equipment repair/replacement/upgrades, etc.) and personnel with authority to allocate budget resources should be involved in the program-planning process to ensure they understand the potential costs and cost savings of a maintenance program.

Understanding the Regulatory Requirements

Familiarize yourself with the maintenance requirements of the authorities having jurisdiction (AHJs) in your area. They are regulatory governmental agencies with the force of law behind them. Pay specific attention to the revision date of the standard(s) they endorse. Most standards are revised on a three-year cycle, but the latest published edition may not be the one that applies in your region of the country. The following is a partial list of agencies that may meet the definition of AHJ for your facility and are accompanied by the standards organizations they typically recognize.

Authorities Having Jurisdiction

Local Fire Marshal or Building Code Inspector

- Have their own written requirements, some of which will direct you to one or more national standards; may also have amendments to those standards.
- May recognize The International Fire Code (IFC), written by the International Code Council (ICC)
- Usually recognizes the National Fire Protection Association (NFPA)
- Occasionally recognizes ASME PVHO (American Society of Mechanical Engineers Pressure Vessels For Human Occupancy)

Department of Health (or the state your facility is in)

- Have their own written requirements, some of which will direct you to one or more national standards
- Usually recognizes The Joint Commission (TJC)
- Usually recognizes the NFPA
- Occasionally recognizes ASME PVHO

- May recognize The American Institute of Architects Health Care Design Standards

Food and Drug Administration

- Have their own written requirements, some of which will direct you to one or more national standards.
- Recognizes the NFPA
- Recognizes ASME PVHO

Centers for Medicare & Medicaid Services (CMS)

- Have their own written requirements, some of which will direct you to one or more national standards.
- Recognizes TJC
- Recognizes the NFPA
- Recognizes ASME PVHO

Standards Organizations

Standards are typically written by technical or safety committees of industry-specific nonprofit organizations. Standards are voluntary until they are adopted by a regulatory governmental agency or other AHJ. They then become a "code" by force of law. What makes this confusing for the public is that some standards are called codes, by custom vs. rule of law. The authorities having jurisdiction, mentioned above, use these standards organizations to fulfill most of their code requirements.

The Joint Commission (TJC)

- 2018 Comprehensive Accreditation Manual for the following: Hospitals (CAMH), Ambulatory Care (CAMAC), Behavioral Health Care (CMABHC), Critical Access Hospitals (CAMCAH), Disease-Specific Care (DSC), Home Care (CAMHC), Laboratories (CAMLAB), Nursing Care Centers (CAMNCC), Office-Based Surgery (CAMOBS), Palliative Care) (PCC)
- Does not prescribe maintenance requirements and frequency. Requires organizations to follow manufacturer's recommendations. In the absence of manufacturer's recommendations, the organization must develop procedures including the elements described in the Environment of Care Chapter, Standard EC.02.04.01.[3]
- Considered an AHJ, for you, if your organization has chosen and passed their accreditation process
- Recognizes the NFPA

- Recognizes Undersea and Hyperbaric Medical Society (UHMS) as a complementary accreditation body

National Fire Protection Association (NFPA)

- *NFPA 99, Health Care Facilities Code, 2018 edition,* Chapter 14: Hyperbaric Facilities
- Other NFPA standards, as applicable, will be referred to in *NFPA 99*
- Recognizes *ASME PVHO*

American Society of Mechanical Engineers (ASME)

- *ASME PVHO-1-2016, Safety Standard for Pressure Vessels for Human Occupancy*
- *ASME PVHO-2-2016, Safety Standard for Pressure Vessels for Human Occupancy In-Service Guidelines For PVHO Acrylic Windows*
- Other ASME standards, as applicable, will be referenced in PVHO-1 and PVHO-2
- Recognizes the NFPA

While familiarizing yourself with the maintenance requirements of the AHJs, you realize some of these organizations' requirements can be difficult to decipher, are general in nature, and can seem to be at odds. Fortunately, the National Fire Protection Association's standard *NFPA 99, Health Care Facilities Code, 2018 Edition* is the most comprehensive standard with a chapter addressing hyperbaric facilities specifically and is recognized by almost all AHJs. The entire document is important, but pay special attention to Chapter 14: Hyperbaric Facilities, Section 14.3: Administrative and Maintenance.[4] Most people think of *NFPA 99* as a standard specific to hospital-based facilities, but its broader scope includes all health care facilities other than home care and veterinary care.[5] Regardless of enforcement, this standard is a great resource for all categories of hyperbaric facilities. Most AHJs have recently become less prescriptive-specific to maintenance and look for the following: a) Do you have a plan? b) Do you follow manufacturer's recommendations? c) Do you have an evolving best practice based on your facility's experiences? and d) Can you articulate why you do what you do, both verbally and through documentation? With few exceptions, by following a – d and the standards in *NFPA 99,* you should meet the requirements of all AHJs.

Maintenance Teams

The Facility Maintenance Team should consist of all hyperbaric staff, with each having their level of responsibility and required skill set. A single individual may take on multiple roles in facilities with limited staff (such as the safety director also serving as maintenance supervisor).

- *Hyperbaric administrative director:* Ensures maintenance program meets minimum regulatory standards through collaboration with the safety director, maintenance supervisor, and all other involved parties. Keeps the person responsible for financial decisions informed of current and projected budget needs. Verifies all staff meet the skill requirements of their assigned role(s).
- *Hyperbaric safety director:* Develops maintenance program to include staff training, with supportive input from all involved parties. Periodically reviews/revises program to improve safety, improve efficiency, address new equipment maintenance needs, and maintain regulatory compliance. This, too, is best done in collaboration with all involved parties. Maintains the skills competency necessary to teach and perform all in-house maintenance. Be competent enough to evaluate the skills of those hired to do the outsourced maintenance. Maintains the vendor list. Knows the responsibilities given by *NFPA 99*, Chapter 14.
- *Hyperbaric maintenance supervisor:* Oversees implementation and documentation of the maintenance program. Maintains the skills competency necessary to perform all in-house maintenance. Actively participates in staff training. Maintains the spare parts and tools inventory.
- *Hyperbaric technical staff:* Maintains the skills competency necessary to perform all routine in-house maintenance. Works toward the goal of skills competency to perform all in-house maintenance. Performs maintenance duties as assigned. Maintains safe practice and use of all equipment assigned. Reports all issues of faulty equipment.
- *Hyperbaric allied health staff:* Maintains safe practice and use of all equipment assigned. Reports all issues of faulty equipment.
- *Hyperbaric nursing staff:* Maintains safe practice and use of all equipment assigned. Reports all issues of faulty equipment.
- *Hyperbaric medical staff:* Maintains safe practice and use of all equipment assigned. Reports all issues of faulty equipment.

The Support Maintenance Team may consist of the following, as assigned by the hyperbaric administrative director, with each having their level of responsibility and required skill set.

- *Biomedical engineering:* Maintains preventive maintenance and repair of all medical equipment to the specifications of the original equipment manufacturer (OEM). May be in-house, outsourced, or a combination of both. Keeps their hyperbaric point of contact informed on the status of all hyperbaric medical equipment.
- *Plant operations:* Maintains preventive maintenance and repair of all facility plant equipment and infrastructure. May be in-house, outsourced, or a combination of both. Works in concert with their hyperbaric point of contact when maintenance and repairs will impact the hyperbaric facility.

- *Environmental services:* Maintains cleanliness of facility. May be in-house, outsourced or a combination of both. Works in concert with their hyperbaric point of contact when their services will impact the hyperbaric facility.
- *Facility safety director:* Maintains the larger facility safety program. May be in-house, outsourced, or a combination of both. Works in concert with their hyperbaric point of contact when appropriate.
- *Third party maintenance contractor:* As assigned by contract or case-by-case request, maintains and/or repairs equipment they have an expertise in (i.e. chamber systems, compressors, process controls, piping, electrical, acrylics, computers, and office equipment). The hyperbaric safety officer verifies that the contractor is qualified to perform the task(s) assigned to the specifications of the OEM. Keeps their hyperbaric point of contact informed on the progress of all assigned tasks. The facility may have a relationship with more than one contractor.

Establishing an Equipment Database

Before collecting data, research and decide how you will organize and implement this data. Data management can range from a simple paper logbook to digital word processing/spreadsheet/calendar files to a complete maintenance software package. If you choose to purchase maintenance specific software, do your homework and make sure it will meet all of your needs. Organize all pertinent information into a word processing file first. You can cut and paste as you go, and it costs nothing if you already have word processing software.

The maintenance program should encompass the inspection, maintenance, and testing requirements for equipment specific to the following:

Plant operations: Heating, ventilation, air conditioning, main power, emergency power, water and sewer, information technology, and housekeeping of the building or a critical portion of the building the hyperbaric chamber and its subsystems are housed in.

Office support: Computers, chairs, desks, phones, copy machines, etc.

Medical support: Wheelchairs, gurneys, weight scale, etc.

Medical devices: Cardiac monitors, infusion pumps, ventilators, defibrillators, etc.

Hyperbaric chamber systems: This category includes more than just the hyperbaric chamber(s). It includes supportive equipment and services that most likely came from a different vendor than the chamber manufacturer, either directly or indirectly. For a monoplace chamber, think of it as a medical device plugged into a "point-of-connection" (POC). Services prior to the POC would fall under plant operations, while devices connected beyond the POC would fall under the hyperbaric chamber system. That means the chamber manufacturer built the chamber, brought it into the room, and connected it to the needed power, medical gases, and grounding source, i.e. the POC. The manufacturer or installer then tested and approved the chamber for use. For a multiplace chamber, you can think of it the same way but with more supportive equipment, more specifications for the POC, and more vendors to deal with. Given the need for dedicated, specialized support equipment of multiplace chambers such as compressors and fire protection systems, there may be a hazy line defining the actual POC. The warranty for either chamber type probably stops at the POC.

Make an equipment list, categorized by subsystem, for each hyperbaric chamber system your facility has. This will help later and reduce the chance of missing something. Review each equipment manual in your inventory to help with this process.

- *Chamber hull:* seals, viewports, relief valves, hull stop valves, piping, lighting, etc.
- *Chamber control system:* process controls, valves, regulators, gauges, piping, etc.
- *Communications:* main unit, speakers, headsets, backup, entertainment system, etc.
- *Closed-circuit monitoring:* viewing screens, cameras, recorder, etc.
- *Chamber compression and exhaust system:* compressors, filtration, air storage tank, valves, piping, gas monitor, etc.
- *Breathing gas system:* gas cylinders, liquid oxygen tanks (LOX), manifolds, valves, regulators, piping, gas analyzers, breathing circuits, etc.
- *Fire suppression system:* flow controls, valves, enunciator panel, pump(s), deluge tank, hand-line tank, etc.
- *Medical equipment interfaces:* hull penetrators, monitors, signaling cables, power, etc.

Note: Depending on the type of chamber system(s) you have, some of these items may not be applicable.

Take inventory of all equipment in each category above subdivided by responsibility. For those items that you are not responsible for, get the inventory list from the contractor or responsible party. Fill in the below information on each item. You will quickly discover how organized and complete your facility maintenance library is. Obtain needed documents to fill in all data points. Search out the more critical missing information, i.e. manufacturer's suggested maintenance requirements. Go to the manufacturer's website or call for a public copy of the user's manual. Your network of industry contacts can also be helpful in the hunt for missing information. As you get the needed information, make sure you update your facility maintenance library. For items whose maintenance is outsourced, knowing some data points may not be necessary.

Outsourced doesn't mean out of mind, so choose wisely what is not necessary to list.

- Manufacturer
- Serial number
- Responsible maintenance party
- Date purchased/installed
- Location of all reference materials (user's manuals, maintenance manuals, pictures, drawings, parts lists, etc.)
- Parts that make up that piece of equipment
- Manufacturer's suggested maintenance requirements (from manufacturer provided manuals)
    - List of suggested tasks, in sufficient detail to ensure quality and completeness of each task; include the safety precautions
    - Frequency of each task (daily, weekly, monthly, quarterly, semi-annually, annually, and other) (the category "other" includes hourly, every two years, etc.)
    - List of needed spare parts and supplies for each task
    - List of competent department staff (for each task done in-house, including documentation of training and competency assessment)
    - List of approved vendors (for each task outsourced)
- Regulatory requirements (see the section Understanding the Regulatory Requirements at the beginning of this chapter)
    - List of required tasks, in sufficient detail to ensure quality and completeness of each task; include the safety precautions
    - Frequency of each task (daily, weekly, monthly, quarterly, semi-annually, annually and other)
    - List of needed spare parts and supplies for each task
    - List of competent department staff (for each task done in-house, including documentation of training and competency assessment)
    - List of approved vendors (for each task outsourced)
- Facility generated requirements (established through your institution's own experiences with past equipment issues, advice from other hyperbaric and non-hyperbaric maintenance staff, and new critical information as it becomes available)
    - List of required tasks, in sufficient detail to ensure quality and completeness of each task; include the safety precautions
    - Frequency of each task. (daily, weekly, monthly, quarterly, semi-annually, annually, and other)

   - List of needed spare parts and supplies for each task
   - List of competent department staff (for each task done in-house, including documentation of training and competency assessment)
   - List of approved vendors (for each task outsourced)
- Spare parts and supplies to be stocked on-site
- Vendor list for stocked and nonstocked parts and supplies

Before moving on to the next step, make sure you keep this newly established equipment database in a safe place. This now becomes your main maintenance database. It is a living document and will need constant updating with new and changing information.

Establishing a Maintenance Schedule

With your equipment database complete and safe, the next step is to establish a schedule for meeting the inspection, maintenance, and testing requirements of each item of equipment. This is the routine and preventive maintenance portions of your program and will focus on tasks that will add years of life to your equipment and minimize operational downtime. It, too, is a timely process, so pace yourself.

Because most of the nonhyperbaric operations related tasks are typically outsourced, you may want to keep them separate under the heading of Facility's Maintenance Schedule. This schedule would be less detailed and easy for your administrative person to track. The types of equipment/services involved would include heating/ventilation/air conditioning, main power, emergency power, water and sewer, information technology, housekeeping, office support equipment, medical support equipment, and biomedical equipment. The hyperbaric operations specific tasks would then go under the heading of Hyperbaric Maintenance Schedule. The size and scope of your facility will usually dictate whether to make one large schedule or two smaller more specific schedules.

Make a COPY of your equipment database: Information from it will be used to populate your maintenance schedule(s). If you are using maintenance-specific software and it has a scheduling function, use it. From this newly made copy, remove all but the manufacturer's suggested requirements, regulatory requirements, and facility generated requirements for each equipment entry. Include the frequency for each maintenance function. Separate each required task for each equipment entry into a list of daily, weekly, monthly, quarterly, semi-annually, annually, and other. The category "other" includes hourly, nonfixed cycle, every two years, etc. For better tracking, assign a letter/number designation to each task, e.g., daily (D-1, D-2, etc.), weekly (W-1, W-2, etc.), etc. for all frequency categories. If a letter/number designation becomes inactive, save it in archive for later retrieval. New tasks should be assigned their own new designation.

Make sure you add to the schedule needed tasks that may not be in the equipment database to include predictive maintenance measures.

- Periodic review/revision of the maintenance program. Typically done annually and should be a team approach focusing on the goal of improving safety, improving efficiency, and maintaining regulatory compliance. The experiences of the previous year and the changes in equipment inventory will also impact the list of tasks to be added, deleted, and modified.
- Special consideration should be made for equipment that has been in service for five years or more. Make it part of your schedule to closely inspect all systems and subsystems at least every five years. Some systems require, by manufacturer recommendation, overhaul or in-depth inspection every 10 years.
- Cleaning must be seen as part of routine maintenance. If no schedule for cleaning is stated, specific to a piece of equipment, one should be assigned by the safety director.
- For areas with wide environmental changes between summer and winter, there should be season-specific tasks.
- Some centers find that putting routine tasks not typically found in the equipment database on their daily or weekly maintenance schedule helpful, e.g., complete staff exposure log, clean sink area, thin patient reading library, etc.
- The safety director will review and vet newly recommended tasks or changes to maintenance schedules needing inclusion before the next review cycle before being added to the maintenance program. These additions or changes are typically due to unacceptable frequency of unscheduled downtime. Equipment breakdowns indicate your preventive and predictive maintenance schedule needs to be modified and may also point out issues with design or reliability of components that should be addressed with suppliers. Less critical tasks may wait for review at the next scheduled meeting of the facility maintenance team.
- Predictive maintenance is a lesser-known component of a modern preventive maintenance strategy. It goes against the theory of, "Don't fix it if it's not broke." You want to fix it before it breaks so the task is done at a time of your choosing. Knowledge of equipment failure patterns, i.e. early warning signs and the use of forecasting tools, are essential in anticipating breakdowns and scheduling repairs in advance. Some of these tools include vibration analysis, lubrication analysis, thermography, and ultrasonics. Knowing which parts of a piece of equipment are prone to breakdown soonest is also helpful. Keeping track of the progression of these early warnings is a must in deciding when it's time to rebuild or replace the piece of equipment in question. Sometimes, just making minor adjustments fixes the problem.

Note: As new maintenance tasks are added, assign them a letter/number designation specific to their needed frequency, add them to the global maintenance schedule, and add them to the appropriate tracking form.

Having a prenotification system is a good idea in general and can be a great help for staying on schedule with complex tasks by giving you additional time to assemble all needed resources. It can also be a needed reminder for upcoming tasks in the "other" category that may otherwise be missed.

It is now time to shuffle the tiles so all tasks are accomplished within the required timeline but without overloading the staff on any one given month and leaving other months' workload extremely light. For example, not all annual tasks need to be done in January. If you have 18 tasks, assign one to each even numbered month and two to each odd numbered month. The same goes for quarterly. Assign some to a January-April-July-October schedule and others to a February-May-August-November schedule. Lump like tasks together in the same month. Look at what months are light operationally and consider slightly increasing your maintenance load on those months. Awareness of historical treatment loads can allow scheduling of major maintenance items to reduce disruption of the facility's clinical operations.

Once you have a global schedule, you will need a scheduler to orchestrate the completion of each task. For example, A-1 is assigned for January but by whom and on what day and time? Scheduling should be coordinated by a staff member who is experienced and familiar with the operational tempo of the facility. Things that the scheduler needs to keep in mind are the following:

- Can it be done without impacting operations? If not, include administration in deciding the best available date and time that limits operational downtime.
- What qualified labor resources are appropriate? Hyperbaric staff, facility staff, vendor under contract or noncontract vendor?
- What is the normal lead time for the scheduling of labor, parts and supplies to complete this task?
- Know how long the task typically takes. Block out extra time to allow for unforeseen issues.
- Make sure the scheduled date and time does not conflict with anything else occurring at the facility.
- Don't use labor resources during overtime hours unless you have to.

Corrective Maintenance

Nothing lasts forever. Over time, equipment will wear out and need to be repaired or replaced. Corrective maintenance is not a bad word if it occurs as a result of findings during the preventive maintenance process. The corrective action of repair is then done at a time of your choosing. When something breaks at an inopportune time and impacts safety and the otherwise smooth flow of operations, then "corrective maintenance" becomes a bad word. If this occurs, it means the following:

- The routine, preventive and/or predictive maintenance schedule may need modification.

- Staff may need further education on how to identify subtle changes in the performance of equipment and reporting it to the maintenance supervisor.
- Maintenance management personnel should track failures to determine whether a failure is an isolated event or point to a potential problem with component design or manufacturing.
- Senior staff may need to adjust to how they react to input from staff on subtle changes in the performance of equipment.

The maintenance scheduler will oversee the timeliness of any needed corrective maintenance, keeping in mind the six bullet points mentioned at the end of the Establishing a Maintenance Schedule section. Equipment downtime events will take priority and the hyperbaric safety officer should be notified. The scheduler should ask the person doing the corrective maintenance to inspect the surrounding supportive/attached equipment for signs of needed preventive maintenance. If found, doing the work now could avert a safety issue and/or additional unscheduled downtime later. Once the corrective action has taken place, appropriate testing and documentation must occur. If the failure results in an actual or potential staff or patient injury, the investigation will be more thorough and should also involve the facility's risk management department.

Documentation

If it isn't documented, it didn't happen. Beyond the more formal/legal reasons, documentation helps track what has been done, predict trends, and becomes a reliable historical record. For those required to follow *NFPA 99*, Chapter 14: Hyperbaric Facilities, note that the hyperbaric facility safety director must sign-off on all maintenance actions.

Tracking Forms

These forms may be part of the permanent record or be worksheets that a data entry person uses to place into an electronic record/maintenance program.

- Daily inspection/maintenance schedule (Table 1)
  - Start-up checklist
  - Shutdown checklist
- Compressor and gas record. With sign-off for start-up and shutdown, acrylic window inspections may be included in this record or in the daily inspection maintenance schedule checklist (Table 2)
- HP gas resupply log (Table 3)
- Weekly maintenance schedule (Table 4)
- Monthly, quarterly, semi-annual, annual, and other maintenance schedule (Table 5)
- Annual maintenance schedule for quarterly, semi-annual, and annual (Table 6)
- Maintenance record (Table 7)

- › Use record as is for preventive, corrective, testing, and new install
- › Modify record. Have known data preprinted on a separate form for each monthly, quarterly, semi-annual, annual, and other task. Give sufficient detail to ensure quality and completeness of each task. Results are then manually entered for each scheduled task.

- Master maintenance log (Table 8)
  - › Maintained for each piece of equipment.
  - › Provide a quick overview of routine and corrective maintenance activities.
  - › Allow review to determine the full scope of work performed.
  - › Include documentation of the safety director's approval of the equipment's return to service, if that documentation is not included on the service report.

Table 1.

Daily Inspection/Maintenance Schedule	
Task #	Detailed Description
D-1	
D-2	
D-3	

Used for start-up and shutdown procedures. Sign-off is done on next example form.

Table 2.

Compressor and Gas Record								
Month ______								Year ______
DATE	Start-Up INT	Comp #1 HRS	Comp #2 HRS	LOX PSI	HP 02 PSI	MED AIR PSI	DEL AIR PSI	Shut-down INT
1								
2								
3								
31								

Full version has 31 rows.

Table 3.

HP Gas Resupply Log Year ______							
DATE	GAS TYPE	Cyl #	FULL PSIG	DATE empty	EMPTY PSIG	Snooped and Analyzed	02 %

* Please remember to rotate bottles from back to front with the newest in back and complete all requested information above.

Table 4.

Weekly Maintenance Schedule					
Month ______________ Year _______		Week of Month			
Task #	Detailed Description	1	2	3	4
W-1					
W-2					
W-3					
					Initial when complete

Table 5.

Monthly Maintenance Schedule	
Task #	Detailed Description
M-1	
M-2	
M-3	
	Fill in Maintenance Record when completed

Use same format, but replace monthly with quarterly, semi-annual, annual, and other. Under task #, replace "M" with Q, S, A ,and O respectively.

Table 6.

Annual Maintenance Schedule Year _______									
January	Q-1	Q-3	Q-7	Q-10	S-1	S-3	A-1		
February	Q-2	Q-4	Q-8	Q-11	S-2	S-4	A-2		
March	Q-5	Q-6	Q-9	Q-12	S-5	S-6	A-3		
April	Q-1	Q-3	Q-7	Q-10	S-7	S-8	A-4		
May	Q-2	Q-4	Q-8	Q-11	S-9	S-10	A-5		
June	Q-5	Q-6	Q-9	Q-12	S-11	S-12	A-6		
July	Q-1	Q-3	Q-7	Q-10	S-1	S-3	A-7		
August	Q-2	Q-4	Q-8	Q-11	S-2	S-4	A-8		
September	Q-5	Q-6	Q-9	Q-12	S-5	S-6	A-9		
October	Q-1	Q-3	Q-7	Q-10	S-7	S-8	A-10		
November	Q-2	Q-4	Q-8	Q-11	S-9	S-10	A-11		
December	Q-5	Q-6	Q-9	Q-12	S-11	S-12	A-12		
Fill in maintenance record and cross out when completed.									

Table 7.

Maintenance Record			
Type of work	Routine [ ] Preventive [ ] Date _______ Testing [ ] Corrective [ ] New Install [ ]		
Task #		(e.g., M-1, Q-1, S-1, A-1, H-1, N/A)	
Reason for work			
Work performed			
Results			
Part #1		Qty	Vendor
Part #2		Qty	Vendor
Part #3		Qty	Vendor
Part #4		Qty	Vendor
Part #5		Qty	Vendor
Person(s) doing work			Man-hour
			Man-hour
			Man-hour
Contractor			Attach work order / invoice
Safety Officer			Date

Table 8.

Equipment Maintenance Master Log	
Device _______________ Serial # _______	
Date	Description of Activity

Facility Maintenance Library

Having a set place to keep maintenance-specific reference materials makes sense. Consider making it part of your bigger facility library.

- Equipment manuals (operations, maintenance, and repair)
- Equipment data sheets
- Equipment drawings/schematics
- Facility drawings
- Registration cards (register for manufacturer updates and recalls)
- Copy of maintenance specific requirements from all applicable AHJs
- Training material (manufacturer provided, in-house, etc.)
- Safety data aheets (SDS) for materials used in maintenance activities

Vendor List

Know who your service, repair,and parts and supply vendors are and have a relationship with them before they are needed. Know which ones are contracted vs. fee- for-service. It's good to have more than one contact for any given need. This list will continue to change based on changing needs, change in contracts, quality of past experience with a vendor, changing fees, etc. In addition to the typical information in an address book, a notes section is helpful to keep more detailed information, e.g., service technician, supervisor, accounts payable person, etc. Keep it current and cross-referenced to your main equipment database.

- Service and repair vendors
    - Hyperbaric chamber manufacturer (preventive maintenance beyond the scope of in-house staff, systems repair, upgrades, and overhauls)
    - Third-party hyperbaric services (preventive maintenance beyond the scope of in-house staff, systems repair, upgrades, and overhauls)
    - Air compressor services (preventive maintenance beyond the scope of in-house staff and systems repair or replacement)
    - Medical gas suppliers (LOX and HP cylinder rentals)

- › Air testing labs (supply air lab for you to take samples or testing on-site)
- › Housekeeping services
- › Electricians (preventive maintenance and repair)
- › Plumbers (preventive maintenance and repair)
- › Heating/ventilation/air conditioning services (preventive maintenance and repair)
- › Biomedical engineering (preventive maintenance and repair)

Note: The above companies would not typically be used for routine tasks, i.e., daily or weekly checks or inspections. This would include such things as checking compressor oil levels, logging of gas pressures, light cleaning, etc.

- Parts and supply vendors

Spare Parts and Tools Inventory

When something breaks down, it is not the time to realize you do not have the needed part to make a simple repair or that it comes from overseas and will take two weeks to get here. The initial list should be developed by the hyperbaric safety officer and the hyperbaric maintenance supervisor. Like most of the maintenance program, it should always be evolving. Example inventory is as follows and keep an inventory list for all parts on hand, with their minimum par level:

- Parts used routinely, year after year, to complete preventive maintenance, such as air filters, oil filters, etc.
- Commonly used rebuild kits
- Commonly used hard-to-get parts, such as pressure gauge, depth gauge, fittings, nuts and bolts, communications head-set, etc.
- Parts that have a shorter service life than the piece of equipment they are in, such as hoses, tubing, O-rings, gaskets, washers, lamps, fuses, door seals, oxygen analyzer cells, check valves, etc.
- Supplies, such as compressor oil, sodasorb, oxygen compatible lubricants, etc.
- Sufficient hand and power tools to adequately and safely perform in-house maintenance

Establishing a Training Program

The fundamentals of a maintenance training program are no different than any other training program. For ease of organization, integrate maintenance training into your main facility training program. The modules will need to be developed by your in-house maintenance experts and are usually a collaboration between the safety director and the maintenance supervisor.

- The less you outsource, the larger and more comprehensive your maintenance training program needs to be.
- For new hires, start out small by orienting to routine daily/weekly maintenance duties first.
- To train someone fully to be competent at all in-house tasks will take time. Make each maintenance project a hands-on learning experience for those not yet signed off. Once they've shadowed a competent person several times, on a specific task, have them assessed for sign-off by the maintenance supervisor.
- Ensure staff understands the importance of red-tagging a piece of equipment that is inoperable, unsafe, or is currently offline due to maintenance or any other reason.
- Ensure staff understands the importance of maintaining the cleanliness of the system, especially the components exposed to oxygen and/or high pressure.
- Ensure staff understands the safety issues with the utilization of high-pressure gases.
- Housekeeping staff who clean the hyperbaric facility must be trained in their specific duties (what they clean and what the hyperbaric staff will be responsible for cleaning) and training is documented. Recurrent training for housekeeping staff should be coordinated to ensure trained staff are available.
- Staff should read safety warnings at the front of each equipment user's manual, maintenance manual, and data sheet.
- Staff should have the equipment specific reference materials with them when doing maintenance on any piece of equipment.
- Encourage staff to do in-services on new equipment.
- Make time for in-service modules on common maintenance.
- Experts have determined that a cultural approach is better than just a "put a guard on it" approach when trying to keep staff safe. An effective safety program is behavior driven.

Quality Improvement

Most facilities have a quality improvement (QI) program. Include your maintenance activities into this QI program. Use the same principles and practices already in place, with the added list of indicators being maintenance-specific. Your safety director should be involved in the choosing of these indicators. As is typical in QI, look for indicators specific to high volume, high risk, and identified problem areas. Look in the areas of documentation, timeliness of completing a given scheduled task, frequency of corrective maintenance, frequency of equipment downtime, etc. Rotate out those indicators that are not an issue and add fresh indicators to look at.

Maintenance Budget

There are several things that impact the size of a maintenance budget, but it starts with the complexity of your chamber system(s). Example costs are as follows:

Fixed costs:

- Maintaining the routine and preventive maintenance program
  - In-house labor
  - Contracted labor
  - Maintenance contract(s)
  - Parts and supplies
- In-house staff training (little variability)

Variable costs:

- Corrective maintenance
  - In-house labor
  - Contracted labor
  - Maintenance contract(s)
  - Parts and supplies

  Note: Frequency increases exponentially with the age and complexity of the chamber system(s)
- Equipment down time

  Note: Lost revenue. Frequency is a function of luck and the quality of your predictive maintenance.
- Specialized staff training
- Equipment upgrades/modifications/new technology
  - Communications
  - Entertainment
  - Process controls system
  - Low-pressure air system (compressor, filtration, etc.)
  - Gas delivery system
  - In-chamber seating
  - Painting of chamber(s)
  - Fire suppression system
  - Manufacturer recommended overhaul (each 5-10 years)

  Note: Add associated labor costs. Frequency increases exponentially with the age and complexity of chamber system(s).

- Equipment replacement
  - New acrylic window(s) (each 10-20 years)
  - New air compressor(s) (each 10-15 years)
  - New deluge tank(s)
  - New tools

Note: Add associated labor costs. Frequency increases exponentially with the age and complexity of chamber system(s).

Manufacturers' Examples of Scheduled Chamber Maintenance

Monoplace Hyperbaric Chamber Maintenance Schedule Example

The following example is an edited overview of the maintenance requirements outlined in the user's manual for a Sechrist model 3300H/HR, 3600H/HR, and 4100H/HR hyperbaric chamber.[6] The information provided is for educational purposes only—other chamber models may have substantially different requirements. Always adhere to the full maintenance schedule and instructions outlined in the maintenance and/or operations manual for your specific make and model of chamber.

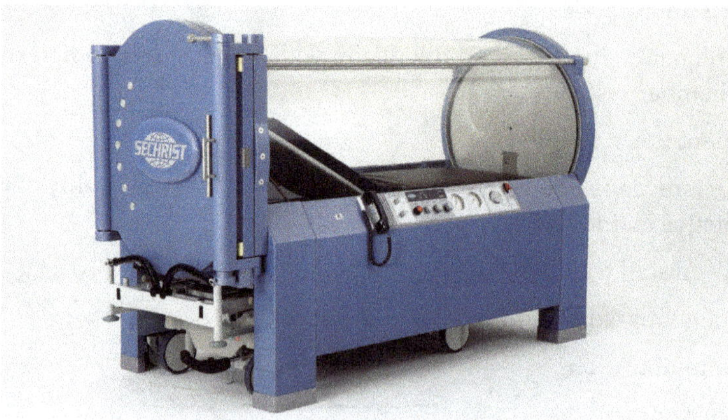

Figure 1. Photo and user's manual excerpt provided courtesy of Sechrist Industries, Inc.

User's Manual, Chapter 7: Maintenance and Service

Caution: Do not attempt to perform maintenance or repairs other than those described in this manual without instructions from Sechrist Industries. Do not make modifications to interface equipment to the chamber unless authorized by Sechrist Industries.

Sechrist Industries hyperbaric chambers are designed for durability and reliability. A regular program of inspections, performance verifications, and factory-authorized preventive maintenance will keep your chamber in optimal condition. Daily, weekly, and annual performance verifications are recommended. Keep written records of all performance verifications and maintenance. Sechrist Industries recommends factory-authorized preventive maintenance to be performed once a year.

Warning: If any Sechrist Industries monoplace hyperbaric chamber fails to perform as outlined, remove the chamber from service and contact a Sechrist Industries authorized service technician. The chamber should not be used until proper performance has been verified.

Daily Inspection and Performance Verification

Prior to beginning treatments, the following inspections should be performed daily.

- Ensure that the supply pressure is between 50.0 and 70.0 PSI.
- Visually inspect the acrylic cylinder for scratches and signs of crazing. *Warning:* If major scratches (.110" deep or deeper), or signs of crazing are present, immediately contact Sechrist Industries. Deep scratches or crazing can cause the acrylic cylinder to rupture. DO NOT USE the chamber in this condition.
- Visually inspect the chamber interior and exterior for cleanliness.
- Visually inspect the door gasket for damage and cleanliness. Replace or clean as required.
- Check the chamber ground and patient ground by utilizing the methods described in Section 4.
- Inspect chamber supply and vent hoses for kinks and loose connections. Ensure proper function before use.
- Perform a visual inspection of the complete chamber for damage, loose knobs, etc.
- Inspect and verify the functionality of the intercommunication system.
    - Lists a nine-step process

Weekly Performance Verification

- Check for proper function of the ventilation flow rate control.
    - The ventilation flow rate is the rate at which gas exhausts from the chamber during treatment. The ventilation flow rate control adjusts the flow rate from approximately 80 liters per minute (lpm) to 400 lpm (when the chamber pressure is set at 15 PSI).
- Check for proper function of the emergency vent system by depressurizing rapidly using the emergency vent button. Before pressing the emergency vent button, turn the master valve to the emergency vent position.
- Check for proper function of the emergency shutoff and automatic vent system depressurizing rapidly by moving the emergency shutoff toggle valve to the up position. After check has been completed, return the emergency shut-off and automatic vent toggle to the "off" position.

- Check for proper function of the safety lockpin device.
  - With the chamber door closed and locked, turn the master valve to the "on" position. The chamber should pressurize to an idle pressure of approximately 1.5 PSI during which time the safety lockpin should slide into the hole at the base of the swing arm assembly.
  - Turn the master valve to the "off" position. The safety lockpin will retract when the chamber pressure is under 1.0 PSI.

  Note: describes *actions to take if safety lockpin becomes jammed*

Semi-Annual Performance Verification

- Check the calibration of the rate set control on a semi-annual basis.
  - Exhaust Line: Check the end of the exhaust line on the exterior of the building. Make sure the screen on the end of the exhaust line is not occluded.
  - Rate Set Verification: lists a twelve-step process

Annual Factory Authorized Preventive Maintenance

- This annual maintenance may be accomplished within three months of the annual maintenance date, i.e. between 9 and 15 months of service. It is very important that the filters and various mechanisms in the chamber are kept clean and as free as possible of hydrocarbons. Sechrist Industries provides annual service contracts for preventive maintenance as well as for all service and repairs. A field-based technician is scheduled into each area of the country once a year to perform preventive maintenance.

Ten-Year Factory Overhaul

- As a manufacturer of the equipment, it is strongly recommended that Sechrist hyperbaric chambers receive a mechanical refurbishment when they reach either 10 years from the date of fabrication or have reached 10,000 cycles, whichever comes first.
  - The acrylic cylinder minimum design life expectancy per the *ASME PVHO-1* Standard is 10 years, 10,000 cycles or 40,000 hours, whichever occurs first. After refurbishment and overhaul, the chamber is reassembled, pressure tested, and verified in compliance with ASME code and PVHO safety standards.

Additional Maintenance Considerations

- Cylinder Replacement
  - In accordance with *ASME PVHO-2 Safety Standard for Pressure Vessel In-Service Guidelines* that address acrylic window service life, when a chamber with an acrylic cylinder for medical use reaches the maximum

usage period of 20 years or 20,000 cycles, this chamber MUST have the acrylic cylinder replaced as well as the door/endplate gaskets before the chamber can continue in use. Sechrist Industries can replace the acrylic cylinders that have reached this limit during a factory overhaul.

› *Caution:* If not in compliance with *ASME PVHO-2*, the chamber must be taken out of service.

- Care and Cleaning of Acrylic Cylinder
  - *Caution:* Avoid abrasion of the polished acrylic cylinder during cleaning. Use only a damp pure cotton or lined cloth to remove dust. Never allow liquids or solvents to contact the acrylic cylinder. Clean up any spills as soon as possible.
  - *Caution:* Avoid using any oil or alcohol-based substances on the acrylic cylinder.
  - Dust removal: Wipe the cylinder with a soft, 100% cotton, lint-free, water-moistened cloth.
  - General cleaning: Wash the cylinder with soft, 100% cotton, lint-free cloth-moistened with a mild detergent solution. Rinse and dry with soft, 100% cotton, lint free, water moistened cloth.
  - *Caution:* Do not allow water to accumulate on the bottom of the chamber while cleaning. The water could drain into and contaminate the supply piping system.
  - *Caution:* Do not use disinfectants that have not been approved by Sechrist Industries to clean and disinfect the acrylic viewport.
- Care and Cleaning of Chamber and Gurney
  - Disinfect the chamber according to the type of cases being treated and as directed by the medical staff. Refer to the list of acceptable disinfectants available from Sechrist Industries.
  - Wash stretcher, pillows, positioning pads, and mattress surfaces with mild soap.
  - Refer to the *Gurney User Manual* for cleaning instructions.
- Cleaning of Painted and Anodized Surfaces
  - Use the same methods for cleaning as used for the acrylic cylinder.
- General Care of Equipment
  - Always keep the chamber covered with a clean cloth sheet when not in use.
  - Always keep the chamber door closed when not in use.
  - Do not store items near the chamber that could fall on or against it.

- Never allow anyone to lean on the chamber.
- Do not allow unauthorized personnel in the chamber area.
- Keep the door to the chamber facility locked when not in use.
- List of approved chamber disinfectants.

Multiplace Hyperbaric Chamber System Maintenance Schedule Example

The following example is an edited overview of the maintenance requirements outlined in the *Instructions for Use (IFU) Manual* and *Service Manual for a HYPERBARIC MODULAR SYSTEMS, INC.* (HMS), HMS5000, Twelve (12) Patient Rectangular Hyperbaric Chamber System.[7-8] The information provided is for educational purposes only. Other chamber models may have substantially different requirements. Always adhere to the full maintenance schedule and instructions outlined in the maintenance and/or operations manual for your specific make and model of chamber.

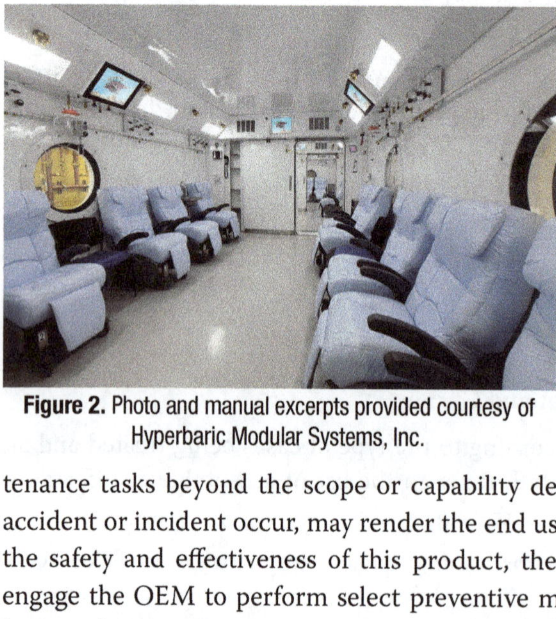

Figure 2. Photo and manual excerpts provided courtesy of Hyperbaric Modular Systems, Inc.

As an OEM of these devices, HMS shall ensure that its hyperbaric chamber(s) are safe, effective, and perform in accordance with the design articulated in its FDA 510(k) premarket notification throughout the operational life of the product. As such, the end user must operate and maintain this device in accordance with the directions supplied by HMS in its operations manual and maintenance manual. Failing to do so, and/or performing maintenance tasks beyond the scope or capability described in these manuals, should an accident or incident occur, may render the end user liable for such action(s). To ensure the safety and effectiveness of this product, the end user is strongly encouraged to engage the OEM to perform select preventive maintenance on a regularly scheduled basis and corrective maintenance on an as required basis.

Excerpts Taken from the *Instructions for Use Manual*

Caution: The hyperbaric chamber system must be checked, maintained, and serviced periodically as specified in a separate manual (refer to Maintenance, Equipment Care, Maintenance, and Performance Verification). A defective device should never be used. Should repair become necessary, contact the OEM, HMS, National City, California. This product should be maintained and repaired by HMS factory-trained technicians or by written instructions provided by HMS. This product should not be modified in any way, except by the OEM's factory trained technicians with prior written approval provided by HMS.

The HMS 5000 Multiplace Hyperbaric Chamber System requires a comprehensive preventive maintenance program recommended by HMS that incorporates daily, weekly, monthly, quarterly, semi-annual, and annual maintenance tasks. Maintenance tasks that exceed the skill level of those performing the maintenance should be referred to HMS. The Preventive Maintenance Program is covered in the *HMS Service Manual for the Twelve (12) Patient Rectangular Hyperbaric Chamber System.*

Excerpts Taken from the Service Manual

Daily/Weekly Maintenance Requirements

To be assigned by facility maintenance officer based on facility specific needs.

- Daily
  - Start-up checklist
  - Compressor log
  - Gas log
  - Daily facility maintenance task log
  - Shutdown checklist
- Weekly
  - Once-a-week tasks
  - Twice-a-week tasks
  - Three-times-a-week tasks

Monthly Maintenance Requirements

- Clean the environmental control system (ECS) housing unit inside and out; check glycol level.
- Take a condensate sample from air receiver and check for contaminants (particles, grit, grime, sheen, etc.).
- Clean compressors inside and outside.
- Check the alternate breathing source for pressure, damage, and wear (check hoses, face mask, and straps for cracks or damage).
- Check/clean compressor filters.
- Clean the top and outside of the chamber.
- Clean the control console.
- Inventor tools.
- Check the analog depth gauges for zero.
- Check flow from all built-in breathing system (BIBS) solenoids.

- Check fluid level on all door reservoirs.
- Remove and clean chamber mufflers.

Quarterly Maintenance Requirements

- Inspect door gaskets for nicks, gouges, and cuts.
- Clean and lubricate all gaskets/O-rings.
- Clean gurneys and wheel chairs, lubricate if needed.
- Check accuracy of the stopwatches.
- Inspect, clean ECS fan, and heat exchanger for debris.
- Inspect chamber paint for chips or coating damage.
- Clean interior of the chamber lighting units.
- Clean headset terminals and plugs.
- Check and tighten all BIBS valve handles.

Semi-Annual Maintenance Requirements

- Test the pressure relief valve.
- Leak-test the chamber.
- Perform an air quality test for water, CO_2, CO, and oil.
- Cycle all valves that are not commonly used.
- Check the ECS glycol level.
- Clean BIBS (Scott masks) regulator parts and hoses. Lubricate their flappers.
- Check chamber ground for continuity.
- Perform fire suppression system (FSS) test.

Annual/Hourly/Other Maintenance Requirements

- Inspect all wiring for wear.
- Inspect the interior of the FSS water tanks for rust, peeling, and pitting
- Inspect the interior of the air receiver tank for rust, peeling, and pitting
- Replace coalescing and particulate filter elements; inspect and clean the water trap.
- Compressor annual maintenance.
- Replace Mister system water filter.
- Review the maintenance program. Done annually by OEM under terms of the service contract.
- Hourly maintenance requirements are identified based upon the type and size of the compressors installed within the hyperbaric system. Hourly maintenance

is found in the manufacturers' manuals that are provided with the purchase of the compressors.

Excerpts Taken from the Service Agreement

Maintenance Requirements Outside the Scope of the Hyperbaric Technician

As the OEM of the HMS 5000, HMS must ensure that its product remains safe and effective for administering HBOT to patients and to operate for the life of the product. As the experts in this hyperbaric chamber's design, manufacture, and installation, HMS has developed the following list of annual preventive maintenance/servicing tasks which are beyond the scope of expertise for the hyperbaric facility's hyperbaric technicians to perform and should be performed annually by its own trained staff in order to maintain the HMS 5000 in a fully operational state of readiness. HMS staff can be retained to accomplishing these tasks annually through execution of a five-year (recommended) service agreement, which includes annual performance of the preventive maintenance tasks, and the additional services specified below.

- Check door locks.
- Check door seals.
- Check pressure relief valve.
- Check chamber ground continuity.
- Check chamber screw torque (as appropriate).
- Check communication system operation.
- Check pressure indicators (analog and digital depth and pressure gauges).
- Check hood/BIBS supply system.
- Check fire suppression system.
- Check pressurization (rate and pressure).
- Check system for leaks.
- Check emergency decompression/depressurization time.
- Review maintenance program and maintenance logs with hospital staff.
- Certification of PVHO-1 Windows for 10-year extension, provided windows are in compliance with PVHO-2.

After the completion of servicing, an HMS factory-trained senior field service representative (FSR) prepares a service report and submits this document to the contracting POC for the facility. The report will indicate the pass/fail status of the aforementioned items and a list of what maintenance actions were performed. For any items identified during the course of performing the service that are beyond the scope of the service agreement, HMS will itemize and present as recommendations to address in a follow-on visit, or if mutually agreed to, performed while its FSR team is still on-site.

Included in the annual service agreement, HMS also offers the following:

- Telephone and e-mail support. HMS will provide 24/7 telephone and e-mail support.
- On-call, on-site visits. In the event of an unplanned maintenance action identified by the customer which requires HMS to send a FSR to the HMS 5000 Multiplace Hyperbaric Chamber System Facility, this will be accomplished at an additional cost under HMS standard rates and terms.
- Remote diagnostics via an Internet connection and software maintenance. HMS will provide 24/7 remote diagnostics support and business hours software maintenance. The purpose of offering this remote diagnostics and software maintenance service is to provide a more effective method of responding to system failures, software "bugs," and/or customer-requested software upgrades or changes. Note: All software changes must be validated by HMS prior to implementation.
- Spares and consumables. Commensurate with the length of the service agreement and size of HMS 5000 hyperbaric chamber.

Conclusion

Having a hyperbaric facility specific maintenance program is a must for many reasons. It is the hope that this chapter has provided you with substantial guidance on your way to a maintenance program that meets your present and future needs.

References

1. bizfluent.com, 2017 posting. How to develop a facility maintenance program. https://bizfluent.com/how-8490445-develop-facility-maintenance-program.html.
2. HyperbaricLink. Hyperbaric Oxygen Therapy Treatment Centers Directory. Cambridge, Massachusetts: HyperbaricLink. www.hyperbariclink.com.
3. The Joint Commission. Comprehensive Accreditation Manual for Hospitals. Oakbrook Terrace, Illinois: The Joint Commission; 2018 Edition.Chapter: Environment of Care, EC.02.04.01.
4. National Fire Protection Association. NFPA 99 Health Care Facilities Code. Quincy, Maryland: National Fire Protection Association; 2018;14.3:99-118.
5. National Fire Protection Association. NFPA 99 Health Care Facilities Code. Quincy, Maryland: National Fire Protection Association; 2018;1.3.1:99-115.

6. Sechrist. User's Manual Monoplace Hyperbaric Chamber: Model 3300H/HR, 3600H/HR, and 4100H/HR Hyperbaric Chamber. Anaheim, California: Sechrist Industries, Inc. Rev. 54, P/N 100383-1, Section 7 Maintenance and Service. 7.0-7.7.
7. Hyperbaric Modular Systems, Inc. Instructions for Use (IFU) Manual for the HMS 5000, Twelve (12) Patient Rectangular Hyperbaric Chamber System. National City, California: Hyperbaric Modular Systems, Inc.
8. Hyperbaric Modular Systems, Inc. Service Manual for the HMS 5000, Twelve (12) Patient Rectangular Hyperbaric Chamber SystemNational City, California: Hyperbaric Modular Systems, Inc.
9. American Society of Mechanical Engineers. ASME PVHO-1 2016, Safety Standard for Pressure Vessels for Human Occupancy. New York, New York: American Society of Mechanical Engineers.
10. American Society of Mechanical Engineers ASME PVHO-2 2016, Safety Standard for Pressure Vessels For Human Occupancy: In-Service Guidelines. New York, New York: American Society of Mechanical Engineers.
11. Centers for Medicare & Medicaid Services. http://www.cms.gov.
12. Colorado Department of Public Health and Environment. Denver, Colorado. https://www.colorado.gov/cdphe.
13. Denver Fire Code. City and County of Denver: Denver, Colorado. http://www.denvergov.org.
14. Centers for Medicare & Medicaid Services. Hospital Equipment Maintenance Requirements. Centers for Medicare & Medicaid Services: Baltimore, Maryland. Update posted 12/20/13. https://www.cms.gov/Medicare/Provider-Enrollment-and-Certification/SurveyCertificationGenInfo/Downloads/Survey-and-Cert-Letter-14-07.pdf.
15. Ottenberg K. Phone conversation about his experiences with AHJ compliance specific to maintenance. 12/16/11. Facility Manager: Bio-Medical Engineering, Aramark Healthcare, Contracted to Presbyterian/St. Luke's Medical Center, Denver, Colorado.
16. Maintenance Programs. Harry Johnston. 2011. http://maintenanceprograms.org.
17. Food and Drug Administration. Medical Devices. Silver Spring, Maryland: Food and Drug Administration. http://www.fda.gov/MedicalDevices/default.htm.
18. National Fire Protection Association. NFPA 99 Health Care Facilities Code. Quincy, Maryland: National Fire Protection Association. 2018 Edition.
19. National Fire Protection Association. NFPA 99 Health Care Facilities Code. Quincy, Maryland: National Fire Protection Association. 2018 Edition, Annex A.
20. National Fire Protection Association. NFPA 99 Health Care Facilities Code. Quincy, Maryland: National Fire Protection Association.

21. National Fire Protection Association. NFPA 99 Health Care Facilities Code: Chapter 14. Quincy, Maryland: National Fire Protection Association. 2018 Edition.
22. Robert Gibson. Phone conversation about his experiences with AHJ compliance specific to maintenance. 12/16/11, Facility Plant Operations Manager, Presbyterian/St. Luke's Medical Center, Denver, Colorado.
23. Standards for Hospitals and Health Facilities 6 CCR 1011-1. Colorado Department of Public Health and Environment: Health Facilities and Emergency Medical Services Division, Denver, Colorado. Chapter 04 General Hospitals, Part 5 Facility Operations: 5.300 Maintenance Services, and 5.302 Programmatic Functions, and (3) Equipment Maintenance.
24. UHMS. UHMS Guidelines for Hyperbaric Facility Operations. North Palm Beach, Florida: UHMS. 2004 Edition.
25. William C. Preisler, CSP, ARM. In person conversation about his experiences with AHJ compliance specific to maintenance. 12/19/11, Facility Safety Officer, Presbyterian/St. Luke's Medical Center, Denver, Colorado.

CHAPTER 9
Decompression Sickness in Inside Attendants

Sean Hardy, MD

Introduction

Hyperbaric oxygen therapy (HBOT) is used in an expanding role to treat a wide variety of illnesses and pathologic conditions, from well-known indications such as decompression illness to more recently investigated conditions such as sudden sensorineural hearing loss. Delivery methods can vary greatly as well, from remote deck decompression chambers (DDC) in the North Sea to sophisticated hospital and research chambers. The common element to these conditions and delivery methods is the delivery of higher partial pressures of oxygen by placing a patient under elevated atmospheric pressure. Much of current hyperbaric oxygen therapy (HBOT) is delivered in monoplace chambers. These chambers are limited to one occupant, are generally pressurized with 100% oxygen, and have a depth limit often of 66 feet of sea water (fsw). Their benefit is in their smaller size, relative simplicity, and lack of need for inside attendants during delivery of therapy. In contrast to the monoplace chamber is the larger multiplace chamber. This type of pressure vessel is larger, holding from two to sometimes 12 people. It is the multiplace hyperbaric chamber environment which we will be dealing with in this chapter.

The Multiplace Chamber Environment

A multiplace hyperbaric chamber is designed to accommodate multiple occupants, generally both patients and necessary inside attendants (IAs). They allow the efficient treatment of multiple patients at a time, generally allow higher treatment pressures for deeper treatment table use, and allow access to critical patients during therapy. They can also be outfitted for delivery of multiple treatment gases, which allows more precise control of patient partial pressure of O_2 (ppO_2) during varied treatment tables. Due to its larger volume, as well as the presence of inside attendants who are not patients, these chambers are generally pressurized with compressed air as opposed to the oxygen environment of the monoplace chamber. Treatment gases are delivered to the patients by means of a tight-fitting mask or hood, which can be removed/turned off during air breaks. Thus, the patients receiving therapy are predominantly breathing oxygen just as in the monoplace chamber. However, one of the benefits of the multiplace environment is the presence of IAs. IAs have a number of roles during therapy, including assisting patients with their oxygen delivery devices, supervising air breaks, patient monitoring, medication administration, respiratory therapy/ventilator management, and many others. These care providers are not breathing treatment gas during the treatment. This is due both to the demands of their duties, as well as to reduce the risk of central nervous system (CNS) oxygen toxicity in the supervising personnel, which could lead to seizure. Since the IAs are predominantly breathing compressed air during the course of the treatment table, they are exposed to increased partial pressures of inert gas, mainly nitrogen. This makes them subject to the general risks of compressed air diving, predominantly decompression sickness (DCS).

Decompression Physiology and Decompression Sickness

To understand the proper administration of multiplace HBOT as well as the risks of inside attendant injury and subsequent treatment, some discussion of decompression physiology and the pathology of decompression sickness must be undertaken. Full description of these entities is beyond this scope of this text, and those interested in a more robust explanation are encouraged to reference any of the excellent primary texts on diving medicine. However, a functional discussion will be provided here in the setting of IA DCS.

Air breathing animals have a level of dissolved inert gases in their blood and tissues which is based on the partial pressure of each inert gas. In the usual air environment, this inert gas is mostly nitrogen, which makes up roughly 79% of the air we breathe. Nitrogen will accumulate in tissues at a rate dependent on its fractional percentage of the breathing gas, the environmental pressure, the vascular supply to the tissue, and the solubility of the gas. Any increase or decrease in the percentage of nitrogen or the ambient pressure will result in nitrogen moving into or out of the tissues in an attempt to reach a new balanced state. This process takes time and is different for the various types of tissues in the body. How fast nitrogen accumulates or leaves a tissue is generally expressed in terms of a half-life. This number, usually in minutes, is the amount of time it takes for nitrogen or other inert gas in tissue to change its value by half. Thus, a tissue with a short half-life will accumulate or offload inert gas at a faster rate than a tissue with a longer half-life. A tissue is generally considered to have fully saturated or fully desaturated after a period of six half-lives. Thus, significant differences can result in how fast the tissues of the body take on and give off inert gas.

The uptake and elimination of nitrogen or other inert gas as pressure changes through a typical multiplace chamber treatment or in-water dive can be followed to illustrate the normal physiology of inert gas transfer as well as the pathology which occurs when this process is disrupted. We can follow the chronological changes in inert gas transfer through a dive profile and discuss the importance of proper application and more importantly reduction in partial pressure of inert gas. As an IA or diver is pressurized, the increase in pressure results in elevated partial pressure of inert gases, primarily nitrogen. This results in a diffusion gradient, which drives nitrogen into the blood and tissues above the prior surface levels. Tissues begin to accumulate nitrogen based on their respective half-life and the partial pressure of the gas. This process will continue as long as the IA or diver remains at an elevated pressure and breathing inert gas. As the ambient pressure is reduced during ascent, or if the fraction of inert gas in the breathing mix is reduced (such as a switch to an elevated oxygen blend or pure oxygen), the partial pressure of nitrogen in the lungs and therefore the blood begins to drop. Thus, nitrogen begins to leave the tissues in an attempt to restore the resting state. Again, the speed of this process is determined by the pressure of nitrogen, circulation to the tissue, and the half-life of the tissue. As nitrogen leaves the tissues, it will generally enter the bloodstream and be carried to the lungs in a dissolved state, where it is able to be exhaled. If this process continues in this fashion, generally no harm results. However, there is a limit to the amount of nitrogen which can be removed from a tissue and dissolved into the blood without formation of bubbles. If the amount of nitrogen leaving the tissues is too great, bubbles will form and this can begin the process by which tissue injury and pathology occurs.

Decompression sickness is a spectrum of injury caused by the formation of bubbles in blood and/or tissues beyond a critical level. Bubble formation itself does not always correlate with clinical illness, but the formation of bubbles is generally felt to be necessary for decompression sickness to occur. Bubbles can cause damage in several ways. They can displace and disrupt tissue if they form directly in the tissues themselves. Bubbles in the bloodstream can also accumulate in smaller vessels downstream and block blood flow, causing ischemia. Bubbles themselves cause damage to blood vessel endothelium and result in inflammation of the vessels and surrounding tissues. At high volume, they can inhibit blood flow through the lungs and cause decreases in oxygen delivery and blood return to the heart. Thus, signs and symptoms of DCS can vary greatly based on the location and volume of bubble formation.

The process by which persons can be removed from elevated pressure environments without causing harmful levels of bubble formation has been the basis for the development of decompression tables in both commercial and recreational dive settings. While approaches have varied, the common element has been limiting time at elevated partial pressures of inert gas and specifying a rate at which pressure can be reduced to avoid pathologic formation of bubbles. The most common method of decompression schedule formation has been based on the early work of Haldane,[1] whose initial observations and research led to the first decompression schedules for use in both caisson and diving operations. Haldane used the concept of tissue half-times explained above combined with practical observations of the limits of decompression from various depths to formulate a method for returning compressed air workers from elevated pressure exposures. Haldane noted that there was a critical ratio of nitrogen pressures in tissue compared to ambient pressure, which if exceeded, resulted in significant bubble formation and called this the supersaturation ratio. He defined this ratio as a 2:1 ratio of tissue nitrogen pressure to ambient pressure. This meant that pressure could be reduced relatively rapidly as long the pressure reduction did not exceed this ratio. He proposed several theoretical tissue types each with their own half-life, and using each tissue and the supersaturation ratio, determined how quickly a person could be brought to the surface from depths. This led to the common approach of staged decompression in which those unable to return directly to the surface are required to make several "stops" at shallower depths while nitrogen leaves tissues so that their ratio remains below two in all tissues. Over the many years since he formulated his first tables, Haldane's approach has been modified to include more than the initial five tissue half-lives as well as to refine the supersaturation ratio. In addition, the model has been fine-tuned based on the actual results of many thousands of dives. These newer tables are referred to as modified Haldane models and make up a large percentage of current dive tables in use in both clinical hyperbaric medicine and diving operations.

Regardless of the model and table used, some method of tracking inert gas and control of the rate of decompression must be used for all those exposed to inert gas at elevated pressures. This is commonly done through the use of dive tables, which specify the maximum time one can be exposed to a given inert gas at a given depth/pressure, and describe the proper manner in which to return to the surface with an acceptable risk of decompression illness. Tables from the United States Navy (USN), the Royal Navy, National Oceanic and Atmospheric Administration (NOAA), civilian scuba organizations such as the Professional Association of Diving Instructors (PADI), as well as commercial diving entities are all in use, and serve to guide the safe return of pressurized gas workers back to surface pressures. Despite the large degree of sophistication of these tables and their successful use in clinical, recreational, and commercial diving environments, they do not, in fact, eliminate risk, but rather aim to reduce it to acceptable levels. Therefore, decompression sickness can result even in the presence of proper adherence to accepted protocols.

Prevalence of DCS in the Inside Attendant Population

Since the introduction of modern diving tables and decompression strategies, recreation and work in a pressurized environment has enjoyed a vastly improved safety record. However, DCS has not been eliminated. Much has been written regarding the incidence of DCS in recreational and working divers, and the risk was generally regarded as low. There has been less reported on the incidence of illness in clinical hyperbaric IAs. This population is important to study given their routine exposure to inert gas loading, modern occupational safety guidelines, and the possible predilection of care-worker injuries to go under reported for numerous reasons. This section will examine some of the more pertinent literature regarding inside attendant DCS, and lessons taken from this review can be applied to later discussions regarding prevention of DCS. In 1964, Anderson and colleagues[2] from Duke University published their initial experience of 666 varied clinical and research dives. A total of 56 people underwent 1,615 exposures to pressure. Of the 56 staff, 52 were available for survey (four had left the system), and reported a total of 10 events which were probable DCS. This represented an incidence of 0.62%. However, this correlates to a cumulative risk of roughly 16%. Later, Dunford et al. from Virginia Mason University reported on their experience of IA DCS from 1979-1990.[3] In that time, 7,910 treatments resulted in 8,424 IA exposures. DCS was noted in 26 cases, representing an incidence of 0.31%. Importantly, they found that the risk of DCS was directly related to the depth of exposure ($P<0.0001$, highly correlated). Following this report, Virginia Mason instituted a number of modifications to the decompression of IAs, including a safety stop during decompression and oxygen breathing by IAs during decompression. Since 2009, they have noted five subsequent cases of DCS in IAs: two following 2.36 ATA profiles, two following USN Treatment Table 6, and one following a 3 ATA exposure.[4]

Unfortunately, fatalities have occurred among inside attendants. In 1991 a tragic series of events led to the death of a female nurse in Panama City, FL, following a 6 ATA hyperbaric exposure.[4-6] As is the case with many serious incidents, numerous individual errors compounded to produce a serious outcome. She had been exposed to a compression earlier in the day, resulting in a residual nitrogen load which persisted to the beginning of the dive in question. The exposure was at a high pressure, 6 ATA, which as reported by Dunford above, directly correlated with increased risk. Additionally, her breathing apparatus was delivering air rather than the required 50:50 nitrox blend required at that depth, significantly increasing her nitrogen load. Lastly, when she began to develop symptoms suggestive of pulmonary DCS during the later stages of decompression, this did not result in evaluation by a physician. This tragic case illustrates several of the principles, which will be discussed later in the chapter, regarding detection and prevention of DCS in IAs.

In 1995, Dietz published a review of IA DCS from the University of Maryland Shock Trauma Center.[7] This retrospective review covered 23 years and included 25,164 hyperbaric exposures among 120 IAs. In the reporting time period, 19 cases of DCS occurred among 13 IAs, for an incidence of 0.076%. This corresponds to a cumulative risk of nearly 15%. Shortly afterward, Brattebo et al.[8] shared their experience with IA DCS in 1997. They reported three cases of cutaneous DCS among 18 IAs over 395 pressure exposures. This represented an incidence of 0.76% and a cumulative risk of 17%. In response, they modified their IA decompression algorithm to include IA oxygen breathing during the final five or 10 minutes while on bottom, as well as during decompression. In the 1,139 exposures which followed, no cases of DCS were noted.

In 2007, Pontani[9] shared the experience of 10,028 dives from a single multiplace chamber in Conroe, Texas. They experienced 15 cases of IA DCS, the majority of which occurred in the early years of operation. They cite a significant reduction in incidence following institution of IA oxygen breathing periods as well as reduced work hours among IAs. The same year, at a different facility, another serious injury to an IA occurred. In this case, a hyperbaric nurse attending an injured diver sustained quadriplegia following decompression.[10]

A number of publications have shown acceptable experiences with IA DCS and have provided some examples of prevention/mitigation strategies. In 2005 Cooper and colleagues[11] shared their 14 year experience with IA pressure exposures. In the period from 1992-2005, they had 6,062 exposures among 155 clinical staff, and no cases of DCS were observed. Several aspects of their operations are worth discussing, which likely contributed to their lack of DCS.

All IAs underwent oxygen breathing during decompression. Additionally, pressure exposures were limited to four days per week and on no more than three consecutive days. As their facility was located in a mountainous area, there were strict restrictions on travel to altitude, even while driving, following hyperbaric exposure. Additionally, Cooper et al.[12] had previously examined their IA exposure profiles using Doppler ultrasound bubble analysis, in the manner described by the Canadian Defense and Civil Institute for Environmental Medicine (DCIEM). Their study examined their standard treatment profile of 2.4 ATA for a maximum of 110 minutes, with IAs breathing oxygen for a minimum of the 20-minute decompression. Time on oxygen could be lengthened for any increased bottom time due to prolongation of the compression phase. In this study, 28 individuals received 1,743 hyperbaric exposures with Doppler ultrasound examination following. They found that 68% of those studied had bubble grades of 0 or 1, which is defined as low risk. Another 22% were grade 2, which is considered intermediate risk. The DCIEM defined acceptable bubble stress as 50% of subjects being grade 2 or below, thus Cooper and colleagues deemed their profile to be acceptable by those independent standards. No episodes of DCS were reported during the study period. Of note, 10% of exposures resulted in high bubble grades (3 and 4), however no clinical DCS occurred. This illustrates the incomplete correlation with bubble grade and clinical manifestations of DCS. Additionally, they noted significant variability in individual IAs in bubble grade following identical profiles over the study period. Though the small numbers did not allow formal statics of these variables, they did note a trend toward higher bubble grades in an IA following illness, injury, or exertion, highlighting the importance of daily assessment of fitness to dive. Further emphasis on compliance with these reduction strategies was illustrated in this same study population, when in 2017, Van den Broek[13] reported two cases of DCS in IAs from this site following the reported study period. In both cases, the prohibition on driving to altitude following hyperbaric exposure was violated.

Two other centers have reported highly positive experiences with IA DCS incidence. In 2011, Uzun et al.[14] published the experience of a single multiplace chamber in Turkey. They retrospectively reviewed 4,532 exposures among 40 IA nurses, with profiles ranging from 2.4–6 ATA. Similar to the Cooper cohort, IAs were limited to three hyperbaric exposures per week, and no more than one per 24 hours. All IAs decompressed on oxygen and were required to breathe oxygen for the final 10 minutes of the isobaric phase. During the study period, there were no reported cases of IA DCS. Lastly, in 2013 Witucki[15] published a 28-year experience of their 2.4 ATA profiles from the University of California San Diego (UCSD). Their center used three different IA decompression profiles for a 2.4 ATA exposure. For bottom times less than 80 minutes, no IA oxygen breathing was utilized, in keeping with USN no-decompression limits. For bottom times between 80 and 119 minutes, IAs breathed oxygen for the final 15 minutes of the isobaric phase prior to decompression. For bottom times over 119 minutes, IAs were given oxygen for the final 30 minutes of the isobaric phase. In the reporting period, no cases of DCS in IAs were diagnosed. It should be noted that this study excluded hyperbaric exposures other than the 2.4 ATA profile, and thus does not represent the full scope of inside attendant exposure, nor those profiles which have been shown to pose the highest risk of DCS to inside attendants.

Treatment of Decompression Syndrome in IAs

As can be seen from the preceding review of the incidence of DCS among IAs, over the course of a career, repeated exposure to hyperbaric conditions does carry with it a cumulative risk of DCS. In cases of a seemingly low incidence of 0.076% for example, an IA making a conservative three dives a week over a 10-year career could statistically experience one or more cases of DCS. Therefore, treatment strategies must be in place.

For illnesses with a low incidence, surveillance and detection is of paramount importance. This is especially true among health care providers in a professional setting, where fears of both personal embarrassment and career impact may impede the reporting of sentinel symptoms. To this end, a departmental culture of safety and surveillance must be created and nurtured. All those exposed to hyperbaric conditions should be evaluated following decompression by a provider familiar with the examination of injured divers to assess for any signs or symptoms of decompression sickness. Individual department policy will dictate the duration of mandatory surveillance. However, considering the time frame for DCS onset, a period of several hours would be reasonable. Any symptoms which may be considered DCS should prompt rapid application of normobaric 100% oxygen while awaiting evaluation by a physician experienced in diving and hyperbaric medicine. This will begin treatment of any early bubble formation through the "oxygen window" of inherent unsaturation. Alternative causes of symptoms, particularly those which have time-dependent interventions such as myocardial infarction and stroke, need to be ruled out as soon as possible. Likewise, injuries which would be DCS mimics, especially those contraindicated to pressurization, would need to be ruled out. Examples of these conditions include inner ear barotrauma as well as baroparesis, a condition in which elevated pressure in the middle ear or sinus can cause unilateral paralysis of the facial nerve, mimicking a stroke.

In the absence of alternative diagnosis and contraindications to recompression, definitive treatment for DCS should be begun as soon as possible. Treatment tables should be selected based on the presenting condition, capabilities of the staff, and equipment present. Likely the most commonly used treatment tables for DCS are those from the US Navy, though alternative tables from the Royal Navy, commercial diving companies, and proprietary tables are also used around the world. A complete discussion of each table is beyond the scope of this chapter, but commonly used treatment tables will be discussed here with emphasis on their intended use, equipment required, and relative risk.

US Navy Treatment Table 5

The USN TT5 is a relatively short 60 fsw oxygen table used primarily for omitted decompression in divers/IAs as well as minimal cases of musculoskeletal DCS. Benefits of this table include its relatively low pressure, shorter duration, and resulting lack of need for specialized treatment gases. Multiplace chambers of all capabilities should be able to provide the 60 fsw depth and 100% oxygen breathing gas required for this table's successful completion. This table can be used in cases where proper decompression of an IA does not occur due to an emergency, such as surfacing the chamber for medical treatment of a patient. IAs without symptoms upon surfacing can be treated with a USN TT5 with a high degree of success in preventing DCS. The USN TT5 can also be used in cases of mild musculoskeletal DCS in which a full neurological exam has ruled out any suggestion of neurological compromise.[16] However, the often subtle presence of neurological signs and symptoms makes confident use of the TT5 difficult in cases of DCS. Additionally, all symptoms must resolve within the first 10 minutes of oxygen breathing for USN TT5 to continue. Otherwise, the longer USN TT6 should be used.[17]

USN Treatment Table 6

The USN TT6 is a 60 fsw oxygen table commonly used for the treatment of musculoskeletal and neurological DCS as well as air gas embolism. This table utilizes oxygen breathing at both 60 and 30 fsw pressure and can be extended 40 additional minutes of oxygen breathing at 60 fsw and 120 minutes of oxygen breathing at 30 fsw.[17] It has shown a high degree of efficacy in treatment of DCS[16] and air gas embolism, and its 60 fsw pressure and oxygen treatment gas make it available to all multiplace centers.

Comex 30

This is a 100 fsw nitrox or heliox table which can be used when symptoms do not respond to compression to the 60 fsw depths of the USN TT6 or similar RN tables. It does require the availability of more specialized treatment gases and will expose IAs to higher nitrogen pressures and loading during the table. Thus, this table will require both more sophistication in chamber equipment as well as a higher degree of experience in treating personnel to avoid complications during its use.

USN TT6A and TT6A modified

These are 165 fsw/6 ATA mixed gas treatment tables generally used for either symptoms refractory to the initial compression to 60 fsw or for significant symptoms primarily from deeper dives.[17] USN TT6A and the later modifications require enriched oxygen blends for breathing at the 6 ATA depths, generally 50:50 nitrox or heliox, as well as 100% oxygen for the shallower depths. This requires a greater degree of both facility and staff sophistication for safe completion. US Navy TT6A can be considered at the appropriate facility when significant symptoms do not respond to the initial compression to 60 fsw on a USN TT6 or similar table or as an initial treatment for serious symptoms following a deep pressure exposure.

USN TT4

This is a deep treatment table which allows longer periods of time for resolution of symptoms when compression to deeper depths is required. It also allows safe exit from tables such as a Comex 30 or USN TT6A if the allowed time at the deeper depths is exceeded. Due to the complexities of this table, it should be reserved for experienced personnel in centers with adequate physical and institutional support.

Post DCS Treatment Care and Evaluation

Following treatment for decompression sickness, staff should be evaluated by a physician knowledgeable in diving and hyperbaric medicine to determine efficacy of treatment, presence of complications, need for possible recurring/tailing treatments, and eligibility to return to work. While use of the standard US Navy treatment tables (and therefore equivalent Royal Navy tables) has shown a >95% efficacy in treatment of DCS when used properly,[16] IAs being treated for DCS should have a thorough evaluation by a hyperbaric physician following completion of their initial treatment table to determine if residual signs and symptoms are present, particularly neurological deficits. Presence of persistent symptoms may warrant recompression, either acutely or in the form of recurring daily treatments. If mild symptoms persist, recurring lower pressure (2.4 ATA) treatments are often prescribed until resolution or a plateau in improvement occurs. Assessment for hyperbaric side effects such as barotrauma and oxygen toxicity should also be made. Finally, at the conclusion of all therapy, an evaluation of the attendant's fitness to return to duty needs to be made. This will encompass an assessment of the risk for future decompression illness and may include evaluations for patent foramen ovale and other predisposing conditions. It will also document any residual signs and symptoms which may make diagnosis of a future DCS event difficult. The attendant's emotional response to both the injury and the prospect of returning to the environment in which the injury occurred will also need to be addressed.

Prevention of IA DCS

Given the repetitive decompression stresses inherent in the performance of IA duties, it is important to examine ways in which the risks of DCS can be minimized. In the examination of DCS incidence earlier in this chapter, several areas of possible improvement have been identified. In addition, there are other interventions which could also yield important improvements in the cumulative risk of IA DCS. The first area to examine is the obvious contribution of depth and time to nitrogen loading and decompression stress. As was shown in the report by Dunford,[3] treatment depth has a direct relationship to risk of DCS in IAs. Thus, every effort should be made to treat at the lowest appropriate depth based on patient condition. While most indications for HBOT have relatively narrow treatment guidelines, there is some variation in the tables used. Choosing the lowest appropriate treatment pressure will help to limit IA DCS risk. Likewise, there is variability of treatment duration among many centers. Department policy on the use of treatment tables should take into account the safe and appropriate minimization of exposure time within clinical guidelines. Further, if the treatment depth and duration cannot be changed, then limiting the IA exposure can be accomplished by the use of more than one tender during therapy. Rotation of IAs allows the exposure time to be divided among more than one person, thus reducing time at pressure and risk of DCS. It can have an added safety benefit in the case of an emergency decompression of the chamber due to patient deterioration or environmental emergency. If this occurs later in the treatment profile, a tender who entered the chamber later will have a lower inert gas load and a lower risk of decompression illness. However, this measure does require a larger staffing pool, which may be difficult in many centers.

The risk of IA DCS can also be reduced through the implementation of IA oxygen breathing during portions of the treatment profile. In the reports reviewed earlier, those centers who reported a 0% incidence of DCS in their IAs universally employed oxygen breathing by IAs at some time during their chamber time.[11,14-15] Oxygen breathing while at depth, either during the isobaric phase or during decompression, dramatically reduces arterial nitrogen partial pressure, and therefore, begins the rapid elimination of nitrogen accumulated in tissues. Hyperbaric oxygen exposure can also serve to eliminate any subclinical bubble formation which may be occurring during decompression through the effect of inherent unsaturation. As the study by Cooper[12] showed, bubble formation occurs even in those who show no clinical signs of illness. Oxygen breathing periods can be implemented at several times during a treatment profile, during decompression, as well as the later minutes of the isobaric phase. An approach similar to that reported by both Uzun[14] and Wituke[15] can be employed, with oxygen breathing by IAs during decompression, as well as during later stages of the isobaric phase based on the bottom time. As it is important to minimize the risk of IA central nervous system oxygen toxicity and resulting seizure, oxygen breathing periods should not be during periods of increased tender activity. Additionally, delivery masks should not be secured to the face so that in the event of convulsion, the oxygen delivery device will spontaneously separate, returning the IA to normal air breathing and reducing oxygen partial pressure.

Special consideration should be given during the use of deeper and longer treatment tables, as these have been shown to carry a greater risk of decompression illness for IAs. The previously discussed findings by Dunford[3] supported increased risk for deeper tables. In addition, in the years following their institution of IA oxygen breathing, five cases of IA DCS occurred, of which 60% were during a USN TT6 or 3 ATA table.[4] In hyperbaric medical practice, several treatment tables can be considered higher risk based on their depth and duration. Common examples of these will be USN TT6 and 6A used for decompression illness, carbon monoxide tables, as well as gas gangrene treatment tables. These all involve treatment pressures at or above 2.8 ATA and longer treatment times, which impose greater nitrogen loading on IAs. As an illustration of the increased risk of these tables, Thalmann[18] published the DCS risk of IAs on a USN TT6 in 1996 during review of US Navy recompression tables. The risk of DCS to an IA without supplemental oxygen breathing during a USN TT6 was 6.2%. This nearly doubled to 11.1% if the table was extended. In contrast, these numbers were cut in half if the attendants breathed oxygen for the 30-minute decompression and reduced to nearly zero if they were provided oxygen for the final 60 minutes at 30 fsw in addition to during decompression. These findings led to the revision of IA decompression during US Navy treatment tables. This highlights the importance of IA oxygen breathing, particularly in deeper and longer tables. For the US Navy tables, guidelines for IA oxygen breathing are given in the respective tables and should be strictly followed to reduce the risk of DCS to an acceptable level.

It is generally accepted that increased activity while at elevated pressures can result in increased tissue inert gas loading.[19] IAs may be required to exert themselves while at depth, and this increased activity could result in higher tissue nitrogen loading and increased risk of DCS. Examples of such activity could be lifting or moving patients, restraint of combative patients, cardiopulmonary resuscitation (CPR), fire extinguishment, etc. A decompression profile which has previously shown a low risk for attendant DCS may benefit from the addition of oxygen breathing or the increase in oxygen breathing time, in the case of significant IA physical exertion while at depth.

Another possible risk reduction strategy is the use of oxygen prebreathing prior to compression, as was suggested in the recent article by Clarke.[5] This strategy is well established in the high altitude aviation and space literature and has been shown to reduce the risk of altitude decompression illness in both pilots and astronauts. Possible benefits of this approach are the reduction in tissue nitrogen loading as well as the elimination of preexisting inert gas microbubbles which may serve as nuclei during decompression stress. Oxygen prebreathing has also been shown to reduce bubble formation in scuba divers. Castagna[20] studied divers conducting a series of two dives each to 100 fsw for 30 minutes. They were separated by a two-hour surface interval. Study participants received either no oxygen, 30 minutes of oxygen prebreathing before the first dive, 30 minutes of oxygen breathing before the second dive, or oxygen prebreathing before both dives. All combinations of oxygen prebreathing showed reduction in Doppler bubble grade compared to the control group. Balestra[21] also showed reduced bubble grade following oxygen prebreathing in divers. Incorporation of IA oxygen prebreathing could be a low impact intervention in circumstances where risk of decompression sickness was felt to be elevated, such as in the deeper and longer treatment tables. Normobaric high-flow oxygen breathing could be undertaken by the IA as the patient and chamber are being prepared for the treatment and would not require specialized equipment or safety procedures. As oxygen partial pressure would not exceed one ATA, risk of CNS oxygen toxicity would not be significantly increased.

Proper postdecompression procedures should be followed to further reduce the risk of DCS among IAs. As is recommended for other pressurized gas workers, avoidance of activity which may lead to bubble formation or bypass of the pulmonary filter is important following decompression from elevated inert gas pressures. IAs, even if they decompressed on oxygen, have a residual inert gas load following decompression to surface pressures. This must be allowed to properly exit the tissues and be eliminated through the lungs. Numerous conditions can interfere with this process and expose the IA to increased risk of pathologic bubble formation or allow bubbles to bypass the lungs and enter the arterial circulation. First, significant reduction in ambient pressure must be avoided, as this will reduce the partial pressure of nitrogen in the blood and increase bubble formation. Most commonly, this will occur on ascent to altitude. IAs should avoid flying or ascending to altitude for a minimum of 18-24 hours following any hyperbaric exposure in which they breathed inert gas. This mirrors current US Navy repetitive diving table recommendations,[17] as well as those of several recreational diving organizations. The importance of this prohibition is evident in the experience outlined earlier by Van den Broek[13] in which IAs experienced DCS following ascent to altitude after undergoing a profile with a previously described high safety record. Significant physical activity, particularly which involves Valsalva or straining should also be avoided. Such activity can risk passage of asymptomatic venous bubbles to the arterial circulation through a previously undetected patent foramen ovale or other shunt.[22] Significant physical exertion is also felt to increase nitrogen release from tissues, and though there remains some discussion of its relative risk to DCS, significant physical activity following inert gas loading is generally not recommended.[19]

Finally, the proper screening and selection of IAs prior to their exposure to the rigors of hyperbaric conditions will help to reduce the incidence of DCS among IAs. The hyperbaric environment places unique demands on staff, which are not encountered in other areas of the health care environment. Thus, initial selection of IAs should seek to identify those with any conditions which may predispose to decompression sickness or other complications of hyperbaric exposure. A full discussion of fitness to dive is beyond the scope of this chapter. However, commonly accepted guidelines from such sources as the US Navy, the Association of Diving Contractors, the UHMS, and recreational diving societies such as the British Sub Aqua Club can provide guidance for the proper evaluation of prospective IAs. Assessment of fitness to work in a pressurized environment should be performed by providers experienced in UHM. Finally, ongoing assessment of staff at periodic intervals should be undertaken to identify any changes in the medical status of IAs, which may disqualify them from work at pressure.

Conclusion

Hyperbaric IAs are exposed to decompression stresses as part of the routine performances of their duties. The degree of this stress is determined greatly by the depth and time of the treatment tables being used at their place of employment. While tables in common use have generally been subject to rigorous evaluation to ensure that they impart a minimal risk of decompression sickness, this risk is not zero. Even a small risk of injury on an individual dive can correlate with an unacceptable cumulative risk over a career as an IA. Thus, every effort should be devoted to ensuring that the risk of DCS is minimized for those working in the delivery of HBOT. This effort should cover all aspects of the IAs' work environment, including the selection of prospective providers, the treatment tables being used, the addition of IA oxygen breathing, surveillance of staff, proper postdive activity, and ongoing incident analysis. IAs should be carefully evaluated for any signs or symptoms suggestive of DCS, and any resulting cases treated promptly with current industry-accepted treatment tables. Treatment should be performed in accordance with the capabilities of the facility, and the knowledge and experience of the supervising physician. Periodic review of these procedures should be undertaken to ensure the chaotic experience of a provider becoming a patient at their own chamber is handled in the best possible manner. Lastly, it is the hope of the author and others tasked with the provision of and education in hyperbaric medicine that hyperbaric facilities and providers share their experiences in this area so that the field can advance together toward a goal of zero injuries.

References

1. Boycott AE, Damant GCC, Haldane JS. Prevention of compressed illness. *J Hyg.* 1908;8:342-443.
2. Anderson B, Whalen RE, Saltzman HA, et al. Dysbarism among hyperbaric personnel. *JAMA.* 1964:190(12):87-89.
3. Dunford RD, Hampson NB. Gender-related risk of decompression sickness in hyperbaric chamber inside attendants: a case control study. *Undersea Biomed Res.* 1992;19(SUPPL):37.
4. Clarke R. Health care worker decompression sickness: incidence, risk, and mitigation. *UHM.* 2017;44(6):509-519.
5. Hyperbaric nurse dies of decompression sickness: unit gets OK. *Hosp Secur Safe Manage.* 1992;13(5):3.
6. District Court of Appeal of Florida, First District. No 94-549 Harley L Vause v Bay Medical Center & Douglas L. Stringer. December 30, 1996.
7. Dietz SK, Myers RA. Decompression illness in HBO inside tenders: a review of 23 years of exposures. *Undersea Hyperb Med.* 1995;22(Suppl):57.

8. Brattebo G, Aanderud L, Riseberg J, et al. Incidence of decompression illness among HBO nurses. Proceedings: 23rd Annual Scientific Meeting EUBS 1997.
9. Pontani BA, Alexander K, Geiger J, Williams RL. 10,000 dives: A review of inside attendant decompression events in a multiplace hyperbaric chamber. Abstract of the Undersea and Hyperbaric Medical Society, Inc. Annual Scientific Meeting June 14-16, 2007. Ritz-Carlton Kapalua Maui, Hawaii.
10. OSHA. *www.osha.gov/pls/imis/accidentsearch.accident_detail?id=170902555.*
11. Cooper PD, Van Den Broek C, Smart DR, et al. Hyperbaric chamber attendant safety II: 14 year health review of multiplace chamber attendants. *Diving Hyperb Med.* 2009;39(2):71-76.
12. Cooper PD, Van Den Broek C, Smart DR, et al. Hyperbaric chamber attendant safety I: Doppler analysis of decompression stress in multiplace chamber attendants. *Diving Hyperb Med.* 2009;39(2):63-70.
13. Van den Broek C. Two cases of decompression sickness in nurse attendants due to a lapse in protocols. XIX International Congress on Hyperbaric Medicine, May 2017 Belgrade, Serbia.
14. Uzun G, Mutluoglu M, Ay H, et al. Decompression sickness in hyperbaric nurses: retrospective analysis of 4500 treatments. *J Clin Nurs.* 2011;20(11-12):1784-1787.
15. Witucki P, Duchnick J, Neuman T, et al. Incidence of DCS and oxygen toxicity in chamber attendants: a 28 year experience. *Undersea Hyperb Med.* 2013;40(4):345-350.
16. Green JW, Tichenor J, Curley MD. Treatment of Type I decompression sickness using the US Navy treatment algorithms. *Undersea Biomed Res.* 1989;16:469-470.
17. US Navy Diving Manual Revision 7, December 2016. Wash DC: Superintendent of Documents, U.S Government Printing Office; 2016.
18. Thalmann ED. Principles of US Navy recompression treatments for decompression sickness. In: Moon RE, Sheffield PJ editors. Treatment of decompression illness. 45th UHMS workshop. Kensington, MD: Undersea and Hyperbaric Medical Society. 1996:75-95.
19. Vann RD. Mechanisms and risks of decompression. In: Bove, AA, editor. Bove and Davis's Diving Medicine, 4th Ed. Philadelphia: Saunders. 2003;141-143.
20. Castagna O, Gempp E, Blatteau JE, et al. Pre-dive normobaric oxygen reduces bubble formation in scuba divers. *Eur J Appl Physiol.* 2009;106(2):167-172.
21. Balestra C, Theunissen S, Papadopoulou V, Le Mener C, Germonpre P, et al. Pre-dive whole body vibration better reduces decompression-induced vascular gas emboli than oxygen or a combination of both. *Front Physiol.* 2016;7:586.
22. Dear GD, Kisslo JA, Adams DB, et al: The effect of immersion and exercise on right-to-left shunt through a patent foramen ovale. *Undersea Hyper Med.* 1993;20(suppl):82.

CHAPTER 10
Clinical Hyperbaric Facility Accreditation —Process Improvement in Action

Wilbur T. Workman, BS, MS, CAsP, CHT-A, FAsMA, FUHM

Author's Note: This chapter was originally published in *Hyperbaric Medicine Practice, 4th Edition,* H.T. Whelan, Editor, Best Publishing Company, 2017.[1] It has been updated as required.

Introduction

In the late 1970s, there were fewer than 30 hyperbaric facilities operational in the United States. Most were military, commercial, or highly specialized research facilities. It is estimated that there are now around 1,350 programs operating in hospitals and hospital-affiliated facilities.[2] Over the years, the primary role of hyperbaric facilities has transitioned from the treatment of diving-related disorders to providing an important primary and adjunct treatment modality for multiple medical conditions. Refined research efforts will no doubt validate continued efficacy and support new indications. The location of facilities is expanding from hospital-based to nonaffiliated outpatient settings, some with appropriate medical supervision, others without. In the past decade, certification in hyperbaric technology and hyperbaric nursing has become a staffing requirement in growing number of programs. After years of dedicated efforts by many of their members, the Undersea and Hyperbaric Medical Society (UHMS), the American Board of Preventive Medicine, the American Board of Emergency Physicians, and the American Osteopathic Association have established board certification for physicians in Undersea and Hyperbaric Medicine. Minimum recommended staffing and training standards were first presented in the UHMS' *Operations Committee Report* in 2000.[3] These recommendations are now an important part of a more comprehensive set of guidelines and recommended practices. *The UHMS Guidelines for Hyperbaric Facility Operations, 2nd Edition* set these foundational standards of practice for hyperbaric medicine.[4]

Each of these milestones reflect a continuing maturation and professional recognition of clinical hyperbaric medicine in the United States. As in any growth process, success has not come easy. There are still many challenges that must be faced. There have been many in the field of hyperbaric medicine that felt an appropriate response to these challenges was to create an external means of quality assurance and performance improvement: a formal clinical hyperbaric facility accreditation program. Programs that evaluate the adequacy of the facility and equipment, the appropriateness of the staff and their training, quality of care, and patient safety have proven useful to professional organizations in ensuring that quality is maintained within their specialty. In 2000, the UHMS accepted this challenge and established a professional, comprehensive clinical hyperbaric facility accreditation program.

The UHMS believes that such a program is the most efficient method to ensure the following:

- Clinical hyperbaric facilities are staffed with the proper specialists who are well-trained.
- Clinical hyperbaric facilities are using quality equipment that has been properly installed and maintained and being operated with the highest level of safety possible.
- Clinical hyperbaric facilities are providing high quality of patient care.
- Clinical hyperbaric facilities are maintaining the appropriate documentation of informed consent, patient treatment procedures, physician involvement, etc.[5]

Background

At the present time, there are approximately 18 different organizations in the United States that have some level of interest in the practice of hyperbaric medicine.[2] They range from federal agencies such as the Centers for Medicare and Medicaid Services (CMS/Medicare), the Food and Drug Administration (FDA), and codes and standards organizations like the National Fire Protection Association (NFPA) to professional groups like the UHMS, the American College of Hyperbaric Medicine (ACHM), the Baromedical Nurses Association (BNA), and the National Board of Diving & Hyperbaric Medicine (NBDHMT). With the exception of the professional medical groups, there is little effort to coordinate among these organizations to foster a greater understanding of our community and on matters important to us.

Many advantages can result from accreditation and thus impact the regulatory environment, individual hyperbaric facilities and programs, and the specialty of hyperbaric medicine. Of immediate importance is the community response to the regulatory climate. In October 2000, the Office of the Inspector General (OIG) of the Department of Health and Human Services released a report on "Hyperbaric Oxygen Therapy: Its Usefulness and Appropriateness."[6] Among its findings, the OIG reported that a lack of testing and treatment monitoring raised a variety of quality of care concerns and that the Health Care Finance Administration (HCFA) (now CMS) guidance to the field of hyperbaric medicine was limited. Specific OIG recommendations were for HCFA to initiate a national coverage decision policy for HBO_2, improve policy guidance (e.g., practice guidelines and physician attendance policy), and improve oversight by requiring contractors to initiate edits and consistent medical review procedures and by exploring the creation of a national registry of facilities and/or physicians. This report laid the foundation for increased government involvement and intervention. By creating a national clinical hyperbaric facility accreditation program, the UHMS responded proactively to the OIG findings and recommendations. This action was a sign to the various regulatory agencies that the organized hyperbaric medical community was concerned with our current situation. It responded to the recognized need to promote, achieve, and maintain quality of care and patient safety across the continuum of clinical hyperbaric facilities.

Equally important are the advantages that an accredited clinical hyperbaric facility may realize. Though not all-inclusive, some of the more immediate are the following:

- Improved quality of care
- Enhanced patient safety
- Increased efficiency at the facility level
- More effective risk management programs
- Outward symbol of code compliance and adherence to recognized standards of practice
- Possibly lower liability insurance premiums
- Staff motivation and esprit de corps
- Maximized public relations and marketing efforts
- Ability to recruit and retain quality staff
- Develop alliances with other provider groups
- Establish credibility of legitimate nonaffiliated outpatient facilities among their professional referral base

Achieving the regulatory and facility level advantages provides the foundation for significant advancements in the acceptance and credibility of hyperbaric medicine as a growing, recognized medical specialty thus enhancing professional organizations such as the UHMS, the ACHM, the BNA, and the NBDHMT, who are at the forefront of the field. Further, a successful accreditation program brings hyperbaric medicine in-line with many other specialties such as radiation oncology and rehabilitative medicine, each who sponsors specific accreditation programs for their respective specialty and will help establish nationally recognized standards of practice for clinical hyperbaric medicine.

Program Design

The focus areas of the UHMS accreditation program are a compilation of national codes and standards that relate to hyperbaric medicine and facilities as well as common quality of care improvement areas as defined by accrediting organizations such as The Joint Commission (TJC), Commission on Accreditation of Rehabilitation Facilities (CARF) and Det Norske Veritas-Germannishcer Lloyd (DNV-GL). Central to the areas that represent compliance to national codes and standards are referenced from the National Fire Protection Association's (NFPA) *Health Care Facilities Code (NFPA 99)*; the NFPA's *Life Safety Code (NFPA 101); the American Society of Mechanical Engineers' Code for Pressure Vessels for Human Occupancy (ASME PVHO-1* and *ASME PVHO-2);* the Compressed Gas Association, and others. The focus areas related to staff, training, certification, physician credentialing, supervision, continuing education, etc., are adopted from the *UHMS Guidelines for Hyperbaric Facility Operations, 2nd Edition.*

The above compilation is represented in 24 concentration areas:[5]

- Governance
- Administration
- Operations
- Maintenance
- Facility Construction
- Hyperbaric Chamber Fabrication
- Hyperbaric Chamber Ventilation
- Hyperbaric Chamber Fire Protection
- Hyperbaric Chamber Electrical Systems and Services
- Hyperbaric Gas Handling
- Patient Rights
- Patient Assessment
- Patient Care
- Environment of Care
- Patient Education
- Quality Improvement
- Professional Improvement
- Leadership
- Human Resources
- Information Management
- Infection Control
- Medical Staff
- Teaching and Publication
- Clinical Research

Surveys are conducted by a voluntary team of three highly experienced members: a hyperbaric physician, board-certified hyperbaric nurse, and board-certified technologist. Each survey is two full days to allow the team sufficient time to evaluate compliance to all concentration areas noted above. Each facility is provided a written report of the assessment and recommended improvement areas are identified.

The survey teams do not make the determination for accreditation; that responsibility resides with the UHMS Accreditation Council (AC). Membership of the AC is comprised of a cross-section of UHMS members representing physicians, nurses, and technologists. The AC responds to each survey report in the following manner:

- Accredit (valid for three years)
- Accredit with a written plan of action
- Accredit after a written plan of action has been completed
- Accredit with distinction (valid for four years)
- Do not accredit

Status

As of June 30, 2018, the UHMS had accredited a total of 262 hyperbaric medicine programs, four of which are international. Of the remaining 258, eight were facilities that were not affiliated with a health care system, resulting in approximately 20% of the hospital-affiliated hyperbaric medicine programs in the country being accredited.[2]

This figure is impressive since, with few exceptions, participation is voluntary. There are two notable exceptions. Beginning in 2006, the Utah Medicaid Management Office mandated UHMS-specific accreditation in order for facilities to receive Medicaid funding for hyperbaric oxygen therapy. In 2014, the third-party payor Mohawk Valley Physicians (MVP) began requiring facility accreditation for their beneficiaries in upstate New York, Vermont, and New Hampshire who required hyperbaric oxygen therapy (HBOT). More specifically, MVP stipulated that physicians, in order to receive payment, must be on staff at an accredited facility.

Hyperbaric facility accreditation has not gone unnoticed by Medicare. In a 2013 draft Local Coverage Determination (LCD) for HBOT published by Novitas-Solutions, Inc., a major Medicare Administrative Contractor (MAC) with jurisdiction in 11 states, proposed that UHMS hyperbaric facility accreditation be a mandate for Medicare reimbursement.[7] While this requirement was not retained in what was to be the final LCD, it represented a major acknowledgement of the program and its potential link to Medicare reimbursement on a broad scale. Many believe this is a sign of things to come.

There are those who recognize there are a variety of issues common to the hyperbaric medicine community regardless of the country of operation. This is especially true when you consider those related to hyperbaric facility safety. This is one common bond that ties the international hyperbaric community together. As a result, the UHMS has been honored to have been asked by international facilities to evaluate their programs for accreditation. Thus, the UHMS has accredited programs in Brazil, Canada, Singapore, and Thailand.

Opportunities for Improvement

Preparing for an accreditation survey is a lot of work. There are those who might question if the effort is worth it. If the process does not add value, then why bother? After 18 years of effort, the UHMS can say the process has merit and demonstrated success in improving the quality of care and patient safety elements in those facilities that have accepted the challenge. Equally important, it has identified a number of areas where opportunities for improvement are most evident. Several of these areas are quite surprising.

The biggest surprise is related to the privileging process for physicians. UHMS accreditation surveyors frequently discover weak or nonexisting policies regarding the granting of physician privileges specifically for hyperbaric medicine. Surveyors have even documented instances in which hyperbaric physicians were not credentialed for hyperbaric medicine at all yet they were routinely supervising the treatment of hyperbaric patients! An even more egregious omission was one hospital allowing physicians to practice hyperbaric medicine with no formal training in the specialty! This is not acceptable.

Given the significant growth in the number of clinical hyperbaric facilities over the recent past, it is difficult for new programs to start out initially with a fully trained and experienced staff. Simply completing a recognized 40-hour introductory course in hyperbaric medicine does not make one a physician, nurse, or technical hyperbaricist! They have only begun their journey to become one. Programs operating with an inexperienced staff should recognize this limitation and be especially observant and supportive of each other to minimize the potential for an operational or clinical misstep.

In the ideal world, once a program is fully staffed with experienced personnel, the staff complement would stabilize. Unfortunately, this is not the case as people come and go as their situation dictates. Staff turnover has proven to be a challenge to most facilities. Surveyors rarely find a process to proctor physicians new to the specialty and/or facility for a period of time before they are granted full unsupervised privileges. Credentialing bodies seem to be receptive to allowing a physician who has just completed a recognized 40-hour introductory course in hyperbaric medicine to independently supervise patients. This, too, is not acceptable.

Currency of continuing medical education (CME) related to hyperbaric medicine is also lacking. It is common to survey a facility in which physicians have been practicing for 20 years and have not had a hyperbaric related CME since their initial course. Can they be considered current in the specialty? I suggest not.

While these opportunities for improvement are prevalent, the UHMS has found that medical staff offices are very receptive to guidance that the UHMS can provide. An excellent source for such guidance is the *UHMS Guidelines for Hyperbaric Facility Operations, 2nd Edition*[4] which includes a complete section on recommendations for credentialing, etc.

With regard to nurses and allied health care providers such as respiratory therapists, etc., specialty-specific board certification is not yet the norm. While improvements have been made in recent years in the number of nurses and allied health care providers who are board-certified as a certified hyperbaric registered nurse (CHRN) or a certified hyperbaric technologist (CHT), there is still much upside potential. For example, as of October 1, 2018, there were 1,402 active CHTs and 611 active CHRNs.[8] Hospitals are strongly encouraged to make board certification a requirement for employment. Proactive hospitals occasionally require certification within two years of employment. This is a reasonable goal.

From an operational safety perspective, one of the biggest concerns is the failure of the designated hyperbaric safety director to assume the responsibilities of the position as outlined in the current *NFPA 99, Health Care Facilities Code.*[9] When the NFPA first established hyperbaric facility safety standards in 1968, they recognized the importance of a hyperbaric facility safety director and stipulated that one be designated at each facility. This requirement went largely ignored until the UHMS implemented their accreditation program in 2000 and surveyors began assessing this requirement. While hyperbaric safety directors are now common in hospital-based or affiliated programs, they are scarce in nonaffiliated, freestanding centers.

Even though safety directors are now being designated in the hospital setting, many are not fulfilling their obligations with regard to creating and managing a comprehensive hyperbaric safety program. An all-too- common finding is the failure to conduct recurring medical and operational emergency drills so that the entire staff is competent in their execution. For many, conducting emergency drills stop at participating in hospital-directed fire drills. The practice of emergency procedures related to loss of chamber pressure, loss of power, communications, contaminated gas, etc., have been absent.

Closely related to the lack of safety director involvement is the availability of additional training to provide the safety director with the added knowledge and tools in order to better fulfill his/her responsibilities as a safety director. Over 18 years ago, there was any additional training that focused on the added skills necessary to be an effective safety director. Today, there are courses designed to do just that. All hyperbaric facilities, regardless of location or governance, should place this supplemental training on the highest priority for their safety director.

While examples of opportunities for improvement can be provided from each of the 24 hyperbaric facility accreditation concentration areas, those described here are trending as the most obvious.

External Recognition

The value of hyperbaric facility accreditation is not only evident from within the hyperbaric medicine community. The process is also recognized by organizations like The Joint Commission (TJC). TJC has a special program called The Cooperative Agreement Program, which was established to recognize alternative accrediting bodies representing medical specialties for which TJC surveyors might not have sufficient expertise or experience to allow them to conduct a meaningful assessment. Many of these specialties include a highly specialized technical component. For hyperbaric medicine, that specialized component is the hyperbaric chamber itself. The UHMS is very proud that their accreditation program is one of four such programs that have been formally endorsed by TJC as a complementary accrediting body.[10]

Equally important to the external awareness of added value for the hyperbaric medicine community is the parallel acknowledgment of compliance to time-honored, internationally recognized management principles of process improvement and the implementation of quality systems control. The UHMS Clinical Hyperbaric Facility Accreditation Program enjoys the singular distinction of being the only ISO 9001-2015 certified hyperbaric facility accrediting program in the world.[2]

International Expansion

Prior to 2000 and the creation of the UHMS program, there was only one other international effort to implement a meaningful facility accreditation program. This process, which was initially conceived by Dr. John Ross of Aberdeen, Scotland, was developed and managed by the British Hyperbaric Association (BHA). This watershed event, along with the unparalleled success of the UHMS program, has stimulated significant interest within the greater international hyperbaric medicine community. Programs now exist, or are under strategic development, in South Africa, Brazil, Canada, and the United Kingdom.

In countries where professional hyperbaric medicine societies and hyperbaric specific codes or standards do not exist, program leaders are beginning to seek accreditation through the UHMS. As an international medical society, the UHMS has successfully demonstrated that their process is easily tailored to a specific country's need and that the program standards can be equitably applied to their need. Thus far, the UHMS has accredited programs in Brazil, Canada, Singapore, and Thailand and are working with programs in Saudi Arabia to further expand the program to be truly international.

Summary

Over 18 years ago, meaningful hyperbaric facility accreditation did not exist. Today, it is quickly becoming the gold standard throughout the world as an outward symbol of quality of care and patient safety. Facilities that spend the energy to prepare for an accreditation survey and can demonstrate compliance to high quality and safety standards, are rewarded with the pride that comes along with mastering such a lofty standard. It is clear that staffs of accredited facilities take their responsibilities to their patients seriously and are playing an important role in improving the quality of care and safety one facility at a time. As each new program is added to the growing list of accredited facilities, quality of care and safety of the hyperbaric patient is raised across the entire hyperbaric medicine community. Equally important is that with each newly accredited program, the community is proactively addressing the findings of the infamous OIG report. In spite of accomplishments to date, opportunities for improvement remain numerous. While many believe that facility accreditation will eventually be linked to reimbursement by others beside Utah and Mohawk Valley Physicians, there is still reluctance from many to seek accreditation. There are others who believe the program has clear value and is the right thing to do. I stand with those who believe it is the right thing to do.

References

1. Workman WT. Clinical Hyperbaric Facility Accreditation-Process Improvement In Action, *Hyperbaric Medicine Practice, 4th Edition,* H.T. Whelan, Editor. North Palm Beach, FL: Best Publishing Company; 2017.
2. Undersea & Hyperbaric Medical Society. Hyperbaric Facility Accreditation Office. North Palm Beach, FL: UHMS.
3. Kimbrell PN, ed. Operations committee report. Kensington, MD: Undersea & Hyperbaric Medical Society; 2000.
4. Workman WT, ed. Guidelines for hyperbaric facility operations, 2nd Edition. North Palm Beach, FL: Best Publishing Company; 2015.
5. UHMS. Clinical hyperbaric facility accreditation manual, 4th edition. North Palm Beach, FL: UHMS; 2018.
6. Department of Health and Human Services, Office of the Inspector General. Hyperbaric oxygen therapy: its use and appropriateness. October 2000, OEI 06-99-00090.
7. Draft Local Coverage Determination (LCD) for Hyperbaric Oxygen (HBO) Therapy (L34794). Novitas Solutions, Inc.; January 16, 2014.
8. National Board of Diving & Hyperbaric Medical Technology. Columbia, SC. Email communication dated October 1, 2018.
9. National Fire Protection Association. NFPA 99, health care facilities code, 2018, chapter 14, hyperbaric facilities. Quincy, MA: National Fire Protection Association. 2018;99-121.
10. The Joint Commission. Oak Brook Terrace, IL. Available from https://www.jointcommission.org/facts about the cooperative accreditation initiative/ September 26, 2018.

Bibliography

1. Safety Standard for Pressure Vessels for Human Occupancy (ANSI ASME PVHO-1: 2016). NY: American Society of Mechanical Engineers; [cited 2018 October 1]. Available from: http://www.asme.org.
2. Safety Standard for Pressure Vessels for Human Occupancy In Service Guidelines (ANSI ASME PVHO-2: 2016) NY: American Society of Mechanical Engineers; [cited 2018 October 1]. Available from: http://www.asme.org.

CHAPTER 11
Safety in Animal Hyperbaric Oxygen Systems

Dennis Geiser, DVM, CHT-V and Shelena Hoberg, CHT, CHT-V

Introduction

Safety in the use of hyperbaric chambers for animal care is of primary importance and a major focus area for every hyperbaric program. Personnel and patient safety should be the primary focus. Prevention of incidents and emergencies should be the first consideration. Prevention is accomplished through adequate and proper personnel training, established operational protocols, and the use of certified equipment that is installed and housed in accordance with established safety standards.

A good hyperbaric safety program includes proper program oversight, knowledge, leadership, adherence to laws, standards and guidelines, adequate facilities, equipment constructed to accepted standards, personnel training and retraining, and the establishment of a risk assessment plan and emergency protocols.

Resources for Regulatory Guidance

An abbreviated list of governing and guiding bodies can be found in Table 1. At the writing of this chapter, work was still being done on defining more specific standards and guidelines for animal hyperbaric oxygen (HBO_2) therapy (HBOT). All standards are subject to periodic changes and it is the responsibility of the hyperbaric facility to keep up with the latest editions. Many of the standards and guidelines for human hyperbaric therapy also apply for its use in animals. Guidance for the production, inspection and certification of animal hyperbaric chambers should follow the same parameters as those used for human chambers [American Society of Mechanical Engineers (ASME) publishes the *Boiler and Pressure Vessel Code* (*BPVC*, 2017) and *ASME Pressure Vessels for Human Occupancy PVHO 1&2*, 2016].[1-2] Any alteration of the original pressure boundary requires retesting of that boundary before the chamber can be certified for use. The responsibility for maintenance and inspection of acrylic interfaces lies with the chamber user. The National Fire Protection Association's (NFPA) *NFPA 99, Health*

Care Facilities Code, NFPA 50, Standards for Bulk Oxygen Systems, and *NFPA 101, Life Safety Code* each contain information on the use of HBO_2 in humans. *NFPA 99,* Chapter 14 (2018) pertains to hyperbaric facilities and contains brief references to safety for Class C animal chambers. A separate standards document exists for fire and life safety in animal facilities (*NFPA 150, Fire and Life Safety in Animal Housing Facilities Code,* 2019). This document does not currently address the inclusion of a hyperbaric system in an animal facility. The Compressed Gas Association (CGA) publishes guidelines for the use of and handling compressed gases, gas containers, gas purity, and gas identification. These guidelines apply to the use of compressed gas regardless of the type of facility (industrial, medical, recreational, etc.). The Occupational Safety and Health Administration (OSHA) oversees facilities, equipment, and operations with regard to personnel safety. The Food and Drug Administration (FDA) considers a hyperbaric chamber as a Class II medical device. However, there is little oversight of chambers used for clinical hyperbaric therapy in animals. Other resources that provide guidance for the hyperbaric facility include the Veterinary Hyperbaric Medicine Society (VHMS), the Undersea and Hyperbaric Medical Society (UHMS), the National Board of Diving and Hyperbaric Medical Technology (NBDHMT), and the American Society for Testing and Materials (ASTM). They also provide information on material oxygen compatibility and device and system design for oxygen service.

Table 1. Governing and Guiding Organizations

Organization	Acronym
American Society of Mechanical Engineers	ASME
National Fire Protection Association	NFPA
Food and Drug Administration	FDA
American Society for Testing and Materials	ASTM
Compressed Gas Association	CGA
Resources	**Acronym**
Undersea and Hyperbaric Medical Society	UHMS
National Board of Diving and Hyperbaric Medical Technology	NBDHMT
Veterinary Hyperbaric Medicine Society	VHMS
International Hyperbaric Medicine Association	IHMA

Figure 1. Hyperbaric program oversight.

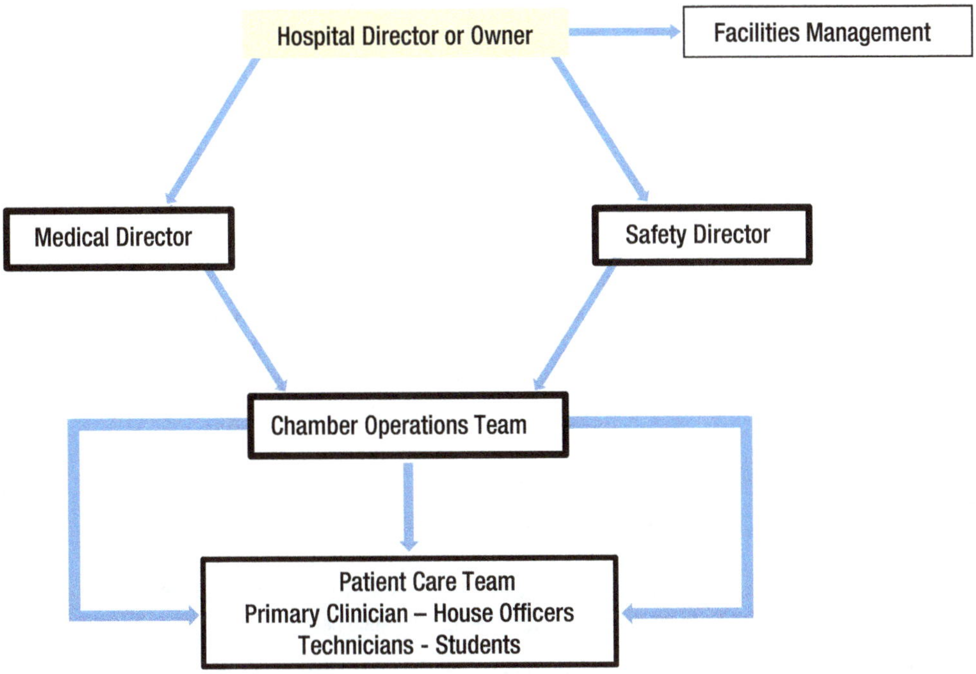

Clinical Hyperbaric Medicine Program – Oversight

The oversight of an animal hyperbaric medicine program and facility should follow the same basic template as that used in human hyperbaric programs, whether that program resides in a small veterinary practice or in a multiveterinarian referral center. The difference would be the scale. Management of the facility is critical in developing and deploying an effective safety program. Figure 1 summarizes the ideal hyperbaric program oversight scheme. This suggested scheme should not discourage the small center from providing animal hyperbaric services and managing a hyperbaric program. Often the roles mentioned here may be assumed by one person even though the team approach is ideal because it provides levels of checks and balances.

The responsibilities of medical director, safety director, and chamber operation team should include completion of a quality basic hyperbaric medicine course. In addition, the role of safety director connotes additional training in a quality safety director certificate course. Table 2 lists some of the responsibilities of each team responsible for the patient before, during, and after hyperbaric oxygen therapy. Although multiple roles can be assumed by one individual, there should be adequate redundancy in training so coverage of the hyperbaric treatment program is consistent. For example, appropriate coverage by adequately trained individuals occurs when someone is on vacation, ill, etc. This is important in maintaining continuity in the safety program for each facility.

Table 2. Responsibilities for Hyperbaric Patient Care and Safety

Position	Responsibilities
Hospital Director	• Manages all hospital operations – financial, facilities, personnel, communications, etc. • Might be the owner of a practice
Hyperbaric Medical Director	• Veterinarian • Working knowledge of HBOT • Knowledge of the side effects, contraindications, and their prevention/management • Makes recommendations concerning the efficacy of HBOT in patients in consultation with the primary care team • Recommends HBOT protocols for patients • Works in collaboration with the safety director to assure patient and personnel safety
Hyperbaric Safety Director	• Recognition of hazards • Policies and procedures development • Oversight of safety training and education • Analysis/problem solving – decision-making and risk assessment • Equipment and facilities maintenance needs
Chamber Operations Team	• Day-to-day chamber operation • Patient management • Chamber maintenance and hygiene
Primary Patient Care Team	• Works with HBOT medical director in making decisions for HBOT for each patient • All other care associated with the patient outside of HBOT, which includes treatments, diagnostics, etc. • Directs and coordinates other members of the primary care team

Animal HBO_2 Treatment Systems and Facilities

The following is a list of known animal-specific hyperbaric chamber manufacturers/distributors and a brief description of their product. Some of these distributors are no longer actively supplying vessels; however, their products are still in use. Note that different products will vary in design and operation, thus it is important that relevant in-service training be provided by the chamber manufacturer/distributor at time of purchase/installation.

VHO (veterinary hyperbaric oxygen, formerly equine oxygen therapy): US distributor of small and large animal chambers (manufactured in the United States initially by Gulf Coast Engineering). This chamber is pressurized using 100% O_2. As such, there are no other breathing apparatuses or inlet lines required. The chamber should be housed in a temperature-controlled room for patient comfort and safety. This chamber console operates pneumatically (operated by air). A separate compressed air supply is required to power the chamber control system. The console uses standard power supply for the LCD screen and other electric components. This chamber also has real time O_2% and inside chamber temperature and humidity readings. Electricity supplies the chamber lights and monitoring cameras. Later models from this company have a digital screen lock so power is required to pressurize. A backup battery provides power in the event of an outage. Decompression is possible with no power supply. The door is fully manual and requires nothing other than muscle to operate.

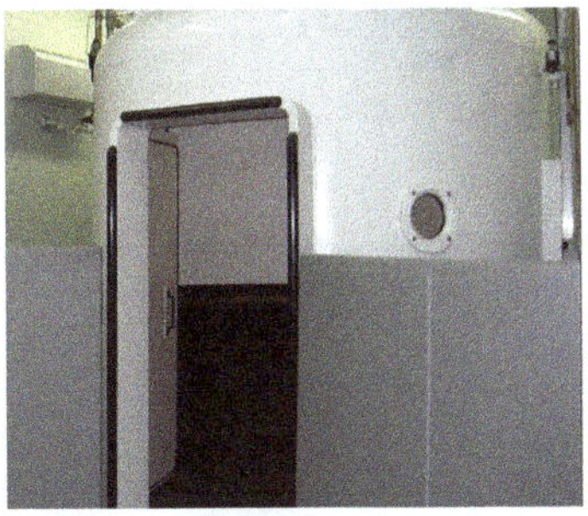

Figure 2. Veterinary hyperbaric oxygen (VHO) large animal chamber. Photo courtesy of S. Hoberg.

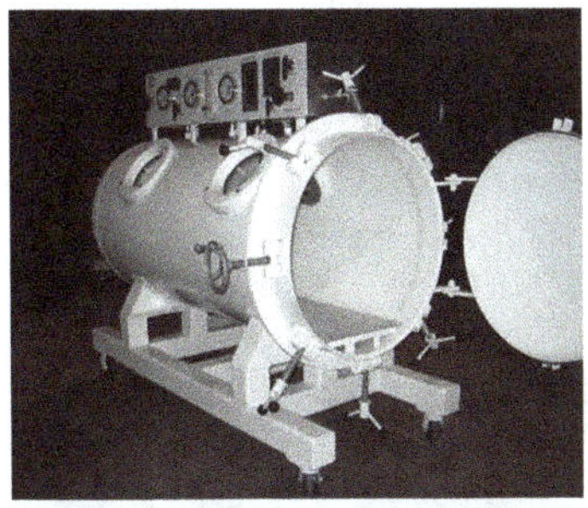

Figure 3. Veterinary hyperbaric oxygen (VHO) small animal chamber. Photo courtesy of S. Hoberg.

The purpose-built, steel-with-acrylic windows, small animal chamber offered by VHO is also compressed with O_2 and the controls are fully pneumatic using the O_2 supply. This chamber has real time O_2% and inside chamber temperature and humidity readings. Power is required externally for the lighting source. The door is fully manual. These chambers have minimal operational components and all operations are manual (including decompression).

MEHOT (mobile equine hyperbaric oxygen therapy): US provider of HBOT-vessels manufactured by Fink Engineering. The system is entirely self-contained, with the chamber and supporting plant assembled into a custom design standard width trailer which can easily be transported to where it is needed. Patients breathe 100% oxygen via masks while the chamber is pressurized with air. The chamber is constantly flushed with air throughout the treatment, providing ventilation and preventing the buildup of oxygen inside. The vessel can house two patients with the animals standing side by side as in a two-horse trailer.

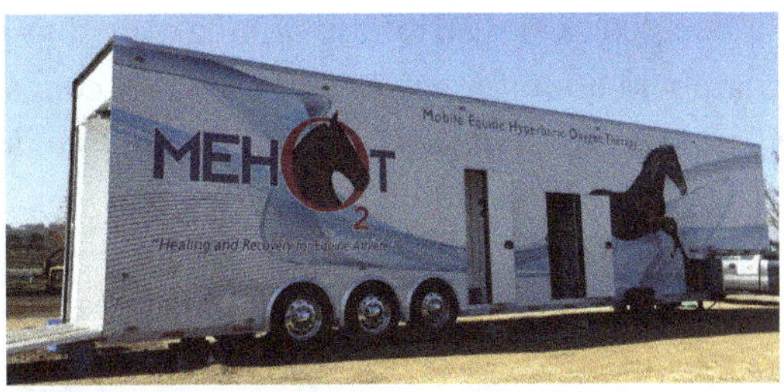

Figure 4. Mobile equine HBOT chamber. Photo courtesy of MEHOT.

HVM (hyperbaric veterinary medicine): US distributor of small animal chambers. This is a purpose-built, small-animal steel construction chamber with two viewing ports and video monitoring. Pressurized with 100% O_2, this chamber has real-time O_2% and temperature and humidity readings. Console controls are pneumatic using the O_2 supply with external power supplying lights, viewing cameras, and monitor. The door has a manual single-lock closure with safety pin that must be closed to allow pressurization.

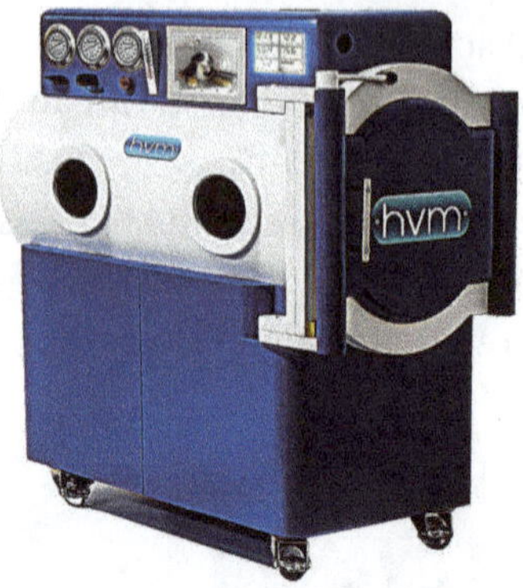

Figure 5. Hyperbaric veterinary medicine chamber. Photo courtesy of HVM.

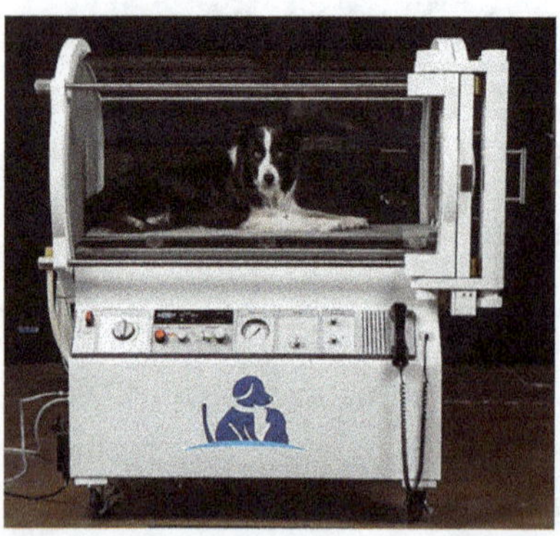

Figure 6. Sechrist animal hyperbaric chamber. Photo courtesy of Sechrist.

Sechrist: US distributor of human hyperbaric chambers, this company now offers chambers for veterinary use that have an acrylic cylindrical vessel with hyperbaric and enhanced O_2 dual modes.

Pet pressure: US distributor of inflatable low-pressure chambers. Low-pressure, fabric chambers do not meet ASME or NFPA codes even though FDA has approved them as Class II medical devices for the treatment of acute mountain sickness.

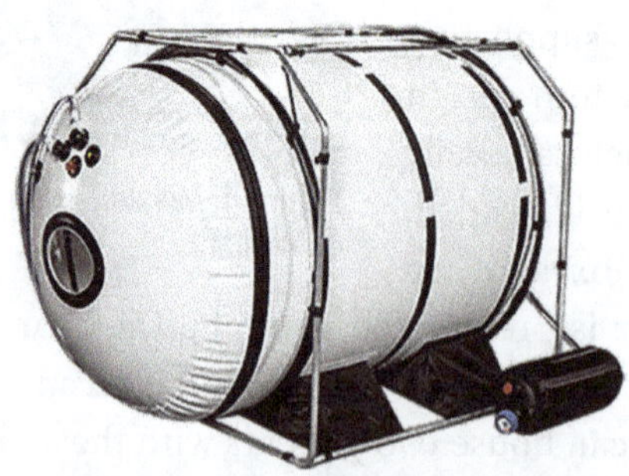

Figure 7. Pet pressure animal chamber.

The major components of all high-pressure animal chambers are similar. All clinical chambers require an oxygen supply, and for large volumes, this is usually a liquid O_2 (LOX) supply. LOX is a cryogenic liquid that may be stored in large fixed tanks or in smaller portable dewars. To convert the liquid to gaseous oxygen, an evaporator/heat exchanger is required to allow the liquid to warm and expand into gas while passing from the storage tank into the chamber. Other smaller dewar tanks are designed to store smaller volumes of LOX than fixed systems, are portable, and contain integral vaporizers. Low-pressure chambers or small volume designs typically utilize smaller, high-pressure (2,000 pounds per square inch [PSI]) gas-only O_2 tanks.

There are many other chambers in use for animals including research-style chambers (size suits small animals) and repurposed human chambers. Buyers should ensure the chamber they are considering for purchase is one that is built to the required standards of the country in which the chamber is used, and that it has not been decommissioned from previous use.

Hyperbaric chambers for clinical use on animals are located in a variety of facilities around the world. The United States currently has four universities with small animal chambers and one with both an equine and small animal chamber. These universities have and will continue to allow the next generation of veterinary students to be exposed to HBOT, ensuring the field continues to expand. Other facilities include full-service veterinary hospitals, specialty centers, rehabilitation clinics, and private equine breeding farms. At the time of this publication, the authors estimate 100+ animal hyperbaric locations across the United States, two in New Zealand, one in England, two in Australia, one in Israel, two in Mexico and an unaccounted number in China, Taiwan, and Japan.

Maintenance of Animal Hyperbaric Systems and Facilities

As with all human hyperbaric systems and facilities, maintenance programs should be established according to chamber supplier recommendations in conjunction with the facility maintenance coordinator. (See Operational Safety section for more information on maintenance and example maintenance protocols.)

Fire Safety

Fire prevention is a primary safety goal during hyperbaric operations. In order to be effective at achieving this goal, it is important to understand the nature of fire. Fire is the result of a chemical reaction when oxygen, combining with fuel, in the presence of energy (heat) produces more energy (fire). This is a self-sustaining reaction as long as there is a constant supply of O_2 and fuel.

According to *NFPA 99* (2018) Chapters 14 and 16, the key points for fire prevention are to do the following:[3-4]

1. Eliminate or tightly control ignition sources in the chamber (no potential spark-generating materials, steel shoes, or materials that may produce heat; chemical agents; and electrical equipment).

2. Control the type of fuel sources in the chamber (no flammable materials, oils, grease, alcohols, or other products that may produce vapors).
3. Limit the total quantity of fuel sources inside the chamber (If it is not necessary, leave it out. For example, bandages, dressings, etc.).

Burn rates are dramatically increased under hyperbaric oxygen conditions; therefore, fires in a hyperbaric chamber can quickly become catastrophic. This, combined with a quick escape not being possible, means prevention is the frontline approach to fire safety. Reducing the risk of fire is achieved by following the NFPA guidelines of ELIMINATE, CONTROL, LIMIT any products or equipment inside the chamber. With equines and other animals, this will include shoes (no steel), blankets (none), bandages, dressings, topicals (limited to only necessary and allowable products), and grooming products (none). Having animals as patients means we do not have to be concerned about them trying to take anything inside the chamber. However, the potential risk is the lack of the education of owners who may have applied something to their animal. Operators are encouraged to "feel and smell" patients to check for products that may be a concern. Essential oils, grooming sprays, etc. may prove volatile in the HBO_2 environment.

NFPA 99 does not require but does permit automatic fire suppression and flame detection systems in hyperbaric facilities. NFPA requires fire extinguishing systems inside all multiplace chambers (chambers that permit multiple patients and are pressurized with air). US hyperbaric facilities covered by *NFPA 99* (this also includes France, Italy, and Poland) require deluge or water spray systems in multiplace chambers. Deluge systems are not required by NFPA in chambers pressurized with oxygen.[5]

Operational Safety Procedures

A sound operational safety program is woven into every aspect of the total hyperbaric program. Facilities should be constructed according to recommendations laid out in *NFPA 99*.[5] Requirements may differ depending on the location of the chamber in the veterinary hospital or clinic or in a separate building. Chambers should be constructed and certified according to human standards and guidelines (ASME and PVHO).[1-2] The layout of the hyperbaric facility should allow for safe ingress and egress of patients and personnel and should include at least two, clear exit points. Attention should be paid to local codes as well as fire wall construction that protects the chamber facility and clinic/hospital. Other considerations include the access to an adequate oxygen source and the safe venting of exhausted oxygen. Each facility should have access, on site, to standards and guideline resources (e.g., *NFPA 99*).

Proper facility oversight is crucial in the deployment of a successful safety program (See Clinical Hyperbaric Medicine Program-Oversight section). There are four essential responsibilities that should be covered by the management team: medical director, safety director, chamber operations team, and primary patient care team. In small veterinary clinics and hospitals, multiple oversight responsibilities may be shouldered by one individual, but ideally these responsibilities should be shared for a better system of checks and balances. There should be more than one person trained in the actual chamber operations, so that treatment and safety consistency can be maintained in the absence of one or more personnel.

It is recommended that at least one individual be a certified veterinary hyperbaric technologist (CHT-V) by the National Board of Diving and Hyperbaric Medical Technology and that the safety director complete a basic safety director course. The medical director and safety directors should have basic knowledge of hyperbaric medicine. The medical director should have veterinary medical knowledge and the safety director advanced knowledge in hyperbaric systems and operations. The two work together to ensure patient and personnel safety. For example, the safety director makes decisions about what can and cannot accompany a patient into the chamber, whereas the medical director would make more decisions about the patient's suitability to withstand the hyperbaric environment. The chamber operations team conducts the daily treatment protocols and should have a basic working knowledge of animal behavior, effects of hyperbaric therapy, side effects and their prevention/management, as well as a sound working knowledge of chamber operation. There should be sufficient operations personnel to provide consistent coverage when one or more people are absent. The patient primary care team are the people responsible for the entire patient management from history, physical exam, diagnosis, and treatment. They work closely with the hyperbaric medical director, safety director, and the treatment team to ensure safety with each hyperbaric treatment.

Training and retraining is the foundation of a quality safety program. Everyone involved with the delivery of hyperbaric oxygen therapy should have completed an approved basic training course that contains basic physics, physiology, application, indications, and side effects, including animal-related information in these areas. Most basic hyperbaric information applies across mammalian species, including man and domestic animals. However, there are differences in the various species of animals, and it is important for hyperbaric teams to be aware of those differences. It is also extremely important that hyperbaric personnel have animal experience and a knowledge of animal behavior and management. One unique challenge in animal hyperbaric therapy lies in the number of species veterinarians care for and there are significant challenges in applying this therapy in exotic and nontraditional animal species. It is preferred to have at least one individual trained and board-certified in animal hyperbaric therapy (CHT-V; NBDHMT) on staff. The hyperbaric medical director and the safety director should complete a basic course and the safety director an approved safety course. Technical training for operating the chamber is usually provided by the individual chamber manufacturers. This training does not include the theory and practice of hyperbaric medicine.

At a minimum, personnel should have annual operational and safety refresher training and updating. Valuable, additional training can be found in the areas of chamber acrylics and maintenance.

All training should be documented. A log should be maintained for all training sessions which includes date, type of training provided, provider, and attendees. Each attendee should receive a training certificate indicating that they completed the training. Chamber operations staff should have documented initial and recurrent competency testing covering basic operations, maintenance, and emergency procedures.

Chamber operation protocols are specific to each chamber. A copy of the operation manual should be readily available to all hyperbaric personnel. A laminated copy of the step-by-step operation of the chamber should be maintained at the chamber. All emergency protocols should also be available at the chamber, and the chamber operations team should have firsthand knowledge of the procedures. As part of the annual training exercises, staff should be refreshed with all standard and emergency protocols and be asked to run through all procedures and discuss various potential common emergency situations.

Chamber maintenance is an important aspect of the safety program. Proper chamber performance is critical in day-to-day normal operations. Proper function and reliability is crucial when an incident or emergency occurs. It is the responsibility of the individual hyperbaric programs to establish a consistent maintenance protocol for all chambers. Chamber maintenance should also include following the chamber manufacturer's recommended maintenance schedule designed for their specific chamber. The maintenance protocol may include daily, weekly, monthly, semiannual, and annual inspections, testing, certifications, test pressurizations, cleaning and disinfection, as well as maintenance of the chamber area and accessory equipment. All conducted maintenance procedures, inspections, and repairs should be dated and documented, with approval given by the safety director for the chamber's return to service. A sample list of chamber testing is included in Table 3.

Table 3. Maintenance, Inspection, and Testing

Routine Frequent Inspection and/or Testing			
Chamber/Equipment	Frequency	Minimum Frequency *	
Oxygen Sensor	At each treatment	14 days	
Temperature/humidity	At each treatment	14 days	
Door seal	At each treatment	14 days	Leak testing
Penetrations/ports	At each treatment	14 days	Leak testing
Acrylic ports	At each treatment	14 days	Leak testing
Acrylic tubes	At each treatment	14 days	
Routine Less Frequent Inspection/Testing			
Over pressure relief valve (PRV)	Annual	Annual	Pressure check and certification
Fire suppression system	Annual	Annual	Test

* when chamber is used infrequently

Risk Management

Risk management is a systematic process of identifying and evaluating the potential risks that may be involved in a projected activity or undertaking. Risk assessment identifies and analyzes events that may negatively impact patients, personnel, assets, and/or the environment and makes a determination of an acceptable level of risk. This evaluation is followed by a coordinated application of resources to eliminate, minimize, and control probability and impact of an unfortunate event. Although risk management sounds like a daunting process, it actually something done every day.

The ultimate goal is the prevention of an incident or emergency. Risk assessment in the delivery of animal hyperbaric therapy is focused on two specific aspects: assessing risk involving the patient and assessing the chamber environment.

Patient Safety

Each patient is selected for treatment based on the efficacy of HBOT in treating the patient's current diagnosis.[7] The patient's medical history, diagnosis, current physical and behavioral statuses, and current therapies are evaluated to ensure no contraindications exist and that there is a reasonable assurance the patient can tolerate the high-pressure, high-oxygen environment. It is imperative that the hyperbaric treatment team have a knowledge of the indications and contraindications for HBOT and the potential side effects of the high-pressure environment. The risk for seizure during therapy and barotrauma are among the most common complications. The goal is the prevention of untoward side effects and injury to the patient while in the chamber. The patient should have a basic physical examination prior to hyperbaric treatment, regardless of how many exams have been done previously.

For example, a fever can develop in a patient in a very short period of time and may not have been detected since the last physical examination. Each patient is then assessed for risks involved in providing the treatment. The medical director, safety director, and primary patient care teams should interact to ensure the patient's safety, but ultimately the safety director makes the final decision on whether to treat or not. The patient must also be assessed based on the current therapies being administered. A knowledge of drugs and other substances that may have the potential to create complications for the patient while in the chamber is important. If substances have been used that might cause an untoward event, a risk assessment should be done to determine if the drug/substance is critical to a positive outcome and how much risk it might create versus the benefits of hyperbaric treatment.

In animals, a temperament and behavior evaluation is important. The placement of animals into a strange environment, such as a hyperbaric chamber, may cause undesirable behavioral changes that could endanger the patient as well as create a problem in the chamber environment. For example, an anxious two-year-old Thoroughbred stallion unwilling to enter the chamber and kicking periodically should be considered for sedation for his treatment. If wearing shoes, he is a good candidate to become irritated in the chamber and potentially injure himself as well create a spark with the contact of his shoes with the chamber wall.

Most animals are quiet in the chamber, but some have to be managed with additional restraint or sedation.

Chamber Environment

The second consideration in assessing risk is the chamber environment and how it might be altered to create potential risks. The evaluation of substances and devices associated with the patient or requested to accompany the patient into the chamber is part of the risk assessment process. Unlike human HBOT, our patients do not consciously carry unacceptable items into the chamber. However, there may be substances placed on the patient by the owner or primary treatment team that pose a high risk in the pressurized hyperbaric environment. Examples might include petroleum jelly around a wound or draining lesion, Velcro collar or boot, essential oils, external fracture fixator, etc. If such a substance or device is present, a risk vs. benefit analysis should be performed. If there is a high risk, is there an alternative low risk option? Can the risk be eliminated and still have an optimum patient outcome? Should the hyperbaric treatment be postponed or cancelled? The primary concern in a high-oxygen, high-pressure environment is the risk for fire. (See Fire Safety section.) Elimination of ignition sources and reduction of fuel sources are the two main goals. There is one innate risk that accompanies most of our domestic mammal patients and that is the presence of hair. Hair is very flammable in the presence of high oxygen and pressure. The management of this risk begins with the elimination of any potential ignition source in the chamber. This is especially critical in the majority of the animal chambers, since they are pressurized with 100% oxygen and some (large animal) contain a large volume of gas. Steps that should be taken to eliminate ignition from static electricity include maintenance of chamber humidity at levels 50% or greater, moistening or wetting the patient, application of a grounding system or strap that may be integrated into the restraint devices or floor of the chamber, and removal of any devices that can produce an electrical current or spark. High humidity aides in reducing static electricity. Often the medical grade oxygen entering the chamber is very dry and tends to reduce humidity as does a very dry environmental scenario.

There are many visual aids that help remind staff of the need for vigilance and continual evaluation. Examples of these aids are provided in Figures 8-10. A "Go–No Go" list contains common items, drugs, topicals, conditions, etc. which can or cannot go into the chamber. It is impossible to cover every possibility in such a list, but it usually contains the most common or frequently encountered items. This list will vary between facilities and programs. The list is also fluid and can change frequently as new information is uncovered about various items. The risk assessment tree can be used as a guide for evaluating items/procedures/devices that are not on the Go–No Go list. Figure 8 is a sample decision tree that utilizes the Go–No Go list to make decisions. Also helpful is the risk assessment guide for need assessment. (See Figure 9.)

Because of the large volume of our large animal chambers and the fact that we use 100% oxygen to pressurize most of our chambers (large and small animal), a prudent philosophy is one of *conservatism*.

Figure 8. Sample go-no go list.

Go-No Go List
Equine Hyperbaric Therapy

GO

MATERIALS & EQUIPMENT

- Cotton halters/brass hardware
- Cotton ropes
- Cotton wraps
- Elastikon
- Cotton gauze
- Polyethylene tubing, IV sets
- IV catheters–must be capped appropriately
- Heimlich valves, chest drains
- 100% cotton towels

MEDICATIONS

- Alpha-2 agonists
- Diazepam
- Other medications

Consult hyperbaric technician, safety officer for materials not on the GO list and materials not commonly placed in the chamber. Need and risk assessments must be performed and documented.

NO GO

MATERIALS & EQUIPMENT

- Nylon/polyester anything
- Electrical devices including battery-operated
- Heating devices, patches, chemical warmers
- Anything that might produce a spark
- Steel metal horseshoes
- Velcro
- Vet wrap or comparable
- Horse blankets, noncotton blankets

MEDICATIONS/TOPICALS

- Alcohol, including alcohol preps
- Petroleum-based products
- Baby oil
- Petrolatum
- Ointments
- Fly sprays, other topicals
- Hoof packing, hoof paints

MEDICATIONS - RELATIVE CONTRAINDICATIONS

- Cis platinum
- Disulfram
- Doxorubicin
- Mafenide acetate
- Opiates

CONDITIONS - ABSOLUTE CONTRAINDICATION

- Untreated pneumothorax

CONDITIONS - RELATIVE CONTRAINDICATIONS

- Upper-respiratory obstruction
- Fever
- History of seizure
- Uncontrolled hemorrhage

Figure 9. Risk assessment decision tree.

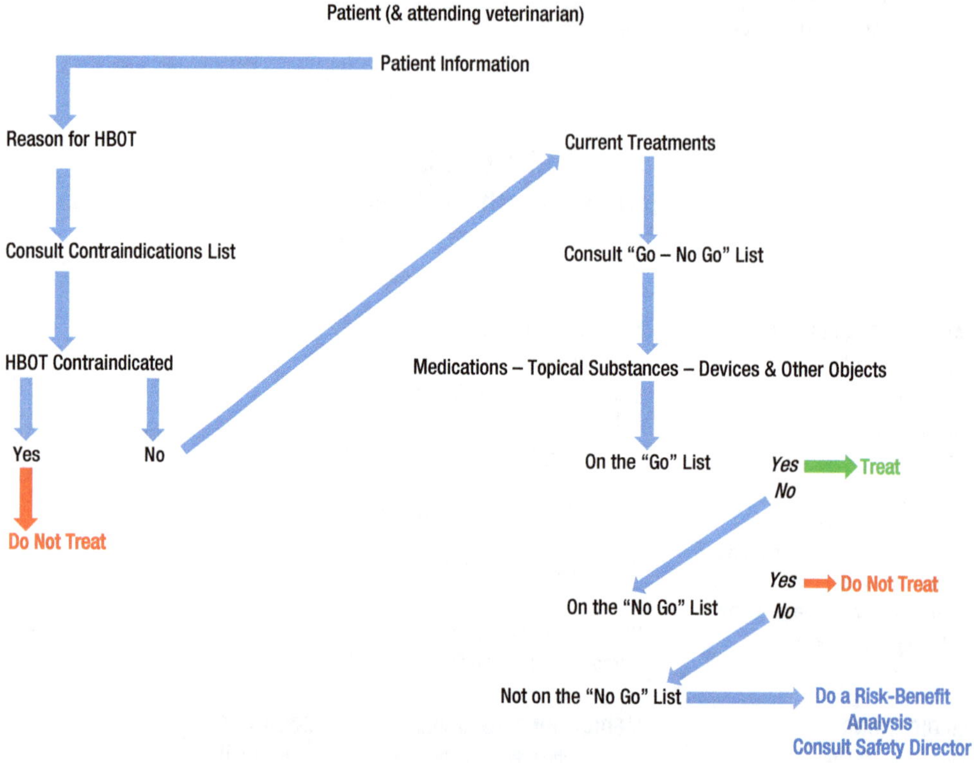

Figure 10. Sample guide for assessment of need.

If the item has no effects on the medical outcome of the patient, then don't place it in the chamber.

If the item is needed for a positive medical outcome for the patient, then assess the risk of placing it in the chamber.

If the item has a high risk, ask if there is an alternative with low or no risk.

Frequency of placement in the chamber doesn't matter if there is not or very low risk. Must evaluate risk vs. benefit.

Low cost is preferable, but safety, outcome, and comfort take precedent over cost.

In general, simple items are easier to evaluate risk than complex items, but safety and outcome take precedent over complexity and simplicity.

Alternatives that are safe or no/low risk should be considered, if required, for a positive medical outcome and comfort.

Safety and Patient Evaluation – Preparation

Proper patient evaluation and preparation is a critical part of the safety protocol in any hyperbaric medicine program. As previously mentioned, the evaluation of the patient includes a review of the following: patient history; current diagnosis and medical/surgical problem list; current therapies; pretreatment physical examination; and temperament evaluation. A patient evaluation checklist is often useful for completeness and consistency and serves as a part of the hyperbaric medical record. A risk level can also be assigned to each patient. (See Tables 4 and 5.)

The goal of patient preparation is to eliminate/reduce potential fuel sources and to eliminate any ignition sources. Patient preparation begins with grooming to make sure that the hair coat is clean and free of any debris. During this examination, make sure there are no topicals present that might be contraindicated or not previously evaluated. This is also a good time to evaluate the hair coat, particularly if it is extensive, for static electricity and the potential need for wetting the hair coat. The environmental humidity and temperature should also be taken into account especially in dry environments and colder times of the year. At a minimum, horses should have the mane and tail wetted and the body wiped with a wet towel. A maneuver that may also help increase humidity includes placement of wet towels or a tray of water in the chamber. Large animal chambers may also be thoroughly wetted down and water left in the floor drain reservoir.

Grooming includes cleaning the hooves of large animals to remove bedding, manure, and hoof packing that might be present. When topicals are identified that cannot go into the chamber, removal by bathing the entire patient and/or cleaning the area may be necessary (e.g., petroleum jelly around a wound). All horses should have steel shoes removed to eliminate potential contact with the metal of the chamber leading to the creation of a spark. All devices on the patient should be evaluated and removed if not needed. Collars and halters should be removed. Only cotton halters are allowed, if required. If devices cannot be removed, then covering them may be prudent, even though oxygen is very penetrating (e.g., covering external metal fixators with cotton and Elastikon). Never place a substance in the chamber that can produce excessive heat (e.g., a fiberglass cast that is still curing). Make sure that no electrical, battery-run devices are on the patient. Check the chamber for any devices that may have been dropped by personnel (e.g., cell phones). Vascular devices should be securely capped. Catheters with air-filled cuffs should have the cuffs deflated or the cuffs filled with a liquid substance (saline). A thorough examination and common sense are important in preparing the patient. A conservative approach is ideal in animal hyperbaric therapy.

Table 4. Example Patient Checklist

Patient Management Checklist

Item	√	Comments
Patient Evaluation		
Review medical history and signalment		
Review diagnosis		
Review current treatments		
Red Flags	Yes	
	No	
Patient Examination		
TPR completed		
Auscult cardiopulmonary system		
Upper respiratory exam/signs		
Temperament evaluation		
Red Flags	Yes	
	No	
Patient Preparation		
Evaluate for potential ignition sources		
Evaluate for reduction of fuel sources		
Red Flags	Yes	
	No	
Groom		
Bathe		
Cover devices		
Remove substances		
Wet the patient		
Evaluate for the need for sedation		
Determine need for physical restraint		
Documentation		
Complete general hyperbaric record – Update daily		
Determine current barometric pressure and record		
Complete hyperbaric patient monitoring form for each treatment		
Determine need for pre- and postpictures, video etc.		
Risk Level		

Table 5. Example Criteria for Patient Risk Level

Risk Level Criteria

Level	Evaluation Criteria
1	Nothing in the medical history that would contraindicate treatment in high-pressure, high-oxygen environment No current treatments that preclude the use of HBOT No absolute or relative contraindications present in this patient Pretreatment examination is within normal limits, no respiratory complications Nothing present that is listed on the "No-Go" list No devices, substances, medications, etc. that require a risk assessment No potential ignition or heat sources present on the patient Excellent-to-good temperament
2	History may contain information that could result in complications Primary reason for HBOT is a respiratory problem Disease present that has produced systemic compromise, requires risk assessment Nothing present that is on the "No-Go" list No absolute contraindication present in this patient Relative contraindication present that may be manageable in the hyperbaric oxygen environment Presence of treatment/substances (topicals etc.) that could be a fuel source or minor risk assessment, requires removal and bathing Presence of devices that cannot be removed and may require covering
3	One or more of the following is present: Item present which is on the "No-Go" list Significant pulmonary system disease or alteration Presence of an absolute contraindication High fever, multiple relative contraindications Treatments that would predispose the patient to the development complications Devices, substances, medications etc. that have an unknown response to high oxygen/high pressure and will require a significant risk assessment Things present that would/could result in ignition or heat generation

Emergency Protocols

Every effort should be made to prevent the occurrence of incidents and emergencies. However, being properly prepared for the possibility of an emergency occurrence will aid in the prevention of personnel and patient injury and the damage of equipment and facilities. Each hyperbaric program should develop their own emergency protocols and tailor them to their specific program. The first step in the prevention of an emergency is the posting of proper signage in the chamber facility and associated areas. The signage should include the following:

- Oxygen in use . . . no smoking or other ignition sources allowed

- Remember chamber oxygen is usually vented to the outside
- Reminding people that human occupancy/treatment in an animal chamber is not allowed
- Improper operation of this device (chamber) can cause serious injury and even death to patients in the chamber and to people operating and/or in the vicinity of the chamber
- Step-by-step procedures for fire outside the chamber, fire inside the chamber, rapid decompression, and decompression rates. All common potential emergency protocols should be described and placed in a folder which is located chamber side.
- Bulleted, step-by-step procedure list for various scenarios visible on the chamber or wall makes it convenient for chamber operators to refer to it during an emergency situation

The development and written description of a rapid decompression protocol may be useful in many common emergency situations. The speed of decompression will depend on the individual chamber. The tolerance of various animal species for rapid decompression is not known and extrapolation from the human diving community can be used as a rule of thumb. Using the base rate of 0.5 ft/sec, the total time from a pressure of 2 atmospheres absolute (ATA), 2.5 ATA, and 3.0 ATA would be 1 minute, 1.5 minutes and 2.2 minutes, respectively. Some chambers may not be able to achieve these fast rates, some patients may not tolerate these rates, and more time may be required.

Fire is one of the main emergencies that should be addressed in any hyperbaric emergency management program. There are five general principles/maneuvers that should be considered in managing this type of emergency: 1) determination of the location of the fire, inside or outside of the chamber; 2) use of fire suppression systems; 3) discontinuation of oxygen flow into the chamber; 4) exhaust of existing oxygen in the chamber; and 5) depressurization.

A fire protocol will vary slightly depending on the location of the fire. For example, a fire in the immediate area of the chamber may be handled different than one outside of a two-hour fire door or wall. A fire inside the chamber will be managed slightly differently than one outside of the chamber. Those chambers with deluge systems should have the system activated in the instance of an internal chamber fire. Figures 11 and 12 are examples of protocols for emergency shutdown procedures in the case of fire. They may not be appropriate for all chamber types and facilities but merely indicate some of the components of such a protocol.

Other potential incidences that may require emergency-type maneuvers or rapid shutdown include loss of electrical power, patient seizure or other major patient complications, loss of oxygen supply, and loss of compressed gas supply. Preparedness for these scenarios will decrease operator stress and improve response efficiency.

Documentation of the activation of an emergency protocol is imperative. This documentation should include the emergency or incident, protocol initiated, outcome, date, and time. *Remember anything not recorded did not occur.*

Figure 11. Example of an emergency shutdown procedure. Procedures are chamber-specific and the following are only examples of what a protocol might look like.

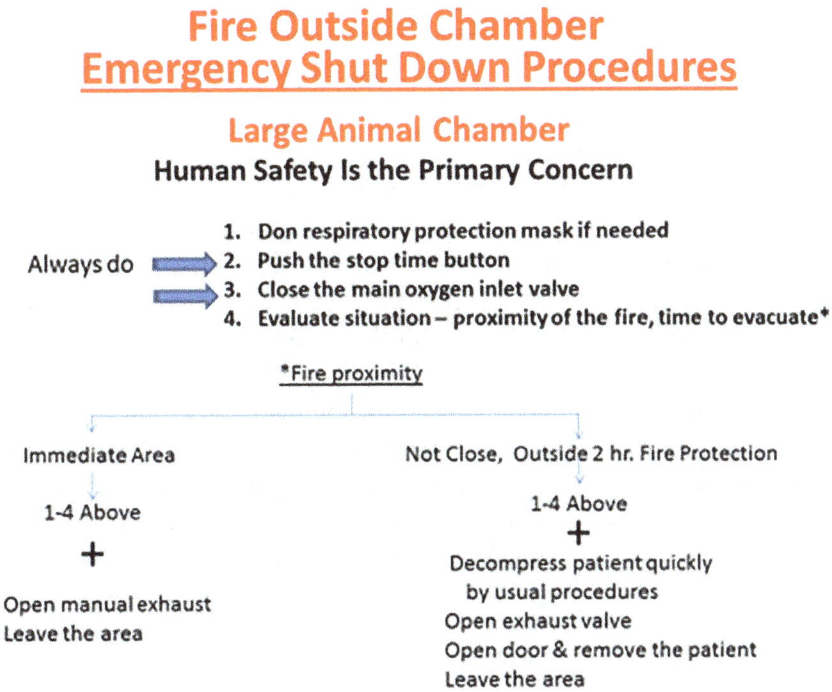

Figure 12. Example of an emergency shutdown procedure.

Fire Inside the Chamber

Emergency Shut Down Procedures

1. Turn chamber oxygen inlet valve to "off"
2. Turn set pressure valve to 1 ATA
3. Turn off main oxygen inlet valve
4. Open the manual exhaust valve
5. Leave the area

Summary

Safety touches all aspects of a quality animal hyperbaric oxygen treatment program. *Prevention* is key and is woven into every aspect of the development and deployment of clinical hyperbaric oxygen therapy. The standards and codes are there to guide us. Oversight provides a system of checks and balances and supports team development for consistency of patient care and safety. In this equipment-laden discipline, proper maintenance of equipment and facilities is crucial to the safety program. Paramount to following the mantra of prevention is a knowledge of the effects of HBO_2 on the patient and on the treatment environment (chamber). Basic and advanced training followed by consistent retraining is ideal to maintain a proper level of expertise and knowledge. Most historical incidences and emergencies, both in human and animal HBOT, have occurred due to human error. A thorough and consistent evaluation coupled with proper preparation of the patient are frontline procedures that are crucial in the prevention of incidences and emergencies. On a daily basis we are evaluating risk and making decisions concerning the elimination or reduction in those things that might ultimately lead to an unsafe treatment environment. The development and deployment of a sound safety program will significantly reduce the need for the initiation of emergency protocols. However, even with the best of safety programs, unexpected incidences can happen and therefore the presence of and training in emergency procedures is important. Documentation is the last important aspect of the safety program. Documentation includes treatment logs, maintenance, training, and incidence occurrences.

References

1. American Society of Mechanical Engineers (ASME) Safety Standard for Pressure Vessels for Human Occupancy, 2016 Edition (ASME PVHO-1). New York, NY; 2016.
2. American Society of Mechanical Engineers (ASME) Safety Standard for Pressure Vessels for Human Occupancy: In Service Guidelines, 2016 Edition (ASME PVHO-2). New York, NY; 2016.
3. National Fire Protection Association (NFPA) 99 Health Care Facilities Code, Chapter 14, Hyperbaric Facilities, 2018 Edition. National Fire Protection Association: Quincy MA; 2018;108-121.
4. National Fire Protection Association (NFPA) 99 Health Care Facilities Code, Chapter 16, Features of Fire Protection, 2018 Edition. National Fire Protection Association: Quincy MA; 2018;142-145.
5. National Fire Protection Association (NFPA) 99 Health Care Facilities Code, 2018 Edition. National Fire Protection Association: Quincy, MA; 2018.

6. National Fire Protection Association (NFPA) 150, Fire Safety and Life Safety in Animal Housing Facilities Code, 2019 Edition. National Fire Protection Association, Quincy, MA; 2019.
7. Birnie GL, Fry DR, Best MP. Safety and tolerability of hyperbaric oxygen therapy in cats and dogs. *J Am Anim Hosp Assoc.* 2018 Jul/Aug; 54(4):188-194.

INDEX

www.ingramcontent.com/pod-product-compliance
Lightning Source LLC
LaVergne TN
LVHW081330021026
849161LV00008BA/1827